Dietary Reference Intakes (DRIs): Recommended Intakes for Individuals, Vitamins

Food and Nutrition Board, Institute of Medicine, National Academies

Life Stage Group	Vit A (μg/d)[a]	Vit C (mg/d)	Vit D (μg/d)[b,c]	Vit E (mg/d)[d]	Vit K (μg/d)	Thiamin (mg/d)	Riboflavin (mg/d)	Niacin (mg/d)[e]	Vit B_6 (mg/d)	Folate (μg/d)[f]	Vit B_{12} (μg/d)	Pantothenic Acid (mg/d)	Biotin (μg/d)	Choline[g] (mg/d)
Infants														
0–6 mo	400*	40*	5*	4*	2.0*	0.2*	0.3*	2*	0.1*	65*	0.4*	1.7*	5*	125*
7–12 mo	500*	50*	5*	5*	2.5*	0.3*	0.4*	4*	0.3*	80*	0.5*	1.8*	6*	150*
Children														
1–3 y	**300**	**15**	5*	**6**	30*	**0.5**	**0.5**	**6**	**0.5**	**150**	**0.9**	2*	8*	200*
4–8 y	**400**	**25**	5*	**7**	55*	**0.6**	**0.6**	**8**	**0.6**	**200**	**1.2**	3*	12*	250*
Males														
9–13 y	**600**	**45**	5*	**11**	60*	**0.9**	**0.9**	**12**	**1.0**	**300**	**1.8**	4*	20*	375*
14–18 y	**900**	**75**	5*	**15**	75*	**1.2**	**1.3**	**16**	**1.3**	**400**	**2.4**	5*	25*	550*
19–30 y	**900**	**90**	5*	**15**	120*	**1.2**	**1.3**	**16**	**1.3**	**400**	**2.4**	5*	30*	550*
31–50 y	**900**	**90**	5*	**15**	120*	**1.2**	**1.3**	**16**	**1.3**	**400**	**2.4**	5*	30*	550*
51–70 y	**900**	**90**	10*	**15**	120*	**1.2**	**1.3**	**16**	**1.7**	**400**	**2.4**[i]	5*	30*	550*
>70 y	**900**	**90**	15*	**15**	120*	**1.2**	**1.3**	**16**	**1.7**	**400**	**2.4**[i]	5*	30*	550*
Females														
9–13 y	**600**	**45**	5*	**11**	60*	**0.9**	**0.9**	**12**	**1.0**	**300**	**1.8**	4*	20*	375*
14–18 y	**700**	**65**	5*	**15**	75*	**1.0**	**1.0**	**14**	**1.2**	**400**[i]	**2.4**	5*	25*	400*
19–30 y	**700**	**75**	5*	**15**	90*	**1.1**	**1.1**	**14**	**1.3**	**400**[i]	**2.4**	5*	30*	425*
31–50 y	**700**	**75**	5*	**15**	90*	**1.1**	**1.1**	**14**	**1.3**	**400**[i]	**2.4**	5*	30*	425*
51–70 y	**700**	**75**	10*	**15**	90*	**1.1**	**1.1**	**14**	**1.5**	**400**	**2.4**[h]	5*	30*	425*
>70 y	**700**	**75**	15*	**15**	90*	**1.1**	**1.1**	**14**	**1.5**	**400**	**2.4**[h]	5*	30*	425*
Pregnancy														
14–18 y	**750**	**80**	5*	**15**	75*	**1.4**	**1.4**	**18**	**1.9**	**600**[i]	**2.6**	6*	30*	450*
19–30 y	**770**	**85**	5*	**15**	90*	**1.4**	**1.4**	**18**	**1.9**	**600**[i]	**2.6**	6*	30*	450*
31–50 y	**770**	**85**	5*	**15**	90*	**1.4**	**1.4**	**18**	**1.9**	**600**[i]	**2.6**	6*	30*	450*
Lactation														
14–18 y	**1,200**	**115**	5*	**19**	75*	**1.4**	**1.6**	**17**	**2.0**	**500**	**2.8**	7*	35*	550*
19–30 y	**1,300**	**120**	5*	**19**	90*	**1.4**	**1.6**	**17**	**2.0**	**500**	**2.8**	7*	35*	550*
31–50 y	**1,300**	**120**	5*	**19**	90*	**1.4**	**1.6**	**17**	**2.0**	**500**	**2.8**	7*	35*	550*

NOTE: This table (taken from the DRI reports, see www.nap.edu) presents Recommended Dietary Allowances (RDAs) in **bold type** and Adequate Intakes (AIs) in ordinary type followed by an asterisk (*). RDAs and AIs may both be used as goals for individual intake. RDAs are set to meet the needs of almost all (97 to 98 percent) individuals in a group. For healthy breastfed infants, the AI is the mean intake. The AI for other life stage and gender groups is believed to cover needs of all individuals in the group, but lack of data or uncertainty in the data prevent being able to specify with confidence the percentage of individuals covered by this intake.

[a] As retinol activity equivalents (RAEs). 1 RAE = 1 μg retinol, 12 μg β-carotene, 24 μg α-carotene, or 24 μg β-cryptoxanthin. The RAE for dietary provitamin A carotenoids is twofold greater than retinol equivalents (RE), whereas the RAE for preformed vitamin A is the same as RE.

[b] As cholecalciferol. 1 μg cholecalciferol = 40 IU vitamin D.

[c] In the absence of adequate exposure to sunlight.

[d] As α-tocopherol. α-Tocopherol includes *RRR*-α-tocopherol, the only form of α-tocopherol that occurs naturally in foods, and the *2R*-stereoisomeric forms of α-tocopherol (*RRR*-, *RSR*-, *RRS*-, and *RSS*-α-tocopherol) that occur in fortified foods and supplements. It does not include the *2S*-stereoisomeric forms of α-tocopherol (*SRR*-, *SSR*-, *SRS*-, and *SSS*-α-tocopherol), also found in fortified foods and supplements.

[e] As niacin equivalents (NE). 1 mg of niacin = 60 mg of tryptophan; 0–6 months = preformed niacin (not NE).

[f] As dietary folate equivalents (DFE). 1 DFE = 1 μg food folate = 0.6 μg of folic acid from fortified food or as a supplement consumed with food = 0.5 μg of a supplement taken on an empty stomach.

[g] Although AIs have been set for choline, there are few data to assess whether a dietary supply of choline is needed at all stages of the life cycle, and it may be that the choline requirement can be met by endogenous synthesis at some of these stages.

[h] Because 10 to 30 percent of older people may malabsorb food-bound B_{12}, it is advisable for those older than 50 years to meet their RDA mainly by consuming foods fortified with B_{12} or a supplement containing B_{12}.

[i] In view of evidence linking folate intake with neural tube defects in the fetus, it is recommended that all women capable of becoming pregnant consume 400 μg from supplements or fortified foods in addition to intake of food folate from a varied diet.

[j] It is assumed that women will continue consuming 400 μg from supplements or fortified food until their pregnancy is confirmed and they enter prenatal care, which ordinarily occurs after the end of the periconceptional period—the critical time for formation of the neural tube.

Reprinted, by permission, from National Academies Press, 2006, Dietary reference intakes: Recommended intakes for individuals, vitamins. In *Dietary reference intakes: The essential guide to nutrient requirement* © 2006 by the National Academy of Sciences, Washington, D.C.

Sport Nutrition
for Health
and Performance

— Second Edition —

Melinda M. Manore, PhD, RD, CSSD, FACSM
Oregon State University

Nanna L. Meyer, PhD, RD, CSSD
University of Colorado

Janice Thompson, PhD, FACSM
The University of Bristol

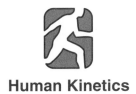

Human Kinetics

Library of Congress Cataloging-in-Publication Data

Manore, Melinda, 1951-
  Sport nutrition for health and performance / Melinda M. Manore, Nanna
L. Meyer, Janice Thompson. -- 2nd ed.
      p. ; cm.
  Includes bibliographical references and index.
  ISBN-13: 978-0-7360-5295-5 (hard cover)
  ISBN-10: 0-7360-5295-X (hard cover)
  1. Athletes--Nutrition. 2. Physical fitness--Nutritional aspects. I.
Meyer, Nanna L. II. Thompson, Janice, 1962- III. Title.
  [DNLM: 1. Nutritional Physiological Phenomena. 2. Sports
Medicine--methods. 3. Exercise--physiology. 4. Food. 5. Nutritional
Requirements. 6. Physical Fitness--physiology. QT 261 M285s 2009]
  TX361.A8M37 2009
  613.2'024796--dc22
                                    2009004396

ISBN-10: 0-7360-5295-X (print)
ISBN-13: 978-0-7360-5295-5 (print)

The Web addresses cited in this text were current as of January 2009, unless otherwise noted.

Acquisitions Editor: Michael S. Bahrke, PhD; **Developmental Editor:** Amanda S. Ewing; **Assistant Editors:** Christine Bryant Cohen, Nicole Gleeson, and Casey A. Gentis; **Copyeditor:** Joyce Sexton; **Proofreader:** Joanna Hatzopoulos Portman; **Indexer:** Nancy Ball; **Permission Manager:** Dalene Reeder; **Graphic Designer:** Joe Buck; **Graphic Artist:** Dawn Sills; **Cover Designer:** Keith Blomberg; **Photographer (cover):** Corey Rich/Aurora Photos; **Photo Asset Manager:** Laura Fitch; **Photo Production Manager:** Jason Allen; **Art Manager:** Kelly Hendren; **Associate Art Manager:** Alan L. Wilborn; **Illustrator:** Keri Evans; **Printer:** Edwards Brothers Malloy

Printed in the United States of America   10 9 8 7 6

The paper in this book is certified under a sustainable forestry program.

Human Kinetics
Web site: www.HumanKinetics.com

United States: Human Kinetics
P.O. Box 5076
Champaign, IL 61825-5076
800-747-4457
e-mail: humank@hkusa.com

Canada: Human Kinetics
475 Devonshire Road Unit 100
Windsor, ON N8Y 2L5
800-465-7301 (in Canada only)
e-mail: info@hkcanada.com

Europe: Human Kinetics
107 Bradford Road
Stanningley
Leeds LS28 6AT, United Kingdom
+44 (0) 113 255 5665
e-mail: hk@hkeurope.com

Australia: Human Kinetics
57A Price Avenue
Lower Mitcham, South Australia 5062
08 8372 0999
e-mail: info@hkaustralia.com

New Zealand: Human Kinetics
P.O. Box 80
Torrens Park, South Australia 5062
0800 222 062
e-mail: info@hknewzealand.com

E3147

To our mothers and families for your
constant love and support, unflagging
faith, and endless patience. We thank you.

To our colleagues and students in sport
nutrition for your interest, encouragement,
and enthusiasm for a topic we love.

Contents

Contributors

Jaclyn Maurer Abbot, PhD, RD, CSSD
Nutrition consultant
Department of Nutrition Sciences
University of Arizona
Tucson, AZ

Hawley Almstedt, PhD
Assistant professor
Department of Natural Science
Loyola Marymount University
Los Angeles, CA

Katherine A. Beals, PhD, RD, FACSM
Associate clinical professor
Division of Nutrition & Department of Family & Preventive Medicine
University of Utah
Salt Lake City, UT

Melissa Hayman, MS
Doctoral student
Department of Exercise & Sport Science
University of Utah
Salt Lake City, UT

Linda Houtkooper, PhD, RD, FACSM
Associate director, programs, Cooperative Extension
College of Agriculture & Life Sciences
Professor, Department of Nutritional Sciences
University of Arizona
Tucson, AZ

Nancy Rodriguez, PhD, RD, CSSD, FACSM
Professor, Department of Nutritional Sciences
Director, Sports Nutrition Programs
University of Connecticut
Storrs, CT

Kristine Spence, MS, RD
Sports Dietitian, TOSH Sport Science
The Orthopedic Specialty Hospital
Salt Lake City, UT

Stacie L. Wing-Gaia, PhD, RD, CSSD
Assistant professor, Division of Nutrition
Director of Coordinated Master's program, Sports Dietetics Emphasis
University of Utah
Salt Lake City, UT

Preface

The first edition of this textbook was the result of many years of hard work and dedication. In 1993, Drs. Melinda Manore and Gail Butterfield developed the idea for an advanced sport nutrition textbook that would be appropriate for students who had already completed courses in nutrition and exercise physiology. As an advanced-level textbook did not exist, these two pioneers in sport nutrition set forth on an adventure to develop a book that would serve as an instructive guide, including the most recent references and research findings in sport nutrition. Joined by their colleague, Dr. Janice Thompson, and with support from Human Kinetics, they developed the first edition of this textbook. Although Gail Butterfield was not a primary author, she provided inspiration, advice, moral support, and invaluable editorial input throughout the writing period. Sadly, Gail passed away on December 27, 1999, of a brain tumor. Although she did not live to see this textbook in print, she was able to write the foreword for the first edition. Gail's contributions to the concept of this book and to the field of sport nutrition are immeasurable. Her indomitable spirit and undying passion for science have served as an inspiration to all who have been blessed to work with her. As authors of this textbook, we want to formally recognize Gail's significant contribution to getting this book off the ground. The second edition of the textbook was written with the help of a new colleague and an expert in the field, Dr. Nanna Meyer, who is also enthusiastic about sport nutrition and the role of nutrition and exercise in health.

Now, more than ever, there is an increased demand for accurate sport nutrition information. For everyone from the elite athlete attempting to win an Olympic gold medal to the recreational athlete trying to improve a personal best, nutrition can play a vital role in helping active individuals achieve their health, fitness, and performance goals. Nutrition can help them maximize performance, prevent injury, enhance recovery from exercise, achieve and maintain optimal body weight, improve daily training workouts, and maintain overall good health.

For the health, nutrition, or fitness professional working with active individuals, keeping up with sport nutrition information can be an overwhelming task. Currently, consumers get their sport nutrition information from a variety of sources, including magazines, television, advertisements, product labels, peers, and the Internet. Unfortunately, some of this information has little or no scientific basis. Thus, our goal in writing this text was to provide you with a clear, concise, authoritative review of current exercise and nutrition research. We hope this book will help you sort fact from fiction and give you a scientific foundation from which to evaluate future claims and make sound sport nutrition recommendations.

WHO THE BOOK IS FOR

This book is written for the variety of professionals who work to guide athletes or active individuals through the sport nutrition maze. Thus, we assume that the reader has a basic understanding of nutrition, exercise science, physiology, and metabolic pathways used in the metabolism of fuel substrates. The following are the primary audiences for this text:

- Undergraduate and graduate students in either nutrition, exercise physiology, health, or wellness programs with a strong science background and an interest in nutrition as it relates to sport, exercise, and fitness
- Athletic trainers or physical therapists who are working with athletes or athletic teams, or who are teaching future athletic trainers or therapists
- Dietitians who have completed an undergraduate or graduate degree in nutrition or dietetics and are interested in sport nutrition
- Health fitness specialists, personal trainers, fitness practitioners, and physical therapists working in spas, gyms, or fitness and rehabilitation facilities—these individuals frequently provide nutrition information to clients
- Sports medicine specialists who are working with athletes or athletic teams

UPDATES TO THIS EDITION

This second edition has been thoroughly revised and updated to reflect the latest issues, guidelines, and recommendations for active individuals. All macronutrient and micronutrient chapters have been entirely rewritten, and all chapters have been revised to reflect the latest Dietary Reference Intakes, USDA Food Guide Pyramid, Food Pyramid for Athletes, Dietary Guidelines for Americans, and physical activity recommendations from various organizations, including the 2008 Physical Activity Guidelines by USDHHS. Some of the current topics discussed in the text include the following:

- Carbohydrate recommendations for athletes before, during, and after exercise, including changes in substrate oxidation as either the diet or the supplement used are altered

- Protein requirements of athletes based on the latest research, including amount of protein required for different types of athletes, and timing of protein intake for enhanced recover from exercise

- Updated evaluation of the fat needs of athletes and the role of fat loading as a technique for increasing fat oxidation during exercise to improve performance

- Complete update on energy balance, including the new guidelines for estimating energy expenditure and the role of nonexercise activity thermogenesis (NEAT) on body weight

- An evidence based reexamination of various diets and techniques used for weight loss, including low calorie diets, low-carb and high-protein diets, the volumetric diet, and weight loss supplements in the market

- New research on body composition assessments and standards

- New research on fluid balance including the latest evidence based position papers on exercise and fluid replacement, exertional heat illness and the prevention of cold injuries during exercise

- The latest on controversial nutrition issues such as the role of protein, vitamin D, and energy in bone health and new criteria for assessing bone health in young adults

- New nutritional and fitness assessments, questionnaires, and methods for measuring energy expenditure, including a review of the new technology in energy expenditure devices

- Update on the issues of the active female, including new research on the Female Athlete Triad and a recent position paper published on this topic

- Updated information on ergogenic aids, including new supplement resource list, World Anti-Doping Agency Codes (WADA), list of third party supplement evaluation programs, techniques for evaluating supplements by the Australian Institute of Sport, and updated information on creatine and anabolic steroids

TOPICS COVERED

This text begins with an overview of sport nutrition and the role that good nutrition can play in sport and exercise. We think it is important that sport nutrition recommendations be consistent with general nutrition recommendations made to all individuals for good health. We then cover the macronutrient requirements of sport and the roles that carbohydrate, fat, and protein play in fueling the system at rest and during exercise (chapters 2-4). Special attention is given to the metabolic pathways used during exercise and the ways in which these pathways are altered with exercise intensity, duration, and training. Understanding these metabolic pathways, and how exercise changes them, will also help professionals working in this area evaluate the myriad performance-enhancing and weight loss products marketed to active individuals.

We have also covered in detail the topics of energy balance, methods for achieving an optimal body weight, and body composition measurements (chapters 5-7). It is rare to find an athlete or any active individual who is not concerned to some extent about body weight and composition. Because many sports "demand" a certain body shape or size, weight control issues frequently plague athletes in lean-build or aesthetic sports. The various components of energy balance are discussed in detail, and factors that may alter each of these are addressed. In addition, we present specific guidelines for helping an active individual either gain or lose weight, as well as reviewing the body composition issues associated with weight change. Since assessment of body composition is becoming more common, it is important that athletes understand how these data are derived and what they mean.

Poor fluid balance, especially dehydration, is a major nutritional concern of any active individual. We have provided the most recent information related to the physiology of fluid and electrolyte balance and make recommendations for maintaining good fluid balance before and during exercise and for rehydrating after exercise is over (chapter 8). Chapters 9 through 13 detail the vitamin and mineral concerns most frequently associated with sport and exercise. The micronutrients are grouped according to their functions. For example, chapter 12 deals with the nutrients involved in blood formation. The other functional groups included in these chapters are vitamins important in energy metabolism, antioxidant nutrients, nutrients for bone health, and minerals. This functional grouping of the micronutrients provides an easy framework for understanding how these nutrients can influence exercise performance and good health. In addition, this framework helps to improve one's ability to remember the functions and interactions of these micronutrients.

The final section of the book covers the practical side of working with a recreational or elite athlete or an athletic team. Topics covered in this section include nutrition and fitness assessment (chapter 14), nutrition and exercise issues specific to the active female (chapter 15), and evaluation of ergogenic aids (chapter 16). The appendix provides a variety of helpful resources and references frequently used by people working with active individuals. These resources include the Dietary Reference Intakes (DRIs), various ethnic food guide pyramids, equations for determining energy expenditure, prediction equations for resting metabolic rate, nutrition assessment tools, energy costs of various activities, commonly reported clinical blood biochemical values, and methods for assessing energy expenditure.

UNIQUE FEATURES

One way we have provided you with additional insights into the nutrition and exercise research is through our chapter "highlights." These highlights will give you in-depth information on a topic or help you to critically evaluate issues surrounding a myth or controversy in sport nutrition. To facilitate understanding of the topics presented, each chapter begins with the key points to be covered and ends with a summary of the key points. Key terms are boldfaced throughout the text, and each chapter ends with a listing of that chapter's key terms along with the number of the page on which each term is defined. For readers who may want more in-depth information on a specific topic, additional helpful readings are listed at the end of each chapter. Finally, this book bridges the gap between the scientific literature and the practical application of research information to the athlete or active individual. Numerous charts, figures, sidebars, and tables give information that you can use to help athletes and active individuals make decisions regarding daily intakes of food and supplements. For example, we have provided information on the nutrient content of various sport foods, diet composition recommendations for athletes at various energy intakes, when to use nutritional supplements, and how to evaluate an ergogenic aid.

In addition, an image bank is provided for instructors. The image bank includes most of the art, tables, and content photos from the book in easy-to-use PowerPoint files. Instructors can take these items and use them to facilitate lectures, create handouts, or provide other learning tools for students. A blank PowerPoint template is also provided, and this blank template matches the design of the image bank, helping instructors more easily create a cohesive presentation. The image bank is available to instructors at www.HumanKinetics.com/SportNutritionforHealth andPerformance.

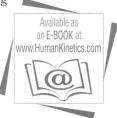

Available as an E-BOOK at www.HumanKinetics.com

Acknowledgments

Writing a book is no small task, especially when our days are already too busy. Although it was a long and arduous process, we were able to complete this book due to the contributions and support of many people. First, we would like to thank the Human Kinetics publication team, especially Mike Bahrke and Amanda Ewing, who constantly urged us on with encouraging words, unbelievable patience, and good humor. Second, we would like to thank the following contributing authors:

- Dr. Nancy Rodriguez, a leader in the area of sport nutrition and an expert in protein metabolism, revised the chapter on protein and exercise (chapter 4).

- Dr. Linda Houtkooper graciously agreed to write the body composition chapter (chapter 7) along with Dr. Jaclyn Maurer Abbot. As experts in this area, these authors have presented the most current body composition research along with practical recommendations.

- Dr. Katherine Beals, an expert in eating disorders and nutrition issues of active women, agreed to help Dr. Manore revise the chapter on minerals and exercise (chapter 11).

- Dr. Hawley Almstedt, with research expertise in bone and exercise, agreed to help revise the chapter on nutrients for bone health (chapter 13).

- Dr. Stacie L. Wing-Gaia, with research expertise in antioxidants and dietary supplements, revised both the chapter on antioxidant nutrients (chapter 10) and the chapter on ergogenic substances (chapter 16).

- Dr. Nanna Meyer, one of the coauthors, had help from two of her former nutrition graduate students in the revision of some chapters. Ms. Kristine Spence, a sport dietitian, helped revise the introductory chapter (chapter 1) and Ms. Melissa Hayman, a doctoral student in exercise science, helped revise the nutrition and fitness assessment chapter (chapter 14).

These individuals certainly made our lives a lot easier.

Third, we would like to thank our many students, who read through our chapters, pointed out our mistakes, and made wonderful suggestions. Fourth, we would like to thank the many active individuals, including athletes and research participants, who have taught us so much over the last 15 to 25 years about the topic we love. Finally, we would like to thank our families, friends, and colleagues, as they listened to us complain, gave us valuable advice, edited our work, encouraged us to finish, and continually asked, "When is your book going to be revised?" We can finally say, "We are *finished!*"

CHAPTER 1

Introduction to Nutrition for Exercise and Health

Chapter Objectives

After reading this chapter you should be able to

- understand the role of nutrition in exercise and sport,
- identify the essential nutrients and the dietary recommendations for these nutrients,
- describe the various methods used in evaluating the diets of active individuals, and
- discuss the role of nutrition and exercise in the prevention of disease.

The goal of this book is to promote optimal health and sport performance by linking together information about nutrition and exercise. For competitive athletes this may mean determining fluid, nutrient, and energy needs during times of intense training and competition. It may also mean determining the appropriate food, fluids, and supplements required for various exercise situations or environmental conditions. For individuals who exercise for fitness or recreation, it may mean learning to eat to promote good health, maintain or decrease weight, and fuel exercise. No matter what one's fitness or exercise goals, good nutrition can help improve exercise performance, decrease recovery time from strenuous exercise, prevent exercise-associated injuries due to fatigue, provide the fuel required during times of high-intensity training, and control weight. Combining good nutrition with exercise can also help reduce the risk of numerous chronic diseases such as diabetes, cardiovascular disease, hypertension, obesity, osteoporosis, and some cancers; moreover, physicians often recommend nutrition and physical activity to treat individuals who already have these diseases. Learning how nutrition and exercise work together for optimal health is essential for health, nutrition, or fitness professionals who must teach the public how to maintain good health and reduce risks of chronic disease. This chapter briefly outlines the various guidelines and tools that nutritionists and dietitians use to evaluate dietary intakes and to determine an individual's nutrient and energy needs. Knowing these general guidelines will help set the stage for the information covered later in this text. The more detailed guidelines for active individuals and athletes, discussed later in this book, are usually modifications—specific to the individual, sport, and environment—of these general nutrition recommendations.

ROLE OF NUTRITION IN EXERCISE AND SPORT

Research on the role of nutrition in exercise and sport has increased dramatically over the last 20 years. Today there is no doubt that nutrition plays a vital role in exercise performance and training. Chapter 2 shows that carbohydrates are important for endurance exercise performance and during periods of high-intensity training. Chapter 8 discusses the role that fluid intake plays in both short-term and endurance exercise. There is no question that competitive athletes can benefit from adequate energy, nutrient, and fluid intakes. Good nutrition can also help competitive or recreational athletes recover from strenuous physical activity: Refueling and rehydrating the body, while providing nutrients to build and repair muscles, enable individuals to engage in the next bout of physical activity without adverse effects. This is especially important for athletes during sport tournaments, or for individuals who engage in strenuous physical activity on a daily or more than daily basis. For example, a triathlete may do an hour swim in the morning and a 3 h cycle workout in the afternoon. Between these workouts, the athlete must replenish the body's glycogen stores, repair muscle tissue, and consume adequate fluid to ensure optimal exercise performance. Chapter 14 discusses methods for assessing both diet and fitness levels so that individual recommendations can be made to improve energy and nutrient intakes based on activity levels.

Well-fueled and well-hydrated athletes reduce their risk of injury during exercise—a risk that increases as individuals become fatigued and lose their ability to concentrate, and as they deplete the substrates that fuel exercise. For example, as discussed in chapter 15, health problems develop in female athletes who lack the energy and nutrients to fuel their activity. Proper nutrition can help speed the healing process for injured athletes; recovery from muscle or bone injuries or from surgery requires extra energy and nutrients, including protein, vitamins, and minerals. These points are discussed in detail in chapter 4 (protein), chapter 9 (energy nutrients), chapter 10 (antioxidants), chapter 11 (minerals), chapter 12 (blood nutrients), and chapter 13 (bone health). These chapters consider the roles that nutrients play in exercise and the issue of whether exercise increases the need for specific nutrients.

Nutrition also plays an important role in weight control and body composition. Few individuals today are happy with their weight, body fat levels, or body shape. Helping active individuals develop *realistic* approaches to weight maintenance (or weight loss or gain) can significantly improve health and reduce stress levels. For many active persons, weight control is a primary concern. Chapter 3 (fat), chapter 5 (energy and macronutrient balance), chapter 6 (achieving optimal weight), and chapter 7 (body composition) address these issues. If concerns about weight and body image become overwhelming, an individual is at increased risk for disordered eating or even for developing a clinical eating disorder. Chapter 15 deals with these issues in women.

As interest in sport nutrition increases, the number of products purported to lead to improved exercise performance, gains in muscle strength, quick weight loss, and changes in body composition increases exponentially—which makes it difficult to sort fact from fiction. You cannot pick up a popular fitness, nutrition, or health magazine without being bombarded with advertisements for various nutrient supplements, ergogenic aids, and sport foods. When these advertisements are combined with the myriad advertisements for weight loss or weight gain, it is not surprising that the public is confused and distrustful. Since nutrition and exercise research is still in its infancy, there are many unanswered questions. Chapter 16 presents ways to critically evaluate sport nutrition supplements and ergogenic aids.

ESSENTIAL NUTRIENTS AND DIETARY RECOMMENDATIONS

Over the last 80 years, nutrition research has identified a number of specific nutrients in foods that are essential to good health. Various organizations and governments have used this information to make dietary recommendations to ensure the health of their citizens. These dietary recommendations can also be used as general guidelines in designing diets for active individuals. We should not forget, however, that energy and nutrients are found in foods—and that learning to select, prepare, and eat healthy foods can be one of life's great pleasures. Ultimately, we eat foods, not nutrients.

Essential and Nonessential Nutrients

The concept of essential nutrients evolved from observations that certain diseases occurred in populations that consumed poor diets, and evidence that including certain foods in the diet could correct or prevent the diseases (Carpenter and Harper 2006). Food constituents that prevent diseases or health problems were classified as indispensable or essential nutrients. Nutrients that could be deleted from the diet with no adverse health effects were classified as dispensable or nonessential nutrients. These concepts are sometimes confusing because a nutrient can be *physiologically* essential for the body but classified as nonessential for the diet since the body can synthesize it. Many nutritionists therefore prefer the terms indispensable (essential) and dispensable (nonessential). Although all nutrients

Nutrients Essential for Humans

Water
Amino acids (L-isomers)
  Histidine
  Isoleucine
  Leucine
  Lysine
  Methionine
  Phenylalanine
  Threonine
  Tryptophan
  Valine
Vitamins
  Ascorbic acid
  Vitamins A, D, E, K
  Thiamin
  Riboflavin
  Niacin
  Vitamin B_6 (pyridoxine)
  Pantothenic acid
  Folic acid
  Biotin
  Vitamin B_{12} (cobalamin)

(Choline[2])[a]
Energy sources
Fatty acids
  Linoleic acid
  α-Linolenic acid
Minerals
  Calcium
  Phosphorus
  Magnesium
  Iron
  Zinc
  Copper
  Manganese
  Iodine
  Selenium
  Molybdenum
  Chromium
Electrolytes
  Sodium
  Potassium
  Chloride
Ultratrace elements[b]

[a] In experimental animals, choline is a conditional nutrient that is useful when methionine is not present in adequate amounts as a "methyl" donor, and this may also be true for humans. [b] None have so far been proven by adequate studies to be essential for humans, but it remains possible that one or more may be found to be essential in exceedingly small amounts.

Reprinted from K.J. Carpenter and A.E. Harper, 2006, Evolution of knowledge of essential nutrients. In *Modern nutrition in health and disease*, edited by M.E. Shils et al. (Baltimore, MD: Williams & Wilkins), 5.

are important for growth and good health, they need not all come from the diet. Classification of a nutrient as essential or indispensable clearly requires careful and extensive scientific examination. By the 1950s, a number of nutrients had been identified as essential (indispensable) (see "Nutrients Essential for Humans" p. 3). However, as the science of human nutrition has developed, classifying nutrients as either essential or nonessential has proved difficult at times. A nutrient is classified as essential if its absence from the diet results in signs and symptoms characteristic of a deficiency disease and if these signs can be prevented only by the nutrient itself or by a precursor to the nutrient (Carpenter and Harper 2006). All of the nutrients listed in the Recommended Dietary Allowances and the Dietary Reference Intakes are currently accepted as essential for humans (see upcoming section).

Conditionally Essential Nutrients

Animal research of the 1920s and subsequent research with premature infants showed that the body could synthesize some "essential" nutrients from precursors; this led to the understanding that interactions between nutrients could alter requirements, and that some disease states or genetic defects altered essential nutrient needs (Carpenter and Harper 2006). A third category, **conditional essentiality,** has therefore been suggested. For example, a premature infant may require certain nutrients not required in a full-term infant. In order for the premature infant to grow and thrive, these nutrients must be added to the diet even if they are not classified as essential nutrients for full-term infants. Rudman and Feller (1986) proposed three criteria, all of which must be present to establish the conditional essentiality of a nutrient:

1. The plasma concentration of the nutrient declines into the subnormal range, although the body should be able to synthesize the nutrient.

2. Chemical, structural, or functional abnormalities appear that are associated with low blood concentrations of the nutrient.

3. Dietary supplementation of the nutrient returns plasma concentrations to normal and corrects the chemical, structural, or functional abnormalities seen when blood concentrations are low.

Desirable and Beneficial Nutrients

In the last 20 years, the science of nutrition has taken a new direction. Nutritionists no longer focus only on preventing deficiency diseases—they now recognize many nutrients that, although not classified as essential nutrients, are important for good health and disease prevention. This has prompted researchers to suggest a fourth nutrient category called **desirable or beneficial for health** (Carpenter and Harper 2006). Nutrients that might fit into this category are fiber, various phytochemicals, carotenoids, and amino acid derivatives. While many of these nutrients are now recommended for good health, they are not classified as essential or conditionally essential nutrients. As the science of nutrition progresses, we may see this fourth category of nutrients evolve with specific inclusion criteria, which would then stimulate the rigorous research required for their inclusion.

Recommended Dietary Allowances and Dietary Reference Intakes

The Institute of Medicine (IOM), Food and Nutrition Board (FNB) of the National Academy of Sciences has revised the manner in which it makes nutrient recommendations to the population. The **Dietary Reference Intakes (DRIs),** a family of nutrient recommendations, has replaced the Recommended Dietary Allowances (RDAs). The new DRIs were developed jointly by Canadian and United States scientists to reflect the growing body of scientific evidence showing that chronic diseases may alter nutrient requirements. Figure 1.1 shows the evolution of the dietary guidelines from the RDAs to the more elaborate DRI system (which includes RDAs) as a series of reports grouped by nutrient function and classification. The DRIs include a family of reference values: the Estimated Average Requirement (EAR), the RDA, the Adequate Intake (AI), and the Tolerable Upper Intake Level (UL). These values are designed not only to prevent nutrient deficiency diseases, as was the goal with the previous RDAs, but also to reduce the risk of chronic diseases and offer guidance for both group and individual meal planning.

The following were the goals of the IOM, FNB in setting up the DRIs:

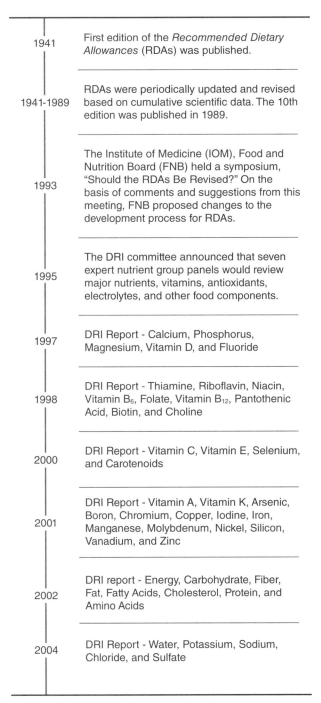

1941	First edition of the *Recommended Dietary Allowances* (RDAs) was published.
1941-1989	RDAs were periodically updated and revised based on cumulative scientific data. The 10th edition was published in 1989.
1993	The Institute of Medicine (IOM), Food and Nutrition Board (FNB) held a symposium, "Should the RDAs Be Revised?" On the basis of comments and suggestions from this meeting, FNB proposed changes to the development process for RDAs.
1995	The DRI committee announced that seven expert nutrient group panels would review major nutrients, vitamins, antioxidants, electrolytes, and other food components.
1997	DRI Report - Calcium, Phosphorus, Magnesium, Vitamin D, and Fluoride
1998	DRI Report - Thiamine, Riboflavin, Niacin, Vitamin B_6, Folate, Vitamin B_{12}, Pantothenic Acid, Biotin, and Choline
2000	DRI Report - Vitamin C, Vitamin E, Selenium, and Carotenoids
2001	DRI Report - Vitamin A, Vitamin K, Arsenic, Boron, Chromium, Copper, Iodine, Iron, Manganese, Molybdenum, Nickel, Silicon, Vanadium, and Zinc
2002	DRI report - Energy, Carbohydrate, Fiber, Fat, Fatty Acids, Cholesterol, Protein, and Amino Acids
2004	DRI Report - Water, Potassium, Sodium, Chloride, and Sulfate

Figure 1.1 Recommended Dietary Allowance (RDA) and Dietary Reference Intake (DRI) time line.

Adapted from the International Food Information Council 2002 and the IOM Dietary Reference Intakes 1997-2005.

• Develop a comprehensive set of reference values for dietary nutrient intakes for the healthy population in the United States and Canada. These values replace the RDAs for the United States and the Recommended Nutrient Intakes (RNIs) for Canada.

• Clearly document the derivation of the reference values, with emphasis on nutrient function.

• Consider the evidence concerning prevention of disease and developmental disorders in addition to prevention of nutrient deficiency.

• Examine data on nutrients that had not been previously considered essential nutrients.

• Make recommendations for future research to fill the identified knowledge gaps.

As reference values, the DRIs are quantitative estimates of nutrient intakes to be used for planning and assessing diets for healthy people (IOM 2006). Think of the DRIs as an umbrella term that includes the following specific definitions.

• **Recommended Dietary Allowance (RDA):** The intake that meets the nutrient requirement of almost all (97.5-98%) of the healthy individuals in a specific age and gender group. The RDAs can help people achieve adequate nutrient intake in order to decrease risks of chronic disease. Values for RDAs are estimates of average requirements plus increases to account for variations within a particular group. Available scientific evidence allowed DRI committees to calculate RDAs for vitamin A, vitamin C, vitamin E, phosphorus, magnesium, copper, iron, iodine, molybdenum, selenium, zinc, thiamin, riboflavin, niacin, vitamin B_6, folate, and vitamin B_{12}.

• **Adequate Intake (AI):** Empirical intake levels of healthy people, used when sufficient scientific evidence is not available to estimate RDAs. The AI values derive from experimental or observed intake levels that appear to sustain a desired indicator of health, such as calcium retention in bone, for most members of a population group. For example, the average observed nutrient intake of populations of breast-fed infants defined AIs for infants through 1 year of age. Individuals should use AIs as goals for intake where no RDAs exist. To date, DRI committees have set AIs for vitamin D, vitamin K, fluoride, pantothenic acid, biotin, choline, calcium, chromium, manganese, potassium, sodium, and chloride.

• **Estimated Average Requirement (EAR):** The nutrient intake value that is estimated to meet the requirement of half of the individuals in a specific group. This figure is used as a basis for developing the RDA. Makers of nutrition policy used EARs to evaluate the adequacy of nutrient intakes of a group and to plan how much the group should consume. For example, the RDA for a particular nutrient is calculated as follows: $RDA = EAR + 2\ SD_{EAR}$ where SD_{EAR} is the standard deviation of the EAR. If data about the variability in requirements are insufficient to allow calculation of a standard deviation (SD), a coefficient of variation (CV) for the EAR of 10% is ordinarily assumed.

• **Tolerable Upper Intake Level (UL):** The maximum intake by an individual that is unlikely to pose risks of adverse health effects to almost all healthy individuals in the general population. As intake increases above the UL, the risk of adverse effects increases. This figure is not intended to be a recommended level of intake. There is no established benefit for individuals to consume nutrients at levels above the RDA or AI. For most nutrients, the UL refers to total nutrient intake from food, fortified food, and nutrient supplements. The term "tolerable intake" was chosen to avoid implying a possible beneficial effect from this level of the nutrient.

• **Acceptable Macronutrient Distribution Ranges (AMDRs):** Ranges that have been established for fat, including essential fatty acids, protein, and carbohydrate. Acceptable ranges vary by age and gender. In addition to acceptable range values, carbohydrate and protein have established RDA values based on age and gender, while daily water intake, total fiber, and essential fatty acids have established AI values. The total water recommendation includes all water contained in food, beverages, and drinking water.

Figure 1.2 graphically describes the relationships among the preceding terms and shows where they fall on an intake continuum. Tolerable Upper Intake Levels have been established for vitamins A, C, D, E, B_6, niacin, and folate, as well as choline, boron, calcium, copper, fluoride, iodine, iron, magnesium, manganese, molybdenum, nickel, phosphorus, selenium, vanadium, zinc, sodium, and chloride.

ROLE OF EATING A BALANCED DIET

What does it mean to eat a balanced diet? Do active individuals need a different balanced diet from that of sedentary individuals? What does a "balanced diet" mean if you are a vegetarian?

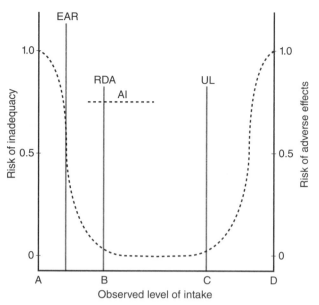

Figure 1.2 Dietary Reference Intakes. This figure shows that the Estimated Average Requirement (EAR) is the intake at which the risk of inadequacy is 0.5 (50%). The Recommended Dietary Allowance (RDA) is the intake at which the risk of inadequacy is very small—only 0.02 to 0.03 (2% to 3%). The Adequate Intake (AI) does not bear a consistent relationship to the EAR or the RDA because it is set without benefit of the ability to estimate the requirement. At intakes between the RDA and the Tolerable Upper Intake Level (UL), the risks of inadequacy and of adverse effects are both close to zero. The UL is the highest level of daily nutrient intake that is likely to pose no risks of adverse health effects to almost all individuals in the general population. At intakes above the UL, the risk of adverse effects increases. A dashed line is used because the actual shape of the curve has not been determined experimentally. The distances between points A and B, B and C, and C and D may differ much more than depicted in this figure.

Although the term "balanced diet" is frequently used by nutritionists and dietitians, most consumers have no clue as to its meaning or how to change their diet so that it is more "balanced." To help provide consumers with dietary guidelines and a simple way of evaluating their diets, the U.S. Department of Agriculture (USDA) and the Department of Health and Human Services

(USDHHS) developed the Dietary Guidelines for Americans and the Food Guide Pyramid. Similarly, the Canadian government has developed Canada's Guidelines for Healthy Eating (Health and Welfare Canada 1989) and Canada's Food Guide to Healthy Eating (1992). European countries, Australia, and New Zealand have developed similar guidelines. For example, in Switzerland, the Society for Nutrition (Schweizerische Gesellschaft für Ernährung) developed the Swiss Food Guide Pyramid, which formed the basis for a newly designed pyramid geared toward active individuals and athletes (Walter et al. 2007).

Dietary Guidelines for Americans

The Dietary Guidelines for Americans have evolved over the last 15 to 25 years in an attempt to answer the question "What should Americans eat to stay healthy?" (Kennedy 1998) (see table 1.1). The Dietary Guidelines—targeting healthy Americans age 2 years and older—provide advice about food choices that promote health, decrease the risk of chronic disease, meet nutrient requirements, and support active lives (Kennedy et al. 1996). The guidelines were developed by a panel

Table 1.1 Dietary Guidelines for 1980-2005

1980	1985	1990	1995	2000	2005
Eat a variety of foods.	Eat a variety of foods.	Eat a variety of foods.	Eat a variety of foods.	Let the pyramid guide your food choices.	Make smart choices from every food group.
Maintain ideal weight.	Maintain desirable weight.	Maintain healthy weight.	Balance the food you eat with physical activity—maintain or improve weight.	Aim for a healthy weight; be physically active each day.	Find your balance between food and physical activity.
Avoid too much fat, saturated fat, and cholesterol.	Avoid too much fat, saturated fat, and cholesterol.	Chose a diet low in fat, saturated fat, and cholesterol.	Choose a diet low in fat, saturated fat, and cholesterol.	Choose a diet that is low in saturated fat and cholesterol and moderate in total fat.	Know your fats: Look for foods low in saturated fats, trans fats, and cholesterol.
Eat foods with adequate starch and fiber.	Eat foods with adequate starch and fiber.	Choose a diet with plenty of vegetables, fruits, and grain products.	Choose a diet with plenty of grain products, vegetables, and fruits.	Choose a variety of fruits and vegetables daily.	Mix up your foods within each food group.
Avoid too much sugar.	Avoid too much sugar.	Use sugars only in moderation.	Choose a diet moderate in sugars.	Choose beverages and foods to moderate your intake of sugars.	Get the most nutrition out of your calories.
Avoid too much sodium.	Avoid too much sodium.	Use salt and sodium only in moderation.	Chose a diet moderate in salt and sodium.	Choose and prepare foods with less salt.	Reduce sodium; increase potassium.
If you drink alcohol, do so in moderation.	If you drink alcoholic beverages, do so in moderation.	If you drink alcoholic beverages, do so in moderation.	If you drink alcoholic beverages, do so in moderation.	If you drink alcoholic beverages, do so in moderation.	If you choose to drink alcohol, do so in moderation.

Reprinted from E. Kennedy, L. Meyers, and W. Layden, 2005, "The 1995 dietary guidelines for Americans: An overview," *Journal of American Dietetic Association* 96: 234-237; Adapted from Dietary guideline for Americans, 2005. Available: www.health.gov/dietaryguidelines/.

of experts based on current science as well as on input from the public and from government agencies. The 2005 Dietary Guidelines differ in scope from previous versions in that they synthesize comprehensive scientific analyses of individual food components and nutrients into recommendations for a pattern of eating. The language and messages of the guidelines are directed toward policy makers, health care providers, nutritionists, and nutrition educators who can translate the information into specific messages for the public (Dietary Guidelines for Americans 2005). Yet while the Dietary Guidelines in table 1.1 present general goals for all Americans (including active individuals), they do not provide the specific methods for achieving the goals. The newly released **Food Guide Pyramid** (2005), called MyPyramid, offers personalized recommendations for translating the message of the Dietary Guidelines into specific daily dietary suggestions (see the next section). Since the Dietary Guidelines were designed to convey dietary recommendations and not medical advice, it is the job of health professionals to help clients interpret and implement these guidelines within their own lifestyles. The key recommendations of the 2005 Dietary Guidelines for the general population are listed here followed by suggestions on how the guidelines can be translated into practical eating behaviors, attitudes, and healthy lifestyle changes (USDHHS and USDA, "Finding Your Way to a Healthier You" 2005).

1. **Feel better today, stay healthy for tomorrow.** This guideline reflects the message that food can be used to help prevent and manage chronic diseases in addition to meeting nutrient needs. Making healthy food choices now not only establishes a foundation for a lifetime of healthy behaviors; these choices also affect the composition of the body and future health.

2. **Make smart choices from every food group.** Making smart choices means emphasizing fruits and vegetables, whole grains, and low-fat dairy products for their nutrient density while limiting unhealthy fats and refined, added sugars. Remember that fat-containing foods are not inherently bad, though we do want to choose more monounsaturated and polyunsaturated fats (the type of fat found in foods like nuts, vegetable oils, and fish) while cutting back on saturated fats and *trans* fats (fats traditionally found in animal products, some margarines, and prepackaged and fast foods). Choosing what to eat and making smart food choices mean planning for all occasions—choosing appropriate foods at the grocery store,

at restaurants, when eating on the go, and while at work or at school. Making smart food choices involves making a plan and sticking to it.

3. **Mix up your choices within each food group.** Variety is what helps ensure that our body gets all of the important nutrients, phytochemicals, vitamins, and minerals that it needs to function and run efficiently. The key messages of the Dietary Guidelines emphasize choosing fats wisely for health, choosing and preparing foods with little salt, and making carbohydrate choices that promote good health. The following "catch phrases," also reflected in MyPyramid.gov, may be used to help apply these ideas.

- Focus on fruits
- Vary your veggies
- Get your calcium-rich foods
- Make half your grains whole
- Go lean with protein
- Know the limits on fats, salt, and sugar

4. **Find your balance between food and physical activity.** Following the trend of the 1995 recommendations, the 2005 Dietary Guidelines continue to emphasize that both diet and physical activity are important for weight control. The new pyramid schematic also reflects the importance of physical activity with the activity of stair climbing. The guidelines recommend being physically active for at least 30 min most days of the week to reduce chronic disease risk and reap other health benefits. Because lack of time is often cited as the biggest barrier to physical activity, the guidelines emphasize that short, 10 min bouts of activity can also be advantageous. It is the total accumulated time that is most important. To prevent weight gain, an additional 30 min of moderate- to vigorous-intensity exercise may be necessary. For maintaining weight loss in previously overweight or obese individuals, 60 to 90 min of physical activity per day is recommended. Children and teenagers are encouraged to engage in regular physical activity and to limit sedentary activities (Dietary Guidelines for Americans 2005). More information concerning physical activity recommendations can be found later in this chapter in the section "Physical Activity and Public Health."

5. **Get the most nutrition out of your calories.** For each person, there is an appropriate number of calories—the number that he or she needs to consume daily in order to stay in energy balance and maintain current body weight. The Dietary Guidelines recognize that it is easy to use up this

allotment on a few high-calorie food items, but that these foods rarely contain the nutrients needed to support body functions. Instead, choosing nutrient-dense foods ensures that vitamin and mineral needs are met. Choosing foods like fruits and vegetables, whole grains, and lean proteins helps ensure that both nutrient and energy needs are met.

6. **Nutrition: Know the facts—use the label.** The 2005 Dietary Guidelines stress the importance of learning to understand and use the nutrition labels on foods "to make smart food choices quickly and easily." The guidelines offer the following tips:

- Check servings and calories: Look at the serving size and at how many servings you are actually consuming.
- Make your calories count: Look at the calories on the label as well as the nutrients the food provides.
- Don't sugarcoat it: Since sugars contribute calories with few if any nutrients, look for foods and beverages low in added sugars. Some names for added sugars are sucrose, glucose, high-fructose corn syrup, corn syrup, maple syrup, and fructose.
- Know your fats: Look for foods low in saturated fats, *trans* fats, and cholesterol to reduce the risk of heart disease.
- Reduce sodium (salt), increase potassium: Research indicates that eating less than 2300 mg of sodium (about 1 tsp) per day can reduce the risk of high blood pressure. This recommendation may not apply to very physically active individuals and athletes exercising in hot climates, since they can lose large amounts of sodium through sweating (see chapter 8). Keep in mind that most of the sodium we consume comes from processed foods, whereas foods high in potassium are whole and unprocessed items such as fresh fruits and vegetables.

7. **Play it safe with food.** The new Dietary Guidelines emphasize food safety and stress the importance of knowing how to prepare, handle, and store foods to prevent food-borne illnesses and diseases. The guidelines recommend washing hands thoroughly before handling food, cleaning food surfaces, and separating meats from vegetables during food preparation. Cooking meat thoroughly and reheating dishes to appropriate internal temperatures will help prevent potential illnesses from microorganisms, and chilling perishable food promptly will keep it fresh and safe to eat.

8. **If you drink alcoholic beverages, do so in moderation.** Although the wording of this guideline is the same as in the 1990 edition, there are slight changes in the text accompanying it (Kennedy et al. 1996). The guideline acknowledges that current research associates moderate drinking with lower risks of heart disease and that many societies use alcoholic beverages to enhance the enjoyment of meals. The guidelines define moderation as one drink a day for women and up to two drinks for men. However, there is still a strong emphasis on the negative effects of high levels of alcohol intake, which can increase risks of high blood pressure, stroke, heart disease, certain cancers, accidents, violence, suicides, birth defects, cirrhosis of the liver, inflammation of the pancreas, and overall mortality (deaths). High alcohol intake also increases the risk of malnutrition, because the energy in alcohol may replace other more nutritious foods. Finally, the guidelines include a listing of individuals who should not drink.

Food Guide Pyramids

The USDA first released the Food Guide Pyramid in 1992, intending to translate the Dietary Guidelines recommendations on nutrient intake into practical recommendations for food intake (Cronin 1998; Welsh et al. 1992; Nestle 1998). The most recent version, **MyPyramid,** was released in 2005 and was designed to apply to a wide range of ages and activity levels for both men and women (Britten et al. 2006). MyPyramid retained the five primary food groups from the original pyramid: Fruits; Vegetables; Bread, Cereal, Rice, and Pasta; Meat, Poultry, Fish, Dry Beans, Eggs, and Nuts; and Milk, Yogurt, and Cheese (Britten et al. 2006). Based on the nutrient guidelines of MyPyramid and the 2005 Dietary Guidelines, adult men and women need to increase fruit consumption by 100%, increase vegetable consumption by 50%, and nearly quadruple whole grain consumption (e.g. replace processed grains with whole grains); women should double their intake of dairy products to meet current recommendations (Britten et al. 2006).

The MyPyramid diagram is shown in figure 1.3; however, an interactive and comprehensive Web site (MyPyramid.gov) provides custom recommendations based on age, gender, and activity level (entering weight and height is optional). This Web site also gives users the opportunity to track food intake and activity (MyPyramid Tracker) to

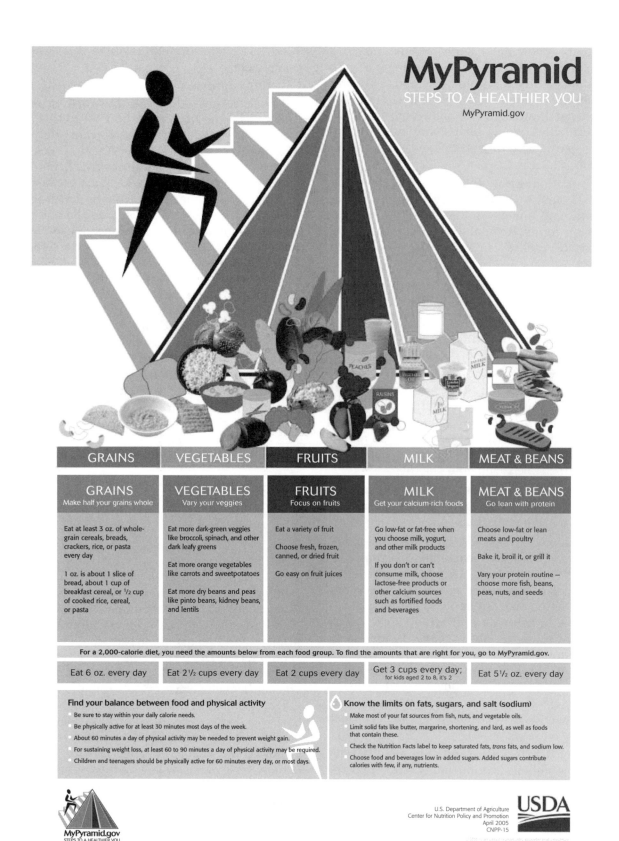

Figure 1.3 USDA MyPyramid.
U.S. Department of Agriculture and the U.S. Department of Health and Human Services or USDA and USDHHS.

identify energy (calorie) and nutrient intake and energy expenditure. The Web site has a section for children and a modified graphic to instruct kids on the importance of making good food choices, and a new feature provides information specific to pregnant and lactating women. According to the USDA's Center for Nutrition Policy and Promotion, "The plan for the USDA MyPyramid Food Guidance System included a new graphic and slogan, clear and concise nutrition messages, and a variety of materials and tools to help motivate and educate consumers to follow a healthful diet. The MyPyramid.gov Web site was developed to provide a range of tools and information to meet the needs of varied audiences" (Haven et al. 2006,

p S153). Canada's Food Guide was revised in 2007, and like the MyPyramid eating plan, contains a personalized section to help consumers make individualized choices regarding servings and portions from each food group. It was designed to translate the science of nutrition into a healthy eating pattern that emphasizes physical activity and good nutrition ("Eating Well with Canada's Food Guide," www.healthcanada.gc.ca/foodguide).

Using MyPyramid

A key to using MyPyramid is understanding what constitutes a serving size for each of the food groups and how many servings from each group should be consumed. Figure 1.4 and table 1.2

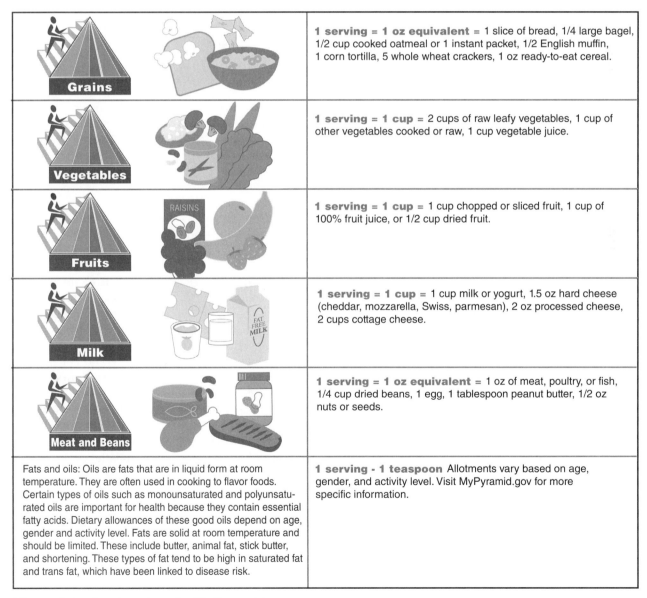

Grains	**1 serving = 1 oz equivalent** = 1 slice of bread, 1/4 large bagel, 1/2 cup cooked oatmeal or 1 instant packet, 1/2 English muffin, 1 corn tortilla, 5 whole wheat crackers, 1 oz ready-to-eat cereal.
Vegetables	**1 serving = 1 cup** = 2 cups of raw leafy vegetables, 1 cup of other vegetables cooked or raw, 1 cup vegetable juice.
Fruits	**1 serving = 1 cup** = 1 cup chopped or sliced fruit, 1 cup of 100% fruit juice, or 1/2 cup dried fruit.
Milk	**1 serving = 1 cup** = 1 cup milk or yogurt, 1.5 oz hard cheese (cheddar, mozzarella, Swiss, parmesan), 2 oz processed cheese, 2 cups cottage cheese.
Meat and Beans	**1 serving = 1 oz equivalent** = 1 oz of meat, poultry, or fish, 1/4 cup dried beans, 1 egg, 1 tablespoon peanut butter, 1/2 oz nuts or seeds.
Fats and oils: Oils are fats that are in liquid form at room temperature. They are often used in cooking to flavor foods. Certain types of oils such as monounsaturated and polyunsaturated oils are important for health because they contain essential fatty acids. Dietary allowances of these good oils depend on age, gender and activity level. Fats are solid at room temperature and should be limited. These include butter, animal fat, stick butter, and shortening. These types of fat tend to be high in saturated fat and trans fat, which have been linked to disease risk.	**1 serving - 1 teaspoon** Allotments vary based on age, gender, and activity level. Visit MyPyramid.gov for more specific information.

Figure 1.4 Serving sizes for MyPyramid.

U.S. Department of Agriculture and the U.S. Department of Health and Human Services or USDA and USDHHS.

Table 1.2   Sample Diet for a Day at Four Different Energy (kcal) Levels

Food group	Tip	1600 kcal/day	2200 kcal/day	2800 kcal/day	3200 kcal/day
Grains	Make at least half your grains whole.	5 oz equivalents	7 oz equivalents	10 oz equivalents	10 oz equivalents
Vegetables	Try to have vegetables from several subgroups each day.	2 cups	3 cups	3.5 cups	4 cups
Fruits	Make most choices fruit, not juice.	1.5 cups	2 cups	2.5 cups	2.5 cups
Milk	Choose fat-free or low-fat most often.	3 cups	3 cups	3 cups	3 cups
Meat and beans	Choose lean meat and poultry. Vary your choices—more fish, beans, peas, nuts, and seeds.	5 oz equivalents	6 oz equivalents	7 oz equivalents	7 oz equivalents
Physical activity	Build more physical activity into your daily routine at home and work.	At least 30 min of moderate to vigorous activity a day, 10 min or more at a time	At least 30 min of moderate to vigorous activity a day, 10 min or more at a time	At least 30 min of moderate to vigorous activity a day, 10 min or more at a time	At least 30 min of moderate to vigorous activity a day, 10 min or more at a time

U.S. Department of Agriculture and the U.S. Department of Health and Human Services or USDA and USDHHS.

provide this information. (Figure 1.5 is a worksheet that can be used to track food intake and compare actual with the desired intake.) Table 1.2 also outlines some of the specific food and nutrition messages carried in the MyPyramid diagram—the primary messages being the importance of dietary variety, dietary fat and sugar awareness, balance (serving size and number of servings within each food group), and physical activity. As a health professional, you can decide which of these specific messages you want to emphasize with your client. The pyramid provides an excellent way to quickly review individuals' dietary intake and to recommend dietary changes that combine their food preferences with their specific energy and nutrient needs (see "Building Your Own Food Guide Pyramid" p. 15).

Variations of Food Guide Pyramids

Many countries have their own nutrition organizations that develop dietary guidelines, reference intakes, and food guide pyramids to meet the dietary needs of the particular population, taking into consideration cultural aspects related to food, eating patterns, and lifestyle factors. One of the most often referenced food guide pyramids is the Mediterranean Food Guide Pyramid, designed for most of the Mediterranean countries, from the Atlantic coast (Portugal) to the Mediterranean Sea (Italy, France, Spain, Greece) to the eastern countries, including Turkey, Lebanon, and Israel. Considering the range of countries, it should become apparent that the Mediterranean diet has many variations; however, it is mainly characterized by an increased consumption of fruit and vegetables, fish, whole grains and legumes, red wine, nuts, olive oil, some cheeses, eggs, and yogurt, with a much lower intake of meat, especially red meat. The Mediterranean diet has been simplified over the years, and Manios and colleagues (2006) have recently highlighted the original diet of the island of Crete. In addition to the foods just listed, the original diet of Crete included an abundance of locally grown wild greens and herbs, walnuts, figs, and snails—all foods rich in omega-3 fatty acids. Previous research has described the health benefits of the Mediterranean diet (Giugliano and Esposito 2008; Lairon 2007; Renaud et al. 1995; Tavani et al. 1995), particularly with respect to the lower risk for cardiovascular disease.

MyPyramid.gov
STEPS TO A HEALTHIER YOU

MyPyramid Worksheet
Check how you did today and set a goal to aim for tomorrow

Food Group	Tip	Goal Based on a 2400 calorie pattern.	Write in Your Choices for Today / List each food choice in its food group*	Estimate Your Total
GRAINS	Make at least half your grains whole grains	**8 ounce equivalents** (1 ounce equivalent is about 1 slice bread, 1 cup dry cereal, or ½ cup cooked rice, pasta, or cereal)	_____ _____ _____	_____ ounce equivalents
VEGETABLES	Try to have vegetables from several subgroups each day	**3 cups** Subgroups: Dark Green, Orange, Starchy, Dry Beans and Peas, Other Veggies	_____ _____	_____ cups
FRUITS	Make most choices fruit, not juice	**2 cups**	_____ _____	_____ cups
MILK	Choose fat-free or low fat most often	**3 cups** (1 ½ ounces cheese = 1 cup milk)	_____ _____	_____ cups
MEAT & BEANS	Choose lean meat and poultry. Vary your choices—more fish, beans, peas, nuts, and seeds	**6 ½ ounce equivalents** (1 ounce equivalent is 1 ounce meat, poultry, or fish, 1 egg, 1 T. peanut butter, ½ ounce nuts, or ¼ cup dry beans)	_____ _____	_____ ounce equivalents
PHYSICAL ACTIVITY	Build more physical activity into your daily routine at home and work.	At least **30 minutes** of moderate to vigorous activity a day. 10 minutes or more at a time.	_____	_____ minutes

*Some foods don't fit into any group. These "extras" may be mainly fat or sugar—limit your intake of these.

How did you do today? ☐ Great ☐ So-So ☐ Not so Great

My food goal for tomorrow is: _____

My activity goal for tomorrow is: _____

Figure 1.5 MyPyramid worksheet.
U.S. Department of Agriculture and the U.S. Department of Health and Human Services or USDA and USDHHS.

13

The Mediterranean diet can also fit an active lifestyle: It is high in nutrient-dense carbohydrates and fruit and vegetables, and moderate in protein. The Mediterranean diet is relatively high in fat (contains ~40% fat as opposed to the recommended 20-35% fat in the U.S. diet), mainly from sources such as olive oil, nuts, and fish. This higher fat content makes this diet an ideal dietary approach for endurance athletes recovering from prolonged exercise training and events such as marathons and ultra-endurance events. These highly trained athletes oxidize more fat for a given relative and absolute intensity than untrained individuals, particularly from fats stored in muscle (intramuscular triglycerides; see chapter 3). Research has shown that 50% of these fats are typically depleted after 2 h of submaximal exercise and that an athlete on a traditionally low-fat diet will not replace these fats during a 48 h period (Van Loon et al. 2003). Thus, eating more fat at the right time may help in the recovery process, as long as the fats are from sources such as nuts, seeds, olive oil, and fish. The Mediterranean diet can also be modified to fit athletes with lower energy requirements who need to eat a nutrient-dense diet. They can simply reduce the total amount of fat from olive oil, cheese, and nuts but maintain the high intake of vegetables, whole grains, and lean sources of protein. Appendixes A.1 through A.4, pp. 501-504, illustrate the Mediterranean Food Guide Pyramid along with other food guide pyramids. Most pyramids are somewhat similar in that all are based on the same building blocks—grains, vegetables, and fruit (Kennedy 1998; Nestle 1998)—and all include daily physical activity. Before recommending these modifications of the Food Guide Pyramid to your clients, however, be sure you understand how your clients are interpreting the messages in these pyramids (Crotty 1998a, 1998b; Gifford 1998; Nestle 1998; Wilson 1998). As with any general nutrition guideline, you can adapt information from any of the pyramids for use with a specific individual. In general, the pyramids provide a visual educational tool that can help consumers make wise daily food choices.

Few pyramids exist that specifically address athletes. Houtkooper (1994) modified the standard 1992 U.S. Food Guide Pyramid and included fluids as a new food category at the base of the pyramid, underlining the importance of adequate hydration for athletes. The new U.S. Food Guide Pyramid is more easily adapted to fit athletes' dietary needs; however, the recommendations and available worksheets (as shown in figure 1.5) apply only up to 3000 kcal/day, and these guidelines were not developed specifically to fit the athlete's energy and nutrient needs. Recently, the Swiss Forum for Sport Nutrition designed a Food Pyramid for Athletes, which is discussed next.

The Food Pyramid for Athletes

The Swiss Forum for Sport Nutrition designed the Food Pyramid for Athletes, which builds on the foundation of the Basic Food Pyramid used in Switzerland, originally designed for normally active (physical activity level, PAL = 1.4) healthy adults and published through the Swiss Society for Nutrition. The additional guidelines for athletes illustrated in the Food Pyramid for Athletes cover the extra energy and nutrient requirement incurred by the demands of daily exercise training (figure 1.6 on pp. 16-17).

Multiple steps were involved in the design of the Food Pyramid for Athletes. The first step was to define the additional energy requirement for exercise. For this purpose, the energy requirement of different sports performed at various intensities was considered (Ainsworth et al. 2000), and an additional average requirement of 0.4 kJ (~0.1 kcal) per minute of exercise and kilogram of body mass was defined. This represents running at approximately 8 km/h (5 mph), cycling at 2 W/kg body mass on a bicycle ergometer, or the "stop and go" nature of most intermittent and team sports such as an average ice hockey match, soccer game, or tennis match.

Following the integration of volume and intensity of various sports, the additional energy requirement was divided into the different food groups of the pyramid, with the macronutrient recommendations for sport taken into consideration (Burke et al. 2004; Tipton and Wolfe 2004). Consideration was also given to the extra servings added to each food group for the athlete and to the issue of whether such quantities are feasible in a real-life setting. Additional sport-specific foods and fluids such as sport drinks, energy bars, or recovery products were also integrated. The issue of different energy needs relative to body mass was solved through adjustment of the serving sizes originally established for the Basic Food Pyramid. Consequently, it is the duration of daily exercise training that determines the number of extra servings, whereas the athlete's body mass determines the serving size.

As a final step, the validation of the Food Pyramid for Athletes involved examining whether a simulated practical implementation of the pyramid's recommendations led to the desired energy

Building Your Own Food Guide Pyramid

Encourage your clients to build their own food guide pyramid. The new MyPyramid Web site provides opportunity for individuals to create a personalized eating plan. Visit MyPyramid.gov; click on the MyPyramid Plan; and enter age, sex, weight, height, and physical activity level for an estimate of energy (kcal) needs. This is a good place to start and provides a general overview of the number of servings one would need from each food group to meet daily energy needs. The Web site also offers a MyPyramid Tracker function that enables users to keep a food log and enter daily activities. The general recommendations can be somewhat low for athletes, so using this tool and the Pyramid for Athletes (figure 1.6) can help point your clients in the right direction. Eating smart and exercising are not just for today; they are lifetime commitments. The following are some guidelines for helping clients make gradual changes in diet and exercise that will translate into a lifetime of positive health behaviors. Get them to start building their pyramid now!

1. **Modify food choices gradually.** This is easier than overhauling your whole diet at once. For example, begin selecting 1% or 2% milk instead of whole milk. When the time is right, you can make the big jump to nonfat milk or stay with 1% milk. This substitution will help reduce both fat and energy intake. Another easy change is to substitute whole wheat bread for white bread or to add beans to a meal. These changes will help improve micronutrient and fiber intakes.

2. **Choose foods from the five major food groups on a daily basis.** If you are vegetarian, choose beans, legumes, tofu, or other high-protein foods instead of meat. Learn to build your pyramid from the bottom up—with plenty of whole grains, fruits, and vegetables! Use the Food Guide Pyramid to help make meal selections. If it is dinnertime and you have not eaten any vegetables yet, this would be a great time to have a big salad or a bowl of stir-fried vegetables instead of a hamburger. Remember that fat is not the enemy. Choosing healthful monounsaturated and polyunsaturated fats, especially as replacements for saturated and *trans* fats, can go a long way toward improving health and reducing disease risk.

3. **Use moderation as your goal.** Do not set out to eliminate all your favorite foods. This will not work and may cause you to binge on these foods after days of deprivation. Try to eat foods lower in fat and sugar more often than foods high in these components. Work to keep your meals and snacks in balance. Learn to pack healthy snacks with you to help reduce the urge to eat from the vending machine. Pick low-fat milk, juice, and water over soda pop.

4. **Spice up your life.** Try new foods. Besides the nutritional benefits, a variety of foods adds interest to meals and snacks. For example, add new vegetables to your shopping list, try new menu items in restaurants, or add the seasonal fruits to your diet. If you are really adventurous, try adding a new recipe each week to your standard menu. This can make eating more interesting for everyone sitting around your dinner table. If you do not cook, start. You may find that you love the adventure.

5. **Drink lots of fluids.** Water is an important nutrient we often forget about. Learn to drink water throughout the day and at mealtimes. In addition, consuming fruits, vegetables, soups, coffee, tea, and fruit juices adds fluid to the body. Remember that in young athletes, thirst is not always a good indicator of fluid needs. They should drink even when they are not thirsty, especially on hot days. Sport beverages are a great way to keep hydrated when exercising.

6. **Evaluate your lifestyle.** Are you active? Is your weight stable? Do you want to gain or lose weight? Consider the amount of energy (kcal) and food you need to maintain your current lifestyle. Then from each food group, eat enough servings—at least the minimum—to reach or stay at your healthy weight.

7. **Get active.** For athletes, getting active is usually not a problem. If you are not already active, however, begin adding physical activity to your day. For example, take the stairs instead of the elevator; walk briskly on your next errand instead of driving the car; work in the yard; briskly walk the dog; take a walk on your lunch hour; or try exercising in front of the TV. If you are already physically active, try increasing the intensity at which you exercise, adding a new sport or activity to your exercise routine, or beginning strength training. Exercise helps keep your muscles toned, burns calories, and makes you feel great! Remember, weight is maintained when you burn all the calories consumed each day.

and nutrient supply. A total of 168 days of simulated meal plans were developed for athletes of differing body mass (range: 50-85 kg, 110-187 lb) training 1 to 4 h/day. All meal plans were evaluated indi- vidually and compared with reference values. The reference values for energy were calculated using the formula for the Estimated Energy Require- ment (EER) of the Dietary Reference Intake (DRI)

Food Pyramid for Athletes

For athletes exercising ≥5 hours per week

Based on the Food Pyramid for healthy adults of the Swiss Society for Nutrition

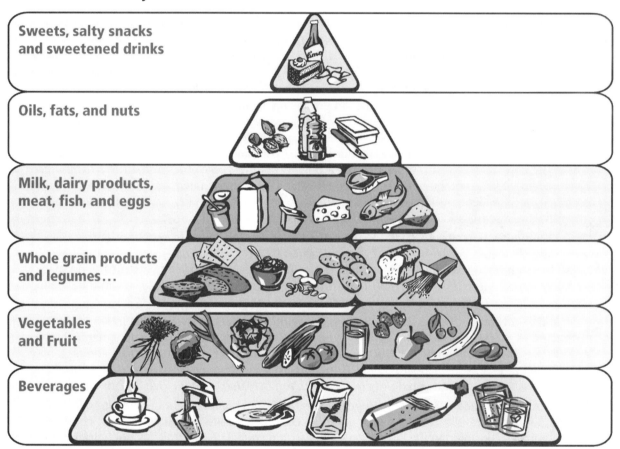

Sweets, salty snacks and sweetened drinks

Oils, fats, and nuts

Milk, dairy products, meat, fish, and eggs

Whole grain products and legumes...

Vegetables and Fruit

Beverages

© 2005 Swiss Society for Nutrition SSN

The Food Pyramid for Athletes is based on the Food Pyramid designed and developed by the Swiss Society for Nutrition (Schweizerische Gesellschaft für Ernährung) for healthy adults, which for the purpose of this chapter will be referred to as the Basic Food Pyramid. This Basic Food Pyramid has been expanded to cover the energy and nutrient needs for daily exercise typically performed by athletes and active individuals.

The Food Pyramid for Athletes is aimed at healthy adults exercising on most days of the week for at least one hour or more per day at moderate intensity, totaling at least 5 hours of exercise per week.

Moderate intensity represents continuous activities such as swimming (2.5 km/h), running (8 km/h) or cycling (2 watts per kg body mass) or the "stop and go" of most intermittent and team sports such as an

ice hockey match, a soccer game or tennis match. The Basic Food Pyramid reflects balance in food choice, and the same applies to the recommendations for athletes. Both pyramids ensure sufficient energy and nutrient supply for their target population. All foods are allowed, but it is important that a variety of foods are chosen from each section, that produce is chosen seasonally, and all foods are processed gently. The regular intake of vitamin and/or mineral-fortified

Figure 1.6 Food Pyramid for Athletes. This pyramid is for athletes exercising ≤ 5 h per week. A free version of the Food Pyramid for Athletes, in color, can be downloaded from the Web site of the Swiss Forum for Sport Nutrition at www.sfsn.ch. *(continued)*

for adult men and women (Institute of Medicine, 2005). A physical activity level (PAL) of 1.4 (corresponding to a physical activity coefficient value of 1.11 and 1.12 for men and women, respectively, in the EER formula [Institute of Medicine, 2005]) was used for a sedentary lifestyle (zero hours of exercise), as the basic pyramid is designed for this PAL (Walter, Infanger et al., 2007). The previously defined additional energy requirement for exercise of 0.1 kcal·kg^{-1}·min^{-1} was added to the sedentary lifestyle energy requirement to get the reference energy intake for one, two, three, and four hours of exercise per day. The evaluation of these meal plans showed that the energy requirement was fulfilled by 97%. The carbohydrate supply was 4.7, 6.4, 7.5, and 8.6 g/kg body mass, and the protein

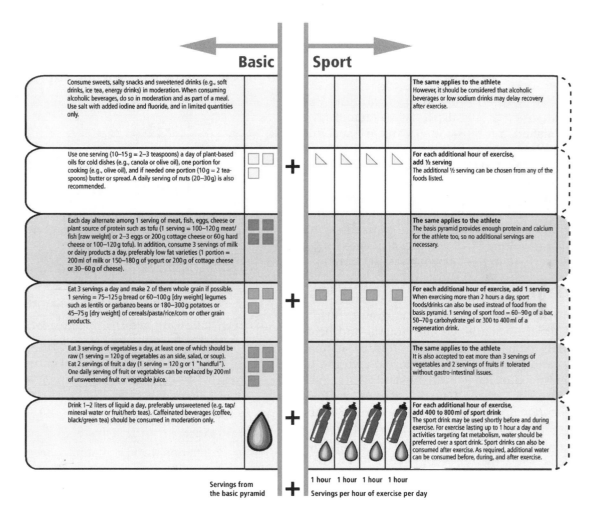

Version 1.0 © 2008 Swiss Forum for Sport Nutrition, www.sfsn.ch, in collaboration with ETH Zurich and Federal Office of Sport FOSPO

foods and beverages or the use of dietary supplements may exceed the upper tolerable intake level.

Adherence to the Food Pyramid for Athletes offers a solid foundation for long-term, successful performance capability. In contrast to the Basic Food Pyramid, where the recommendations do not have to be followed strictly on a daily basis, it is suggested that athletes meet the guidelines consistently to ensure optimal regeneration and performance capability. The additional requirement to cover exercise training includes a volume of 1 to 4 hours of moderate intensity exercise per day. For high-intensity exercise and/or greater volumes, the energy and nutrient requirements will be higher. For athletes, the serving sizes depend on body mass. Small servings apply to a body mass of about 50 kg, whereas the largest serving sizes apply for an athlete weighing about 85 kg. Intermediate serving sizes apply to an athlete of corresponding intermediate body mass (e.g. medium serving size for 67 kg). Quantification of the serving sizes can be found in the pyramid.

Figure 1.6 *(continued)*

supply was 1.6, 1.7, 1.8, and 1.9 g/kg body mass for 1, 2, 3, and 4 h of exercise training per day, respectively. The average micronutrient supply exceeded 100% of DRIs (IOM 1997, 1998, 2000, 2001) for all micronutrients; and at an energy supply of 14 MJ/day (3344 kcal/day) or higher, the micronutrient provision covered between 200% and 400% of DRIs for nearly all micronutrients. Based on this validation, it can be concluded that the Food Pyramid for Athletes is a well-founded food guide pyramid applicable to athletes.

ROLE OF NUTRITION AND EXERCISE IN DISEASE PREVENTION

The role that nutrition and physical activity play in reducing chronic disease risk factors is well established. Yet most Americans are sedentary, overweight, and eat too many calories that are high in saturated fat and sugar as well as too few whole fruits, vegetables, grains, and low-fat proteins. In order to communicate positive nutrition and physical activity messages to all Americans, various public and private organizations have jointly developed diet and physical activity goals as described in the following two sections.

Healthy People 2010

Healthy People 2010 is a national initiative designed to challenge individuals and professionals to take necessary steps toward sustaining long and healthy lives. Developed with the best scientific knowledge available and the resources of the 1979 *Surgeon General's Report on Disease Prevention and Health Promotion,* the 1980 report *Promoting Health/Preventing Disease: Objectives for the Nation (1980),* and most recently *Healthy People: 2000,* Healthy People 2010 sets forth 467 specific objectives in 28 different focus areas to achieve two primary goals: (1) to increase quality and years of healthy life and (2) to eliminate health disparities.

Encouraged by the lessons learned from the Healthy People 2000 initiative, namely that the health of our nation can be influenced and altered in a relatively short period of time, Healthy People 2010 hopes to address, among other issues, chronic disease, mental disorders, violence and abusive behaviors, obesity, and the increasing lack of physical activity in the United States. The specific objectives serve as a guide for public

health professionals working toward the goals of Healthy People 2010 at the individual, community, state, and national levels. In late 2006, a midcourse review was published that allowed researchers to reorganize objectives, drop unproductive objectives, and track progress (*Healthy People 2010: Midcourse Review* 2007). Halfway through the decade, progress was noted toward the end goal for 70% of the 507 trackable objectives and subobjectives. Tracking progress will allow the initiative to continue to develop in the most productive and sustainable way possible (see "Healthy People 2010: Goals and Focus Areas"). Appendix A.5 also provides a complete list of public and private organizations involved in developing and implementing the objectives—agencies, among others that, by the year 2010, expect to publish even newer objectives for Healthy People 2020.

Healthy People 2010: Goals and Focus Areas

Healthy People 2010 establishes two primary goals, at which 28 focus areas and 467 specific objectives are aimed.

> Goal 1: Increase Quality and Years of Healthy Life
>
> Goal 2: Eliminate Health Disparities

The following are the specific focus areas related to nutrition and exercise:

> Arthritis, osteoporosis, and chronic back conditions
>
> Cancer
>
> Chronic kidney disease
>
> Diabetes
>
> Educational and community-based programs
>
> Environmental health
>
> Food safety
>
> Heart disease and stroke
>
> Maternal, infant, and child health
>
> Nutrition and overweight
>
> Physical activity and fitness

For a full list of objectives related to each of these focus areas, visit www.healthypeople.gov.

From U.S. Department of Health and Human Services.

Physical Activity and Public Health

The greatest emphasis in the Healthy People 2010 objectives is on getting the American population more physically active. The American College of Sports Medicine (ACSM) is the largest sports medicine and exercise science organization in the world and routinely publishes recommendations for physical activity and public health. Recently, the college updated the recommendations for physical activity, health promotion, and disease prevention. In addition, the USDHHS released its *Physical Activity Guidelines Advisory Committee Report* in 2008. This was the first time the United States had issued a specific report for the American public on the health benefits of physical activity and a summary of the science to support these recommendations. Listed next are the most current recommendations for exercise targeting healthy adults aged 18 to 65 years (Haskell et al. 2007). These recommendations are also in accordance with the American Heart Association (AHA) (2007) and the USDHHS Physical Activity Guidelines (2008).

Aerobic Activity

- Perform moderate-intensity aerobic physical activity for a minimum of 30 min at least five days per week.
- OR perform vigorous-intensity aerobic physical activity for a minimum of 20 min at least three days per week.
- Combinations of moderate- and vigorous-intensity activity can be performed to meet this recommendation.

Muscle-Strengthening Activity

- Perform activities that maintain or increase muscular strength and endurance for a minimum of two days a week (two nonconsecutive days).
- Eight to 10 exercises should be included to target all the major muscle groups.
- A weight should be used that allows 8 to 12 repetitions resulting in volitional fatigue.

It should also be noted that these guidelines are recommended in addition to daily living activities of light intensity (e.g., cooking, cleaning, casual walking or shopping) or activities lasting less than 10 min in duration (e.g., walking around the house, or from the parking lot). Individuals looking for further improvements in their physical health and decreased disease risk may exceed the minimum recommendations. In addition, people trying to lose weight or prevent unhealthy weight gain may have to exceed these recommendations. To achieve energy balance, individuals must take into consideration level of physical activity, food intake, and other factors that may affect their body weight. To achieve negative energy balance for weight loss, it has been consistently demonstrated that weight loss and weight maintenance are most successful if daily activity accompanies healthy food choices such that the nutrition and exercise components both contribute to a daily calorie deficit appropriate for moderate and sustainable weight loss (Jakicic et al. 2001).

The recommended amounts of physical activity can be accumulated in short bouts of activity throughout the day. Although exercising at a greater intensity and for a longer duration will certainly improve physical fitness and provide definite health benefits, people can gain most of the health benefits by performing moderate physical activity. Moreover, most people are more likely to work toward accumulating 30 min of total activity each day than to achieve 30 min of activity in one session. Table 1.3 provides examples of moderate-intensity activities. One of the reasons for the current low participation in physical activity may be that individuals assume they will reap health benefits only if they engage in vigorous continuous activity for 30 to 60 min. We now know this is not true. Health benefits gained from increased physical activity depend on one's initial activity level. Sedentary individuals realize the most benefit from increasing their activity to recommended levels. Ideally, a fitness program should include an aerobic (cardiorespiratory) component and muscle strength, endurance, and flexibility components (see chapter 14).

Despite the well-documented benefits of physical activity, many individuals have barriers to starting a fitness program, or excuses for why they cannot start a fitness program, or both. The highlight "15 Great Reasons to Get More Active" on p. 21 tells why your clients should start performing exercise, including aerobic, strength, and balance activities. Give this list to your clients to help encourage them to get motivated.

CHAPTER IN REVIEW

Diet and exercise play an important role in health, sport performance, and the reduction of chronic disease risk factors. Numerous government and

Table 1.3 Examples of Common Physical Activities for Healthy U.S. Adults

Light (<3.0 METs or <4 kcal/min)	Moderate (3.0-6.0 METs or 4-7 kcal/min)	Hard or vigorous (>6.0 METs or >7 kcal/min)
Walking	**Walking**	**Walking, jogging, and running**
Walking slowly around the house, store, or office = 2.0 METs	Walking 3.0 mph = 3.3 METs Walking at a very brisk pace (4 mph) = 5.0 METs	Walking at a very, very brisk pace (4.5 mph) = 6.3 METs Walking or hiking at moderate pace and grade with no pack or light pack (<10 lb) = 7.0 METs Hiking at steep grades and pack of 10-42+ lb = 7.5-9.0 METs Jogging at 5 mph = 8.0 METs Jogging at 6 mph = 10.0 METs Running at 7 mph = 11.5 METs
	Household and occupation	
Sitting, doing computer work at desk, using light hand tools = 1.5 METs Standing, performing light work such as bed making, washing dishes, ironing, preparing food; or working as store clerk = 2.0-2.5 METs	Cleaning—heavy: washing windows, washing car, cleaning garage = 3.0 METs Sweeping floors or carpet, vacuuming, mopping = 3.3-3.5 METs Carpentry—general = 3.5 METs Carrying and stacking wood = 5.0 METs Mowing lawn—walking power mower = 5.5 METs	Shoveling sand, coal, and so on = 7.0 METs Carrying heavy loads such as bricks = 8.0 METs Heavy farming such as baling hay = 8.0 METs Shoveling, digging ditches = 8.5 METs
	Leisure time and sports	
Arts and crafts, playing cards = 1.5 METs Billiards = 2.5 METs Boating—power = 2.5 METs Croquet = 2.5 METs Darts = 2.5 METs Fishing—sitting = 2.5 METs Playing most musical instruments = 2.0-2.5 METs	Badminton, recreational = 4.5 METs Basketball, shooting around = 4.5 METs Bicycling, on flat, light effort (10-12 mph) = 5.0 METs Dancing, ballroom, fast = 4.5 METs Fishing from river bank and walking = 4.0 METs Golf—walking, pulling clubs = 4.3 METs Sailing boat, wind surfing = 3.0 METs Leisurely swimming = 6.0 METs Table tennis = 4.0 METs Tennis doubles = 5.0 METs Volleyball, noncompetitive = 3.0-4.0 METs	Basketball game = 8.0 METs Bicycling, on flat, moderate effort (12-14 mph) = 8.0 METs; fast (14-16 mph) = 10.0 METs Skiing cross country, slow (2.5 mph) = 7.0 METs; fast (5.0-7.9 mph) = 9.0 METs Soccer, casual = 7.0 METs; competitive = 10.0 METs Swimming, moderate/hard = 8-11.0 METs Tennis singles = 8.0 METs Volleyball, competitive at gym or beach = 8.0 METs

Activities are classified according to kilocalories (kcal) per minute. The METs (metabolic equivalents: work metabolic rate/resting metabolic rate) are multiples of the resting rate of oxygen consumption during physical activity. One MET represents the approximate rate of oxygen consumption of a seated adult at rest, or about 3.5 mL · kg^{-1} · min^{-1}. The equivalent energy cost of 1 MET in kcal/min is about 1.2 for a 70 kg person, or approximately 1 kcal · kg^{-1} · h^{-1}.

Adapted from B.E. Ainsworth et al. 2000, "Compendium of physical activities: An update of activity codes and MET intensities," *Medicine and Science in Sports and Exercise* 32: S498-S504.

professional agencies have identified essential dietary nutrients, recommended appropriate nutrient intakes, and defined goals for nutrition and exercise for all North Americans. They have also developed educational tools to help implement these recommendations in people's daily lives. The goal now is to learn how to motivate individuals to make positive diet and exercise changes. While this is a tremendous challenge, this book will give you the knowledge, understanding, and tools necessary to help you teach your clients how to make healthy lifestyle changes.

Highlight: 15 Great Reasons to Get More Active

1. Helps maintain a healthy body weight and reduces abdominal fat.

2. Helps prevent weight regain if weight has been lost due to dieting.

3. Helps increase muscle mass, strength, power, and neuromuscular activation.

4. Helps maintain bone health and improve joint function.

5. Helps reduce the risk of hip fracture by 36% to 68% and the risk of falls in older adults by 30%.

6. Reduces risk of cardiovascular disease, coronary heart disease, and stroke by 20% to 35%.

7. Reduces risk of hypertension and high blood lipids.

8. Reduces risk of diabetes and metabolic syndrome by 30% to 40%.

9. Reduces risk of colon cancer by 30% and risk of breast cancer by 20%.

10. Improves posture and decreases risk of lower back pain.

11. Reduces risk for depression, distress, and dementia by 20% to 30%.

12. Improves sleep.

13. Reduces risk of all-cause mortality by 30%.

14. Improves self-esteem and feelings of energy.

15. Improves overall quality of life.

Adapted from Physical Activity Guidelines Advisory Committee, 2008, *Physical Activity Guidelines Advisory Committee Report, 2008* (Washington, DC: U.S. Department of Health and Human Services).

Key Concepts

1. Understand the role of nutrition in exercise and sport.

Good nutrition can improve exercise performance, decrease recovery time from strenuous exercise, prevent exercise injuries due to fatigue, provide the fluid and fuel required during times of high-intensity training, and help maintain an appropriate body weight and composition for one's sport. Optimal energy, fluid, and nutrient intakes also help keep athletes healthy, which in turn helps them perform at their best in training and competition. Finally, combining good nutrition with exercise can help reduce the risk of chronic diseases such as diabetes, cardiovascular disease, hypertension, obesity, osteoporosis, and some cancers.

2. Identify the essential nutrients and the dietary recommendations for these nutrients.

Food constituents that prevent disease or health problems are classified as essential nutrients, while nonessential nutrients are those that can be deleted from the diet without adverse effects on growth or health. The RDAs and the DRIs are dietary guidelines that help determine the amount of an essential nutrient required for good health.

3. Describe the various methods used in evaluating the diets of active individuals.

The United States, Canada, and a host of other countries and regions have developed dietary guidelines for healthy eating. These guidelines provide advice about food choices that promote health, decrease the risk of chronic disease, meet nutrient requirements, and support active lives. The U.S. MyPyramid and MyPyramid.gov interactive Web site and Canada's Food Guide for Healthy Eating were developed to help translate these guidelines into everyday eating behaviors. These tools allow individuals to monitor their food selections to improve overall nutrient intakes.

4. Discuss the role of nutrition and exercise in the prevention of disease.

The roles of nutrients and exercise in disease prevention are well documented in scientific literature. Appropriate levels of exercise combined with a healthy diet can help reduce the risk of coronary heart disease, stroke, hypertension, diabetes, osteoporosis, and cancer as well as help maintain a healthy body weight and composition throughout life. Diet and exercise affect these diseases by lowering blood pressure, improving blood lipid profiles, improving blood glucose and insulin levels, improving cardiac function, improving bone mineral density, and helping to maintain a healthy body weight. Physical activity also helps maintain muscular strength, endurance, and flexibility—which in turn help preserve independence in older adults.

Key Terms

Acceptable Macronutrient
  Distribution Range (AMDR) 6
Adequate Intake (AI) 5
conditional essentiality 4
desirable or beneficial for health 4
Dietary Guidelines 7
Dietary Reference Intakes (DRI) 4
dispensable nutrient 3
essential nutrient 3

Estimated Average Requirement (EAR) 5
Food Guide Pyramid 8
Healthy People 2010 18
indispensable nutrient 3
MyPyramid 9
nonessential nutrient 3
Recommended Dietary Allowance
  (RDA) 5
Tolerable Upper Intake Level (UL) 6

Additional Information

Physical Activity Guidelines (2008) www.health.gov/PAGuidelines

The U.S. Department of Health and Human Services recently released the first-ever physical activity guidelines for Americans designed to provide guidance and recommendations for individuals aged 6 years and over. The documents emphasize both the immediate and long-term health benefits of a lifetime of physical activity.

American College of Sports Medicine (ACSM): www.acsm.org

The ACSM is the largest sports medicine and exercise science organization in the world and routinely publishes recommendations for physical activity, nutrition, public health, and performance.

American Dietetic Association (ADA): www.eatright.org

The ADA is the world's largest organization of nutrition professionals. This site provides food and nutrition recommendations, access to current research, and resources for students and health professionals.

Australian Institute of Sport (AIS): www.ausport.gov.au/ais

The AIS is internationally recognized as a terrific model for its holistic and government-supported approach to elite athlete development, support, and research.

Ainsworth BE, Haskell WL, Whitt MC et al. Compendium of physical activities: an update of activity codes and MET intensities. Med Sci Sports Exerc 2000;32:S498-504.

"Compendium of Physical Activities" is a comprehensive resource on the caloric expenditure of various activities related to both daily living and sport. Professionals can use this as a tool when developing nutrition and exercise programs for clients and for research protocols.

Healthier US: www.healthierus.gov

Healthier US is a national initiative focused on improving people's lives through reduced disease and healthier living. The site provides resources for individuals and professionals regarding healthy eating, physical exercise, and preventive screening.

Healthy People 2010: www.healthypeople.gov

Healthy People 2010 is a national initiative designed to challenge individuals and professionals to take necessary steps toward sustaining long and healthy lives. This site is a good resource for professionals who wish to find research related to the development of the program and its progress.

MyPyramid: www.mypyramid.gov

Introduced with the 2005 Dietary Guidelines for Americans, MyPyramid.gov provides a means of personalizing governmental nutrition recommendations based on age, gender, and activity level. The site also provides a menu planner, a way of tracking intake, and information for pregnant and breast-feeding mothers.

Swiss Forum for Sport Nutrition: www.sfsn.ch

This site provides access to the Food Pyramid for Athletes.

USDA Food and Nutrition Information Center http://fnic.nal.usda.gov/nal_display/index.php?info_center=4&tax_level=1&tax_subject=242

The Food and Nutrition Information Center is a great resource for dissemination of information, providing resources for health professionals and consumers on a variety of topics including food labeling, dietary supplements, nutrition assistance programs, and nutrition and chronic disease.

References

Ainsworth BE, Haskell WL, Whitt MC et al. Compendium of physical activities: an update of activity codes and MET intensities. *Med Sci Sports Exerc* 2000;32:S498-S504.

Britten P, Marcoe K, Yamini S, Davis C. Development of food intake patterns for the MyPyramid food guidance system. *J Nutr Educ Behav* 2006;38:S78-S92.

Burke LM, Kiens B, Ivy JL. Carbohydrates and fat for training and recovery. *J Sports Sci* 2004;22:15-30.

Canada's food guide to healthy eating. Ottawa: Minister of Supply and Services Canada, 1992.

Carpenter KJ, Harper AE. Evolution of knowledge of essential nutrients. In: Shils ME, Shike M, Ross AC, Caballero B, Cousins RJ eds. Modern nutrition in health and disease. Baltimore: Williams & Wilkins, 2006;3-9.

Cronin FJ. Reflections on food guides and guidance systems. *Nutr Today* 1998;33:186-188.

Crotty P. The Mediterranean diet as a food guide. *Nutr Today* 1998a;33:227-232.

Crotty P. Point/counterpoint: Response to K. Dun Gifford. *Nutr Today* 1998b;33:224-245.

Dietary guidelines for Americans, 2005. Executive summary. Washington, DC: U.S. Department of Health and Human Services, U.S. Department of Agriculture, 2005.

Food and Nutrition Board (FNB), Institute of Medicine. Recommended dietary allowances, 10th ed. Washington, DC: National Academy Press, 1989.

Gifford D. The Mediterranean diet as a food guide: the problem of culture and history. *Nutr Today* 1998;33:233-243.

Giugliano D, Esposito K. Mediterranean diet and metabolic diseases. *Curr Opin Lipidol* 2008;19:63-68.

Haskell WL, Lee IM, Pate RR et al. Physical activity and public health: updated recommendation for adults from the

American College of Sports Medicine and the American Heart Association. *Med Sci Sports Exerc* 2007;39:1423-1434.

Haven J, Burns A, Herring D, Britten P. MyPyramid.gov provides consumers with practical nutrition information at their fingertips. *J Nutr Educ Behav* 2006;38:S153.

Health and Welfare Canada. Nutrition recommendations. A call for action: summary report of the Scientific Review Committee and Communications/Implementation Committee. Ottawa: Minister of Supply and Services Canada, 1989.

Houtkooper L. Winning sports nutrition training manual. Tucson: University of Arizona Cooperative Extension, 1994.

International Food Information Council (IFIC) Foundation. Dietary Reference Intakes: An Update. Washington, DC: IFIC Foundation: 2002.

Institute of Medicine (IOM), Food and Nutrition Board. Dietary reference intakes: calcium, phosphorus, magnesium, vitamin D, and fluoride. Washington, DC: National Academy Press, 1997.

Institute of Medicine (IOM), Food and Nutrition Board. Dietary reference intakes: thiamin, riboflavin, niacin, vitamin B-6, folate, vitamin B-12, pantothenic acid, biotin, and choline. Washington, DC: National Academy Press, 1998.

Institute of Medicine (IOM), Food and Nutrition Board. Dietary reference intakes for vitamin C, vitamin E, selenium and carotenoids. Washington, DC: National Academy Press, 2000.

Institute of Medicine (IOM), Food and Nutrition Board. Dietary reference intakes for vitamin A, vitamin K, arsenic, boron, chromium, copper, iodine, iron, manganese, molybdenum, nickel, silicon, vanadium and zinc. Washington, DC: National Academy Press, 2001.

Institute of Medicine (IOM), Food and Nutrition Board. Dietary reference intakes: water, potassium, sodium, chloride and sulfate. Washington, DC: National Academy Press, 2004.

Institute of Medicine (IOM), Food and Nutrition Board. Dietary reference intakes for energy, carbohydrate, fiber, fat, fatty acids, cholesterol, protein and amino acids. Washington, DC: National Academies Press, 2005.

Institute of Medicine (IOM), Food and Nutrition Board. Dietary reference intakes research synthesis. Washington, DC: National Academies Press, 2006.

Jakicic JM, Clark K, Coleman E, Donnelly JE, Foreyt J, Melanson E, Volek J, Volpe SL; American College of Sports Medicine. American College of Sports Medicine position stand. Appropriate intervention strategies for weight loss and prevention of weight regain for adults. Med Sci Sports Exerc 2001;33:2145-2156.

Kennedy E. Building on the pyramid—where do we go from here? Nutr Today 1998;33:183-185.

Kennedy E, Meyers L, Layden W. The 1995 dietary guidelines for Americans: an overview. J Am Diet Assoc 1996;96:234-237.

Lairon D. Intervention studies on Mediterranean diet and cardiovascular risk. Mol Nutr Food Res 2007;51:1209-1214.

Manios Y, Detopoulou V, Visioli F, Galli C. Mediterranean diet as a nutrition education and dietary guide: misconceptions and the neglected role of locally consumed foods and wild green plants. *Forum Nutr* 2006;59:154-170.

Nestle M. In defense of the USDA food guide pyramid. *Nutr Today* 1998;33:189-197.

Physical Activity Guidelines Advisory Committee. Physical Activity Guidelines Advisory Committee report, 2008. Washington, DC: U.S. Department of Health and Human Services, 2008.

Renaud S, de Lorgeril M, Delaye J et al. Cretan Mediterranean diet for prevention of coronary heart disease. *Am J Clin Nutr* 1995;61:1360S-1367S.

Rudman D, Feller A. Evidence for deficiencies of conditionally essential nutrients during total parenteral nutrition. *J Am Coll Nutr* 1986;5:101-106.

Tavani AJ, Negri E, La Vecchia C. Calcium, dairy products, and the risk of hip fracture in women in northern Italy. *Epidemiology* 1995;6:554-557.

Tipton KD and Wolfe RR. Protein and amino acids for athletes. *J Sports Sci* 2004;22:65-79.

U.S. Department of Agriculture. The food guide pyramid. Washington, DC: Human Nutrition Information Service, Home and Garden Bulletin no. 252, 1992.

U.S. Department of Health and Human Services. Healthy people 2010: Midcourse Review 2007.

U.S. Department of Health and Human Services and U.S. Department of Agriculture. Dietary guidelines for Americans, 2005, 6th ed. Washington, DC: U.S. Government Printing Office, Jan 2005.

U.S. Department of Health and Human Services and U.S. Department of Agriculture. Finding your way to a healthier you: based on the dietary guidelines for Americans 2005. www.healthierus.gov/dietaryguidelines.

Van Loon LJ, Schrauwen-Hinderling VB, Koopman R, Wagenmakers AJ, Hesselink MK, Schaart G, Kooi ME, Saris WH. Influence of prolonged endurance cycling and recovery diet on intramuscular triglyceride content in trained males. *Am J Physiol Endocrinol Metab* 2003;285:E804-E811.

Walter P, Infanger E, Mühlemann P. Food pyramid of the Swiss Society for Nutrition. Ann Nutr Metab 2007;51:15-20.

Welsh S, Davis C, Shaw A. Development of the food guide pyramid. *Nutr Today* 1992;Nov/Dec:12-23.

Wilson CS. Mediterranean diets: once and future? *Nutr Today* 1998;33:246-249.

CHAPTER 2

Carbohydrate as a Fuel for Exercise

Chapter Objectives

After reading this chapter you should be able to

- describe the function, classification, and dietary sources of carbohydrate,
- discuss carbohydrate metabolism during exercise,
- discuss carbohydrate reserves and dietary intake,
- describe recommendations for carbohydrate feeding before exercise,
- describe recommendations for carbohydrate feeding during exercise,
- describe carbohydrate feeding recommendations for postexercise and during training periods, and
- explain the concept of muscle glycogen supercompensation.

It is common knowledge that carbohydrate is important for athletic performance. High levels of stored glycogen before endurance exercise can help prevent fatigue during exercise. Carbohydrate intake during exercise, especially exercise lasting longer than 1 h, can help increase performance and prolong time to fatigue. After exercise, diets high in carbohydrate help replenish muscle glycogen levels, enhancing recovery. For active people, it appears prudent to consume a diet high enough in carbohydrate to replace muscle glycogen used during exercise. Unfortunately, many athletes and active people consume inadequate levels of carbohydrate. Optimum dietary carbohydrate levels depend on total energy intake; body size; health status; and the duration, intensity, frequency, and type of exercise in which an individual participates.

FUNCTION, CLASSIFICATION, AND DIETARY SOURCES OF CARBOHYDRATE

Carbohydrates are a primary source of energy and they provide the substrate (glucose) necessary for glycogen replacement. When consumed during exercise, they help maintain blood glucose levels and help prevent premature fatigue. Athletes in moderate training are encouraged to eat carbohydrate diets that supply ~5 to 7 g carbohydrate per kilogram body weight and up to 10 g carbohydrate per kilogram body weight during periods of heavy training (Burke 2007). Athletes should also use carbohydrate-containing sport beverages and foods to supplement their diet as needed.

We can classify dietary carbohydrates in a number of ways—according to the type of carbohydrate in the food, the level of commercial processing the food has undergone, or the blood glucose or glycemic responses to the carbohydrate within the body. In the past, carbohydrate-containing foods comprising long complex chains of sugars linked together were frequently termed **complex carbohydrates.** Initially, it was thought that these long chains of sugar digested more slowly than the simple carbohydrates described next. We now know this is not true (see section on glycemic index next), so the term 'complex carbohdyrate' only refers to the structure of the carbohydrate and not to any digestive properties. Nutritionists still use the term "complex carbohydrate" for carbohydrate-containing foods such as fruits, vegetables, whole grains (breads, cereals, pasta), and legumes (beans, peas, lentils) because they are good sources of vitamins, minerals, and fiber. The dominant digestible carbohydrate in these foods is starch, except in the case of fruits that contain primarily simple sugars. Carbohydrates from processed foods (sweetened cereals, breakfast bars) or foods high in sugar (candy, sodas, and desserts) are frequently termed **simple carbohydrates.** These foods contain primarily glucose, sucrose, fructose, and high-fructose corn syrup and are generally low in vitamins, minerals, and fiber unless they are fortified.

In general, complex carbohydrates have a more complex chemical structure, are less processed, and contain more nutrients and fiber than simple carbohydrates. Although this classification of carbohydrates (complex vs. simple) has been used with reference to the body's glycemic response to these carbohydrates, this categorization is no longer appropriate. Research shows that the glycemic responses to both simple and complex carbohydrate foods can vary greatly, and that some complex carbohydrates (i.e., foods high in starch) can be hydrolyzed and absorbed as quickly as simple sugars (Cummings and Englyst 1995; Foster-Powell et al. 2002).

As shown in "Glycemic Index of Some Common Foods" (see p. 27), we can now classify foods as producing a high, moderate, or low glycemic response. Foods that produce a high glycemic response—a large and rapid rise in blood glucose and insulin—increase muscle glycogen more than foods that produce a low glycemic response (Burke et al. 1998). See "Calculating the Glycemic Index" on p. 29 for more information.

The "Primary Carbohydrates and Sugars in the Diet" are listed on p. 28. Foods generally classified as simple carbohydrates are made up of mono-, di-, and oligosaccharides, while foods generally classified as complex carbohydrates are made up of starch and fiber (e.g., grains, cereals, and legumes). Most of these carbohydrates occur naturally in foods, while others, such as high-fructose corn syrup, are produced commercially and used as sweeteners in processed foods. The rate at which the various forms of carbohydrate can be absorbed and oxidized within the body varies and will be discussed later in this chapter.

The various types of dietary carbohydrate listed on p. 28 should not be confused with low-calorie sweeteners, which do not add significant amounts of energy or carbohydrate to the diet and are used solely to enhance flavor. Artificial sweeteners are found in a number of foods marketed as reduced calorie or reduced fat. Appendix B.1 describes the most common low-calorie sweeteners used or proposed for use in the United States. Some of these sweeteners, such as sorbitol and xylitol, can cause gastrointestinal distress if used in large quantities. Some people may need to avoid these sweeteners.

CARBOHYDRATE METABOLISM DURING EXERCISE

Muscles require carbohydrate as a fuel source during exercise. The amount of carbohydrate required depends on the frequency, intensity, duration, and type of the exercise and the environmental conditions in which the exercise is per-

Glycemic Index of Some Common Foods*

High Glycemic Index Foods (GI > 85)

Cream of Wheat	Cornmeal	English muffin	Sport drinks
Shredded Wheat	Croissant, doughnut	Mashed potatoes	Soft drinks
Total cereal	Rice cakes	Carrots	Hard candy
Crispix cereal	Pop-Tarts	Watermelon	Jelly beans
Corn Flakes, Rice Krispies, Bubbles	Angel food cake	Raisins	Syrups or sucrose
	White bread or bagel	Pretzels	Glucose, maltose
Cheerios	Soda crackers	Couscous	Molasses
Corn Chex cereal	Corn chips	Gnocchi	Fruit Roll-Ups
Grape-Nuts	Waffles, pancakes	Vanilla wafers	Dates

Moderate Glycemic Index Foods (GI = 60-85)

100% whole wheat bread	Brown or wild rice	Popcorn	Grapes
Rye kernel bread	Cracked barley	Sponge cake	Grapefruit juice
7-grain bread	White rice (long grain)	Linguine, durum	Orange (whole or juice)
Pita bread, white	Buckwheat	Sweet corn	Fruit cocktail
Oat bran cereal	Basmati rice	Oat bran	Mango or papaya
Bran Chex cereal	Wheat, cooked	Oatmeal	Kiwi fruit
Special K cereal	Bulgur	Marmalade or honey	Cranberry juice
All-Bran Cereal	Parboiled rice	Ice cream, low-fat	
		Sweet potato	

Low Glycemic Index Foods (GI <60)

Barley kernel bread	Fettuccini, egg	Beans (all types)	Apples (whole or juice)
Wheat kernels	Apricots (dried)	Peaches or pears (fresh)	Power bar
Tomato soup	Rice bran	Fructose	Oat bran bread
Cherries, plums	Soy milk or drink	Hummus	Lentils
Milk (whole or nonfat)	Dried peas	Peanuts	Grapefruit
Yogurt (all types)	Banana		Peanut M&Ms
	Barley		

*White bread (50 g) was used as the reference food.

formed (Jeukendrup 2003). Figure 2.1 illustrates how carbohydrate use changes with exercise intensity. The carbohydrate used during exercise can come from any of the following sources:

- Endogenous production of glucose by the liver (gluconeogenesis)
- Blood glucose
- Muscle and liver glycogen stores
- Carbohydrate consumed during exercise (e.g., exogenous carbohydrate)

The amount of gluconeogenesis that occurs during exercise depends on the available carbohydrate reserves before exercise begins; the amount of carbohydrate provided during exercise; the type, duration, and intensity of the exercise bout; the exercise environment (e.g., temperature, altitude); and level of endurance training. Thus, the total amount of carbohydrate used during exercise (as well as the source of this carbohydrate) depends on a number of factors, some of which can be manipulated with

Primary Carbohydrates and Sugars in the Diet

Monosaccharides (glucose, fructose, galactose) are the simplest form of sugar.

- Glucose: The main carbohydrate in the blood and the substrate required to make the glycogen stored in the liver, muscles, and other organs; the main carbohydrate energy source in the cell. Rapidly absorbed from the gut through the sodium-dependent glucose transporter.

- Fructose: The simple sugar found primarily in fruit and honey. Fructose is sweeter than common table sugar (sucrose). It is absorbed from the gut through the glucose transporter 5 (GLUT5) and must be transported to the liver for conversion to glucose.

- Galactose: The simple sugar found in milk.

Disaccharides (sucrose, lactose, and maltose) are sugars made up of two simple sugars.

- Sucrose: Common table sugar. It is made up of one glucose and one fructose unit. Sucrose is extracted from sugar cane and beet sugar. Sucrose is the most common disaccharide in our diet. It is converted to glucose and fructose in the gut, and each is absorbed through the specific transport system previously mentioned.

- Lactose: Sugar found in milk products and made up of one glucose and one galactose unit. Many adults, especially Asians, Native Americans, Hispanics, and blacks, cannot digest this sugar and are termed lactose intolerant because they are lacking the lactase enzyme.

- Maltose: Sugar made up of two glucose units. This sugar is made from the breakdown of starch. Rapidly digested to glucose and absorbed quickly into the body. Absorption rate is similar to that with feeding glucose.

Oligosaccharides are short chains of 3 to 10 monosaccharides linked together.

- Maltodextrin: A glucose polymer manufactured as long starch units are broken into smaller groups. This sugar is found frequently in sport drinks and many processed foods. As with maltose, maltodextrins are rapidly digested to glucose and absorbed.

- Corn syrup: A sweet syrup made up of glucose and short-chain glucose polymers produced by enzymatic hydrolysis of corn starch. As with maltodextrins, corn syrup is rapidly digested, and the glucose units are absorbed.

- High-fructose corn syrup: An especially sweet corn syrup in which 45% to 55% of the carbohydrate is enzymatically hydrolyzed to the simple sugars glucose and fructose. High-fructose corn syrup is less viscous than traditional corn syrup, yet has nearly twice the concentration of mono- and disaccharides found in regular corn syrup. It is currently the predominant sweetener found in commercially sweetened foods.

Polysaccharides are foods that contain starch and fiber. These foods are often called complex carbohydrates.

- Starch: Found in plants, seeds, and roots. Starch is made up of straight chains of glucose polymers called amylose and some branching chain polymers called amylopectin. Complex carbohydrates are composed primarily of starch and fiber, and the starch is digested into glucose. The extent of starch digestion in the small intestine is variable, and some starch escapes digestion in the small intestine and enters the colon. Starches high in amylopectins are more rapidly digested and absorbed than starches high in amylase.

- Dietary fiber: A part of the plant that cannot be digested by human gut enzymes. Dietary fiber passes through the small intestine to the colon, where it is expelled as fecal material or fermented and used as a food source for gut bacteria. Thus, some fibers are broken down in the colon. Diets high in fiber generally increase the amount of fecal material and flatulence produced.

Adapted, by permission, from A.F. Jeukendrup and R. Jentjens, 2000, "Oxidation of carbohydrate feedings during prolonged exercise," *International Journal of Sports Medicine* 29(6): 204-424.

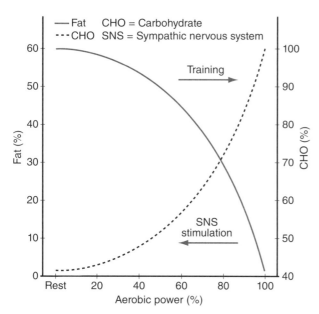

Figure 2.1 The crossover concept of fuel use during exercise. At low- to moderate-intensity exercise, carbohydrate (CHO) and lipids both play major roles as energy substrates. However, when relative aerobic power output reaches 60% to 65%, CHO becomes increasingly important and lipids become less important. Because of the crossover phenomenon, in most athletic activities glycogen stores provide the greatest fuel for exercise. Lipids become important energy sources during recovery.

Reprinted from G.A. Brooks, T.D. Fahey, and K.M. Baldwin, 2005, *Exercise physiology. Human bioenergetics and its applications*, 4th ed. (Boston, MA: McGraw-Hill Companies), 143. © The McGraw-Hill Companies.

exogenous carbohydrate intake either before or during exercise.

Endogenous Glucose Production During Exercise

The substrates for **gluconeogenesis** during exercise are lactate, alanine, glycerol, and pyruvate. In general, these substrates come primarily from the muscle, with small amounts of glycerol coming from adipose cells. These substrates are transported to the liver for glucose production. Figure 2.3 on p. 31 reviews the gluconeogenic pathway.

The primary source of lactate during exercise is from the metabolism of glucose to lactate, through glycolysis, in both the working and nonworking muscle. (See figures 2.4 and 2.5 on pp. 32-33 for a quick review of intermediate metabolism and **glycolysis**.) The lactate is transported to the liver for glucose production through the **Cori cycle** (figure 2.6), or it may be used directly by adjoining cells as an energy source. As glycogen is depleted in the working muscle, the nonworking muscles can give up some of their stored carbohydrate by releasing lactate. This phenomenon was first demonstrated in humans by Ahlborg and Felig (1982). They showed that lactate release from the arms increased both during and after 3.0 to 3.5 h of leg exercise (cycling), providing substrate for gluconeogenesis.

A second major gluconeogenic precursor is alanine. Alanine is the primary amino acid released by working muscle during exercise. One of the first studies to demonstrate this was done by Felig and

Highlight

Calculating the Glycemic Index and Glycemic Load of a Food or Meal

The term **glycemic response** refers to the body's increase in blood glucose and insulin after consumption of a given food or combination of foods. The glycemic response is determined by measuring the area under the glucose curve using sophisticated computer software. The greater the blood glucose response to a particular carbohydrate food, the greater the area under the glucose response curve. For example, what would be the glucose response to feeding an individual two very different carbohydrates such as white bread or lentils? This point is demonstrated in figure 2.2. Because blood sugar rises higher and stays elevated longer with white bread compared to lentils, white bread is said to produce a greater glycemic response.

To standardize the glycemic response, researchers have categorized foods using the **glycemic index (GI)**. The GI is determined for any particular food or combination of foods by feeding 50 g of

(continued)

Calculating the Glycemic Index and Glycemic Load   *(continued)*

the food and determining the blood glucose response over a 2 h period. The GI is then calculated using the following formula (Burke et al. 1998):

> Glycemic index (GI) = [(Blood glucose area of test food) / (Blood glucose area of reference food)] × 100.

In the example here,

> GI = (Blood glucose area, lentils) / (Blood glucose area, white bread) × 100.

The reference food is typically white bread and has a GI of 100, although sometimes glucose is used as the reference food (GI = 100). (See figure 2.2 for an example of the blood glucose response to a high and a low glycemic index food, and "Glycemic Index of Some Common Foods," p. 27, for common foods and their GI values.) The GI of a meal or of a total diet can be calculated from the weighted means of the GI values for the component foods of the meal or diet (Wolever et al. 1991). The weighting is based on the proportion of the total carbohydrate provided by each food within the meal. Thus, if a food represents 60% of the carbohydrate consumed in the meal, the contribution of this food to the total GI of the meal is the food GI multiplied by 60%. After this calculation is done for each carbohydrate-containing food in the meal, the values are added to give a total meal GI.

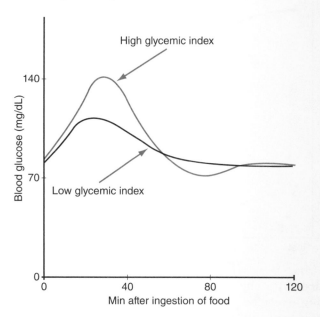

Figure 2.2 Blood glucose concentrations following the ingestion of a food with low (e.g., lentils) or high (e.g., white bread) glycemic index.
Reprinted, by permission, from P.C. Champe, R.A. Harvey, and D.R. Ferrier, 2008, *Lippincott's illustrated reviews: Biochemistry*, 4th ed. (Philadelphia, PA: Lippincott Williams & Wilkins), 366.

The concept of **glycemic load (GL)** was introduced to help determine the glycemic effect of meals and diets, and it accounts for both the amount and source of the carbohydrate in a meal. For example, Wolever and colleagues (2006) tested 14 different meals that varied in energy content, protein, fat, available carbohydrate, and GI. They found that together the carbohydrate content and GI of a meal accounted for 88% of the variation in glycemic response ($P < 0.0001$) in normal subjects. You can calculate the GL as follows:

> Glycemic load (GL) = Glycemic index (GI) of a food or meal × g available carbohydrate in the food or meal.

Wahren (1971), who showed that the rate of alanine appearance increased 60% to 96% after 40 min of strenuous exercise. Alanine is synthesized as nitrogen (released from the breakdown of amino acids in the muscles) and is combined with pyruvate (see chapter 4). Alanine is transported to the liver, where it is broken back down into pyruvate and nitrogen. This pathway is called the **glucose-alanine cycle** (figure 2.7 p. 34). The pyruvate can be used as a gluconeogenic substrate, while the

nitrogen is converted into urea and eliminated through the kidneys.

The third gluconeogenic precursor the liver uses is glycerol, the three-carbon backbone of triglyceride (also called triacylglycerols). When adipose tissue or muscle triglycerides are broken down, they yield three fatty acids and glycerol (see chapter 3). The fatty acids from the adipose tissue can be transported to the muscles for energy production, but glycerol is transported to

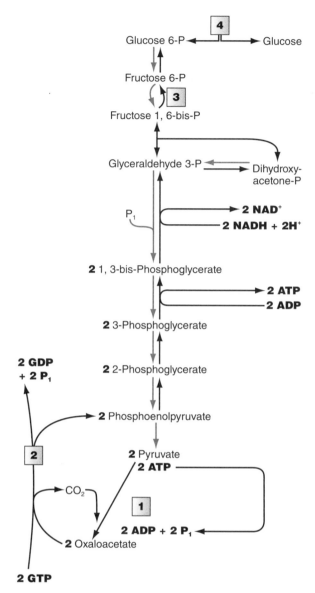

Figure 2.3 Gluconeogenesis pathway shown as a part of the essential pathways of energy metabolism. Blue arrows show the direction of gluconeogenesis. Numbered reactions are unique to gluconeogenesis.

Reprinted, by permission, from P.C. Champe, R.A. Harvey, and D.R. Ferrier, 2008, *Lippincott's illustrated reviews: Biochemistry*, 4th ed. (Philadelphia, PA: Lippincott Williams & Wilkins), 121.

the liver for gluconeogenesis. Finally, some pyruvate leaks from the working cells into the blood and is transported to the liver. Like glycerol, this three-carbon compound can be used by the liver to make glucose.

During prolonged exercise, especially when no exogenous carbohydrate is provided, gluconeogenesis is a major source of glucose for the work-

ing muscles. Ahlborg and Felig (1982) estimated that after 3 h of endurance exercise (58% $\dot{V}O_2$max), the uptake of lactate, pyruvate, and glycerol by the liver accounts for 60% of the glucose output.

The amount of lactate coming from working muscle during prolonged exercise decreases as muscle glycogen is depleted. The body then must rely on lactate from nonworking muscles and from amino acid metabolism to make glucose (Ahlborg 1985; Ahlborg and Felig 1982). Thus, an increase in gluconeogenesis late in exercise requires that the body use amino acids from the breakdown of protein as an energy substrate. The amount of protein used for energy during exercise depends on a number of factors, including the amount of carbohydrate stores available at the beginning of exercise; whether exogenous carbohydrate is provided during exercise; and the type, intensity, and duration of the exercise bout (see chapter 4).

Another source of blood glucose during exercise is the breakdown of liver glycogen (liver glycogenolysis). **Glycogenolysis** is the chemical process by which glucose is freed from glycogen. Unlike the situation with muscle glycogen, glucose from liver glycogen can be released directly into the bloodstream, thus helping to maintain blood glucose levels during exercise. Like muscle glycogen, liver glycogen can be depleted if exercise is strenuous and of long duration. As both liver and muscle glycogen become depleted, blood glucose levels fall, and the body must rely on gluconeogenesis to maintain blood glucose levels.

Finally, remember that the rate of endogenous glucose production as just discussed will be altered if exogenous carbohydrate (e.g., sport or energy drink, carbohydrate-containing foods, or gels) is provided during exercise. When this occurs, the body can utilize this exogenous carbohydrate as an energy source, and the need to synthesize new glucose from gluconeogenic precursors such as protein will be reduced.

Hormonal Control of Carbohydrate Metabolism During Exercise

During exercise, a number of hormonal changes signal the body to break down stored energy for fuel, which can then be used by the working muscles for energy. The list on p. 35 outlines these hormonal responses, which depend on a variety of factors including the intensity and duration of the exercise and the individual's level of physical

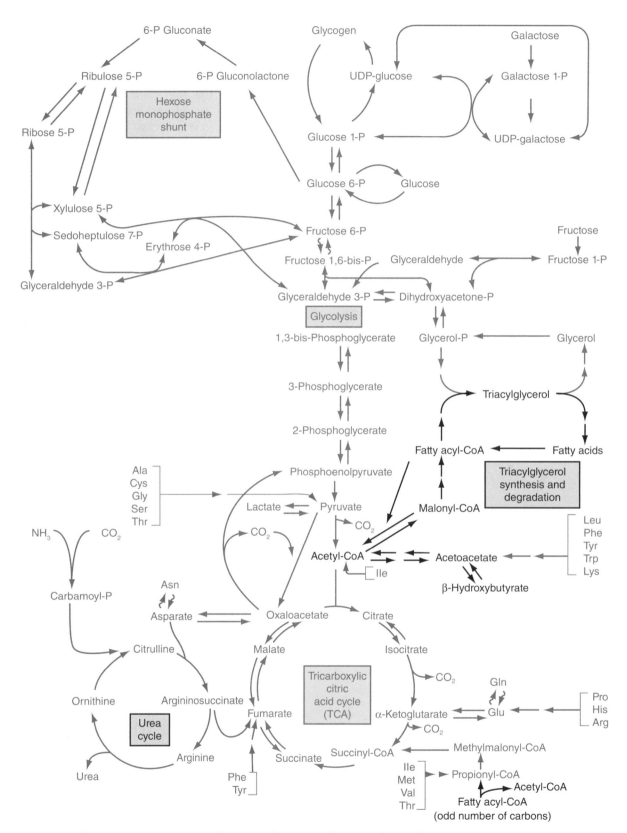

Figure 2.4 Important reactions of intermediate metabolism. Curved reaction arrows indicate forward and reverse reactions that are catalyzed by different enzymes. Straight arrows indicate forward and reverse reactions that are catalyzed by the same enzyme. Blue text = intermediates of CHO metabolism; black text = intermediates of lipid metabolism; gray text = intermediates of protein metabolism.

Reprinted, by permission, from P.C. Champe, R.A. Harvey, and D.R. Ferrier, 2008, *Lippincott's illustrated reviews: Biochemistry*, 4th ed. (Philadelphia, PA: Lippincott Williams & Wilkins), 92.

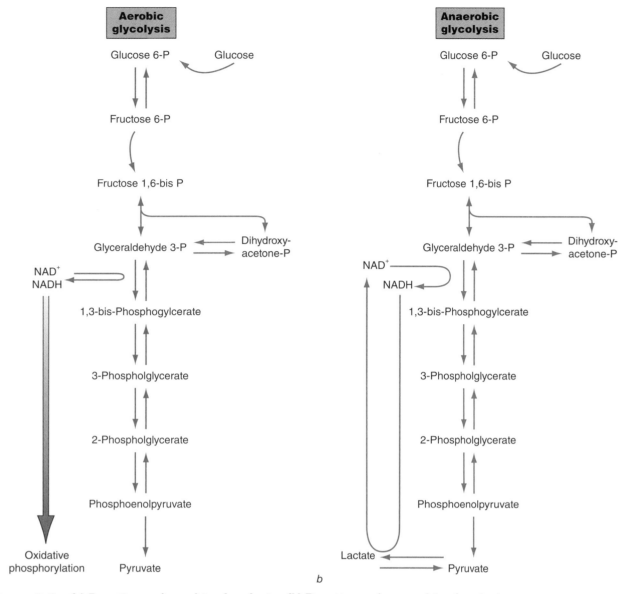

Figure 2.5 *(a)* Reactions of aerobic glycolysis. *(b)* Reactions of anaerobic glycolysis.

Reprinted, by permission, from P.C. Champe, R.A. Harvey, and D.R. Ferrier, 2008, *Lippincott's illustrated reviews: Biochemistry*, 4th ed. (Philadelphia, PA: Lippincott Williams & Wilkins), 96.

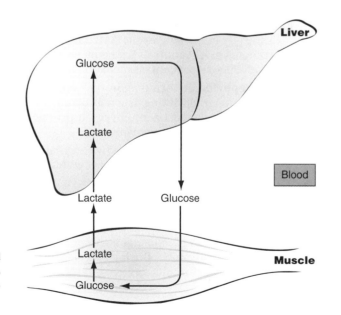

Figure 2.6 The Cori cycle.

Reprinted, by permission, from P.C. Champe, R.A. Harvey, and D.R. Ferrier, 2008, *Lippincott's illustrated reviews: Biochemistry*, 4th ed. (Philadelphia, PA: Lippincott Williams & Wilkins), 118.

fitness. Thus, trained individuals may have different responses than untrained individuals.

Blood levels of norepinephrine and epinephrine rise dramatically within minutes of the initiation of exercise (Coker and Kjaer 2005). These hormones stimulate the breakdown of stored fat (in both adipose and muscle tissue) and carbohydrate (both liver and muscle glycogen), making these fuels available to the working muscles. Insulin levels decrease or are maintained at a low con-

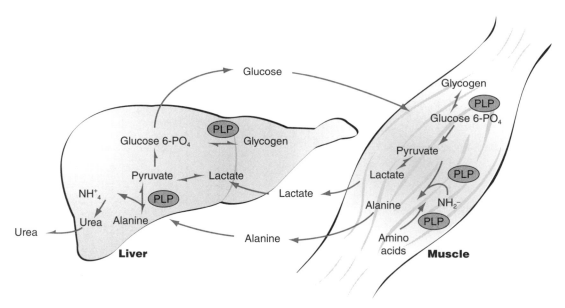

Figure 2.7 The glucose-alanine cycle and the involvement of vitamin B_6 (PLP) in glucose and alanine metabolism. PLP = pyridoxal phosphate (the active form of vitamin B_6).

Reprinted from J.E. Leklem, 1985, Physical activity and vitamin B-6 metabolism in men and women: Interrelationship with fuel needs. In *Vitamin B-6: Its role in health and disease,* edited by R.D. Reynolds and J.E. Leklem, (New York, NY: Alan R. Liss), 222. By permission of J.E. Leklem.

Effect of Various Hormones on Fuel Production During Exercise

Cortisol: A hormone produced in the adrenal cortex that stimulates gluconeogenesis and helps to mobilize free fatty acids and amino acids.

Epinephrine: A hormone produced mainly by the adrenal medulla that produces effects on target tissues by increasing cyclic AMP (adenosine monophosphate) concentrations in the cells. It promotes glycogenolysis in the muscle and liver, activates lipolysis in adipose tissue, and raises blood glucose concentrations and fatty acid levels.

Norepinephrine: A hormone produced in the adrenal medula and released in response to nerve stimulation, thus acting as a neurotransmitter. Norepinephrine stimulates the breakdown of stored fat and glucose for energy. It produces metabolic effects on peripheral tissues similar to those evoked by epinephrine.

Glucagon: A hormone secreted by the α-cells of the pancreas. Glucagon responds to low levels of blood glucose by activating cyclic AMP in the liver, stimulating both gluconeogenesis and glycogenolysis.

Insulin: A hormone secreted by the β-cells of the islets of Langerhans in the pancreas that enhances the uptake of glucose by the peripheral tissues and helps maintain blood glucose within normal limits (65-110 mg/dL). Insulin also increases the synthesis of glycogen from glucose, decreases gluconeogenesis, and promotes lipogenesis in the fat cell. Thus, insulin acts as an anabolic hormone. During exercise, insulin levels are low because the body needs fuel to be released, not stored.

Hormonal Changes That Stimulate the Breakdown of Stored Energy During Exercise

Increased With Exercise

Cortisol

Epinephrine

Norepinephrine

Glucagon

Decreased With Exercise

Insulin

centration during exercise, while glucagon levels increase. Glucagon, released from the pancreas in response to the low blood glucose levels that may occur with exercise, is a potent stimulator of glycogenolysis and gluconeogenesis. Both of these metabolic processes play a significant role in maintaining blood glucose levels by increasing the release of glucose into the blood (Coker and Kjaer 2005). Exercise, both acute and chronic, also increases the sensitivity of the skeletal muscle to the action of insulin. Muscle contractile activity has an "insulin-like" effect on the muscle, increasing the uptake of glucose without the need for insulin (El-Sayed et al. 1997). This occurs as exercise stimulates the translocation of GLUT4, a glucose transporter, to the surface of the muscle cell. Thus, adequate glucose can be delivered to the muscle in spite of the lower blood insulin levels usually observed during exercise.

All of these hormonal changes create an optimal environment for the breakdown and oxidation of both fat and carbohydrate for energy during exercise. In many ways, the acute hormonal response to exercise is similar to that seen in fasting. In both exercise and fasting, the body must provide energy to working muscles from the body's energy reserves: Body energy reserves must be broken down and provided to cells and tissues that require energy.

CARBOHYDRATE RESERVES AND DIETARY INTAKE

During exercise the primary sources of energy are carbohydrate (glucose) and fat (fatty acids). The relative amounts of each of these substrates used depend on exercise intensity and duration

(see figure 2.1). Compared to protein and fat stores, the body's carbohydrate reserves are severely limited—the total amount of energy stored as glycogen ranges from ~800 to 2000 kcal, depending not only on diet and on the size and the fitness level of the individual, but also on the time of day. Dietary recommendations for active people usually focus on making sure that the diet is adequate in carbohydrate to replace these limited and easily depleted reserves. Carbohydrate may also be consumed during exercise to supplement these reserves.

Muscle and Liver Glycogen

The body's carbohydrate reserves are primarily in liver and muscle glycogen. Glycogen concentrations are highest in the liver—the amount in the typical liver (about 1.5 kg) after an overnight fast is ~4% of the liver's total weight, or 60 g. After a meal, the amount of glycogen can double to ~8% of the liver's weight, or 120 g (Flatt 1995; Champe et al. 2008). Thus, the amount of carbohydrate stored in the liver ranges from 60 to 120 g (250-500 kcal), depending on the time of day and the amount of carbohydrate in the last meal consumed. Liver glycogen plays a major role in maintaining blood glucose levels throughout the night. A morning meal helps replenish glycogen stores.

The amount of carbohydrate stored in muscle is lower than that in the liver; deliberate carbohydrate loading is required to increase the amount to more than 2% of fresh weight of rested muscle (~400 g) (Champe et al. 2008). Since muscle typically accounts for 20% to 30% of total body weight, the absolute amount of glycogen stored in the muscle can range from roughly 300 to 400 g (1200-1600 kcal) in a person weighing 154 lb (70 kg) (Maughan 2003). Muscle glycogen levels can be dramatically increased under certain conditions, however, such as by consumption of a high-carbohydrate meal after exercise has depleted the stores of muscle glycogen (see "Muscle Glycogen Supercompensation," p. 60).

The body's total glycogen reserve (that found in liver, muscle, and other organs) is not much greater than the amount of carbohydrate usually consumed each day (Flatt 1995). For people consuming 2000 kcal/day with 50% of the energy coming from carbohydrate, this represents approximately 250 g of carbohydrate. Maintenance of glycogen stores within a desirable range requires that the body balance carbohydrate oxidation to carbohydrate intake (Flatt 1995). After a typical meal, about one fourth to one third of the carbohydrate consumed is converted to liver glycogen; about one third to one half is converted to muscle glycogen; and the remainder is oxidized for energy in the hours after eating (Flatt 1995).

Use of muscle glycogen during exercise will depend on a number of factors including the amount of glycogen available before exercise begins, the exercise intensity and duration, the environmental conditions, and whether or not endogenous carbohydrate is consumed (Hargreaves 2004). As illustrated in figure 2.1 (p. 29), a major determinant of muscle glycogen use during exercise is the intensity of an exercise bout, with more carbohydrate in the form of glycogen being oxidized for energy at higher intensities (Maughan 2003). For example, the rate of glycogen breakdown is 0.7, 1.4, and 3.4 mmol $\cdot$ kg^{-1} $\cdot$ min^{-1} at 50%, 75%, and 100% of $\dot{V}O_2$max, respectively (Sherman 1995). Higher-intensity exercises use muscle glycogen more quickly, since the availability of fat for fuel is limited. In exercise events lasting greater than 90 min at intensities of 65% to 85% $\dot{V}O_2$max, fatigue usually occurs concurrently with the depletion of glycogen stores. For example, in cycling at 70% $\dot{V}O_2$max, the time to fatigue is associated with the depletion of glycogen in the quadriceps muscles (Maughan 2003). Thus, a person with higher glycogen stores at the beginning of an endurance event will fatigue later than someone who begins the event with poor glycogen stores, assuming that other factors affecting carbohydrate use are equal. The pattern of muscle glycogen use during exercise appears to be curvilinear—the highest rate of glycogenolysis occurs during the first 20 to 30 min of an exercise bout lasting 60 min at an intensity of 75% $\dot{V}O_2$max (Sherman 1995). Remember, however, that muscle glycogen depletion is not the only factor involved with the onset of fatigue during exercise. Other physiological, psychological, and environmental factors also have significant effects (Jeukendrup 2004).

Dietary Carbohydrate Intakes of Active Individuals

Active men and women usually report carbohydrate intakes similar to those of weight-matched inactive individuals: 45% to 55% of total energy generally comes from carbohydrate (~5-6 g/kg body weight per day) (Hawley et al. 1995; Joubert and Manore 2008). For recreational or fitness athletes, these intakes may be adequate to meet the carbohydrate demands of exercise for 1 h or

less per day (Dolins et al. 2003). These carbohydrate intake levels may be too low, however, for endurance athletes who are engaging in daily intense training and whose glycogen stores need to be replenished rapidly (Burke 2006; Burke et al. 2006).

If intake of energy is reduced for any reason, carbohydrate intake may be dramatically reduced (e.g., when energy intake is restricted for weight loss). For active women, energy intakes less than 1800 to 1900 kcal/day provide carbohydrate intakes (~3-5 g/day) below recommended levels (Manore 2002); these low carbohydrate intakes are not adequate to replenish the glycogen used during endurance exercise. During intense daily training, the carbohydrate needs may be up to 10 g of carbohydrate per kilogram body weight for men and 6 to 8 g/kg for women. Of course, if activity increases, energy intake usually increases also, allowing more carbohydrate to be consumed.

CARBOHYDRATE FEEDING BEFORE EXERCISE

The positive association between dietary carbohydrate intake, muscle glycogen levels, and the ability to perform endurance exercise is now well known (Hawley et al. 2006). For this reason, most athletic trainers and sport dietitians recommend that athletes consume a high-carbohydrate diet during periods of intense training, including the days before an exercise competition. While these general recommendations differ little from those for the general population (45-65% of energy from carbohydrate) (Institute of Medicine 2002), many athletes want dietary and carbohydrate recommendations specific for the day of competition and for the hours immediately before competition.

Preexercise and Between-Competition Meals

The goals of a preexercise meal, or of any food consumed just before competition, are to promote additional glycogen synthesis, to supply the body with glucose for use during exercise, and to minimize fatigue during exercise. Many active individuals and athletes frequently compete or train after an overnight fast. This fast lowers liver glycogen levels since the liver provides glucose to the body during the sleeping hours. The preexercise meal helps replenish liver glycogen and provides the body with additional carbohydrate to help prevent or delay the onset of fatigue during exercise. Consumption of carbohydrate before exercise can indeed improve performance, especially for individuals who have eaten poorly during the 24 h before competition.

Athletes usually consume their preexercise meal 2 to 4 h before the exercise event, yet in many cases it can be safely eaten as late as 1 h before exercise. The meal should be small, easy to digest, and familiar to the individual; it should contain foods that do not cause gastrointestinal distress; and it should provide carbohydrate to improve glycogen reserves and blood glucose. In addition, consideration should be given to the glycemic index of the preexercise meal. Low glycemic index foods may give a greater feeling of satiety and produce a more stable blood glucose concentrations than a high glycemic index meal (Williams and Serratosa 2006). For these reasons the preexercise meal is usually high in low or moderate glycemic index carbohydrate foods (~150-300 g), moderate in protein, lower in fat and fiber, and moderate in size. Although it takes approximately 4 to 6 h to digest a meal consumed on an empty stomach and for blood hormone levels to return to baseline, current research reveals no reason for individuals to fast this long before an exercise event. There is no evidence that blood glucose and hormone levels need to return to baseline levels before exercise begins. Individuals differ in the volume of food they want in their stomachs during competition. Athletes engaging in early morning competitions may want to schedule a very early morning snack or carbohydrate beverage instead of eating immediately before competition. The timing and amount of food consumed depend on individual preferences and on the type, intensity, and duration of the sport.

Nervousness before an exercise event can cause gastrointestinal distress and loss of appetite. If athletes are too nervous to consume a meal before competition, they can use fruit juices, sport drinks, or glycogen replacement products to provide the energy and carbohydrate needed.

Athletes sometimes must perform more than one exercise event within a 24 h period. The type of food or drink provided in these situations depends on the athlete's preferences, the type of event, and the amount of time between events. If the time is short, water, fruit juices, or sport drinks are most appropriate—they provide the fluid and carbohydrate required to prepare the body for the next exercise bout while they are rapidly absorbed from the gut without having to be digested. People with longer times (1-4 h) between events can consume small meals similar to the preevent meal (see "Key Points to Remember When Feeding Athletes Before Competition" p. 38 and "Practical Dietary Guidelines for Preexercise or Between-Competition Meals" p. 42). In addition, Jentjens and Jeukendrup (2003b) have carefully reviewed the literature on the determinants of glycogen resynthesis when the recovery time between exercise bouts is short (<6 h).

Effects of Preexercise Feedings on Performance and Fatigue

Research examining the effects of feeding carbohydrate before exercise usually focuses on the following questions: Can the preexercise meal enhance exercise performance? Can active individuals eat within 30 to 60 min before exercise without impairing athletic performance?

Research shows that a high-carbohydrate preexercise meal 3 to 4 h before exercise can improve performance (Maffucci and McMurray 2000; Williams and Serratosa 2006). If this meal is then combined with carbohydrate intake during exercise (e.g., a sport drink), the performance improvements are even greater. Wright and colleagues (1991) fed one of four treatments to well-trained male cyclists who exercised at 70% $\dot{V}O_2$max to exhaustion: (1) no carbohydrate (controls), (2) a preexercise carbohydrate meal (3 h before exercise), (3) carbohydrate during exercise, or (4) a combination of carbohydrate feedings before and during exercise. Subjects also completed performance and work production tests. The preexercise meal averaged 333 g of carbohydrate (5 g carbohydrate per kilogram body weight), and an 8% carbohydrate solution was provided during exercise, providing a total of 175 g of carbohydrate. Total work performance during exercise was 19% to 46% higher when carbohydrate was fed. As compared with values in controls, average time to exhaustion was 44% greater when carbohydrate was consumed both before and during exercise, 32% greater when consumed during exercise, and 18% higher when consumed 3 h before exercise. Neufer and colleagues (1987) also reported a 22% improvement in cycling power when carbohydrate was consumed 4 h before exercise (200 g) plus immediately before exercise (43 g). Sherman and coworkers (1989) reported a 15%

improvement in exercise performance time (8.3 min improvement on cycling performance test) when subjects consumed 312 g of carbohydrate 4 h before exercise.

More recent research has examined the combination of a high-carbohydrate breakfast with a sport drink during exercise compared to only breakfast or a placebo breakfast (Chryssanthopoulos et al. 2002). In this study 10 male runners were provided with three treatments before exercise to exhaustion (70% $\dot{V}O_2$max) on the treadmill: (1) a high-carbohydrate breakfast (2.5 g carbohydrate per kilogram body weight) 3 h before exercise and water during exercise, (2) a high-carbohydrate breakfast + a carbohydrate-electrolyte drink during exercise, or (3) a liquid placebo breakfast and water during exercise. All subjects fasted overnight before each treatment. The runners who had the high-carbohydrate breakfast + the carbohydrate-electrolyte drink significantly increased their running time by 9% (125 min) over that with the breakfast-only treatment (112 min) and 21% over that with the placebo breakfast treatment (103 min) ($P < 0.05$). In addition, times with both high-carbohydrate breakfast treatments were significantly longer than those with the placebo and water treatment ($P < 0.05$). Thus, feeding active individuals a preexercise meal high in carbohydrate extends endurance time to exhaustion and improves work output. Complementing this preexercise meal with a sport drink during exercise further improves endurance capacity. Finally, the preexercise meal and the sport drink may be especially helpful for individuals who pay little attention to their diet or who have had a poor diet during the 24 h period before an exercise event.

Carbohydrate Consumption Immediately Before Exercise

Controversy exists over whether carbohydrates eaten immediately before exercise can cause hypoglycemia during exercise. It has been hypothesized that the high blood insulin levels resulting from carbohydrate consumption immediately before exercise (~30-60 min) may cause a decline in blood glucose (hypoglycemia) at the onset of exercise, leading to premature fatigue. Blood glucose decreases because elevated blood insulin levels due to carbohydrate feeding stimulate the uptake of glucose by tissues at the same time that exercise causes an uptake of glucose, and the liver output of glucose may be low. This phenomenon is sometimes referred to in the research literature as rebound hypoglycemia.

Jeukendrup and colleagues at the University of Birmingham have done a series of systematic studies in male cyclists to examine how consuming glucose before exercise affects the development of

---

Highlight

Key Points to Remember When Feeding Athletes Before Competition

- The meal usually should be consumed 2 to 4 h before competition, depending on the athlete's preference and the time of day the competition occurs.

- The meal should be high in carbohydrate, moderate in protein, and lower in fat and fiber. The carbohydrate promotes additional glycogen synthesis before the competition, while lower fat and fiber content helps prevent gastrointestinal distress. Also consider the glycemic index of the preexercise meal. A low glycemic index meal may be more satisfying and keep blood glucose concentrations more stable before exercise.

- The meal should be easy to digest, should be familiar to the athlete, and should not contain foods that cause gastrointestinal distress.

- If an athlete is too nervous to eat before competition, experiment with high-carbohydrate products that are easy to digest, such as juice, sport drinks, meal replacement products, gels, or glycogen replacement beverages. Some sport products and fruit juices fall into the low glycemic index category (see "Glycemic Index of Some Common Foods" on p. 27 for examples).

rebound hypoglycemia and exercise performance (Jentjens and Jeukendrup 2002, 2003a; Jentjens et al. 2003; Achten and Jeukendrup 2003; Moseley et al. 2003). Except for those in the exercise intensity trial, all athletes exercised for 20 min at ~65% to 75% $\dot{V}O_2$max and then underwent a time trial performance test. A number of factors may affect whether consuming glucose before exercise causes hypoglycemia and a subsequent drop in exercise performance. These factors include the type of subjects used (trained vs. untrained), the amount and type of carbohydrate consumed, the timing of the carbohydrate ingestion (how soon before exercise and how often), and the intensity of the exercise performed. The findings were as follows:

- The amount of carbohydrate (0, 25, 75, or 200 g) fed 45 min before exercise did not affect subsequent performance on a time trial (Jentjens et al. 2003).

- The timing of carbohydrate feeding (75 g fed at 15, 45, or 75 min) before exercise did not affect performance or rate of perceived exertion (Moseley et al. 2003). In this study of eight trained male cyclists, two became hypoglycemic (plasma glucose <3.5 mmol/L or 65 mg/dL) when fed 15 min before exercise; three became hypoglycemic when fed 45 min before exercise; and five became hypoglycemic when fed 75 min before exercise.

- The type of carbohydrate fed (75 g glucose, galactose, or trehalose) 45 min before exercise did not alter time trial performance (Jentjens and Jeukendrup 2003a). Ingestion of trehalose and galactose resulted in lower plasma glucose and insulin responses and reduced prevalence of rebound hypoglycemia. Trehalose is a disaccharide made up of two glucose molecules linked by an α-1,1 glycosidic bond, while maltose is a disaccharide made up of two glucose molecules linked by an α-1,4 bond. Glucose and galactose are monosaccharides.

- The various levels of exercise intensity (20 min at 55%, 77%, or 90% $\dot{V}O_2$max [mean values performed]) after the ingestion of 75 g of glucose 45 min before exercise had similar effects on blood glucose and insulin responses (Achten and Jeukendrup 2003).

Overall, Jeukendrup and colleagues found that feeding carbohydrate immediately before exercise did not affect subsequent exercise per-

formance. However, they did observe that some individuals are more prone to hypoglycemia with preexercise glucose feeding regardless of the timing or the amount of carbohydrate fed. To further examine this phenomenon, Jentjens and Jeukendrup (2002) identified individuals as either hypoglycemic (plasma glucose <3.5 mmol/L or 65 mg/dL) or normal glucose after a 75 g preload of glucose 45 min before exercise. They examined the insulin sensitivity of these individuals using an oral glucose tolerance test and found that level of insulin sensitivity did not play a role in rebound hypoglycemia. Figure 2.8 shows the changes in blood glucose in the two groups and the average change in blood glucose over the experiment. In addition, regardless of the group designation, there were no differences in rate of perceived exertion or performance. These results suggest

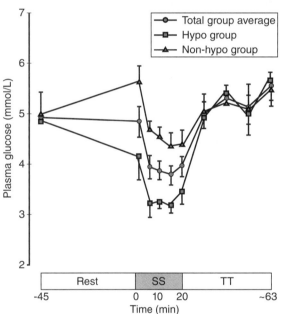

Figure 2.8 Plasma glucose concentrations at rest, during submaximal exercise (SS at 74% $\dot{V}O_2$max), and during a time trial (TT) after ingestion of 75 g glucose 45 min prior to SS. Hypo group: subjects who developed rebound hypoglycemia (<3.5 mmol/L or 65 mg/dL). Non-hypo group: subjects who did not develop rebound hypoglycemia. During SS, the hypo group has significantly lower glucose levels ($P < 0.01$) than the non-hypo group. There were no differences between groups during TT.

Reprinted, by permission, from R.L.P.G. Jentjens and A.E. Jeukendrup, 2002, "Prevalence of hypoglycemia following pre-exercise carbohydrate ingestion is not accompanied by higher insulin sensitivity," *International Journal of Sport Nutrition and Exercise Metabolism* 12: 298-413.

that individuals who experience hypoglycemia do not have decreased exercise performance. In summary, although research indicates that blood glucose declines if carbohydrate is eaten ~30 to 60 min before exercise, there appears to be no adverse effect of this change on exercise performance—in fact, most people do not perceive a change in their blood glucose levels.

Researchers have also examined whether the form of the carbohydrate fed (food vs. beverage) alters blood glucose responses and exercise performance. A number of studies have now addressed these issues and have shown that carbohydrate feeding immediately (30-60 min) before exercise has no adverse effect on performance or perceived exertion. Horowitz and Coyle (1993) fed foods with both moderate (rice, potatoes + margarine, rice + margarine) and high (potatoes, sucrose, candy bars) glycemic indices to nine fit males 30 min before a 75 to 85 min exercise bout. Although blood glucose levels significantly declined with all foods after 20 min of moderate-intensity exercise (60% $\dot{V}O_2$max), the subjects completed each trial without adverse effects, and ratings of perceived exertion were similar among the trials. More recently, Febbraio and colleagues (2000b) fed either a high glycemic index (mashed potatoes, GI = 91), low glycemic index (muesli; GI = 52), or placebo (diet jelly) meal 30 min before exercise (120 min at 70% peak oxygen uptake followed by a 30 s performance cycle) to eight trained male cyclists. They measured the rate of glucose appearance and disappearance and total carbohydrate oxidation, and found that the rates were higher at rest and throughout exercise after the high glycemic index meal compared to the other two treatments ($P < 0.05$), However, there were no differences in work output during the performance cycle among the three groups. The authors also measured muscle glycogen levels before, during (at 20 min), and after the 120 min submaximal exercise bout and found no significant differences between the trials, although there was a tendency for the high glycemic index meal to stimulate more glycogen use ($P = 0.07$). Other researchers (Alberici et al. 1993; Devlin et al. 1986; Neufer et al. 1987) also have found either no difference or improved performance in treatment groups fed carbohydrate (e.g., candy bars) immediately before exercise compared with the control groups.

In summary, feeding carbohydrate, either as food or as a solution, immediately before exercise appears to have little adverse effect on performance. In some cases performance is enhanced.

The carbohydrate fed 30 to 60 min before exercise is most likely oxidized by the muscle during endurance exercise. This exogenous carbohydrate may be especially beneficial for people who have low glycogen stores at the beginning of the exercise. Because individuals differ in their preference for food in their stomach while they exercise, feeding this close to exercise may be more of an individual decision.

CARBOHYDRATE FEEDING DURING EXERCISE

It has long been recognized that individuals fatigue when they engage in moderate exercise (60-80% $\dot{V}O_2$max) of long duration (>90 min)—a result, in part, of a decrease in blood glucose and a depletion of muscle and liver glycogen stores. Depletion of these stores requires increased reliance on liver gluconeogenesis to provide the glucose necessary to sustain exercise. Ingestion of exogenous carbohydrate can delay fatigue but cannot prevent it. Researchers hypothesized that exogenous carbohydrates during exercise may reduce fatigue and improve performance through a number of mechanisms. These include sparing muscle glycogen, maintaining blood glucose and oxidation of carbohydrate, synthesizing glycogen during low-intensity exercise, a direct effect of carbohydrate intake on the brain, or some combination of these mechanisms (Jeukendrup 2004). In addition, the mechanisms may vary depending on the intensity and duration of the exercise bout. Finally, individual responses to exogenous carbohydrate during exercise may depend on the nutritional and health status of athletes when they begin exercise.

Studies examining the effect of exogenous carbohydrate ingestion on muscle glycogen use during exercise have produced mixed results. Some have shown that carbohydrate use during exercise spares muscle glycogen (Erickson et al. 1987; Leatt and Jacobs 1989; van Hamont et al. 2005), while others have not (Angus et al. 2002; Bosch et al. 1994; Claassen et al. 2005; Coyle et al. 1986, 1991; Fielding et al. 1985; Flynn et al. 1987). However, most studies show an improvement in exercise performance or time to fatigue with carbohydrate ingestion during exercise, regardless of the change in muscle glycogen stores. Studies showing no muscle glycogen-sparing effect with exogenous glucose suggest that the observed improvement in exercise performance may be due to a sparing of liver glycogen and the reduced need for gluconeogenesis during exercise. Bosch and colleagues (1991, 1994) observed a 59% reduction in liver glucose production during prolonged exercise (3 h, 70% $\dot{V}O_2$max) when a 10% carbohydrate drink was ingested. Angus and colleagues (2002) also observed that when an 8% glucose solution was fed to male cyclists at the point of fatigue (after~240 min of exercise), liver glucose output never rose above resting levels, and muscle glycogen accounted for 31% of the energy used during exercise. In addition, exogenous carbohydrate intake helps to maintain blood glucose levels throughout exercise (Carter et al. 2005; Claassen et al. 2005; Coggan and Coyle 1989; Coyle et al. 1986; van Hamont et al. 2005). Exercising muscles rely heavily on blood glucose for energy late in exercise—thus, carbohydrate ingestion during exercise may complement the body's muscle glycogen rather than replacing it (Tsintzas et al. 1996; Febbraio et al. 2000b; Angus et al. 2002). The consumption of carbohydrate during exercise should help maintain blood glucose levels and ensure that the muscles have adequate glucose when muscle glycogen sources are low or depleted.

Figure 2.9 illustrates changes in energy substrate use by working muscles during moderate exercise (65-75% $\dot{V}O_2$max) lasting 4 h with no exogenous carbohydrate provided. The subjects in this study were endurance-trained males who had fasted overnight before the exercise performance test. The figure shows that as muscle glycogen levels decline, the muscles increasingly rely on blood glucose for carbohydrate—by the end of 4 h of exercise, about half of the energy required to sustain exercise is coming from blood glucose. This glucose must be provided by the liver, via gluconeogenesis, or must come from an exogenous carbohydrate source.

Carbohydrate Feeding During Exercise Prevents Hypoglycemia

For some individuals, exhaustive exercise (60-75% $\dot{V}O_2$max for 2.5-3.5 h) without exogenous carbohydrate intake can result in hypoglycemia, a condition in which blood glucose levels decrease to less than 45 mg/dL (<2.5 mmol/L). In the research literature, researchers use different blood glucose cutoff levels for defining hypoglycemia; however, the typical blood glucose level used in a clinical setting for hypoglycemia is 45 mg/dL or <2.5 mmol/L. With hypoglycemia, some people may experience light-headedness,

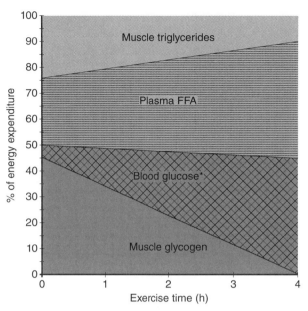

Figure 2.9 Percentage of energy derived from the four major substrates during prolonged exercise at 65% to 75% of maximal oxygen uptake. Initially, fat and carbohydrate each contribute ~50% of the energy. As muscle glycogen concentration declines, blood glucose becomes an increasingly important source of carbohydrate energy for muscles.

*After 2 h exercise, carbohydrate ingestion is needed to maintain blood glucose concentrations and carbohydrate oxidation.

FFA = free fatty acids.

dizziness, inability to concentrate, nausea, irritability, and fatigue. The blood glucose level that corresponds to these symptoms can vary among individuals. For example, one person may have these symptoms when blood glucose drops to 55 mg/dL while another has no symptoms at this same blood glucose level. Coyle and colleagues (1986) found that hypoglycemia leads to a decline in total body glucose oxidation and eventually to exhaustion (figure 2.10, p. 43). In this study, as plasma glucose concentrations decreased, so did total carbohydrate oxidation. Once mean plasma glucose values were between 45 and 54 mg/dL (2.5-3.0 mmol/L), exhaustion occurred and subjects could no longer exercise. It is now well established that feeding carbohydrate during exercise helps to maintain blood glucose levels compared to a placebo, both in normal environmental conditions

Highlight

Practical Dietary Guidelines for Preexercise or Between-Competition Meals

Feeding competitive or recreational athletes before or during competition requires planning and (sometimes) experimentation. The following guidelines will be helpful:

- Provide foods that are familiar to the athlete and that are high in carbohydrate (~150-300 g), moderate in protein, and relatively moderate in fat and fiber. Avoid foods that may cause gastrointestinal distress (e.g., milk products for lactose-intolerant athletes, acidic fruit juices, highly fortified meal replacement beverages or unfamiliar energy bars). Consider the glycemic load of the meal, providing lower-glycemic meals before exercise.

- Meals should be moderate in size. The exact size of the meal will depend on the size of the athlete, the nature of the sport, and the length of time until exercise. For example, the preexercise meal for a football player may provide 1000 to 2000 kcal, while that for a gymnast may provide 400 to 600 kcal. Most athletes do not like to exercise on a full stomach.

- Many athletes like to use drinks containing caffeine (coffee, tea, cola, and energy or sport drinks) before competition. This generally is not a problem as long as the athlete is accustomed to the practice and the quantity is not large enough to cause adverse reactions. In January 2004, the World Anti-Doping Agency removed caffeine from its prohibited list. This change in rules now allows athletes to use caffeine within their usual amounts without fear of sanctions in international competition. The World Anti-Doping Agency is the international independent organization created in 1999 to promote, coordinate, and monitor the fight against doping in sport in all its forms. The role of caffeine in delaying exercise-related fatigue and its inclusion in sport drinks are discussed in more detail in chapter 8.

- The type of meal or snack fed between competitions depends primarily on the amount of time available. If the time is short, replace fluids and carbohydrates by using a sport drink, glycogen replacement product, or fruit juice. High amounts of muscle glycogen synthesis occur when large amounts of carbohydrate (1.2-1.6 $g \cdot kg^{-1} \cdot h^{-1}$) are provided at regular intervals (~every 30 min) (Jentjens and Jeukendrup 2003b). This is a high amount of carbohydrate (~84-112 g carbohydrate for a 70 kg male) in a small amount of time, so athletes should practice with this type of glycogen resynthesis before using it in competition.

- If a second exercise bout is to occur within 6 h, consuming 75 to 90 g of carbohydrate immediately after exercise will help with rapid muscle glycogen restoration (Jentjens and Jeukendrup 2003b). Repeating this level of carbohydrate each hour postexercise with small, moderate-protein, high-carbohydrate, low-fat meals (sandwiches, bagels, cereal) or snacks (fruit, candy bars, energy or sport bars, carbohydrate replacement beverages) will maximize glycogen resynthesis. Smaller adults or children may need to eat small, frequent meals between competitions. Athletes should experiment with between-competition beverages and meals to find out what works best for them. For a complete review of the literature about postexercise glycogen synthesis during short-term recovery (<6 h), see Jentjens and Jeukendrup 2003b.

- Because many athletes have strong preferences about the types of foods they eat before or during competition, it may be convenient to pack a cooler with those preferred foods. If packing a cooler is not possible, check with the sponsoring organization to find out what types of foods will be available to the athletes at the competition.

(Agnus et al. 2002; Claassen et al. 2005; Febbraio et al. 2000a) and in the heat (Carter et al. 2005).

Hypoglycemia occurs during strenuous exercise when glucose output from the liver can no longer keep up with glucose uptake by the working muscles. This point was demonstrated in a study in which subjects consumed only water during exercise versus beverages with two levels

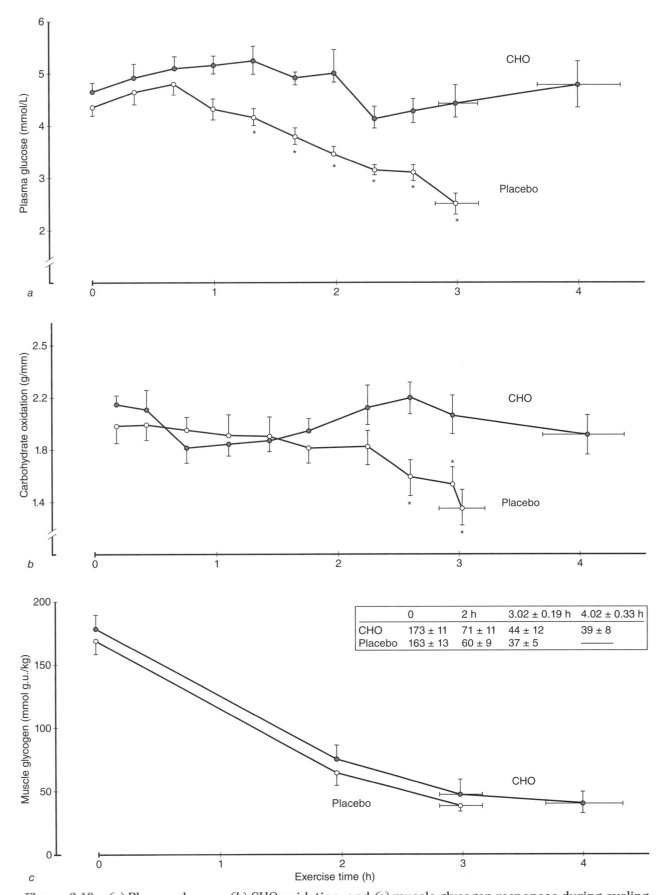

Figure 2.10 *(a)* Plasma glucose, *(b)* CHO oxidation, and *(c)* muscle glycogen responses during cycling at 74% of maximal oxygen uptake and ingesting a placebo (flavored water) or CHO every 20 min. Values are mean ± SE. *Significantly different from CHO; $P < 0.05$; g.u. = glucose used; CHO = carbohydrate.

Reprinted from E.F. Coyle et al., 1986, "Muscle glycogen utilization during prolonged strenuous exercise when fed carbohydrate," *Journal of Applied Physiology* 61(1): 165-172. Used with permission.

of glucose. When only water is provided, the liver must supply the glucose, primarily through gluconeogenesis, to maintain blood glucose. Felig and colleagues (1982) had 19 healthy, active males exercise on a cycle ergometer until exhaustion (~2.5 h, 60-65% $\dot{V}O_2$max while consuming one of three treatments: water, a 5% glucose drink, or a 10% glucose drink. During the water trial, the mean blood glucose decreased from 80 to 60 mg/dL (4.5 to 3.3 mmol/L), with seven subjects developing hypoglycemia (blood glucose levels <45 mg/dL or 2.5 mmol/L). Figure 2.11 depicts the changes in mean blood glucose levels during exercise for each of the three treatments; individual data for each of the subjects who became hypoglycemic are presented in figure 2.12. Ingestion of glucose (either a 5% or a 10% solution) prevented the fall in blood glucose observed during the water-only

period. Exogenous carbohydrate clearly prevented the drop in blood glucose frequently seen with exhaustive exercise. It also decreased the body's reliance on gluconeogenesis for glucose production, thereby possibly sparing body protein.

Carbohydrate Feeding During Exercise Improves Performance and Reduces Fatigue

During prolonged exercise in which no exogenous carbohydrate is provided, the body has difficulty maintaining blood glucose levels within the normal range (65-110 mg/dL or 3.6-6.1 mmol/L). Feeding carbohydrate during prolonged exercise improves performance and lengthens the time an athlete can exercise before becoming fatigued.

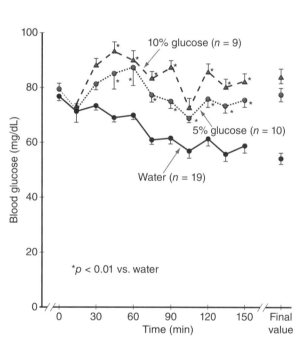

Figure 2.11 Blood glucose response to prolonged exercise with ingestion of either water or glucose (40 to 80 g/h as either a 5% or a 10% solution, respectively). "Final values" refers to the specimens obtained at exhaustion. Bars indicate SEM (standard error of the mean). Figures in parentheses indicate the number of subjects in each group. To convert blood glucose values to millimoles per liter, multiply by 0.05551.

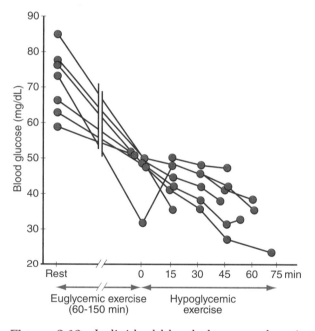

Figure 2.12 Individual blood glucose values in the seven subjects whose blood glucose concentrations fell below 45 mg/dL (~2.5 mmol/L) during the water ingestion phase of the study. "Euglycemic exercise" refers to the period of exercise during which blood glucose levels remained above 50 mg/dL (~2.8 mmol/L). "Hypoglycemic exercise" refers to the duration of exercise after the blood glucose fell below 50 mg/dL (~2.8 mmol/L). To convert blood glucose values to millimoles per liter, multiply by 0.05551.

In early research, Coyle and colleagues (1986) measured plasma glucose and muscle glycogen levels in seven trained cyclists exercising at 70% to 75% $\dot{V}O_2$max to fatigue during two sessions, one with and one without exogenous carbohydrate (figure 2.10). Fatigue was defined as the point when subjects were unable to maintain the designated workload. Muscle biopsies were taken before exercise began, after 2 h of exercise, and 5 min after cessation of exercise. When the subjects consumed only flavored water during exercise (the placebo group), both blood glucose (mmol/L) and carbohydrate oxidation (g/min) declined significantly—and the subjects fatigued 1 h sooner than when they consumed carbohydrate (at 3 vs. 4 h). When a carbohydrate drink was provided during exercise (~400 g carbohydrate over the 4 h period), blood glucose and carbohydrate oxidation remained high and subjects were able to exercise 1 h longer. Thus the consumption of carbohydrate improved exercise time to fatigue by 33% and maintained blood glucose values within normal ranges. Muscle glycogen use was similar between the treatments throughout the study, with minimal muscle glycogen being used during the last hour of the carbohydrate trial—suggesting that blood glucose is a primary fuel substrate during the late stages of exercise when muscle glycogen is depleted.

More recent studies have examined carbohydrate oxidation during exercise with and without carbohydrate feeding. Febbraio and colleagues (2000a) compared glucose kinetics and exercise performance in seven trained cyclists consuming either a carbohydrate solution (6.5%) or a placebo while exercising for 120 min at 63% peak $\dot{V}O_2$ and then performing a time trial. They found that feeding carbohydrate during exercise increased total carbohydrate oxidation and improved performance times compared to those in the placebo group. These results were supported by Angus and colleagues (2002), who examined plasma glucose kinetics during prolonged exercise to exhaustion (232 min) while feeding trained male cyclists an 8% carbohydrate solution (~250 mL every 15 min). They measured plasma glucose kinetics by infusing a labeled glucose solution and adding a different labeled glucose to the carbohydrate solution ingested by the athletes. By using two different labeled glucose solutions, one by infusion and one by ingestion, the researchers could determine how quickly the consumed glucose solution was absorbed and used as an energy source. Throughout the exercise period,

glucose continued to be absorbed and utilized as an energy source, demonstrating that athletes have a high capacity for glucose uptake during prolonged exercise. Glucose was being continually taken up, even at the point of fatigue, which implies that glucose uptake is not a limiting factor in fatigue. In this study, ~31% of the total energy expended and 45% of the total carbohydrate oxidized came from muscle glycogen; thus exogenous carbohydrate feeding did not eliminate the use of muscle glycogen as a fuel source. Based on the studies presented here and an extensive review of this literature by Jeukendrup (2004), it appears that carbohydrate feeding during exercise can improve exercise times in endurance events.

There is also evidence that carbohydrate feeding during shorter (~1 h), more intense exercise sessions (>75% of $\dot{V}O_2$max) can improve performance (Below and Coyle 1995; Davis et al. 1997). Early work by Below and Coyle (1995) showed that when male cyclists consumed a carbohydrate drink (providing 78 g of carbohydrate) during 1 h of high-intensity exercise (80-90% $\dot{V}O_2$max), mean exercise time was increased by 6.3% compared to that with water only. Using a stop-and-go high-intensity cycling protocol, Davis and colleagues (1997) measured time to fatigue in men and women consuming either carbohydrate (4 mL/kg) or a placebo every 20 min of exercise. They found that consumption of carbohydrate delayed fatigue by ~27 min, with no differences between genders. However, these studies were done on athletes who had undergone an overnight fast, which reduces liver glycogen stores. The results might have been different if the athletes had been tested in the afternoon, after eating breakfast and lunch.

If exercise is <1 h and of high intensity, the benefits of carbohydrate feeding during exercise are less clear (Walberg-Rankin 2000). A single bout of intense exercise (e.g., typical exercise resistance bout or 30 s sprint) is not limited by muscle glycogen stores, since only a portion of the total muscle glycogen is used for energy. However, repeated bouts of high-intensity exercise can deplete glycogen stores. For these athletes, a moderate- to high-carbohydrate diet should provide enough carbohydrate to replace muscle glycogen stores.

Although most studies documenting the benefit of carbohydrate intake during exercise have been done in the laboratory, there is ample evidence that this works in "real-life" situations. Tsintzas and colleagues (1993) measured performance time in two 18.6-mile (30 km) races with and without exogenous carbohydrate (5% maltodextrin or a placebo of flavored water). The seven subjects were experienced runners, four men and three women, who competed against each other during the races. Diets were controlled before the races, and treatments were randomly assigned so that the runners did not know which drink they were consuming. Performance time for the carbohydrate trial was significantly faster (128.3 min) than that with the placebo trial (131.2 min); and the runners maintained their speed throughout the race in the carbohydrate trial, whereas those receiving the placebo decreased their speed after 15.5 miles (25 km). Another real-life example of the benefits of consuming carbohydrate during exercise was reported in recreational marathon runners (Utter et al. 2002). In this study, the researchers found that carbohydrate feeding during the marathon reduced marathon running times (~16 min shorter) and significantly decreased rate of perceived exertion during the last 10 km (6.2 miles) of the race compared to a placebo drink.

Currently, there is little evidence to indicate that carbohydrate ingestion during low to moderate activity lasting less than 1 h is beneficial for people who are well fed before beginning exercise. Remember, however, that the amount of carbohydrate used during an exercise bout depends on a variety of factors: the intensity, duration, and type of exercise; the environmental temperature; the fitness level of the individual; and the preexercise glycogen stores in the body. The decision to use exogenous carbohydrate during exercise, regardless of duration and intensity, may need to be individually determined; but research evidence indicates that it can be beneficial in improving performance and reducing fatigue (Jeukendrup 2004, 2007).

Timing and Rate of Carbohydrate Feeding During Exercise

Carbohydrate ingestion generally should begin early in an exercise event to ensure that adequate carbohydrate is available during the later stages of exercise. If athletes wait until the onset of fatigue before consuming carbohydrate, they may be unable to absorb it rapidly enough to prevent fatigue. Early research by Coggan and Coyle (1987) demonstrated that the latest an individual can consume carbohydrate and still prevent fatigue is 30 min before the onset of fatigue. Tsintzas and colleagues (1996) found that ingestion of carbohydrate (48 g) during the first hour of an exhaustive exercise bout

increased time to exhaustion by 14% (~13 min more) compared to a water placebo. In general, current research studies typically provide carbohydrate solutions (5-8%) at regular intervals, usually every 15 to 30 min, when addressing the impact of carbohydrate on performance (Angus et al. 2000, 2002; Carter et al. 2005; Davis et al. 1997; Febbraio et al. 2000a).

The goal of carbohydrate feeding during exercise is to provide working muscle with additional carbohydrate. Performance benefits have been observed with feeding as little as 16 to 22 g of carbohydrate per hour (Fielding et al. 1985; Maughan et al. 1996). However, as reviewed by Jeukendrup (2004, 2007), researchers in most studies feed between 40 and 75 g of carbohydrate per hour and observe performance benefits. This level of feeding provides ~1 g of carbohydrate per minute. Any sport drink containing at least 6% to 8% carbohydrate would provide 60 to 80 g of carbohydrate per liter. Thus, consuming 18 to 34 oz (500-1000 mL) per hour of these drinks should provide adequate carbohydrate and fluid. If this rate of carbohydrate (using a 6% solution) and fluid ingestion is followed, one would consume approximately 500 to 1000 mL and 30 to 60 g of carbohydrate per hour, meeting the carbohydrate requirements of most individuals doing moderate activity. If the activity level is very high and the duration is long (e.g., a marathon, ironman race, ultra-endurance event), or if the temperature is extreme (e.g., either hot [>90° F] or cold [<33° F]), additional carbohydrate and fluid may be needed to maintain body temperature and prevent disturbances in fluid homeostasis (Murray 1995; Yaspelkis and Ivy 1991; Sawka et al. 2007). More information on fluid intake during exercise is provided in chapter 8.

Type of Carbohydrate

What type of carbohydrate should be consumed during exercise? Does one type of carbohydrate absorb more quickly than another? All simple sugars, such as glucose, fructose, sucrose, and maltodextrin (e.g., Polycose, glucose polymers, maltodextrins), are absorbed rapidly from the gut. These carbohydrate sources are also equally effective in maintaining blood glucose levels during exercise (Flynn et al. 1987; Jentjens et al. 2003, 2006; Jentjens, Achten et al. 2004; Jentjens, Venables et al. 2004; Jentjens and Jeukendrup 2005; Jeukendrup 2004; Jeukendrup et al. 2006; Murray et al. 1989). As discussed in more detail later, once simple sugars are absorbed, glucose can be used to maintain blood glucose levels immediately, while fructose must first be converted to glucose in the liver. Choosing one source over another depends more on personal preference and the ability of the carbohydrate to be absorbed quickly and transported to the working muscle.

We now know that using a combination of sugars increases the ability of various transport mechanisms to be utilized in the gut, thus increasing the absorption and subsequent oxidation of these sugars (Adopo et al. 1994; Jentjens et al. 2003, 2006; Jentjens, Achten et al. 2004; Jentjens, Venables et al. 2004; Jentjens and Jeukendrup 2005; Jeukendrup 2004; Jeukendrup et al. 2006). Therefore, sport drinks with a combination of sugars are absorbed, transported, and oxidized more quickly during exercise than a single carbohydrate source. Maltodextrins are frequently added to sport drinks and gels because they are less sweet than sucrose or glucose; the lower sweetness level permits a higher concentration of carbohydrate without making the product unbearably sweet. Most sport drinks on the market today use a combination of sugars with glucose, sucrose, fructose, and maltodextrin. Drinks containing 6% to 8% of various carbohydrates plus sodium are generally well absorbed during exercise and provide adequate carbohydrate to maintain blood glucose if 18 to 34 oz (500-1000 mL) of fluid is consumed per hour. Fluid and electrolyte needs during sport are discussed in more detail in chapter 8.

Fructose (usually from high-fructose corn syrup) is absorbed more slowly from the gut than glucose because it is absorbed through facilitated diffusion instead of active absorption. Large doses of fructose can overload the absorption capabilities of the gut and cause gastrointestinal distress, such as cramping and diarrhea. When fructose is consumed in moderate amounts, however, absorption from the gut is rapid and without adverse effects.

Once fructose is absorbed, it is transported to the liver where it is converted to glucose. This process slows the release of glucose into the bloodstream. The glucose response to a fructose load is lower than that to an equal amount of glucose or sucrose, as demonstrated by a study in which subjects consumed different sugar solutions (6% sucrose, 6% glucose, or 6% fructose) during a 2 h period of intermittent cycling (65-80% $\dot{V}O_2$max). Blood glucose responses for glucose and sucrose were similar, while fructose produced very little change in blood glucose (figure 2.13). When a fructose drink (60-85 g) is fed 60 min before exercise, the change in blood glucose during exercise

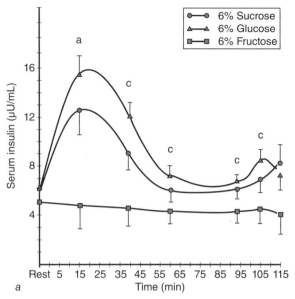

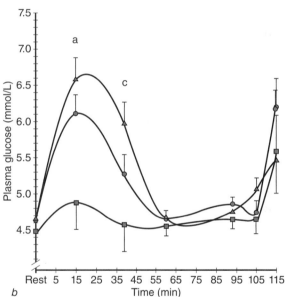

Figure 2.13 Effects of glucose, fructose, and sucrose ingestion during exercise. Data represent (a) insulin and (b) blood glucose values for all subjects. Bars represent SEM. a = glucose and sucrose significantly different from fructose, $p < 0.05$; c = glucose significantly different from fructose, $p < 0.05$.

Reprinted, by permission, from R. Murray et al., 1989, "The effects of glucose, fructose, and sucrose ingestion during exercise," *Medicine and Science in Sports and Exercise* 21:275-282.

is similar to that seen with water only (Okano et al. 1988). Thus, fructose produces no major change in blood glucose levels. While this effect may benefit active people who are sensitive to blood glucose fluctuations before exercise or during the first 15 to 30 min of exercise, fructose alone is not as effective as other sugars in preventing the drop in blood glucose that can occur with exhaustive endurance exercise.

The oxidation rate of fructose fed during exercise is much lower than that of either glucose or glucose polymers (Adopo et al. 1994; Massicotte et al. 1989). However, if fructose is fed in combination with glucose (50 g fructose + 50 g glucose), the oxidation of the combined sugars is significantly higher (25-38% higher) than when a 100 g dose of either fructose or glucose is fed alone (Adopo et al. 1994). More recent research has demonstrated that feeding a combination of glucose and fructose during prolonged exercise raises carbohydrate oxidation rates ~55% higher than when glucose alone is ingested (Jentjens and Jeukendrup 2005). This same phenomenon has been observed with endogenous carbohydrate intake in the heat. Jentjens and colleagues (2006) exercised eight trained male cyclists on three different days for 120 min at 50% $\dot{V}O_2$max in temperatures of ~32° C (~89.6° F). Subjects were fed three different fluids in random order: (1) 1.5 g/min glucose, (2) 1.0 g/min glucose + 0.5 g/min fructose, and (3) water. The authors found that carbohydrate oxidation was significantly higher with the glucose + fructose compared to glucose alone (figure 2.14). Thus, including fructose in combination with other sugars increased the amount of carbohydrate made available for oxidation during exercise.

Fructose does not appear to replace muscle glycogen stores as well as other carbohydrates (e.g., glucose, sucrose, or maltodextrin). Muscle cells do not take up fructose rapidly, and fructose does not stimulate the same glycemic response seen with glucose. This increase in blood insulin stimulates the enzymes involved in glycogen synthesis and enhances the uptake of glucose by muscle cells. Drinks containing only high fructose, therefore, are not recommended during or immediately after exercise. However, fructose works well in combination with other sugars in effectively replacing liver glycogen after exercise.

Although athletes often consume carbohydrate as a liquid during exercise, some prefer solid foods. Researchers have compared the glucose response during exercise using solid (energy or sport bars, whole fruit) and liquid carbohydrate sources (sport drink or blended fruit) with similar amounts of carbohydrate (Mason et al. 1993; Murdoch et al. 1993; Jeukendrup 2004). The studies showed no significant difference in blood glucose levels during exercise with solid versus liquid

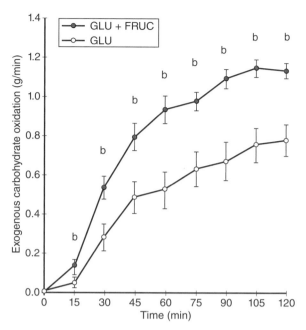

Figure 2.14 Carbohydrate oxidation with ingestion of glucose (GLU) or glucose + fructose (GLU+FRUC). Values are means and SE. *n* = eight trained male cyclists; b = significant differences between GLU+FRUC and GLU (*P* < 0.05). GLU = 1.5 g/min glucose; GLU+FRUC = 1.0 g/min glucose and 0.5 g/min fructose. Exercise was at 50% $\dot{V}O_2$max at ~32° C.
Reprinted from R.L.P.G. Jentjens et al., 2006, "Exogenous carbohydrate oxidation rates are elevated after combined ingestion of glucose and fructose during exercise in the heat," *Journal of Applied Physiology* 100: 807-816. Used with permission.

carbohydrate, which produced similar blood glucose and insulin responses. Thus, the form of carbohydrate consumed during exercise is a matter of availability and personal preference. Since people consuming solid carbohydrate during exercise should drink appropriate amounts of fluid to ensure adequate hydration, use of solid carbohydrates is not always practical during some strenuous activities or sports. Tables 2.1 and 2.2 (pp. 49-50) list various types of energy sources frequently used by athletes before, during, or after exercise.

Practical Guidelines for Carbohydrate Intake During Exercise

The following guidelines may be helpful to active individuals and athletes who consume carbohydrate during exercise. More detail on fluid intake during exercise is provided in chapter 8.

- People respond differently to various types of carbohydrate foods or drinks. To avoid unexpected gastrointestinal disturbances during competition, athletes should use the carbohydrate supplement during training that they will use during competition.

- Athletes should ingest carbohydrate early in an exercise session to prevent the decrease in blood glucose often seen during endurance events. This practice is especially helpful for those who come into an exercise event with poor glycogen stores (e.g., people who are involved in very heavy training or who have followed a low-kilocalorie or a high-fat diet).

- Sport drinks or other carbohydrate-containing drinks should have a concentration of 6% to 8% carbohydrate (60-80 g/1000 mL). Drinks with too high a concentration

of carbohydrate are less absorbed and do not replace lost fluids during exercise as efficiently. An additional advantage to sport drinks is that they contain sodium, which helps in the absorption of carbohydrate across the gut mucosa and helps prevent dehydration and hyponatremia.

- Athletes should drink enough fluid to provide between 40 and 75 g of carbohydrate per hour. Exercise events of long duration or during extreme temperatures may require higher fluid and carbohydrate intakes.

- When using body weight to determine carbohydrate intake during exercise, prescribe 1 to 1.2 g/min (Jeukendrup and Jentjens 2000; Jeukendrup 2007), which provides 60 to 72 g of carbohydrate per hour. The exact amount actually consumed needs to be determined based on an athlete's need.

Table 2.1 Energy and Nutrient Composition of Sport, Energy, and Breakfast Bars

Product (1 serving)*	Energy (kcal/bar)	CHO (g)	Fat (g)	Saturated fat (g)	Protein (g)	Fiber (g)
Balance Bar	200	22	6	1.0-3.5	15	0.5-3.0
Clif Bar	245	44	5	0.5-2.0	10	5
Clif Mojo Bar	205	22	9	2	10	2-3
EAS AdvantEdge Complete	240	27	7	4.5-5.0	17	1-3
Gatorade Energy Bar	260	47	5	0.5	15	2
GeniSoy Soy Protein Bar	240	36	5	2.5-3.0	14	1-2
Harvest PowerBar	245	42	5	0.5-2.5	10	5
Kashi TLC Crunchy Granola	180	26	6	0.5	7	4
Kellogg's All-Bran Bar	130	21	3	0.5	2	5
LARABAR	210	24	11	0-2.5	5	3-5
Luna Bar	180	26	5	0-5-3.0	10	3
Meta-Rx Big 100	380	50	8	1-8	28	2
Myoplex Lite	190	26	5	2.5-3.0	15	4-8
Nature Valley Granola	180	29	6	0.5	4	2
Odwalla Bar	230	41	5	0.5-2.0	5	3-5
PowerBar Performance	230	43	2.5	0	9	2
Slim-Fast Optima Meal	220	35	6	3.0-3.5	5	2-8
ZonePerfect	210	22	7	3.5-5.0	15	0-3

CHO = carbohydrate.

* Indicates average amounts.

Information taken from packages of products sold and from Cooper Clinic Nutrition Department, J. Neily, *Energy and Snack Bar Comparison Chart*, January 2007.

Table 2.2 Examples of High-Carbohydrate Recovery Products (Drinks, Shakes, Gels)

Product	Serving size*	Energy (kcal)	CHO (g)	CHO (% energy)	Protein (g)
Gatorade Nutrition Shake	11 oz	360	54	60	20
Gatorade Protein Recovery Shake	11 oz	270	45	66	20
Gatorade Carbohydrate Energy Formula	12 oz	320	79	100	0
PowerBar Recovery Drink	16 oz	184	40	87	6
PowerBar Recovery Shake	11 oz	250	40	64	13
ClifShot (32 g)	1.1 oz	100	25	100	0
ClifShot Recovery (40 g)	1.4 oz	140	23	67	6
GU Energy Gel (32 g)	1.1 oz	100	25	100	0
PowerGel (41 g)	1.4 oz	110	27	100	0
Carb-BOOM!	1.4 oz	110	27	100	0

CHO = carbohydrate.

*This information is based on the serving size indicated by the manufacturer. All products contain combinations of various forms of carbohydrate (e.g., maltodextrin, dextrose, fructose, brown rice syrup, high-fructose corn syrup, glucose, or some combination of these), and some contain protein.

Nutrition information from manufacturers: Nutrition information varies slightly with different flavors of the same product; one gel pack is typically ~28 to 32 g (~1.1-1.4 oz foil packets).

CARBOHYDRATE FEEDING POSTEXERCISE AND DURING TRAINING PERIODS

After an exercise session, one must replenish muscle glycogen and refuel the body for the next exercise event. Athletes who have 20 to 24 h or more before the next activity can replenish glycogen stores more easily than if they exercise sooner. For many athletes, it is rare for 24 h to pass between exercise sessions; thus postexercise feeding is critical. The types and amounts of food used and the timing of the meals after exercise depend in part on when the next exercise bout will occur. In addition to refueling the body, postexercise feeding should provide the energy and nutrients to repair and strengthen muscle tissue that may have been damaged during the previous exercise session, and should provide fluids to rehydrate the body.

Glycogen Synthesis Postexercise

Glycogen depletion can occur after 2 to 3 h of continuous exercise performed at 60% to 80% $\dot{V}O_2$max, or after high-intensity exercise (90-130% $\dot{V}O_2$max) that occurs intermittently over a shorter time (15-60 min); thus, both endurance exercise (e.g., cycling or running) and intermittent exercise (e.g., tennis, basketball, soccer, swimming) can deplete glycogen stores. After exercise, the majority of glucose for glycogen synthesis will come from oral glucose ingestion. Jentjens and Jeukendrup (2003b) have reviewed the research literature on postexercise glycogen synthesis and report that the rate of muscle glycogen replacement after exercise ranges from 20 to 50 mmol/kg of dry muscle per hour when a carbohydrate supplement is provided postexercise. Normal glycogen levels of trained male athletes on a mixed diet (consuming 6-10 g carbohydrate per kilogram body weight) are ~130 to 160 mmol/kg of muscle, while those of untrained individuals range from ~80 to 110 mmol/kg of muscle. Male athletes who attempt to supercompensate glycogen can increase stored glycogen to ~200 mmol/kg of muscle. Since the amount of glycogen that can be resynthesized within a given period is limited, one goal of postexercise feeding is to provide adequate carbohydrate for liver and muscle glycogen replacement before the next exercise bout.

A number of factors determine the rate of glycogen synthesis, including the degree of muscle glycogen depletion, the degree of insulin activation of **glycogen synthase,** and the carbohydrate content of the postexercise diet. Glycogen resynthesis occurs in two phases: rapid and slow. In the rapid phase of resynthesis (~30-60 min postexercise), the process can proceed without insulin and is optimized with adequate carbohydrate availability. This phase occurs only if muscle glycogen is low (<128-150 mmol/kg dry weight) (Jentjens and Jeukendrup 2003b). The slow phase of glycogen resynthesis is insulin dependent, occurs best when carbohydrate availability and insulin concentrations are high, and lasts for several hours. Without adequate dietary carbohydrate, muscle glycogen cannot be replaced to normal levels. Nearly 90% of the dietary carbohydrate (digested primarily to glucose) consumed postexercise is deposited in muscle glycogen, which predominates over liver glycogen synthesis. Greater muscle glycogen depletion enhances glycogen resynthesis. For example, Bonen and colleagues (1985) found that during the first 4 h after exercise, glycogen synthesis increased 43% after exhaustive exercise (producing an 80% decrease in leg muscle glycogen) compared with only a 13% increase after nonexhaustive exercise (producing a 35% decrease in leg muscle glycogen).

Over the last five to seven years, research in the area of postexercise recovery has exploded (Burke et al. 2006; Jentjens and Jeukendrup 2003b; Williams 2006). Researchers have found that combining some protein or amino acids with carbohydrate can lead to higher muscle glycogen synthesis versus the same amount of carbohydrate without the additional protein (Ivy et al. 2002; van Loon et al. 2000). Ivy and colleagues (2002) measured postexercise muscle glycogen synthesis 4 h after a 2.5 h glycogen-depleting cycling bout in trained male cyclists. Three different treatments were compared: (1) carbohydrate + protein (80 g carbohydrate, 28 g protein, 6 g fat), (2) carbohydrate (80 g carbohydrate, 6 g fat), (3) high carbohydrate (108 g carbohydrate, 6 g fat). The high-carbohydrate treatment was calorically equivalent to the carbohydrate + protein treatment. The supplement was fed immediately after exercise (10 min) and 2 h postexercise. Muscle biopsies were done pre- and 4 h postexercise. Results show that the carbohydrate + protein treatment significantly increased glycogen synthesis (17-26% more) compared to the other two treatments. These results support the need for including both protein and carbohydrate in the postexercise meal.

High-Carbohydrate Diets During Training Improve Performance and Power Output

We have established that high-carbohydrate diets that include protein fed postexercise increase the level of stored glycogen in the body, while high carbohydrate intake during periods of high-intensity training will keep glycogen levels high. The question remains: Do these higher levels of glycogen lead to improved performance?

A tremendous amount of research has been done in the last 10 to 15 years to answer this question. Overall, we know that replacement of glycogen after exercise is important, especially during periods of high training or endurance exercise. But do higher levels of glycogen always translate into increased exercise performance? To examine this question, Simonsen and colleagues (1991) fed male (*n* = 12) and female (*n* = 10) rowers two different carbohydrate levels over a four-week period of intense training that included rowing twice a day. The subjects were randomly assigned to either a high-carbohydrate diet (10 g/kg body weight, 70% of energy) or a moderate-carbohydrate diet (5 g/kg body weight, 42% of energy) (figure 2.15). Dietary protein intake was 2 g/kg body weight (13% of energy) for both groups, and fat intake was adjusted to maintain body weight throughout the period. The subjects exercised daily for 65 min

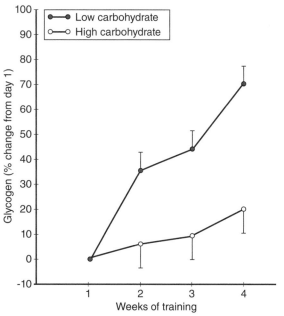

Figure 2.15 Percent change in muscle glycogen from one day of a moderate-carbohydrate diet (5 g/kg body weight per day) and from one day of a high-carbohydrate diet (10 g/kg body weight per day) during four weeks of intense twice-a-day rowing exercise.

Reprinted from J.C. Simonsen et al., 1991, "Dietary carbohydrate, muscle glycogen and power output during rowing training," *Journal of Applied Physiology* 70:1500-1505. Used with permission.

at 70% peak $\dot{V}O_2$ and for 38 min at 90% peak $\dot{V}O_2$. Although muscle glycogen levels increased by 65% in the high-carbohydrate group as compared to the moderate-carbohydrate group, the moderate-carbohydrate group maintained their baseline glycogen levels (119 mmol/kg) throughout the training period. Carbohydrate at 5 g/kg body weight apparently was sufficient to maintain, but not increase, glycogen levels during this period of intense training. However, the mean power output in the time trials increased by 10.7% in the high-carbohydrate group, but by only 1.6% in the moderate-carbohydrate group, after four weeks of intense training. Thus, the high-carbohydrate diet increased glycogen levels and power output when compared to the moderate-carbohydrate diet. These data are supported by Jenkins and colleagues (1993), who found a 5.6% increase in total work done during high-intensity interval cycling when a high-carbohydrate diet was fed for 10 days (83% energy from carbohydrate) versus a moderate-carbohydrate diet (58% from carbohydrate).

Not all studies show improved exercise performance with increased dietary carbohydrate and improved glycogen stores (Hargreaves et al. 1997; Hawley et al. 1997; Sherman et al. 1993). Of course, there are a number of factors that affect performance, and level of stored glycogen is just one factor. For example, Hawley and colleagues (1997) fed six trained cyclists their normal diet (5.9 g carbohydrate per kilogram) or a high-carbohydrate diet (9.3 g carbohydrate per kilogram) for three days. Athletes then performed a 1 h time trial, and muscle biopsies were taken before and after each exercise session. Consuming a high-carbohydrate diet increased muscle glycogen levels by 23% but did not improve time trial performance. Thus, a more moderate level of carbohydrate that maintained muscle glycogen levels at an adequate level for the exercise performed appeared to be adequate. Thus, the level of carbohydrate in the diet needs to match the type of exercises performed and the energy demands placed on the body. When muscle glycogen levels are adequate, increasing levels above normal may not increase exercise performance unless athletes are performing exercise that is strenuous enough to deplete muscle glycogen. However, if athletes are consuming a low-carbohydrate diet, improving carbohydrate intake and subsequent muscle glycogen levels can reduce fatigue and improve power output (Langfort et al. 1997; Johnson et al. 2006).

Type and Amount of Carbohydrate

Glucose, sucrose, maltodextrins, and starch all appear to replace muscle glycogen equally well. To examine both quantity and type of carbohydrate required to restore muscle glycogen after exhaustive exercise, Blom and colleagues (1987) fed carbohydrate immediately after exercise and then at 2, 4, and 6 h postexercise. In one experiment (figure 2.16a), they tested three levels of glucose (high, medium, and low concentrations); in another (figure 2.16b), they tested three types of sugars (glucose, sucrose, and fructose) at equal concentrations (0.7 g/kg body weight). They took muscle biopsies at rest; 5 min after exercise; and 2, 4, and 6 h after exercise. The high- and medium-glucose solutions replaced glycogen equally (~5.7 mmol/kg), as did glucose and sucrose fed at the same concentrations (0.7 g/kg body weight). As one would expect, fructose did not replace muscle glycogen nearly as well as the other sugars. As mentioned earlier, research suggests that fructose is better for the resynthesis of liver glycogen than of muscle glycogen.

Researchers have also examined the effect of meal size on glycogen replacement in the 24 h period following exhaustive exercise. Burke and colleagues (1996) fed eight well-trained triathletes either four large meals ("gorging") or 16 frequent small meals ("nibbling") postexercise. Subjects received the same types of carbohydrate foods, providing 10 g of carbohydrate per kilogram body weight, during each trial. The researchers hypothesized that gorging would elicit a greater glucose and insulin response than nibbling and thus be better at replacing muscle glycogen. There was no statistically significant difference between the groups in muscle glycogen storage over the 24 h period (gorging: 74 ± 8 mmol glycogen per kilogram wet muscle weight; nibbling: 95 ± 15 mmol glycogen per kilogram wet muscle weight). The size of the high-carbohydrate meal apparently had no influence on muscle glycogen levels. This research has practical implications. For many athletes, appetite is frequently suppressed following strenuous exercise, making a large postexercise meal unappealing—yet this is the time when the glycogen storage potential is highest. This research provides a practical solution to this dilemma: Small, frequent postexercise high-carbohydrate snacks can be just as effective at replacing muscle glycogen as large postexercise

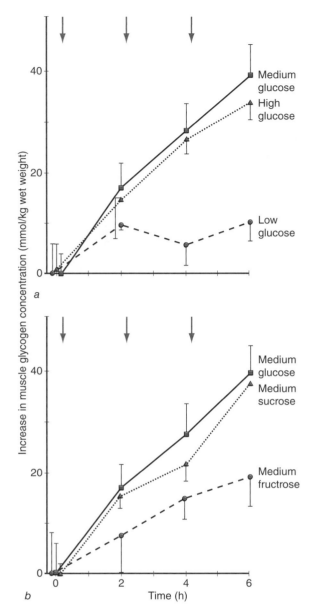

Figure 2.16 Change in muscle glycogen during postexercise recovery when different sugar loads were given. *(a)* Different amounts of glucose. *(b)* Different kinds of sugars. Arrows indicate sugar loads. Mean values are shown; one SEM is indicated by the length of the vertical bar. ● = low glucose (LG) (0.35 g/kg BW); ■ = medium glucose (MG) (0.70 g/kg BW); ▲ = high glucose (HG) (1.4 g/kg BW); ▲ = medium sucrose (MS) (0.70 g/kg BW); ● = medium fructose (MF) (0.70 g/kg BW). Medium glucose appears on both panels. Mean values are shown. One SEM is indicated by the length of the vertical bar. BW=body weight.

Reprinted, by permission, from P.C.S. Blom et al., 1987, "Effect of different post-exercise sugar diets on the rate of muscle glycogen synthesis," *Medicine and Science in Sports and Exercise* 19: 491-496.

meals if one has 24 h or longer in which to replace muscle glycogen.

Most recently, research has examined the use of postexercise protein or carbohydrate–protein combinations (or both) to replace muscle glycogen, improve net protein synthesis, or do both. Here we will focus on the impact of combining protein and carbohydrate in the postexercise meal or beverage to replace muscle glycogen. We address the impact of the protein–carbohydrate combination on postexercise protein synthesis in chapter 4.

When looking at research on glycogen replacement during the postexercise period, it is important to compare the time frames over which muscle glycogen was measured. Did researchers look at it within 6, 12, or 24 h postexercise? This will help you determine what protocol to recommend to an athlete, since what you recommend should be based on the athlete's training routine and competition schedule. One of the first studies to examine the role of protein, carbohydrate, or protein + carbohydrate in muscle glycogen resynthesis was that of Zawadzki and colleagues (1992). They fed nine male cyclists three different treatments immediately after and 2 h after exhaustive exercise. The treatments were (1) carbohydrate = 112 g of carbohydrate (456 kcal); (2) protein = 41 g of protein (164 kcal); and (3) carbohydrate + protein = 112 g of carbohydrate, 41 g of protein (620 kcal). Muscle biopsies were taken immediately after exercise and 4 h postexercise to determine how much glycogen was replaced with each treatment. Glycogen replacement was 28% higher with the carbohydrate–protein combination than with the carbohydrate-only treatment. As expected, the protein-only treatment did a poor job of replacing muscle glycogen. Figure 2.17*a* shows the amount of muscle glycogen replacement for each treatment. The greater amount of glycogen stored with the combination of protein and carbohydrate may have been due to the higher energy content of the combined treatment (more kilocalories were provided in this treatment) versus the carbohydrate and the protein-only treatments. Thus, the amount of glycogen stored after exercise will be a function of total energy intake and the carbohydrate content of the diet.

This question was subsequently addressed by others (Ivy et al. 2002; van Loon et al. 2000). Ivy and colleagues (2002) did an experiment similar to that of Zawadzki and colleagues (1992), but controlled for the differences in energy and carbohydrate intake. They used three treatments:

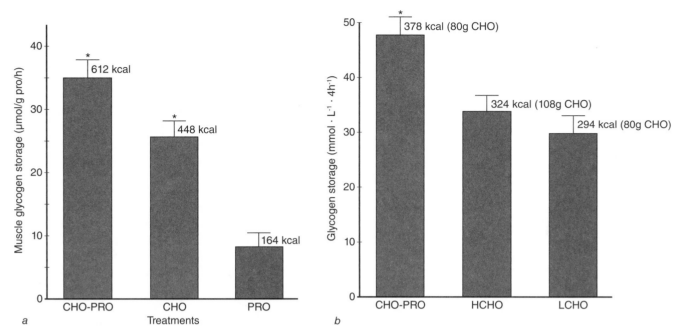

Figure 2.17 *(a)* Rates of muscle glycogen storage during 4 h recovery periods for trained male cyclists receiving 112 g carbohydrate (CHO) + 41 g protein (PRO) after exhaustive exercise; CHO only (112 g); or PRO only (41 g). Supplements were provided immediately and 2 h after exhaustive exercise designed to deplete muscle glycogen. *(b)* Total muscle glycogen storage in the vastus lateralis during 4 h recovery from intense cycling exercise (2.5 h). Treatments were with CHO-PRO (80 g CHO, 28 g PRO, 6 g fat; 378 kcal), High-CHO (equal kilocalories) (108 g CHO, 6 g fat; 324 kcal), and Low-CHO (equal CHO content) (80 g CHO, 6 g fat; 274 kcal) and were provided immediately and 2 h after exercise. *Significantly different from High-CHO and Low-CHO ($P < 0.05$).

Part *a* reprinted from K.M. Zawadzki, B.B. Yaspelkis, and J.L. Ivy, 1992, "Carbohydrate-protein complex increases the rate of muscle glycogen storage after exercise," *Journal of Applied Physiology* 72: 1854-1959. Used with permission. Part *b* reprinted from J.L. Ivy et al., 2002, "Early post-exercise muscle glycogen recovery is enhanced with a carbohydrate-protein supplement," *Journal of Applied Physiology* 93: 1337-1344. Used with permission.

(1) carbohydrate + protein = 80 g carbohydrate + 28 g protein and 6 g fat (378 kcal), (2) high carbohydrate = 108 g carbohydrate + 6 g fat (324 kcal), and (3) low carbohydrate = 80 g carbohydrate = 6 g fat (294 kcal). The first two treatments have equivalent energy content, while treatment 3 has an amount of carbohydrate equivalent to that of treatment 1. Again, the participants were fed immediately after exercise and at 2 h postexercise, and glycogen levels were measured after 4 h. Ivy and colleagues found significantly higher glycogen storage postexercise in the carbohydrate + protein treatment compared to the high-carbohydrate energy-matched treatment (88.8 vs. 75.5 mmol/L, respectively) (figure 2.17*b*). Van Loon and colleagues (2000) did a similar study and measured glycogen levels at 5 h postexercise. They found no differences between the carbohydrate + protein and the energy-matched carbohydrate-only treatments.

Burke and colleagues (1995) addressed this same issue but used a 24 h glycogen replacement protocol and used food instead of drinks. This protocol might more closely reflect the actual dietary behaviors of an active individual or athlete. They randomly assigned three different dietary regimens to eight well-trained triathletes after exhaustive exercise (2 h at 75% peak $\dot{V}O_2$, followed by four 30 s sprints). The diets were fed one week apart. For 24 h after each exercise bout, the athletes were fed one of the following diets:

- High-carbohydrate diet (7 g/kg body weight per day)
- High-carbohydrate diet with added fat and protein (protein: 1.6 g/kg body weight per day; fat: 1.2 g/kg body weight per day)
- Matched energy diet (carbohydrate diet + 4.8 g/kg body weight per day additional carbohydrate)

Overall the researchers found no significant differences between the trials in muscle glycogen storage over a 24 h period. From this study, it appears that as long as carbohydrate and energy intake are adequate, the protein found in a typical diet is enough to enhance glycogen storage. Most athletes have longer than 4 to 5 h to replace muscle glycogen; thus feeding both protein and carbohydrate during the 24 h period following strenuous exercise is recommended. The protein provides the necessary amino acids for building and repairing muscle tissue and for maintaining positive nitrogen balance and also helps in glycogen synthesis, while the carbohydrate provides the substrate for glycogen storage.

Researchers have also examined whether solid or liquid forms of carbohydrate are better at replacing muscle glycogen. In general, it appears that the form of carbohydrate is not as important as the quantity of carbohydrate fed (Jentjens and Jeukendrup 2003b). When solid and liquid carbohydrates are fed at the same rate, muscle glycogen synthesis rates appear to be similar. For example, Reed and colleagues (1989) fed solid and liquid carbohydrate (1.5 g/kg body weight) immediately after exercise and at 2 h intervals after exercise and found similar rates of muscle glycogen synthesis. Thus, it appears that solid and liquid forms of carbohydrate replace muscle glycogen equally well. As discussed in the next section, if quick glycogen replacement is needed, then the postexercise carbohydrate fed, regardless of form, should have a high glycemic index and be adequate in amount (~1-1.2 g of carbohydrate per kilogram body weight each hour). This level of carbohydrate intake is high and may need to be modified to meet individual needs.

Glycogen Replacement Using High Glycemic Index Foods

Most research examining the effects of different types of carbohydrates on muscle glycogen replacement categorizes foods as either simple or complex carbohydrates. This approach assumes that simple carbohydrates (higher in sugar) elicit a large, rapid rise in blood glucose while complex carbohydrates (high in starch) produce a slower, flatter blood glucose response curve. This simplistic approach to classifying carbohydrate foods is incorrect. Carbohydrate foods with quite similar chemical structures (e.g., spaghetti and white bread, which are both high in starch) can produce different blood glucose responses (see "Glycemic Index of Some Common Foods" on p. 27).

If the assumptions cited in the previous paragraph were true, feeding high glycemic index foods postexercise would produce a greater increase in muscle glycogen storage than would low glycemic index foods, even if carbohydrate content was held constant. This hypothesis was tested in the 1990s by researchers. For example, Burke and colleagues (1993) had five well-trained cyclists perform 2 h of exhaustive exercise on two different occasions, one week apart. For 24 h after each trial, the cyclists rested and consumed a high-carbohydrate diet. They consumed a low glycemic index diet in the first trial and a high glycemic index diet for the second. Both diets provided 10 g of carbohydrate per kilogram body weight (730 g carbohydrate; 74% of energy) over the 24 h period, and they were similar in energy content (~3900 kcal/day). Muscle biopsies were taken immediately after exercise and 24 h after consumption of the experimental diets. The degree of muscle glycogen depletion was similar in the two trials (26-34 mmol/kg wet weight). Muscle glycogen content 24 h after recovery was significantly greater with the high-glycemic diet (106 ± 12 mmol/kg wet muscle weight) than with the low-glycemic diet (72 ± 7 mmol/kg wet muscle weight). The authors attributed the higher glycogen content to the significantly higher glucose and insulin response on the high- compared to the low-glycemic diet. It appears that high glycemic index foods are indeed preferable for replacing muscle glycogen immediately after exercise.

Although high glycemic index foods are excellent for replacing muscle glycogen, planning all the meals of an athlete around such foods in the 24 h after exercise may be difficult or impossible—the athlete may be traveling and need to purchase food from restaurants or grocery stores. It may be more practical to provide 100 g of high glycemic index carbohydrate (either food or commercially available product) immediately after exercise and simply to encourage the athlete to eat high-carbohydrate foods for the remainder of the day. "Glycemic Index of Some Common Foods" on p. 27 lists glycemic indices of a number of foods that can be used immediately after exercise. A convenient way to consume a high glycemic index food postexercise is to use glycogen replacement products available on the market. These products are especially convenient for active people who prefer not to eat immediately following strenuous exercise or may wish to eat at times when food is not readily available postexercise. For athletes wanting inexpensive ways to provide small meals containing a known amount of carbohydrate, table 2.3 gives individual foods and combinations of foods that provide either 50 or 100 g of carbohydrate. Finally, many active individuals like the convenience of the energy and sport bars currently on the market. These products usually provide some protein, fat, and micronutrients along with carbohydrate. They are not designed exclusively for glycogen replacement but as a snack to supplement meals. Table 2.1 (p. 49) lists the amount of carbohydrate and energy provided in commonly available sport, energy, and breakfast bars.

Timing and Rate of Postexercise Carbohydrate Feedings

The timing and rate of carbohydrate consumption after exercise can influence the amount of glycogen stored. Glycogen synthesis rates are highest immediately after exercise when the muscle is depleted and glycogen synthase activation is high (Jentjens and Jeukendrup 2003b). Therefore, one goal of postexercise feeding is to get carbohydrate into the system quickly, especially in the first 2 h after exercise. Baker and colleagues (1994) monitored the diets of seven highly trained

Table 2.3   Foods and Combinations of Foods Containing Either 50 or 100 g of Carbohydrate

Food or combination of foods	Amount	Carbohydrate (g)	Energy from carbohydrate (%)	Protein (g)	Fat (g)	Total energy (kcal)
Sweetened applesauce	1 cup	50	97	0.5	0.5	207
Whole wheat bread with Jelly Nonfat milk	1 oz slice 4 tsp 12 fl oz	50	71	16	2	282
Brown rice (cooked) with Tomato sauce	1 cup 1/4 cup	50	83	6	2	242
Spaghetti noodles with Tomato sauce	1 cup 1/4 cup	50	75	8	4	268
Large apple with Saltine crackers	1 8	50	82	3	4	248
Grape-Nuts cereal with Raisins Nonfat milk	1/2 cup 3/8 cup 8 fl oz	100	84	16	1	473
Large bagel with Jelly Nonfat milk	1 (3.5 oz) 8 tsp 8 fl oz	100	81	19	2	494
Brown rice (cooked) with Mixed vegetables Apple juice	1 cup 1/2 cup 12 fl oz	100	88	8	2	450
Large apple with Raisins Saltine crackers	1 1/3 cup 14	100	84	6	6	460
Sandwich/salad						
Whole wheat bread with Chicken breast Whole tomato Loose-leaf lettuce Dressing (low kcal) Pineapple juice	2 slices 2 oz 1 1 cup 1 tbsp 16 oz	104	73	26	4	565

competitive cyclists for three days before and 24 h after exhaustive exercise. Subjects were then given either a flavored high-carbohydrate drink (12% maltodextrin) or a flavored placebo. They completed another exhaustive exercise bout the following day. This protocol was repeated two weeks later until all athletes had completed both the carbohydrate and placebo trials (table 2.4). Athletes receiving the additional carbohydrate after the first exercise session improved their time to exhaustion on the following day by an average of 11%. The athletes' typical diet contained only 4 g of carbohydrate per kilogram body weight, with carbohydrate representing 50% of their total energy intake. The athletes who received the additional high-carbohydrate drink immediately after exercise significantly increased their total carbohydrate intake for the day to 68% of total energy intake (7 g/kg body weight). The additional carbohydrate increased their total energy intake ~500 kcal/day. Thus, the simple addition of a high-carbohydrate replacement drink to the athletes' diet immediately after exercise significantly improved their overall carbohydrate and energy intake, even when the athletes self-selected their diets. High-carbohydrate replacement products like those used in this study are convenient and make it easy to ensure that adequate carbohydrate is provided postexercise. However, they need to be used in combination with nutritious foods and should not replace the postexercise meal.

Since the rate of muscle glycogen synthesis is linear during the first 6 h after glycogen-depleting exercise, most researchers have used this time period to determine the effects of timing on glycogen replacement. Ivy, Katz, and colleagues (1988) found that a 2 h delay in feeding carbohydrate after exercise reduced the rate of glycogen synthesis by 47% compared with feeding carbohydrate immediately after exercise. In a follow-up study, eight male cyclists were fed carbohydrate (either 1.5 or 3.0 g/kg body weight) immediately and 2 h after exhaustive exercise. Muscle biopsies were taken immediately, 2 h, and 4 h after exercise to determine muscle glycogen levels. The authors found that providing >1.5 g of carbohydrate per kilogram body weight resulted in no additional increase in muscle glycogen levels (Ivy, Lee et al. 1988). In another study, Doyle and colleagues (1993) reported that the highest level of glycogen resynthesis (10 mmol $\cdot$ kg^{-1} $\cdot$ h^{-1}) occurred after feeding 0.4 g of maltodextrin per kilogram body weight every 15 min over a 4 h period immediately following exhaustive exercise. This higher glycogen storage may be due to the higher insulin response observed when carbohydrate is consumed more frequently (every 15 min) compared to less frequent feedings (every 1-2 h). Insulin stimulates the uptake of glucose by the cells for glycogen storage and stimulates glycogen synthase. If a 176 lb (80 kg) male consumed the amount of carbohydrate required to achieve the highest level of glycogen replacement (0.4 g of carbohydrate every 15 min for 4 h), he would need to ingest 128 g of carbohydrate per hour or 512 g of carbohydrate in 4 h. This level of carbohydrate intake after exhaustive exercise may be difficult for many athletes to achieve, but certainly could be achieved over a longer time period of 6 to 8 h.

Table 2.4 Energy and Carbohydrate Intake and Cycling Performance Times in Cyclists With and Without Carbohydrate (CHO) Supplementation 24 h Postexercise

	Energy intake on 3-day typical diet (kcal/kg BW)	Energy intake 24 h postexercise (kcal/kg BW)	CHO intake 24 h postexercise (g/kg BW)	CHO intake 24 h postexercise (% energy intake)	Ride time (min)
CHO supplement	34.3 ± 6.3	41.8 ± 9.7	6.8 ± 0.9*	68 ± 6*	72 ± 8**
Placebo	29.3 ± 8.5	34.8 ± 19.2	4.7 ± 2.5	55 ± 5	64 ± 11

CHO supplement = 3.0 g carbohydrate per kilogram body weight; placebo condition = a noncaloric drink.

Subjects performed two exercise tests. After recording their diet for three days, they exercised at 70% $\dot{V}O_2$max to exhaustion and then received either a placebo or a carbohydrate supplement during the next 24 h. The next day they exercised for 1 h of cycling at 70% $\dot{V}O_2$max, then to exhaustion at 85% $\dot{V}O_2$max.

*Diets 24 h postexercise were significantly higher in CHO than self-selected diets before exercise ($P < 0.05$).

**Ride time with the carbohydrate supplement was significantly longer than in the placebo condition ($P < 0.05$). Exercise was 1 h of cycling at 70% $\dot{V}O_2$max, then to exhaustion at 85% $\dot{V}O_2$max.

Reprinted from S.K. Baker, T. Rusynyk, and P.M. Tidus, 1994, "Immediate post-training carbohydrate supplementation improves subsequent performance in trained cyclists," *Sports Medicine, Training and Rehabilitation* 5:131-135. Reprinted by permission of Taylor and Francis, http://www.informaworld.com.

The more frequent feeding (1-2 h) in Doyle and colleagues' (1993) study is comparable to the condition for the "nibblers" (fed every 1.5 h) discussed earlier in this chapter (Burke et al. 1996). However, Burke and colleagues saw no difference in glycogen storage between individuals fed high-carbohydrate diets every 1.5 h versus every 6 h over a 24 h period. The differences in these two studies may be due to the timing of the muscle biopsies done to assess glycogen levels. Burke's group determined glycogen levels 24 h after exhaustive exercise, while Doyle's group did their measurements 4 h after exhaustive exercise. Thus, it appears that as long as adequate carbohydrate is fed within 24 h, glycogen replacement will occur.

Determining Overall Carbohydrate Intake for Individuals

Although it is frequently recommended that athletes consume diets containing 55% to 65% of the energy from carbohydrate, this may be an unrealistic goal for some individuals. Making carbohydrate recommendations based on grams of carbohydrate per kilogram body weight is probably an easier and more realistic approach (see table 2.5). The total amount of carbohydrate consumed in a diet containing 65% of its energy from carbohydrate varies dramatically with the total calories consumed. For example, a 176 lb (80 kg) male athlete consuming 5000 kcal/day with 65% of the energy coming from carbohydrate would

consume 813 g (3252 kcal) of carbohydrate. This is equivalent to ~10 g of carbohydrate per kilogram body weight and more than exceeds the amount of carbohydrate needed to replace glycogen at a maximum rate. For this person, a diet providing 55% of its energy from carbohydrate would still provide 688 g of carbohydrate, or 8.5 g of carbohydrate per kilogram body weight (see the complete diet composition for these two diets in table 2.5). For many male athletes this level of carbohydrate intake would be a more realistic and achievable goal and would easily replace muscle glycogen during heavy training periods.

For many female athletes, who typically report consuming 2200 to 2500 kcal/day, it is almost impossible to consume the 500 to 600 g of carbohydrate per day frequently recommended for adequate glycogen replacement in men. For example, a 121 lb (55 kg) woman who consumed 6 to 7 g carbohydrate per kilogram body weight would need 330 to 385 g of carbohydrate per day (see table 2.5). This is equivalent to 1320 to 1540 kcal just from carbohydrate (or 66-77% of energy coming from carbohydrate based on a 2000 kcal/day diet). This total carbohydrate intake is below the 500 to 600 g/day recommendation for men, but the percentage of energy from carbohydrate is at or above the recommended level. Diets high in carbohydrate prevent the onset of fatigue in active females during exercise. For example, O'Keeffe and colleagues (1989) found that compared to subjects' typical diets (<4.5 g of carbohydrate per kilogram body weight), a diet providing 6 to

Table 2.5 Examples of High- and Moderate-Carbohydrate Diets of Different Energy Levels for Male and Female Athletes

	Male (80 kg) % of energy from carbohydrate				Female (55 kg) % of energy from carbohydrate			
	65%	55%	65%	55%	65%	55%	65%	55%
Energy (kcal/day)	5000	5000	3000	3000	2500	2500	2000	2000
Carbohydrate (%)	65	55	65	55	65	55	65	55
g/day	813	688	488	413	438	344	325	275
g/kg body weight	10.2	8.6	6.1	5.2	7.9	6.3	5.9	5.0
Protein (%)	12	15	12	15	12	15	12	15
g/day	150	188	90	113	75	94	60	75
g/kg body weight	1.9	2.4	1.1	1.4	1.4	1.7	1.1	1.4
Fat (%)	23	30	23	30	23	30	23	30
g/day	128	167	78	100	64	83	51	67
g/kg body weight	1.5	2.1	1.0	1.3	1.2	1.5	0.9	1.2

7 g of carbohydrate per kilogram body weight significantly increased time to exhaustion in female cyclists. Athletes who are dieting may find it easy to consume a high-carbohydrate diet (60-70% of energy from carbohydrate), but the amount of carbohydrate per kilogram of body weight will be low. For example, if a 121 lb (55 kg) woman decided to consume only 1500 kcal/day, a 65% carbohydrate diet would provide only 4.4 g of carbohydrate per kilogram body weight. This level of carbohydrate intake is too low to prevent premature fatigue during prolonged endurance exercise or to adequately replace muscle glycogen on a daily basis during periods of intense exercise training. Carbohydrate recommendations are more accurate when based on grams of carbohydrate per kilogram body weight than when based on percentage of total energy from carbohydrate. This concept is also easier for most athletes to understand and follow since they can readily eat from a recommended list of foods to attain the required carbohydrate intake (see table 2.3 on p. 56).

These points are illustrated by two studies conducted at Ohio State University (Lamb et al. 1990; Sherman et al. 1993): Male athletes consumed either high-carbohydrate diets (80-84% of energy from carbohydrate) or low-carbohydrate diets (42-43% of energy from carbohydrate) for seven to nine days, then either exercised to exhaustion (runners and cyclists) or swam various distances (ranging from 50 m interval sets to continuous 3000 m swims). For the swimmers, there were no differences in mean swim velocities for any interval distances, and mean velocities for all swims were identical on both diets. For the runners and cyclists, there were no differences in time to exhaustion on either diet, although the high-carbohydrate diet maintained a higher muscle glycogen level. The low-carbohydrate diet reduced muscle glycogen by 30% to 36% over the test period. Thus, consuming a lower-carbohydrate diet had no apparent deleterious effects on training capacity or high-intensity exercise performance over the seven to nine days this study was conducted. However, in terms of carbohydrate consumed per kilogram body weight, the low-carbohydrate diet provided 5.0 to 6.5 g of carbohydrate per kilogram body weight while the high-carbohydrate diet provided 10 to 12 g. Thus even the lower-carbohydrate diet (42-43% of energy from carbohydrate, 370 to 470 g carbohydrate per day) appeared to provide adequate carbohydrate to maintain high-intensity work since the subjects were consuming 3600 to 4700 kcal/day. Because the study period was short (seven days), we do not know what effect a "low"-carbohydrate diet such as this would have on muscle glycogen stores over a longer period of time. Would glycogen levels continue to decrease and eventually inhibit exercise performance?

The results of this study might have been very different if active females who were consuming only 2500 kcal/day had been tested. For women with energy needs of 2000 to 2500 kcal/day, a diet containing 43% of energy from carbohydrate would not provide adequate carbohydrate for muscle glycogen replacement. These diets would provide only 215 to 268 g of carbohydrate per day, or 3.9 to 4.8 g of carbohydrate per kilogram body weight for a 121 lb (55 kg) woman. This level of carbohydrate is too low for most active people during periods of intense daily training or competition.

Practical Guidelines for Feeding Carbohydrate Postexercise and During Training Periods

The research described suggests the following recommendations for postexercise carbohydrate feedings. These recommendations assume that the athlete is in training or competition and thus requires maximum glycogen replacement. Athletes frequently train twice a day for a total of 12 to 20 h/week of exercise. Less stringent carbohydrate recommendations are appropriate for recreational or fitness athletes who exercise only 4 to 10 h/week.

- If exercise is to occur again within less than 6 to 8 h, feed approximately 1 to 1.2 g carbohydrate per kilogram body weight immediately after exercise and every 30 to 60 min for the first 5 h after exercise, depending on body size (Williams 2006). Combine this carbohydrate with some dietary protein if possible. This is a high level of carbohydrate intake and may need to be modified for the individual.

- Over a 2 h period, feed ~5 to 7 g of carbohydrate per kilogram body weight for individuals doing moderate training and up to 10 g carbohydrate per kilogram body weight for individuals doing heavy training or fueling up for a competition (Burke 2007). Male athletes consuming more than 3500 kcal/day should be able to consume 500 to 600 g carbohydrate per day. Smaller individuals or those who need fewer calories may find it impossible to consume this much carbohydrate postexercise. A diet providing 6 to 8 g/kg body weight should be adequate for glycogen replacement for these people.

- If you need a more specific postexercise recommendation based on body size, try the following: Feed approximately 1.0 to 1.2 g of carbohydrate per kilogram body weight the first 30 to 60 min after exercise. For a 176 lb (80 kg) man, this would be approximately 80 to 96 g of carbohydrate; for a 121 lb (55 kg) woman, it would be 55 to 66 g. Follow the previously presented guidelines for the recommended 24 h carbohydrate intake.

- Within the first 6 h after exercise, high glycemic index foods or simple carbohydrates (glucose, sucrose, and maltodextrin) provide the best glycogen replacement. These types of foods increase insulin levels in the blood, which stimulate both glucose transport into the cells and glycogen resynthesis.

- Provide a carbohydrate replacement beverage containing 40 to 80 g of carbohydrate per serving (see table 2.2) immediately after exercise if athletes are eating self-selected diets, are unable to eat within 2 h, or do not feel hungry after strenuous exercise. The beverage should provide enough additional carbohydrate to replace muscle glycogen when added to the carbohydrate and protein consumed in the self-selected diet. This recommendation is very useful to coaches or trainers who have little control over athletes' diets, as it promotes adequate glycogen replacement even if athletes have poor diets. Some of the products listed in table 2.2 also contain protein.

- Consider individual athletes' dietary preferences. You can set carbohydrate recommendations and goals, but they will not be achieved if they do not fit well into an individual's daily diet. Your recommendations must be acceptable in relation to the athletes' time and money constraints as well as their cooking abilities. Great diet plans are useless if they are not implemented.

MUSCLE GLYCOGEN SUPERCOMPENSATION

Many endurance athletes know the benefits of maximizing muscle glycogen levels before an exercise event to help prevent fatigue. This practice is called **muscle glycogen supercompensation** or **glycogen loading.** Bergstrom and colleagues (1967) introduced the concept of glycogen loading in 1967 with their "classical" routine, which began one week before an endurance exercise event. On the first three days, athletes ate a low-carbohydrate diet (<10% of energy from carbohydrate) and performed a glycogen-depleting exercise. This was followed by three days of a high-carbohydrate diet (>90% of energy from carbohydrate) with little or no activity. This routine supercompensated the muscles with glycogen and water in preparation for the exercise event that occurred on the seventh day. Because of the adverse side effects associated with this routine (increased risk of injury, irritability, decreased ability to train, dizziness, fluid loss), Sherman and Costill (1984) modified it. The athletes consumed a modified carbohydrate diet (50% of energy from carbohydrate, 353 g carbohydrate per 3000 kcal) for three days, performing a more tapered exercise protocol; then came three days of high carbohydrate intake (70% of energy from carbohydrate, 542 g carbohydrate per 3000 kcal) and little or no exercise. Similar to the classical routine, this routine supercompensated the muscles with glycogen and water for the exercise event on the seventh day. Figure 2.18 compares the modified with the classical glycogen-loading regimen. The two provide similar amounts of muscle glycogen replacement. The modified routine is easier for athletes to follow, however, since eating either an extremely high- or low-carbohydrate diet can be difficult—especially if they are eating meals away from home. The modified routine can also reduce the risk of injury during the first three days of the regimen since it does not totally deplete the athlete of glycogen.

Athletes can maximize muscle glycogen loading by ingesting high-carbohydrate glycemic index foods or liquid carbohydrate supplements during their training period or during the taper period before competition. One advantage of using a liquid carbohydrate supplement is that it may produce less gastrointestinal distress than extreme high-carbohydrate diets (80-90% of energy from carbohydrate) derived solely from food.

Maximizing muscle glycogen levels before an endurance exercise event (>2 h) may improve performance, power, output, and speed. High initial levels of muscle glycogen may increase endurance by postponing muscle glycogen deple-

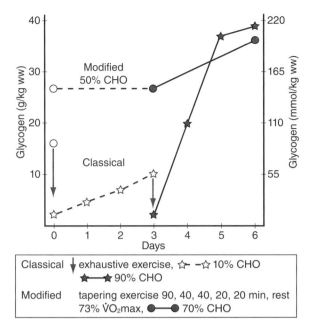

Figure 2.18 Schematic representation of the "classical" regimen of muscle glycogen supercompensation described by Scandinavian investigators and the "modified" regimen of muscle glycogen supercompensation, which elevates muscle glycogen stores to comparably high levels with normal diets and a tapering sequence of exercise.

Reprinted, by permission, from W.M. Sherman and D.L. Costill, 1984, "The marathon: dietary manipulation to optimize performance," *American Journal of Sports Medicine* 12: 44-51.

tion rather than by sparing liver glycogen (Bosch et al. 1993). Although it is assumed that higher glycogen levels will always result in improved performance, research results are mixed. An example of how maximizing muscle glycogen can improve work performance was demonstrated by Rauch and colleagues (1995) in a study using eight well-trained male endurance cyclists (mean peak $\dot{V}O_2$ = 66.3 mL · kg⁻¹ · min⁻¹). Subjects were randomly assigned to one of two experimental treatments (carbohydrate loading or normal carbohydrate) for three days before exercise. They then performed a 2 h submaximal ride (~75% $\dot{V}O_2$ peak) with five 60 s sprints (100% $\dot{V}O_2$ peak) at 20 min intervals. This was then followed by a 60 min performance ride. Order of treatment was randomly assigned, and all subjects completed both treatments with a four-day rest period between each. The carbohydrate-loading trial provided a mean carbohydrate intake of 10.5 g/kg body weight per day, while the normal-carbohydrate trial provided 6.2 g. The carbohydrate-loading trial also provided

significantly more energy (4283 kcal/day) than the normal-carbohydrate trial (3045 kcal/day). The carbohydrate-loading trial significantly increased mean power output (W) by 6% and speed (km/h) by 3% compared with the normal-carbohydrate trial. Simonsen and colleagues (1991) reported similar results: Athletes with higher muscle glycogen levels exhibited significantly improved exercise performance compared to those with lower muscle glycogen levels (figure 2.15, p. 51).

Conversely, in a recent study, Burke and colleagues (2000) failed to see a performance benefit from carbohydrate loading their cyclists before a 100 km (62-mile) ride (~147 min to complete the ride). Either a high-carbohydrate diet (9 g carbohydrate per kilogram body weight) or a moderate-carbohydrate diet (6 g carbohydrate per kilogram body weight) was fed for three days prior to the ride, and a carbohydrate drink was consumed during the ride. The authors hypothesized that the carbohydrate drink provided during exercise may have offset any detrimental effects of performance from the lower preexercise muscle and liver glycogen concentrations.

It should be noted that glycogen loading before exercise does not always improve performance. Some athletes experience extreme gastrointestinal distress, including diarrhea, when attempting to follow this procedure. Because leg muscles become heavier with the addition of extra glycogen and water, many athletes complain that they feel heavy and sluggish, and they may experience a slight weight gain. Athletes should experiment with glycogen loading during practice before trying it for competitions.

CHAPTER IN REVIEW

Carbohydrate is an important component in the diets of active individuals because it is required for glycogen synthesis and for the maintenance of blood glucose levels during exercise. During intense daily exercise training, the diet should provide the following levels of carbohydrate:

- Five to 7 g of carbohydrate per kilogram body weight for individuals during periods of moderate training
- Up to 10 g of carbohydrate per kilogram body weight for individuals during periods of heavy training and competition

This level of carbohydrate should be adequate to replace muscle glycogen and help to optimize exercise performance. The exact level of carbohydrate selected will depend on the athlete, his or her level of energy intake, and body size. Many female athletes will need more moderate amounts. In addition, carbohydrate feedings before and during exercise help improve performance and prevent fatigue, especially in endurance events lasting longer than 1 h. During exercise, carbohydrate-containing drinks with a 6% to 8% concentration will provide optimal gastric emptying and absorption. Finally, carbohydrate or glycogen loading before an endurance event lasting longer than 2 h may help reduce fatigue and improve exercise performance and mood.

Key Concepts

1. Describe the function, classification, and dietary sources of carbohydrate.

Carbohydrate is a primary energy source during exercise, is required for glycogen replacement, and helps maintain blood glucose levels during exercise. Dietary carbohydrates can be classified based on the type of carbohydrate in the food (starch, sugar, or fiber content), the way in which the carbohydrate has been processed, or the glycemic index of the carbohydrate. Complex carbohydrates are higher in starch than simple carbohydrates, which contain more sugar. Carbohydrate foods such as whole grains, breads, cereals, whole fruits, and vegetables contain more vitamins, minerals, and fiber than carbohydrate foods high in simple sugars (candy, desserts, soda). The glycemic index of a carbohydrate food is determined via measurement of the body's glycemic response to the carbohydrate when it is eaten. Foods with a high glycemic index cause a greater rise in blood glucose than foods with a low glycemic index.

2. Discuss carbohydrate metabolism during exercise.

Muscles require carbohydrate as a fuel source during exercise. This carbohydrate will come from exogenous (diet) or endogenous (gluconeogenesis and glycogenolysis) sources or both. The amounts and sources of carbohydrate used during exercise depend on the intensity and duration of the exercise, the athlete's fitness level and overall health, how well fed the athlete is before exercise, and the environmental temperature and conditions. The amount of gluconeogenesis that occurs during exercise depends on the carbohydrate reserves; the amount of carbohydrate provided before and during exercise; and the type, intensity, and duration of the exercise.

3. Discuss carbohydrate reserves and dietary intake.

The body's carbohydrate reserves are primarily in liver and muscle glycogen. The amount of glycogen in each of these pools is limited and will provide <2000 kcal, depending on the level of carbohydrate in the diet, the size of the individual, and total energy intake. Activities that are high in intensity and longer in duration use more glycogen than low-intensity exercise. Although high-carbohydrate diets (55-65% of energy) are generally recommended for athletes, especially endurance athletes, most athletes consume between 45% and 55% of their energy from carbohydrate. It is more practical to make carbohydrate recommendations based on body size than on percent of energy from carbohydrate. During high-intensity training, make carbohydrate recommendations of up to 10 g of carbohydrate per kilogram body weight; lower amounts are recommended for women and for smaller men.

4. Describe recommendations for carbohydrate feeding before exercise.

The goal of the preexercise meal is to promote additional glycogen synthesis, supply the body with glucose for use during exercise, and help minimize fatigue during exercise. The preexercise meal, usually fed 2 to 4 h before exercise, provides ~150 to 300 g of carbohydrate, is moderate in protein, and is lower in fat and fiber. The meal should be easy to digest, should be familiar to the athlete, and should not cause gastrointestinal distress. If possible, lower glycemic index foods are recommended. If food cannot be consumed before exercise, carbohydrate-containing sport beverages are easy to digest and will provide the needed energy.

5. Describe recommendations for carbohydrate feeding during exercise.

Carbohydrate feeding during exercise complements the body's own carbohydrate reserves by providing additional carbohydrate to the working muscles and by helping maintain blood glucose levels—both of which may diminish fatigue. Carbohydrate feeding during exercise should begin early in the exercise event to ensure that adequate carbohydrate is available during the later stages of exercise. Athletes generally should consume ~1 to 1.5 g of carbohydrate per minute during exercise (~60 g/h). This can be provided by a sport beverage containing 60 to 80 g of carbohydrate per liter if athletes consume 4 to 6 oz (120-180 mL) of this fluid every 15 to 20 min. The exact amount fed will depend on the athlete's needs, type of exercise being engaged in, and the environmental conditions.

6. Describe carbohydrate feeding recommendations for postexercise and during training periods.

The purpose of the postexercise feeding period is to replenish muscle glycogen and refuel the body for the next exercise event. The type and amount of carbohydrate fed depend on how soon the next exercise event will occur. How quickly the body replaces muscle glycogen depends on the level of muscle glycogen depletion, the degree to which insulin activates glycogen synthase, and the carbohydrate content of the postexercise diet. In general, athletes should consume 1.0 to 1.2 g of carbohydrate per kilogram of body weight immediately after exercise and every 30 to 60 min for 5 h; within the following 24 h the goal should be ~5 to 7 g/kg body weight for individuals participating in moderate-intensity activity and 8 to 10 g/kg body weight for those who are engaged in heavy training or are fueling for competition. Women may need lower amounts than men depending on body size and sport.

7. Explain the concept of muscle glycogen supercompensation (glycogen loading).

Athletes can maximize muscle glycogen levels before exercise by following dietary and exercise practices that promote muscle glycogen loading. The glycogen-loading routine is followed for six days before competition, with competition occurring on the seventh day. It is now recommended that athletes follow a modified glycogen-loading routine in which they eat a diet containing 55% of the energy from carbohydrate for three days while performing a tapered exercise protocol. For the next three days they should consume a high-carbohydrate diet (70% of energy) and do little or no exercise. Exercise competition occurs on the seventh day.

Key Terms

complex carbohydrates 26
Cori cycle 29
gluconeogenesis 29
glucose-alanine cycle 30
glycemic index (GI) 29

glycemic load (GL) 30
glycemic response 29
glycogen 35
glycogen loading 60
glycogenolysis 31

glycogen synthase 50
glycolysis 29
hypoglycemia 38

muscle glycogen supercompensation 60
simple carbohydrates 26

Additional Information

Coker RH, Kjaer M. Glucoregulation during exercise. The role of the neuroendocrine system. Sports Med 2005;35(7):575-583.

> Provides a detailed review of how glucose is regulated during exercise.

Hawley JA, Tipton KD, Millard-Stafford ML. Promoting training adaptations through nutritional interventions. J Sports Sci 2006;24(7):709-721.

> Exercise training alters the way the body uses macronutrients. This review discusses the training stimulus, responses, and adaptations that occur and how dietary interventions may alter or modify these adaptations.

Jentjens R, Jeukendrup AE. Determinants of post-exercise glycogen synthesis during short-term recovery. Sports Med 2003;33(2):117-144.

> A comprehensive review of the factors that affect glycogen synthesis including regulation, impact of other nutrients, and the physical limitations of muscle glycogen synthesis.

Jeukendrup AE. Carbohydrate intake during exercise and performance. Nutrition 2004;20(7-8):669-677.

> This article reviews the types and forms of carbohydrate needed during exercise, mechanisms whereby carbohydrate improves performance, rate of carbohydrate oxidation during exercise, and bioavailablility of carbohydrate during exercise.

References

Achten J, Jeukendrup AE. Effects of pre-exercise ingestion of carbohydrate on glycaemic and insulinaemic responses during subsequent exercise at differing intensities. Eur J Appl Physiol Jan 2003;88(4-5):466-471.

Adopo E, Peronnet F, Massicotte D, Brisson GR, Hillaire-Marcel C. Respective oxidation of exogenous glucose and fructose given in the same drink during exercise. J Appl Physiol 1994;76(3):1014-1019.

Ahlborg G. Mechanism for glycogenolysis in nonexercising human muscle during and after exercise. Am J Physiol 1985;248(5)Pt 1:E540-545.

Ahlborg G, Felig P. Lactate and glucose exchange across the forearm, legs, and splanchnic bed during and after prolonged leg exercise. J Clin Invest 1982;69:45-54.

Alberici JC, Farrell PA, Kris-Etherton PM, Shively CA. Effects of preexercise candy bar ingestion on glycemic response, substrate utilization, and performance. Int J Sport Nutr 1993;3:323-333.

Angus DJ, Febbraio MA, Hargreaves M. Plasma glucose kinetics during prolonged exercise in trained humans when fed carbohydrate. Am J Physiol Endocrinol Metab 2002;283(3):E573-E577.

Angus DJ, Hargreaves M, Dancey J, Febbraio MA. Effect of carbohydrate or carbohydrate plus medium-chain triglyceride ingestion on cycling time trial performance. J Appl Physiol 2000;88(1):113-119.

Baker SK, Rusynyk T, Tiidus PM. Immediate post-training carbohydrate supplementation improves subsequent performance in trained cyclists. Sports Med Training Rehab 1994;5:131-135.

Below PR, Coyle EF. Fluid and carbohydrate ingestion individually benefit intense exercise lasting one hour. Med Sci Sports Exerc 1995;27(2):200-210.

Bergstrom J, Hermansen L, Hultman E, Saltin B. Diet, muscle glycogen and physical performance. Acta Physiol Scand 1967;71:140-150.

Blom PCS, Hostmark AT, Vaage O, Kardel KR, Maehlum S. Effect of different post-exercise sugar diets on the rate of muscle glycogen synthesis. Med Sci Sports Exerc 1987;19(5):491-496.

Bonen A, Ness GW, Belcastro AN, Kirby RL. Mild exercise impedes glycogen repletion in muscle. J Appl Physiol 1985;58(5):1622-1629.

Bosch AN, Dennis SC, Noakes TD. Influence of carbohydrate loading on fuel substrate turnover and oxidation during prolonged exercise. J Appl Physiol 1993;74(4):1921-1927.

Bosch AN, Dennis SC, Noakes TD. Influence of carbohydrate ingestion on fuel substrate turnover and oxidation during prolonged exercise. J Appl Physiol 1994;76(6):2364-2372.

Bosch AN, Noakes TD, Dennis S. Carbohydrate ingestion during prolonged exercise: a liver glycogen sparing effect in glycogen loaded subjects. Med Sci Sports Exerc 1991;23:S152.

Burke L. Nutrition for recovery and training and competition. In: Burke L, Deakin V eds. Clinical sports nutrition, 3rd ed. Sydney: McGraw-Hill, 2006;415-440.

Burke LM. The IAAF consensus on nutrition for athletes: update guidelines. Int J Sport Nutr Exerc Metab 2007;17:411-415.

Burke LM, Collier GR, Beasley SK et al. Effect of co-ingestion of fat and protein with carbohydrate feedings on muscle glycogen storage. J Appl Physiol 1995;78(6):2187-2192.

Burke LM, Collier GR, Davis PG, Fricker PA, Sanigorski AJ, Hargreaves M. Muscle glycogen storage after prolonged exercise: effect of the frequency of carbohydrate feeding. Am J Clin Nutr 1996;64:115-119.

Burke LM, Collier GR, Hargreaves M. Muscle glycogen storage after prolonged exercise: effect of the glycemic index of carbohydrate feeding. J Appl Physiol 1993;75(2):1019-1023.

Burke LM, Collier GR, Hargreaves M. Glycemic Index—a new tool in sport nutrition? Int J Sport Nutr 1998;8:401-415.

Burke LM, Hawley JA, Schabort EJ, Gibson AS, Mujika I, Noakes TD. Carbohydrate loading failed to improve 100-km cycling performance in a placebo-controlled trial. J Appl Physiol 2000;88:1284-1290.

Burke LM, Loucks B, Broad N. Energy and carbohydrate for training and recovery. J Sports Sci 2006;24(7):675-685.

Carter J, Jeukendrup AE, Jones DA. The effect of sweetness on the efficiency of carbohydrate supplementation during exercise in the heat. Can J Appl Physiol 2005;30(4):379-391.

Champe PC, Harvey RA, Ferrier DR. Lippincott's illustrated reviews: biochemistry, 4th ed. Philadelphia: Lippincott, 2008.

Chryssanthopoulos C, Williams C, Nowritz A, Kotsiopoulou C, Vleck V. The effect of a high carbohydrate meal on endurance running capacity. Int J Sport Nutr Exerc Metab 2002;12(2):157-171.

Claassen A, Lambert EV, Bosch AN, Rodger IM, Gibson AS, Noakes TD. Variability in exercise capacity and metabolic response during endurance exercise after a low carbohydrate diet. Int J Sport Nutr Exerc Metab 2005;15:97-116.

Coggan AR, Coyle EF. Reversal of fatigue during prolonged exercise by carbohydrate infusion or ingestion. J Appl Physiol 1987;63(6):2388-2395.

Coggan AR, Coyle EF. Metabolism and performance following carbohydrate ingestion late in exercise. Med Sci Sports Exerc 1989;21(1):59-65.

Coker RH, Kjaer M. Glucoregulation during exercise. The role of the neuroendocrine system. Sports Med 2005;35(7):575-583.

Coyle EF. Substrate utilization during exercise in active people. Am J Clin Nutr 1995;61(suppl):968S-979S.

Coyle EF, Coggan AR, Hemmert MK, Ivy JL. Muscle glycogen utilization during prolonged strenuous exercise when fed carbohydrate. J Appl Physiol 1986;61(1):165-172.

Coyle EF, Hamilton MT, Alonso JG, Montain SJ, Ivy JL. Carbohydrate metabolism during intense exercise when hyperglycemic. J Appl Physiol 1991;70(2):834-840.

Cummings JH, Englyst HN. Gastrointestinal effects of food carbohydrates. Am J Clin Nutr 1995;61(suppl):938S-945S.

Davis JM, Jackson DA, Broadwell MS, Queary JL, Lambert CL. Carbohydrate drinks delay fatigue during intermittent, high-intensity cycling in active men and women. Int J Sport Nutr Exerc Metab 1997;7:261-273.

Devlin JT, Calles-Escandon J, Horton ES. Effects of preexercise snack feeding on endurance cycle exercise. J Appl Physiol 1986;60(3):980-985.

Dolins KR, Boozer CN, Stoler F, Bartels M, DeMeersman R, Contento I. Effect of variable carbohydrate intake on exercise performance in female endurance cyclists. Int J Sport Nutr Exerc Metab 2003;13:422-435.

Doyle AJ, Sherman WM, Strauss RL. Effects of eccentric and concentric exercise on muscle glycogen replenishment. J Appl Physiol 1993;74(4):1848-1855.

El-Sayed MS, MacLaren D, Rattu AJ. Exogenous carbohydrate utilisation: effects on metabolism and exercise performance. Comp Biochem Physiol A Physiol Nov 1997;118(3):789-803.

Erickson MA, Schwartzkopf RJ, McKenzie RD. Effects of caffeine, fructose, and glucose ingestion on muscle glycogen utilization during exercise. Med Sci Sports Exerc 1987;19(6):579-583.

Febbraio MA, Chiu A, Angus DJ, Arkinstall MJ, Hawley JA. Effects of carbohydrate ingestion before and during exercise on glucose kinetics and performance. J Appl Physiol 2000a;89:2220-2226.

Febbraio MA, Keenan J, Angus DJ, Campbell SE, Garnham AP. Preexercise carbohydrate ingestion, glucose kinetics, and muscle glycogen use: effects of the glycemic index. J Appl Physiol 2000b;89:1845-1851.

Felig P, Cherif A, Minagawa A, Wahren J. Hypoglycemia during prolonged exercise in normal men. N Engl J Med 1982;306:896-900.

Felig P, Wahren J. Amino acid metabolism in exercising man. J Clin Invest 1971;50:2703-2714.

Fielding RA, Costill DL, Fink WJ, King DS, Hargreaves M, Kovaleski JE. Effect of carbohydrate feeding frequencies and dosage on muscle glycogen use during exercise. Med Sci Sports Exerc 1985;17(4):472-476.

Flatt JP. Use and storage of carbohydrate and fat. Am J Clin Nutr 1995;61(suppl):952S-959S.

Flynn MG, Costill DL, Hawley JA et al. Influence of selected carbohydrate drinks on cycling performance and glycogen use. Med Sci Sports Exerc 1987;19(1):37-40.

Foster-Powell K, Holt SHA, Brand-Miller JC. International table of glycemic index and glycemic load values. Am J Clin Nutr 2002;76(1):5-56.

Hargreaves M. Muscle glycogen and metabolic regulation. Proc Nutr Soc 2004;63:217-220.

Hargreaves M, Finn AP, Withers RT, Halbert JA, Scroop GC, Mackay M, Snow RJ, Carey MF. Effect of muscle glycogen availability on maximal exercise performance. Eur J Appl Physiol 1997;75:188-192.

Hawley JA, Dennis SC, Lindsay FH, Noakes TD. Nutritional practices of athletes: are they suboptimal? J Sports Sci 1995;13:S75-S87.

Hawley JA, Palmer GS, Noakes TD. Effects of 3 days of carbohydrate supplementation on muscle glycogen content and utilization during a 1-h cycling performance. Eur J Appl Physiol 1997;75:407-412.

Hawley JA, Tipton KD, Millard-Stafford ML. Promoting training adaptations through nutritional intervention. J Sports Sci 2006;24(7):709-721.

Horowitz JP, Coyle EF. Metabolic responses to preexercise meals containing various carbohydrates and fat. Am J Clin Nutr 1993;58:235-241.

Institute of Medicine, Food and Nutrition Board, National Research Council. Dietary reference intakes for energy, carbohydrate, fiber, fat, fatty acids, cholesterol, protein, and amino acids. Washington, DC: National Academies Press, 2002.

Ivy JL, Goforth HW, Damon BM, McCauley TR, Parsons EC, Price TB. Early post-exercise muscle glycogen recovery is enhanced with a carbohydrate-protein supplement. J Appl Physiol 2002;93:1337-1344.

Ivy JL, Katz AL, Cutler CL, Sherman WM, Coyle EF. Muscle glycogen synthesis after exercise: effect of time on carbohydrate ingestion. J Appl Physiol 1988;64(4):1480-1485.

Ivy JL, Lee MC, Brozinick JT, Reed MJ. Muscle glycogen storage after different amounts of carbohydrate ingestion. Am J Physiol 1988;65(5):2018-2023.

Jenkins DG, Palmer J, Spillman D. The influencc of dietary carbohydrate on performance of supramaximal intermittent exercise. Eur J Appl Physiol. 1993;67:309-314.

Jentjens RLPG, Achten J, Jeukendrup AE. High oxidation rates from combined carbohydrates ingested during exercise. Med Sci Sports Exerc 2004;36(9):1551-1558.

Jentjens RLPG, Cale C, Gutch C, Jeukendrup AE. Effects of pre-exercise ingestion of differing amounts of carbohydrate on subsequent metabolism and cycling performance. Eur J Appl Physiol 2003;88:444-452.

Jentjens RLPG, Jeukendrup AE. Prevalence of hypoglycemia following pre-exercise carbohydrate ingestion is not accompanied by higher insulin sensitivity. Int J Sport Nutr Exerc Metab 2002;12:398-413.

Jentjens RLPG, Jeukendrup AE. Effects of pre-exercise ingestion of trehalose, galactose and glucose on subsequent metabolism and cycling performance. Eur J Appl Physiol 2003a;88:459-465.

Jentjens R, Jeukendrup AE. Determinants of post-exercise glycogen synthesis during short-term recovery. Sports Med 2003b;33(2):117-144.

Jentjens R, Jeukendrup AE. High rates of exogenous carbohydrate oxidation from a mixture of glucose and fructose ingested during prolonged cycling exercise. Br J Nutr 2005;93:485-492.

Jentjens RLPG, Underwood K, Achten J, Currell K, Mann CH, Jeukendrup AE. Exogenous carbohydrate oxidation rates are elevated after combined ingestion of glucose and fructose during exercise in the heat. J Appl Physiol 2006;100:807-816.

Jentjens RLPG, Venables MC, Jeukendrup AE. Oxidation of exogenous glucose, sucrose and maltose during prolonged cycling exercise. J Appl Physiol 2004;96:1285-1291.

Jeukendrup AE. Modulation of carbohydrate and fat utilization by diet, exercise and environment. Biochem Soc Trans 2003;31(6):1270-1273.

Jeukendrup AE. Carbohydrate intake during exercise and performance. Nutrition 2004;20(7-8):669-677.

Jeukendrup A. Carbohydrate supplementation during exercise: Does it help? How much is too much? Sports Sci Exch 2007;20(3):1-5.

Jeukendrup AE, Jentjens R. Oxidation of carbohydrate feedings during prolonged exercise. Sports Med 2000;29(6):407-424.

Jeukendrup AE, Moseley L, Mainwaring GI, Samuels S, Perry S, Mann CH. Exogenous carbohydrate oxidation during ultra-endurance exercise. J Appl Physiol 2006;100:1134-1141.

Johnson NA, Stannard SR, Chapman PG, Thompson MW. Effect of altered pre-exercise carbohydrate availability on selection and perception of effort during prolonged cycling. Eur J Appl Physiol Sep 2006;98(1):62-70.

Joubert LM, Manore MM. The role of physical activity level and B-vitamin status on blood homocysteine levels. Med Sci Sports Exerc 2008; 40(11):1923-1931.

Lamb DR, Rinehardt KF, Bartels RL, Sherman WS, Snook JT. Dietary carbohydrate and intensity of interval swim training. Am J Clin Nutr 1990;52:1058-1063.

Langfort J, Zarzeczny R, Pilis W, Nazar K, Kacuba-Uscitko H. The effect of a low-carbohydrate diet on performance, hormonal and metabolic responses to a 30-c bout of supermaximal exercise. Eur J Appl Physiol 1997;76:128-133.

Leatt PB, Jacobs I. Effect of glucose polymer ingestion on glycogen depletion during a soccer match. Can J Sports Sci 1989;14(2):112-116.

Maffucci DM, McMurray RG. Towards optimizing the timing of the pre-exercise meal. Int J Sport Nutr Exerc Metab Jun 2000;10(2):103-113.

Manore MM. Dietary recommendations and athletic menstrual dysfunction. Sports Med 2002;32 (14):887-901.

Mason WL, McConell G, Hargreaves M. Carbohydrate ingestion during exercise: liquid vs. solid feedings. Med Sci Sports Exerc 1993;25(8):966-969.

Massicotte D, Peronnet F, Brisson G, Bakkouch K, Hilliare-Marcel C. Oxidation of glucose polymer during exercise: comparison of glucose and fructose. J Appl Physiol 1989;66(1):179-183.

Maughan RJ. Nutritional status, metabolic responses to exercise and implications for performance. Biochem Soc Trans Dec 2003;31(Pt)6:1267-1269.

Maughan RJ, Bethell LR, Leiper JB. Effects of ingested fluids on exercise capacity and on cardiovascular and metabolic responses to prolonged exercise in man. Exp Physiol Sep 1996;81(5):847-859.

Moseley L, Lancaster GI, Jeukendrup AE. Effects of timing of pre-exercise ingestion of carbohydrate on subsequent metabolism and cycling performance. Eur J Appl Physiol Jan 2003;88(4-5):453-458.

Murdoch SD, Bazzarre TL, Snider IP, Goldfarb AH. Differences in the effects of carbohydrate food form on endurance performance to exhaustion. Int J Sport Nutr 1993;3:41-54.

Murray R. Fluid needs in hot and cold environments. Int J Sport Nutr Jun 1995;5 suppl:S62-73.

Murray R, Paul GL, Seifert JG, Eddy DE, Halaby GA. The effects of glucose, fructose, and sucrose ingestion during exercise. Med Sci Sports Exerc 1989;2(3)1:275-282.

Neufer PD, Costill DL, Flynn MG, Kriwan JP, Mitchell JB, Houmard J. Improvements in exercise performance: effects of carbohydrate feedings and diet. J Appl Physiol 1987;62(3):983-988.

Okano G, Takeda H, Morita I, Katoh M, Mu Z, Miyake S. Effect of pre-exercise fructose ingestion on endurance performance in fed men. Med Sci Sports Exerc 1988;20(2):105-109.

O'Keeffe KA, Keith RE, Wilson GD, Blessing DL. Dietary carbohydrate intake and endurance exercise performance in trained female cyclists. Nutr Res 1989;9:819-830.

Rauch LHG, Rodger I, Wilson GR et al. The effects of carbohydrate loading on muscle glycogen content and cycling performance. Int J Sport Nutr 1995;5:25-36.

Reed MJ, Brozinick JT, Lee MC, Ivy JL. Muscle glycogen storage post-exercise: effect of mode of carbohydrate administration. J Appl Physiol 1989;66(2):720-726.

Reynolds RD, Leklem JE ed. Vitamin B-6: its role in health and disease. New York: Liss, 1985.

Sawka MN, Burke LM, Eichner ER, Maughan RJ, Montain SJ, Stachenfeld NSCAACoSM. American College of Sports Medicine position stand. Exercise and fluid replacement. Med Sci Sports Exerc Feb 2007;39(2):377-390.

Sherman WM. Metabolism of sugar and physical performance. Am J Clin Nutr 1995;62(suppl):228S-241S.

Sherman WM, Brodowicz G, Wright DA, Allen WK, Simonsen J, Dernback A. Effect of 4 h preexercise carbohydrate feedings on cycling performance. Med Sci Sports Exerc 1989;21(5):598-604.

Sherman WM, Costill DL. The marathon: dietary manipulation to optimize performance. Am J Sports Med 1984;12(1):44-51.

Sherman WM, Doyle JA, Lamb DR, Strauss RH. Dietary carbohydrate, muscle glycogen, and exercise performance during 7 d of training. Am J Clin Nutr 1993;57:27-31.

Simonsen JC, Sherman WM, Lamb DR, Dernbach AR, Doyle AJ, Strauss R. Dietary carbohydrate, muscle glycogen and power output during rowing training. J Appl Physiol 1991;70(4):1500-1505.

Tsintzas K, Liu R, Williams C, Campbell I, Gaitanos G. The effect of carbohydrate ingestion on performance during a 30-km race. Int J Sport Nutr 1993;3:127-139.

Tsintzas OK, Williams C, Wilson W, Burrin J. Influence of carbohydrate supplementation early in exercise on endurance running capacity. Med Sci Sports Exerc 1996;28(11):1373-1379.

Utter AC, Kang J, Robertson RJ, Nieman DC, Chaloupka EC, Suminski RR, Piccinni CR. Effect of carbohydrate ingestion on ratings of perceived exertion during a marathon. Med Sci Sports Exerc 2002;34(11):1779-1784.

van Hamont D, Harvery CR, Massicotte D, Frew R, Peronnet F, Rehrer NJ. Reduction of muscle glycogen and protein utilization with glucose feeding during exercise. Int J Sport Nutr Exerc Metab 2005;15:350-365.

van Loon LJC, Saris WHM, Kruijshoop M, Wagenmakers AJM. Maximizing postexercise muscle glycogen synthesis: carbohydrate supplementation and the application of amino acid or protein hydrolysate mixtures. Am J Clin Nutr 2000;72:106-111.

Walberg-Rankin J. Dietary carbohydrate and performance of brief, intense exercise. Sports Sci Exch 2000;13(4):1-4.

Williams C. Nutrition to promote recovery from exercise. Sports Sci Exch 2006;19(1):1-6.

Williams C, Serratosa L. Nutrition on match day. J Sports Sci 2006;24(7):687-697.

Wolever TMS, Jenkins DJA, Jenkins AL, Josse RG. The glycemic index: methodology and clinical implications. Am J Clin Nutr 1991;54:846-854.

Wolever TMS, Yang M, Zeng XY, Atkinson F, Brand-Miller JC. Food glycemic index, as given in Glycemic Index tables, is a significant determinant of glycemic responses elicited by composite breakfast meals. Am J Clin Nutr 2006;83:1306-1312.

Wright DA, Sherman WM, Dernback AR. Carbohydrate feedings before, during or in combination improve cycling endurance performance. J Appl Physiol 1991;71(3):1082-1088.

Yaspelkis BB, Ivy JL. Effect of carbohydrate supplements and water on exercise metabolism in the heat. J Appl Physiol 1991;71(2):680-687.

Zawadzki KM, Yaspelkis BB, Ivy JL. Carbohydrate-protein complex increases the rate of muscle glycogen storage after exercise. J Appl Physiol 1992;72(5):1854-1859.

CHAPTER 3

Fat as a Fuel for Exercise

Chapter Objectives

After reading this chapter you should be able to

- explain the functions, classifications, and dietary sources of fat,
- compare and contrast the current fat intake of active and inactive individuals,
- understand fat metabolism during exercise and the sources of this fat,
- identify factors that can enhance or inhibit fat oxidation during exercise, and
- discuss the current dietary fat recommendations for active individuals.

Although many people think of dietary fat as something to be avoided, fat is important for athletic performance and good health. Fat and carbohydrate are the primary fuels used by the body during exercise. The two fuels are oxidized simultaneously, with the proportion of energy coming from each substrate dependent on the meal prior to exercise; energy fed during exercise; the duration, intensity, and type of exercise; and one's fitness level. Fat becomes the primary fuel source during endurance exercise events since the body's supply of carbohydrate in the form of glycogen and blood glucose is limited. Although diets high in carbohydrate are necessary to help replenish muscle glycogen levels after exercise, fat should not be eliminated from the diet.

Research has helped us identify the best mix of dietary carbohydrate, fat, and protein for optimal exercise performance and good health. This mix may change depending on individuals' personal food preferences and fitness levels, the sports they participate in, and their general health status—yet all macronutrients are important in the diet.

For active people of all levels, it appears prudent to consume a diet primarily from unprocessed carbohydrates, but also to include adequate amounts of protein and healthy fat. The 2005 Institute of Medicine (IOM) Dietary Reference Intakes for the United States and Canada encourage everyone to eat diets providing between 20% and 35% of energy from fat. Because of the role carbohydrate plays in replenishing glycogen, athletes should consume less fat and more carbohydrate than sedentary individuals. Endurance athletes in training are often encouraged to eat moderate- to low-fat diets (20-25% of energy from fat), while athletes trying to lose weight (body fat) may be also be encouraged to obtain 20% to 25% of kilocalories from fat. But less is not always better. Low-fat foods are not always more nutritious. Ultralow-fat diets (<15% of energy from fat) may not provide additional health or performance benefits over a moderate-fat diet and are usually very difficult to follow (Dreon et al. 1999; Lichtenstein and Van Horn 1998).

This chapter reviews the role of fat in the diet of athletes and active persons and the ways in which fat is metabolized as an energy source during exercise. First, we discuss the function, classification, and dietary sources of fat, including the use of fat-modified foods. This is followed by discussion of the amount of fat typically consumed by all Americans and by active individuals. Next, we review fat metabolism during exercise and describe products and practices used to enhance fat oxidation during exercise. Finally, we provide dietary fat recommendations for active people.

FUNCTION, CLASSIFICATION, AND DIETARY SOURCES OF FAT

Fat plays an important role in the diet of the physically active individual. It is a primary source of energy at rest and during exercise. It is twice as energy dense as carbohydrate or protein, providing 9 kcal/g while carbohydrate and protein provide only 4 kcal/g. This means that 1 tbsp of butter or oil contains ~100 kcal, while it takes 4 cups of chopped broccoli or 1+ slices of whole wheat bread to provide 100 kcal from foods consisting primarily of carbohydrate. Fat also provides the essential fatty acids and fat-soluble vitamins (vitamins A, D, E, and K) our bodies need (see "Essential Fatty Acids"). The **essential fatty acids** (**linoleic** and α-**linolenic acid**) are the precursors for many regulatory compounds within the body,

while fat-soluble vitamins are required for many essential metabolic processes. Fats are a part of the structural component of cell membranes and part of brain and spinal cord tissue. They help keep the skin and other tissues soft and pliable. The body uses fat to store extra energy, which can be used to provide fuel to the working muscles. Fat stored as adipose tissue pads the body and protects the organs. Adipose tissue is also an efficient way to store extra energy in a small space. If all extra energy were stored as carbohydrate (stored glycogen), our bodies would be twice as large as they are. Finally, we can't ignore the role that fat plays in food preparation—fat tastes good! It makes our foods more palatable by adding texture and flavor. In summary, dietary fat is important for good health and for providing energy to the working muscles. Fat should not be eliminated from the diet; instead, healthy fats should be used in moderation.

Fats or lipids are substances that are generally insoluble in water, but soluble in organic solvents (acetone or ether), and are very rich in methyl ($-CH_3$) or methylene ($-CH_2-$) groups (figure 3.1). That they do not mix well with water alters the way they are digested, absorbed, and transported in our bodies (as compared with protein and carbohydrate).

Dietary fats can be classified in a number of ways (see figure 3.1 and "Classification of Dietary Fats," pp. 72-73)—by their structure or chain length (number of carbons in each fatty acid), by their level of saturation (number of hydrogen atoms attached to each carbon atom), by their shape, or by the commercial processing that the fat has undergone. Chain length is important because it helps determine the method of digestion and absorption, the properties of the lipid, and its function within the body. Degree of fatty acid saturation also can determine function within the body, effect on health, and use within food products. The shape of a fatty acid can alter its characteristics and thus its function within the body: A fatty acid that has a **trans** configuration or shape will function differently from the same fatty acid with a **cis** configuration. For example, a *trans* fatty acid may have a negative effect on blood lipids, while the same fatty acid in the *cis* form does not. Finally, processing can change the saturation, chain length, and shape of fats. One of the most common fat-processing methods is **hydrogenation** of oils, wherein the double bonds of fatty acids are broken and extra hydrogen is added, making the fat more saturated. This

Essential Fatty Acids

As with essential vitamins and minerals, the body requires essential fatty acids for good health. Two essential fatty acids have been identified: linoleic acid (C18:2, n-6,9) and α-linolenic acid (C18:3, n-3,6,9). Linoleic is classified as an omega-6 or n-6 fatty acid, while α-linolenic acid is classified as an omega-3 or n-3 fatty acid. Linoleic acid occurs primarily in vegetable oils such as sunflower, safflower, corn, soy, and peanut oil; α-linolenic acid occurs mainly in leafy green vegetables, soy oil and other soy foods, seafood, and canola oil. Fish oils contain two n-3 fatty acids, **eicosapentaenoic acid (EPA)** and **docosahexaenoic acid (DHA)**, which are metabolic derivatives of α-linolenic acid metabolism. Within the body, α-linolenic acid is metabolized to EPA and DHA.

The essential fatty acids are required to make a family of hormone-like substances called eicosanoids, such as prostaglandins, thromboxanes, leukotrienes, and prostacyclins. These substances are important and potent mediators of many biochemical functions and play a critical role in coordinating a number of physiological functions—such as blood clotting, blood pressure, vascular dilation, heart rate, and immune response. Since essential fatty acids are necessary for the normal function of all tissue and cannot be synthesized in the body, deficiencies can develop. Some of the deficiency symptoms associated with poor essential fatty acid intakes are eczema, skin lesions, infertility, reduced growth, increased susceptibility to infection, and abnormal fetal growth and development (especially brain and retinal development) (Jones and Kubow 2006; Heird and Lapillone 2005).

In 2005, the IOM set the Adequate Intake (AI) recommendations for both the n-6 (~5-10% of total energy intake) and n-3 fatty acids (~0.6-1.2% of energy). The specific recommendations for males age 19 to 50 years are 17 g/day of linoleic acid (n-6 fatty acid) and 1.6 g/day of α-linolenic acid (n-3 fatty acid). For women age 19 to 50 years, the recommendations are 12 g/day of linolenic acid and 1.1 g/day of α-linolenic acid. Although there were no specific grams per day recommendations for EPA and DHA acids (n-3 fatty acids), a growing body of evidence suggests that a higher intake of these fatty acids can protect against coronary heart disease (IOM 2005). Currently the mean consumption of α-linolenic is ~1.6 to 1.7 g/day for men and 1.1 g/day for women who are 19 to 50 years of age (IOM 2005). However, intakes of EPA and DHA are very low (<0.03 g/day) (IOM 2005). Thus, one dietary goal should be to increase our intake of n-3 fatty acids, especially EPA and DHA, by incorporating more seafood into our diet. One problem with ultralow-fat diets is that, unless good food choices are made, they may not provide adequate amounts of the essential fatty acids, especially n-3 fatty acids. Table 3.1 (on p. 74) lists various foods and the percentage of total fat kilocalories coming from omega-3 (n-3) and omega-6 (n-6) fatty acids. The list on this page provides the amount of n-3 fatty acids, primarily EPA and DHA, found in various foods, especially seafood.

n-3 Fatty Acid Content Per Serving of Selected Foods

Food item	n-3 fatty acid (g/serving)
Tuna, light in water (3 oz, 85 g)	0.23 g
Canola oil (1 tbsp, 15 mL)	1.27 g
Salmon, smoked Chinook (3 oz, 85 g)	0.50 g
Salmon oil (fish oil) (1 tbsp, 15 mL)	4.39 g
Halibut, fillet, baked (3 oz, 85 g)	0.58 g
Trout, rainbow fillet, baked (3 oz, 85 g)	1.05 g
Shrimp, broiled (3 oz, 85 g)	1.11 g
Crab, Dungeness, steamed (3 oz, 85 g)	0.34 g
Herring, Atlantic, broiled (3 oz, 85 g)	1.52 g
Herring oil (1 tbsp, 15 mL)	1.52 g
Walnuts (1 tbsp, 15 mL)	0.51 g

With the growing interest in n-3 fatty acids for cardiovascular health (Wijendran and Hayes 2004) and the advances in food technology, n-3 fatty acids are being incorporated into many nontraditional food sources. Thus, don't be surprised to see more nonmarine foods in the grocery store (e.g., pasta, cereals, milk, yogurt, eggs, mayonnaise, margarines, and spreads) advertising their n-3 fatty acid content (Whelan and Rust 2006). If the source of n-3 fatty acids in these foods is flaxseed or canola oil, it will increase α-linolenic acid in the blood, but not DHA or EPA (Austria et al. 2008). Increasing DHA and EPA in the blood requires the consumption of n-3 fatty acids from seafood sources.

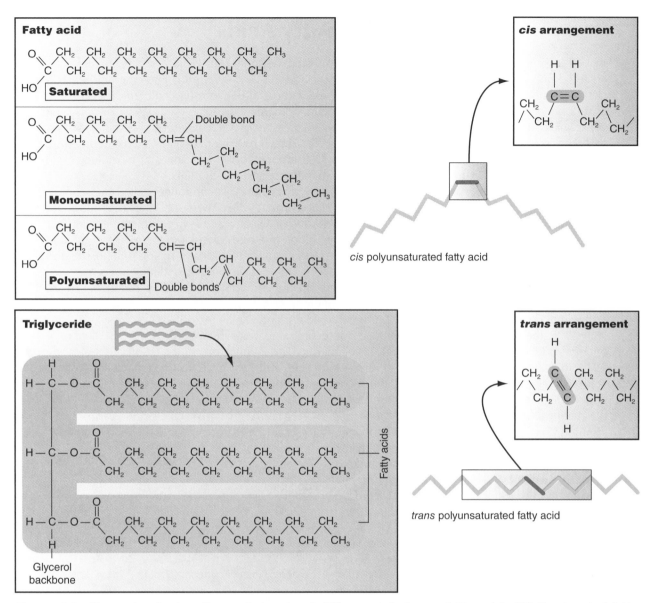

Figure 3.1 Example of saturation and structural differences between fatty acids (16-C saturated fatty acid vs. 18-C monounsaturated fatty acid). Example of a triglyceride (glycerol backbone with three fatty acids attached). Example of differences in shape between *cis* (H on same side) and *trans* (H on different sides) fatty acids. H = hydrogen; C = carbon; O = oxygen.

Adapted, by permission, from J. Thompson, M. Manore and L. Vaughan, 2008, *The science of nutrition* (San Francisco, CA: Benjamin Cummings), 177, 178, 181.

makes the fat more solid at room temperature and converts some *cis* fatty acids to *trans* fatty acids. Corn oil margarine is an example of a partially hydrogenated fat—the double bonds found in the monounsaturated and polyunsaturated fatty acids in the corn oil are broken, and additional hydrogen is added. The more solid the form of margarine, the more hydrogenated the product. Thus, stick margarine has more highly saturated fat than tub or liquid margarine.

Dietary fat is found primarily in the form of triacylglycerols (frequently called triglycerides), where three fatty acids are attached to a **glycerol** backbone (figure 3.1). The **fatty acids (FAs)** can vary in chain length (the number of carbons) and in the degree of saturation. Food also contains other forms of lipids such as cholesterol, phospholipids, and sterols. In general, animal fats provide approximately 40% to 60% of their energy as saturated fats and 30% to 50% as monounsaturated and

Classification of Dietary Fats

Dietary fats can be classified in a number of ways depending on chain length, level of saturation of the chain with hydrogen, and shape. Where each fatty acid is attached to the glycerol backbone to make a triglyceride is also important. The body recognizes and uses dietary fats differently based on these characteristics. The following is a brief overview of how fats are classified in each of these categories.

Chain Length

Fatty acids come in various chain lengths. **Short-chain fatty acids (SCFAs)** are usually less than six carbons in length. **Medium-chain fatty acids (MCFAs)** are 6 to 12 carbons in length, while **long-chain fatty acids (LCFAs)** have 14 or more carbons. Chain length helps determine method of fat digestion, transport, and metabolism. The SCFAs and MCFAs are digested and transported more quickly than LCFAs.

Saturation Level

A fatty acid is considered **saturated** (SFA) if there are no double bonds in the fatty acid chain—all carbon atoms in the fatty acid chain have the maximum number of hydrogen atoms. **Monounsaturated** fatty acids (MUFAs) have one double bond, while **polyunsaturated** fatty acids (PUFAs) have more than one double bond (figure 3.1). Table 3.1 (on p. 74) gives examples of various foods and the distribution of fat kilocalories by SFAs, MUFAs, and PUFAs.

Shape

Fatty acids can be either *trans* or *cis*. These terms refer to the positioning of the hydrogen atom around the double bond (figure 3.1). A *cis* fatty acid has both hydrogen atoms on the same side of the double bond. A *trans* fatty acid has the hydrogen attached to opposite sides of the double bond. *Cis* fatty acids are more common in nature; *trans* fatty acids are rarely found in nature. Most of the *trans* fatty acids in the American diet are due to manipulation of fatty acids during food processing, such as the partial hydrogenation of vegetable oils. Thus, most margarines (excluding those that are not hydrogenated) have more *trans* fatty acids than butter. On the basis of epidemiological data, we know that diets high in *trans* fatty acids increase the risk of coronary heart disease by increasing blood low-density lipoprotein (LDL)-cholesterol levels and lowering blood high-density lipoprotein (HDL)-cholesterol levels (IOM 2005). Because of these findings, the Food and Drug Administration (FDA) legislated in 2003 that manufacturers put the *trans* fatty acid content on the label of conventional foods and some dietary supplements by January 1, 2006 (FDA 2006; Moss 2006). In addition, the IOM (2005) has recommended that we reduce our *trans* fatty acid intake to as low a level as possible. Unfortunately, information about the *trans* fatty acid content of food prepared in restaurants or takeout venues is not generally provided. However, some states are beginning to legislate that restaurants and food establishments provide this information, so in the future it may be available to the consumer. The majority of the *trans* fatty acids in the diet come from cakes, cookies, crackers, pies, and breads (~40%), with the rest coming from animal products (21%), margarines (17%), and fired foods (13%) (U.S. Department of Agriculture [USDA] and U.S. Department of Human Services [USDHHS] Dietary Guidelines for Americans 2005).

Structure of Triacylglycerols

Fatty acids are attached to the glycerol backbone at one of three sites (figure 3.1). The type of fatty acid (either SFA, MUFA, or PUFA) attached at each of these sites determines how the fat is digested, absorbed, and transported.

polyunsaturated FAs; fats from plants provide only 10% to 20% of their energy from saturated FAs with the rest from monounsaturated and polyunsaturated FAs. Table 3.1 lists examples of the primary fat-containing foods in our diet and the composition of the fat in these foods. For example, butter is considered a saturated fat because 65% of its fat is saturated; however, butter still contains some mono- and polyunsaturated FAs. Conversely, olive oil is considered monounsaturated because 74% of its fat is monounsaturated, yet it still contains some saturated and polyunsaturated FAs.

Fat-containing foods such as oils, butter, cream, margarine, or dressings (mayonnaise, salad dressings) are generally termed **visible fats** because almost 100% of the energy (kcal) in the food comes from fat (see table 3.1). These foods are frequently added as condiments to prepared foods, such as butter on toast or mayonnaise on sandwiches, and consumers can clearly see that they are adding additional fat to their food. **Invisible fats** are those incorporated into prepared foods such as cookies, cakes, or casseroles and are not easily discernible as fats. For example, croissants are much higher

Table 3.1 Composition of Common Fat-Containing Foods

Food	% of total kcal from fat	% total fat kcal as omega-3 and -6	Distribution of fat by type		
			% total fat kcal as Saturated Fatty Acids	% total fat kcal as Monounsaturated Fatty Acids	% total fat kcal as Polyunsaturated Fatty Acids
Butter	100	4	65	31	4
Milk, whole 3.3% fat	49	4	63	33	4
Milk, 2% fat	40	4	66	30	4
Milk, nonfat	4	>1	73	30	>1
Beef, ground 16% fat	54	4	45	51	4
Chicken, boneless	35	20	18	44	24
Turkey, boneless	26	28	32	25	35
Tuna, water packed	6	39	32	22	46
Tuna, oil packed	37	36	21	40	39
Salmon, Chinook	33	16	25	48	24
Egg, large	62	13	37	46	16
Canola oil	100	30	7	59	30
Safflower oil	100	74	9	12	74
Corn oil	100	60	13	25	60
Corn oil margarine	100	—	2	27	27
Sesame oil	100	42	15	42	44
Olive oil	100	10	14	74	10
Salmon oil (fish oil)	100	34	20	29	40
Cottonseed oil	100	50	26	20	52
Palm kernel oil	100	2	82	11	2
Coconut oil	100	2	87	6	2
Walnuts	86	63	10	23	64
Cashew nuts	72	17	20	59	17

Data from Food Processor SQL, Version 10.0, ESHA Research, Salem, OR.

in fat (56% of energy per serving from fat) than a slice of bread or a bagel (5-15% of energy per serving from fat)—yet many consumers assume that the fat content of these three "bread" foods is the same. The majority of the fat in most people's diets comes from invisible fat. Foods that can be high in invisible fats are meat and meat products, dairy products, baked goods, and most convenience and fast foods.

Many foods are available with a wide range of fat contents. You can purchase full-fat, low-fat, or fat-free ice cream. The same is true for cookies. Table 3.2 lists a number of full-fat foods (foods as originally produced or found in nature) and their lower-fat alternatives. The latter products may significantly reduce the amount of fat in a person's diet but do not always change total energy intake. For example, buying nonfat milk (86 kcal, 0.5 g of

Table 3.2 Energy and Nutrient Composition of Full-Fat Products and Their Reduced- or Low-Fat Counterparts

Product	Serving size	Energy (kcal)	Protein (g)	Carbo-hydrate (g)	Fat (g)
Milk, whole (3.3% fat)	8 oz	150	8.0	11.4	8.2
Milk, 2% fat	8 oz	121	8.1	11.7	4.7
Milk, 1% fat	8 oz	102	8.0	11.7	2.6
Milk, nonfat	8 oz	86	8.4	11.9	0.5
Cheese, cheddar regular	1 oz	111	7.1	0.5	9.1
Cheese, cheddar low-fat	1 oz	81	9.1	0.0	5.1
Cheese, cheddar nonfat	1 oz	41	6.8	4.0	0.0
Mayonnaise, regular	1 tbsp	100	0.0	0.0	11.0
Mayonnaise, light	1 tbsp	50	0.0	1.0	5.0
Mayonnaise, fat-free	1 tbsp	10	0.0	2.0	0.0
Margarine, regular corn oil	1 tbsp	100	0.0	0.0	11.0
Margarine, reduced-fat	1 tbsp	60	0.0	0.0	7.0
Peanut butter, regular	1 tbsp	95	4.1	3.1	8.2
Peanut butter, reduced-fat	1 tbsp	81	4.4	5.2	5.4
Cream cheese, soft regular	1 tbsp	50	1.0	0.5	5.0
Cream cheese, soft light	1 tbsp	35	1.5	1.0	2.5
Cream cheese, soft nonfat	1 tbsp	15	2.5	1.0	0.0
Crackers, Wheat Thins, regular	18 crackers	158	2.3	21.4	6.8
Crackers, Wheat Thins, reduced-fat	18 crackers	120	2.0	21.0	4.0
Cookies, Oreos, regular	3 cookies	160	2.0	23.0	7.0
Cookies, Oreos, reduced-fat	3 cookies	130	2.0	25.0	3.5
Cookies, Fig Newton, regular	3 cookies	210	3.0	30.0	4.5
Cookies, Fig Newton, fat-free	3 cookies	204	2.4	26.8	0.0
Breakfast bars, regular	1 bar	140	2.0	27.0	2.8
Breakfast bars, fat-free	1 bar	110	2.0	26.0	0.0

The FDA and the USDA have set specific regulations on allowable product descriptions for reduced fat products: The following claims are defined for one serving: *fat free* = less than 0.5 g of fat; *low fat* = 3 g or less of fat; *reduced or less fat* = at least 25% less fat as compared to a standard serving; *light* = one-third fewer calories or 50% less fat as compared with a standard serving size.

Data from Food Processor SQL, Version 10.0, ESHA Research, Salem, OR.

fat per 8 oz, or 240 mL, serving) instead of whole milk (150 kcal, 8.2 g of fat per 8 oz serving) will dramatically reduce both fat and energy intake; buying fat-free Fig Newton cookies (two cookies = 90 kcal, 0 g fat, 1 g fiber) to replace regular Fig Newton cookies (two cookies = 110 kcal, 2 g fat, 0 g *trans* fat, 1 g fiber) reduces fat intake by 2 g per serving but reduces energy intake by only 20 kcal. If you elect to substitute whole wheat Fig Newton cookies for regular Fig Newtons, the fat content does not change; however, fiber increases by 1 g per serving (two cookies = 110 kcal, 2 g fat, 0 g *trans* fat, 2 g fiber).

Unfortunately, many people think that because a product is marked reduced fat or fat-free they can eat as much as they desire (the whole box instead of just two or three cookies). The Calorie Control Council (Atlanta, GA) has been studying U.S. dieting trends for 25 years (CCC 2006). According to a survey the organization did in 2000, 88% of adult Americans use low- or reduced-fat foods and beverages (CCC 2006; www.caloriecontrol.org). Since adult Americans, including active individuals, choose to use reduced-fat products either for weight control or for health reasons, they should understand that while total fat intake may decrease, energy intake may not (Callaway 1998). The Calorie Control Council also asked consumers why they used reduced-fat products (CCC 2006). The following is a list of the responses, with the percentage of consumers who responded "yes" given in parentheses.

- To stay in better overall health (70%)
- To eat or drink healthier foods and beverages (57%)
- To reduce fat (57%)
- To reduce calories (51%)
- To reduce cholesterol (49%)
- To maintain current weight (47%)
- To maintain an attractive physical appearance (43%)
- To reduce weight (38%)
- For refreshment or taste (32%)
- To help a medical condition (31%)

This survey was followed by the 2004 Calorie Control Council National Consumer Survey, in which adults were asked about their regular use (at least once every two weeks) of fat-modified foods (CCC 2006). The results of the survey follow. The reduced-fat products are listed in descending order of popularity. The percentage of consum-

ers who reported using the product at least once every two weeks appears in parentheses.

- Nonfat or low-fat milk (74%)
- Reduced-fat cheese and dairy products (65%)
- Reduced-fat salad dressings, sauces, or mayonnaise (60%)
- Reduced-fat margarine (46%)
- Reduced-fat chips and snack foods (40%)

It is estimated that there are over 7000 different fat-modified foods on the market (Callaway 1998; Sigman-Grant 1997; CCC 2006); however, the degree to which these foods are used by consumers varies dramatically. Consumers appear more likely to use a reduced-fat version of a full-fat product (like milk) from which only the fat has been removed than to replace a full-fat snack (cookie or chips) with a lower-fat alternative in which a fat substitute or a fat replacer may have been used. Fat substitutes and fat replacers are now found in a number of foods, especially snack foods. Appendix B.2 describes the most common fat replacers used in the United States. Some of these products, such as olestra (brand name Olean), may cause gastrointestinal distress if consumed in large quantities. When fat substitutes were introduced into the U.S. marketplace, many people thought they would soon be available in a huge variety of foods and help reduce obesity. This has not occurred, and few products that consumers use on a daily basis contain fat replacers.

BODY FAT RESERVES AND DIETARY FAT INTAKE

During exercise, the primary energy sources are carbohydrate (glucose) and fat (FAs). The relative amounts used of each depend on factors such as exercise intensity and duration, level of physical fitness, composition of the meal prior to exercise, and the energy-containing products consumed during exercise. Compared to protein and carbohydrate stores, the body's fat reserves are almost unlimited. Table 3.3 gives an estimate of the amount of total fat and carbohydrate stored within a 176 lb (80 kg) man. The total amount of energy stored as fat varies with an individual's size and percentage of body fat. For example, a man weighing 176 lb (80 kg) with 15% body fat would have approximately 26 lb (~12 kg) of total body fat or ~100,000 kcal of energy stored as fat. Of course, not all of this fat would be available for

Table 3.3 Estimated Energy Stores of Fat and Carbohydrate for an 80 kg (176 lb) Man With 15% Body Fat

Substrate	Weight (kg)	Energy (kcal)
Carbohydrate		
Plasma glucose	0.02	78
Liver glycogen	0.1	388
Muscle glycogen	0.4	1550
Total (approximately)	0.52	2000
Fat		
Plasma fatty acid	0.0004	4
Plasma triacylglycerols	0.004	39
Adipose tissue	12.0	100,000
Intramuscular triacylglycerols	0.3	2616
Total (approximately)	12.3	106,500

The values given are estimates for a "normal" man of 80 kg (176 lb) and 15% body fat and not those of an athlete, who might be leaner and have more stored glycogen. The amount of protein in the body is not mentioned but would be about 10 kg (22 lb) (40,000 kcal), mainly located in the muscles.

Adapted, by permission, from A.E. Jeukendrup, W.H.M. Saris, A.J.M. Wagenmakers, 1998, "Fat metabolism during exercise: a review," *International Journal of Sports Medicine* 19(4): 231-244.

energy, since 3% to 4% of body fat is biologically essential and incorporated into cell membranes and tissues. Since women typically have higher amounts of body fat than men, their amount of stored energy is usually higher even though body weight is less. A woman weighing 130 lb (59 kg) with 24% body fat would have approximately 31 lb (~14 kg) of body fat, representing ~110,000 kcal of stored energy. Thus, even though the female is on average 46 lb (21 kg) lighter than her male counterpart, she has more stored energy as fat. If we consider that a 130 lb (59 kg) woman may require ~100 kcal to run 1 mile at a moderate pace, this amount of stored fat would be enough for more than 1000 miles!

In addition to adipose tissue fat (subcutaneous fat and deep visceral fat), the body also stores fat within the muscle as intramuscular triacylglycerol. The amount of fat stored here is difficult to estimate and varies with fitness level, daily training time, and dietary fat intake; but it appears that even lean people have plenty of stored energy in the form of adipose tissue. Therefore, dietary recommendations to active people usually focus on making sure that the diet contains an amount of fat that is adequate to replace muscle triacylglycerol stores and to meet energy and essential

FA requirements—but is not excessive. On rare occasions, fat may be consumed during exercise to supplement these reserves. We discuss the pros and cons of this practice later in the chapter.

Dietary Fat Intake in the United States

There appears to be a strong link between high dietary fat intake and risks of obesity, coronary heart disease, and some forms of cancer. Because of these links, the United States and Canadian governments formulated the 2005 Dietary Guidelines for Americans (USDA and USDHHS 2005) and the 2005 Dietary Reference Intakes (IOM 2005). One recommendation in these documents is the reduction of total fat intake to 20% to 35% of total energy intake and the limiting of saturated fat to <10% of total energy intake. Dietitians and nutritionists have been recommending the reduction of dietary fat for a decade. Based on the most recent U.S. governmental data (National Health and Nutrition Examination Survey [NHANES] III and NHANES 1999-2000; Continuing Survey of Food Intake for Individuals 1994-1996, 1999) (IOM 2005; Briefel and Johnson 2004), it appears that relative fat intake (% of energy from fat) decreased from 36% in 1989-1991 to 33% in 1994-1996 for both men and women (figure 3.2). However, the absolute fat consumption (g/day) increased from 73.4 in 1989-1991 to 76.5 g in 1994-1996 (Chanmugam et al. 2003; USDA and USDHHS 2005) (see figure 3.2). Thus, it appears that Americans are reducing their fat intake when one examines percentage of energy from fat; but in reality, total fat intake (g/day) has slightly increased. "How Can One's Percentage of Energy From Fat Decrease While Absolute Fat Intake Increases?" (p. 78) shows calculations that demonstrate how this can occur. Many Americans have not reached the recommended fat goal of ≤35% of total energy intake from fat or the appropriate distribution of this fat (e.g., low saturated and *trans* fat diets).

At the same time that percentage of energy from fat is declining, Americans appear to be getting fatter. A variety of factors contribute to obesity in any one person; high dietary fat intake is but one of many contributing factors, along with physical inactivity and overconsumption of energy, especially from soft drinks, alcohol (e.g., beer), processed food mixtures (e.g., pizza), grain snacks, and pastries (Chanmugam et al. 2003). In general, energy intakes have increased ~200 to 300 kcal/day over the last two decades (Chanmugam et al. 2003; Briefel and Johnson 2004). One cannot assume that only one factor is causing the rise of obesity in the United States. Obesity is a gradual problem that develops over years or decades. Once people become obese, there appear to be powerful metabolic forces that act to maintain the increased body weight. It is difficult to pinpoint a single factor as the major cause of our growing obesity. Obesity is a multifaceted problem that

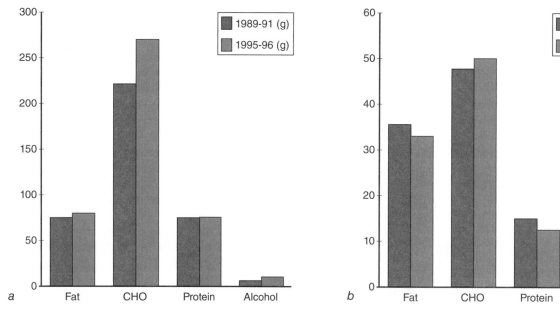

Figure 3.2 *(a)* Change in grams per day and *(b)* % of energy from fat, carbohydrate (CHO), protein, and alcohol from 1989-1991 to 1995-1996 according to the Continuing Survey of Food Intake for Individuals. Data are in grams (g) and percentages (%).

Data adapted from P. Chanmugam et al., 2003,"Did fat intake in the United States really decline between 1989-1991 and 1994-1996?" *Journal of the American Dietetic Association* 103: 8867-8872.

Highlight

How Can One's Percentage of Energy From Fat Decrease While Absolute Fat Intake Increases?

Here is a sample calculation to demonstrate how percentage of energy intake from fat can decrease while absolute total fat intake increases.

Example 1: A diet contains 2250 kcal/day, with 36% of energy coming from fat (90 g of fat/day); the rest of the energy is obtained from protein (15%, 84 g/day) and carbohydrate (49%, 276 g/day).

Example 2: Now increase the diet in example 1 by 300 kcal/day (6 g fat, 12 g protein, 49 g carbohydrate), for a total energy intake of 2550 kcal/day. This diet obtains 34% of its energy from fat (96 g of fat/day), with the rest obtained from protein (15%, 96 g/day) and carbohydrate (51%, 325 g/day).

Notice how the percentage of energy coming from fat has decreased (from 36% to 34%) but the absolute amount of fat has increased (from 90 to 96 g/day). This same scenario appears to be taking place in the United States. Total energy intake is increasing, along with absolute intakes of fat, but relative fat intake (% of energy from fat) is decreasing. Although at first glance it may appear that the American diet is improving, it is not, because both energy and fat intake are increasing. These dietary changes, combined with our abundance of good-tasting food and our inactivity, have contributed to increased obesity in the United States (USDA Center for Nutrition Policy and Promotion 1998).

involves the interactive forces of genetics, physiology, metabolism, and the environment. (See chapter 5 on energy balance for more information about factors contributing to obesity.)

Dietary Fat Intake of Active Individuals

Although active individuals and athletes typically self-report carbohydrate intakes to be approximately 45% to 55% of energy intake (Burke 2006), intakes of fat are much more variable depending on the sport and gender of the athlete. Athletes typically report consuming about 35% of their energy from fat (Hawley et al. 1995). However, athletes in endurance sports, such as runners, cyclists, or cross-country skiers, report lower fat intakes and higher carbohydrate intakes than sprinters and field event athletes (Fogelholm et al. 1992; Hawley et al. 1995; Saris et al. 1989; Onywera et al. 2004). For example, Saris and colleagues (1989) monitored the energy and food intake of five male cyclists during the 22-day race of the Tour de France. Mean energy intake during the race was 5880 kcal/day, with 62% of the energy from carbohydrate, 15% from protein, and 23% from fat. In addition, a recent assessment of the diets of 10 elite Kenyan distance runners (mean = 21 years, 58 kg, 10% body fat, 19.2 body mass index [BMI] [kg/m^2]) during peak training showed that energy intake was 3605 kcal/day, with 77% of energy from carbohydrate, 10% of energy from protein, and only 13% of energy from fat.

Athletes who are concerned about weight, or who participate in sports that require them to "weigh in," have lower fat intakes—especially during periods of energy restriction. For example, Fogelholm and colleagues (1993) examined the diets of wrestlers and judo athletes at baseline and during gradual and rapid weight loss regimens. The gradual weight loss regimen consisted of a three-week period of diet restriction in which subjects reduced energy intake by 1000 kcal/day. The rapid weight loss diet consisted of ~1400 kcal/day for three days. Figure 3.3 shows that both energy intake and the proportion of energy from fat decreased while the proportion of energy from carbohydrate increased. Beals and Manore (1998) also reported that mean fat intake in female athletes with subclinical eating disorders (19% of energy intake, 43 g/day) was lower than that of control athletes (23% of energy intake, 61 g/day). Thus, if athletes are restricting energy intake, distribution of energy as carbohydrate, fat, and protein often compares favorably with recom-

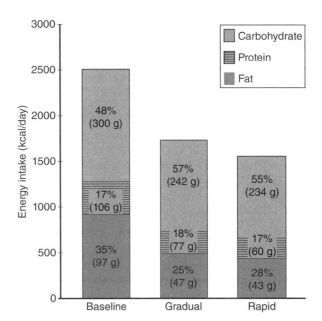

Figure 3.3   Daily energy intake and the proportion of dietary fat, protein, and carbohydrate for 10 male athletes (seven wrestlers, three judo athletes) during weight maintenance (baseline) and during both gradual and rapid weight reduction. Percentage of energy from protein, fat, and carbohydrate is indicated in each column.

Reprinted from M. Fogelholm et al., 1993, "Gradual and rapid weight loss: effects on nutrition and performance in male athlete," *Medicine and Science in Sports and Exercise* 25: 371-377.

mended intakes; yet total energy intake is too low to maintain body weight and rigorous physical activity. Examination of an athlete's diet requires determining total energy intake and distributing energy from each of the macronutrients.

FAT METABOLISM DURING EXERCISE

After reading chapter 2 on carbohydrate, one might feel there is little room for fat in the diet of an athlete or an active individual. Yet fat is a major energy source during exercise, and the ability to mobilize and use stored fat during exercise can improve exercise performance. Fat can be mobilized from any of the following sources: muscle fat, adipose tissue fat, blood lipoproteins, or fat consumed during exercise. A number of factors determine the amount and the source of the fat utilized during exercise:

- Fitness level
- Type of exercise
- Intensity and duration of exercise

Fat and Fatty Acid Nomenclature

Fatty acids are stored in the body in the form of **triacylglycerol** or **triglycerides**, where three FAs are attached to a glycerol backbone. These FAs can vary in their level of saturation and length. If FAs are not esterified to form mono-, di-, or triacylglycerol, they are called non-esterified FAs or **free fatty acids (FFAs)**. However, the term FFA is sometimes ambiguous because the FAs found in the blood are frequently referred to as FFAs, when in actuality they are bound to albumin. There is a very small concentration of true (unbound) FFAs in the plasma (<0.01% of the plasma FA pool) (Jeukendrup et al. 1998a). Because FFAs are not soluble in water, they must be transported bound to some type of transport protein, both within the cell and across cell membranes. However, not all of these transport proteins or carriers have been identified for each step of the fat mobilization and oxidation process. Depending on the article you read, the exact method of FFA transport discussed may vary. Within this chapter, when FFAs are discussed it is assumed that they are not truly free, but are bound to some type of transport or carrier protein. Fatty acid transport proteins are discussed in more detail in review articles by Turcotte and colleagues (1995); Cortright and colleagues (1997); Jeukendrup (2002); and Jeukendrup and colleagues (1998a-c).

- Available fat reserves in the muscles
- Ability to mobilize and transport FAs from adipose tissue to muscles
- Composition of the meal or diet prior to exercise
- Availability of stored carbohydrate or amount of carbohydrate fed during exercise

In the following sections we outline the metabolic processes that stimulate the breakdown, mobilization, and transport of fat from storage to the working muscle for energy during exercise. We also discuss availability of intramuscular fat for energy during exercise. We then briefly review the oxidation of fat within muscle and the numerous factors that can influence this process. Since we cannot discuss the biochemistry of fat metabolism in detail, we suggest the following references as additional readings: Achten and Jeukendrup 2004; Cortright et al. 1997; Jeukendrup 2002; Jeukendrup et al. 1998a, 1998b, 1998c; Spriet 2002; Turcotte et al. 1995; and Westerterp-Plantenga 2004. The nomenclature used in discussing fat is frequently confusing, so see "Fat and Fatty Acid Nomenclature" for a review of terms.

Adipose Tissue Fat

Adipose tissue contains the largest reservoir of stored energy within the body. In order to use this fat as a fuel source during exercise, the body must mobilize and transport it to the working muscle. The use of fat during exercise involves numerous steps:

1. Breakdown of triacylglycerols to FFAs and glycerol
2. Mobilization and transport of FFAs within the fat cell
3. Transport of the FFAs out of the fat cell to the blood
4. Transport of the FFAs in the blood
5. Transport of the FFAs into the muscle cell
6. Transport of the FFAs to the muscle mitochondria
7. Oxidation to energy via the tricarboxylic acid (TCA) cycle

Figure 3.4 illustrates lipolysis and mobilization within the fat cell, as well as the transport of FAs to the muscle cell for oxidation. The breakdown of fat in the adipose or muscle tissue to FFAs and glycerol occurs through a process call **lipolysis.** This metabolic process is initiated when the sympathetic nervous system stimulates production of **hormone-sensitive lipase (HSL)** and **epinephrine.** After exercise begins, blood concentrations of epinephrine rise—which in turn stimulates production of the phosphorylated (active) form of HSL in the adipose cell. Hormone-sensitive lipase is activated when it is phosphorylated by a cyclic adenosine monophosphate (cAMP)–dependent protein kinase. This protein kinase is produced

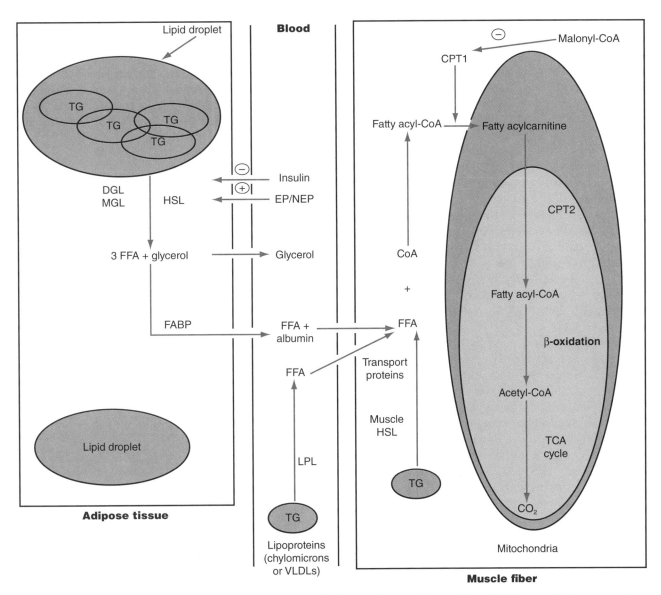

Figure 3.4 Mobilization and oxidation of fatty acids from adipose tissue, blood lipids, and intramuscular fat storage. Adipose tissue: Hormone-sensitive lipase (HSL) cleaves two fatty acids from the triacylglycerol or triglyceride (TG), while the final fatty acid is removed by the enzyme monoglyceride lipase (MGL). Hormone-sensitive lipase is the rate-limiting step of lipolysis. Epinephrine (EP) stimulates the production of active HSL, while insulin inhibits its production. The end product of this lipolysis is three free fatty acids (FFA) and one glycerol molecule. The FFA are transported from the adipose cell via fatty acid binding protein (FABP); a second protein-mediated transport system moves the FFA to the blood where albumin transports the FFA to the muscle tissue. The FFA is then transported across the plasma membrane and into the muscle fiber via additional transport proteins. Glycerol can be transported to the liver for gluconeogenesis. Additional FFA can be released from blood lipoproteins or from fat stored in the muscle fibers. The FFA can now enter the mitochondria for β-oxidation. LPL = lipoprotein lipase; CPT1= carnitine palmitoyl transferase 1; CPT2 = carnitine palmitoyl transferase 2; VLDL= very low-density lipoprotein DGL = diglyceride; NEP=norepinephrine.

in the adipose cell when epinephrine binds to receptors on the cell membrane and activates adenyl cyclase (Champe et al. 2008). Hormone-sensitive lipase splits off two of the FAs attached to the glycerol backbone of the triacylglycerol (FAs at positions 1 and 3), leaving a monoglyceride (glycerol with one FA attached at position 2) (Turcotte et al. 1995). The final FA is removed through the action of the enzyme **monoglyceride lipase (MGL).** Both enzymes, HSL and MGL, are needed for complete breakdown of the triacylglycerol. The end result of lipolysis is three FFA molecules and a glycerol molecule that must be transported across the adipose cell cytosol and the membrane into circulation. Hormone-sensitive lipase is the rate-limiting step in this process; the activity of this enzyme depends on several inhibitory and stimulatory factors (Jeukendrup et al. 1998a; Jeukendrup 2002). These regulatory factors are discussed later.

The glycerol produced by lipolysis cannot be reused by the adipose tissue since the cell does not contain significant amounts of glycerol kinase (Wolfe et al. 1990). Levels of glycerol in the blood are therefore an indirect measure of lipolysis, since one glycerol molecule is produced for each triacylglycerol broken down. Glycerol can then be transported to the liver where it is used as a gluconeogenic precursor.

The FFAs produced through lipolysis must either cross the adipose cell membrane passively or be transported out of the cell by binding proteins such as **fatty acid binding protein (FABP)** or **fatty acid translocase (FAT/CD36)** (Jeukendrup et al. 1998a; Jeukendrup 2002). Free fatty acids released into the blood are bound to albumin and transported to the working muscles. These FFAs are eventually released from albumin and actively transported across the muscle membranes (Cortright et al. 1997; Turcotte et al. 1995). However, not all of the FFAs produced through lipolysis are used for energy. In the triacylglycerol–fatty acid cycle, FAs released during the process of lipolysis are re-esterified if they are not needed for energy. **Re-esterification** can occur within the adipose cell (intracellular recycling) or after the FA is released from the adipose cell (extracellular recycling), in which case the fat is re-esterified elsewhere (e.g., in the liver) (Wolfe et al. 1990). Thus, if the FAs are not needed for energy, they can be re-esterified into triacylglycerols again, either in adipose tissue or in the liver. At rest, re-esterification is high and blood concentrations of albumin-bound FAs are low. During exercise, re-esterification is suppressed at the same time that the rate of lipolysis is accelerated, and blood levels of FFAs bound to albumin increase dramatically (Jeukendrup 2002). Wolfe and colleagues (1990) measured re-esterification at rest and during 4 h of treadmill exercise at 40% $\dot{V}O_2$max. They found that 75% of the FAs were re-esterified at rest, but this value decreased to 25% within the first 30 min of exercise and remained low throughout the exercise period.

Several factors affect the degree of re-esterification. Re-esterification increases if albumin is not available to transport the FFAs away from adipose cells. This may occur if blood levels of albumin are low (during periods of malnutrition or high blood loss), if blood flow through adipose tissue is decreased, or if available transport sites on albumin are full (Jeukendrup 2002). Each albumin molecule can bind only a finite number of FFAs; as albumin becomes saturated with FAs, there is less affinity for the acids. Thus, under any of the conditions mentioned, fewer FFAs are bound and transported away from the fat cell. High lactate levels also decrease FFA mobilization by increasing re-esterification without affecting lipolysis (Turcotte et al. 1995). During prolonged endurance exercise, however, lactate levels usually remain low and probably play a minimal role in regulating FFAs mobilization.

Effect of Exercise on Lipolysis

Exercise stimulates lipolysis sufficiently that the rate of lipolysis usually far exceeds the need for FAs for oxidation by the muscles. At rest, basal level of FFAs after a mixed diet will be ~0.2 to 0.4 mmol/L; during exercise, arterial plasma FFA concentrations can increase 10- to 20-fold over basal levels, depending on the exercise intensity and duration (Achten and Jeukendrup 2004; Jeukendrup et al. 1998a; Wolfe et al. 1990). Figure 3.5 shows the rate of appearance of FFAs and glycerol during 4 h of treadmill exercise at 40% of $\dot{V}O_2$max. The rate of FFA appearance rose dramatically (approximately sixfold) with even low-intensity exercise. The dramatic rise in glycerol appearance indicates an increase in lipolysis within fat cells during exercise. Respiratory exchange ratio also dropped over the 4 h period from 0.92 to 0.83, indicating an increase in fat oxidation (10-fold increase). Immediately after exercise stopped, almost 90% of the FAs released from lipolysis were re-esterified (Wolfe et al. 1990). This study clearly indicates that the best way to mobilize and use stored fat for energy is to exercise. Exercise is the greatest stimulator of fat lipolysis and oxidation currently available to the consumer; however, this stimulant cannot be purchased in a bottle.

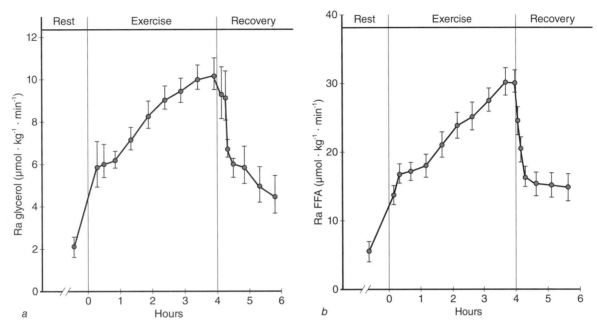

Figure 3.5 Rate of appearance (Ra) of *(a)* glycerol and *(b)* free fatty acids (FFAs) at rest, during exercise (40% V̇O₂max for 4 h on the treadmill), and during recovery in five men. Exercise induced a sixfold increase in FFAs available for oxidation.

Reprinted from R.R. Wolfe et al., 1990, "Role of triglyceride-fatty acid cycle in controlling fat metabolism in humans during and after exercise," *American Journal Physiology* 258: E382-E389. Used with permission.

Hormonal Control of Lipolysis

During exercise, a number of hormonal changes signal the body to break down stored energy to fuel the working muscles. These hormonal responses depend on a variety of factors including the intensity and duration of the exercise, level of physical fitness, and how recently food has been consumed.

The sympathetic nervous system and the catecholamines are the strongest stimulators of lipolysis. The catecholamines stimulate the breakdown of both stored fat (both in adipose and in muscle tissue) and carbohydrate (both liver and muscle glycogen), making these fuels available to the working muscles. Blood levels of the catecholamines, norepinephrine and epinephrine, rise dramatically within seconds of the initiation of exercise and activate cAMP—which then stimulates production of the active phosphorylated form of HSL. Other hormones, such as growth hormone, cortisol, and thyroid stimulating hormone, also stimulate lipolysis (Saltin and Åstrand 1993; Turcotte et al. 1995; Jeukendrup et al. 1998b).

Insulin is the strongest inhibitor of lipolysis. It decreases the amount of active HSL that is produced by blocking cAMP from phosphorylating HSL. During exercise or in times of starvation, when the need for fat as an energy source is high,

insulin is typically low and lipolysis is high. The decrease in insulin concentrations during exercise occurs primarily because epinephrine and norepinephrine inhibit pancreatic insulin release (Jeukendrup et al. 1998b). Insulin is high during times of feeding, when the need for mobilization of energy is low and the stimulation for fat storage is high. Thus, any increase in blood insulin either before or during exercise may inhibit fat lipolysis and oxidation. Horowitz and colleagues (1997) found that feeding either glucose or fructose (0.8 g/kg) 1 h before exercise (1 h of cycling at 44% V̇O₂max) and after an overnight fast significantly increased plasma insulin concentrations compared to fasting. This increase in insulin also significantly decreased whole-body lipolysis and fat oxidation during exercise.

Independent of insulin, any increase in blood glucose concentrations (such as feeding carbohydrate during exercise) suppresses lipolysis and decreases FA turnover within adipose cells. This in turn changes the mix of fuels used for energy during exercise. Carlson and colleagues (1991) demonstrated that a hyperglycemic state in which insulin was held constant decreased FA turnover (i.e., the difference between lipolysis and FFA re-esterification) by 30%. Thus, blood glucose also appears to be a strong regulator of lipolysis and of the availability of FAs for energy during exercise.

Intramuscular Fat

Fat stored within skeletal muscle also appears to be an important source of energy during exercise—although the significance of its contribution to total fat oxidation is still being debated. The initial hypothesis relating to the use of muscle triacylglycerols as a fuel source during exercise came from the observation that the uptake and oxidation of plasma FFAs (albumin-bound FAs) cannot account for all the fat oxidized during exercise (Saltin and Åstrand 1993). One advantage to having triacylglycerols stored within muscle fiber is that the substrate (fat) is close to mitochondria, the site of lipid oxidation and energy production, and does not have to be transported through the blood. However, the exact amount of intramuscular fat stored appears to depend on muscle fiber type, nutritional status, and type of physical activity engaged in (Dyck et al. 1997; Jeukendrup 2002; Jeukendrup et al. 1998c).

The amount of intramuscular fat oxidized during exercise has not been well determined. Depending on the research cited, it is estimated that endurance exercise decreases intramuscular fat concentrations from 25% to 50% (Oscai et al. 1990; Turcotte et al. 1995). Yet the purported contribution of intramuscular fat triacylglycerol breakdown to total fat oxidation during exercise may be 5% to 35%, depending on the study (Hurley et al. 1986; Romijn et al. 1993; Saltin and Åstrand 1993). Differences in estimates of how much intramuscular triacylglycerol is used during exercise most likely stem from differences in subject fitness levels, exercise protocols, and methods used to determine triacylglycerol content. Different types of exercise may recruit different muscle fibers with different fat oxidation rates. Measuring changes in muscle triacylglycerol content is also difficult since fat is not distributed equally within the muscle fibers, and the two major types of muscle fibers oxidize fat differently (Saltin and Åstrand 1993; Turcotte et al. 1995). Exercise intensity and duration may also alter the amount of muscle triacylglycerol used, with higher intensities using more intramuscular fat. Finally, the fitness level of the subjects may alter the amount of intramuscular fat used during exercise since more fit individuals are better fat oxidizers.

The final two of these points are illustrated by two studies that measured changes in muscle triacylglycerol concentrations before and after exercise. In the first, Hurley and colleagues (1986) examined the effect of endurance exercise adaptation on muscle triacylglycerol depletion.

They exercised nine untrained men for 2 h at 65% $\dot{V}O_2$max and measured changes in muscle triacylglycerol and glycogen concentrations. They found a 20% average decrease in muscle triacylglycerol concentration and a 71% decrease in glycogen concentration after the initial test. The subjects were retested after they had trained for 12 weeks. After exercise training, intramuscular triacylglycerol use increased to 41%, twice that in the untrained state; and the amount of glycogen used decreased by nearly 60% (figure 3.6). Thus, exercise training caused a shift in substrate use to more intramuscular fat and less carbohydrate.

Exercise intensity can also change the amount of intramuscular triacylglycerol used on even a short-term basis. Romijn and colleagues (1993) measured substrate utilization at three different exercise intensities in trained male cyclists. The contribution of intramuscular fat was 7%, 26%, and 8% during exercise intensities of 25%, 65%, and 85% $\dot{V}O_2$max, respectively (figure 3.7). Both exercise training and intensity appear to alter the amount of intramuscular fat used during exercise.

However, not all research has demonstrated significant decreases in intramuscular triacylglycerol levels with endurance exercise or exercise training

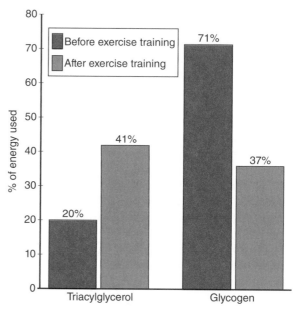

Figure 3.6 Percentage of intramuscular triacylglycerol and glycogen used for energy before and after a 12-week aerobic exercise training program. Subjects were nine men exercising for 2 h at 60% $\dot{V}O_2$max.

Adapted from B.F. Hurley et al., 1986, "Muscle triglyceride utilization during exercise: Effect of training," *Journal of Applied Physiology* 60: 562-567.

(Turcotte et al. 1995). Kiens and colleagues (1993) found no changes in intramuscular utilization with training. In this study they measured changes in muscle triacylglycerol and glycogen before and after training, using knee extensor exercises with one leg only (the other leg was not trained). Figure 3.8 shows no statistically significant change in muscle triacylglycerol concentrations (8% use before training, 12% after training) but significant changes in glycogen after training. The change in muscle glycogen was similar to that reported by Hurley and colleagues (1986). The differences between these two studies and others examining changes in muscle triacylglycerol use during exercise suggest that a number of factors control intramuscular triacylglycerol use. Additional research is needed to identify these regulatory factors and to determine under what exercise conditions muscle triacylglycerol use is high. Finally, differences in the methods used to measure intramuscular fat changes during exercise may also be contributing to the equivocal results. As researchers adopt new standardized methods of measuring intramuscular fat changes, we will have a better idea of the effects that training and exercise intensity have on this fat storage system.

Blood Lipids

Blood lipids, transported in **lipoproteins,** can also contribute to the fat used during exercise (figure 3.4). The two lipoproteins highest in triacylglycerols are chylomicrons and very low-density lipoproteins. If a person is exercising after a meal, chylomicron levels in the blood can be high. **Chylomicrons** are responsible for transporting dietary fat to the tissues of the body for either energy production or storage as fat. Other blood lipoproteins, especially **very low-density lipoproteins (VLDLs),** can also carry triacylglycerols. For a brief description of the definitions, functions, and composition of the various blood lipoproteins, see "Blood Lipoproteins: Synthesis, Functions, and Composition" on p. 86. As with lipolysis in the adipose and muscle tissue, the FAs in lipoproteins must be released from the triacylglycerols before they can enter the muscle cell. The enzyme **lipoprotein lipase (LPL)** is responsible for cleaving the FAs from the triacylglycerol molecules in blood lipoproteins. The FFAs are then available for transport into the muscle cells for energy production or for storage, or into adipose tissue for storage. From a practical standpoint, since most people do not exercise

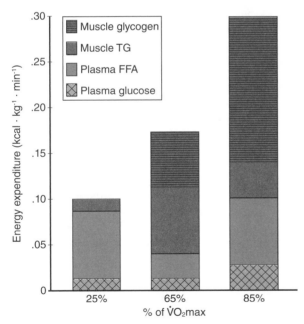

Figure 3.7 Substrate utilization at three different exercise intensities (25%, 65%, 85% V̇O$_2$max) in trained male cyclists after 30 min of exercise. FFA = free fatty acids; TG = triacylglcyerol.

Reprinted from J.A. Romijn, 1993, "Regulation of endogenous fat and carbohydrate metabolism in relation to exercise intensity," *American Journal of Physiology* 265: E380-E391. Used with permission.

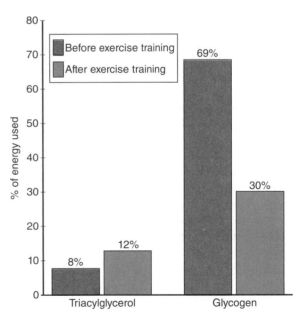

Figure 3.8 Percentage of intramuscular triacylglycerol and glycogen used for energy before and after a 12-week exercise training program using trained and untrained limbs (one-legged knee extensor exercise).

Adapted from B. Kiens et al., 1993, "Skeletal muscle substrate utilization during submaximal exercise in man: effect of endurance training," *Journal of Physiology* 469: 459-478.

Blood Lipoproteins: Synthesis, Functions, and Composition

Lipoprotein	Synthesis	Primary function	Composition
Chylomicrons	Formed in the gut mucosal cell after a meal and released into the intracellular space where they enter the lymph system; eventually they are dumped into the blood at the thoracic duct. Chylomicrons are the largest of the lipoproteins, with the lowest density. While circulating in the blood, chylomicrons can exchange apo-proteins with other lipoproteins, especially HDL. After the triglycerides are removed from this lipoprotein, a chylomicron remnant remains and is taken up by the liver.	Transport dietary fat (exogenous fat) into the blood and to the tissues of the body. Blood chylomicrons are high after a meal, but clear within 4 to 6 h depending on the fat content of the meal.	Triglycerides = 85% Phospholipids = 8% Cholesterol/Cholesterol Esters (CE) = 5% Protein = 2%
Very low-density lipoproteins (VLDL)	Formed in the liver (80% of production) and the intestine (20% of production). As triglycerides are removed, the concentration of cholesterol increases until an intermediate-density lipoprotein (IDL) is formed.	Transport endogenous lipids, especially triglycerides, to the various tissues of the body.	Triglycerides = 50% to 60% Phospholipids = 15% to 18% Cholesterol/CE = 15% to 20% Protein = 10%
Low-density lipoproteins (LDL)	Formed in the blood from VLDL (VLDL → IDL → LDL). As the triglycerides are removed, the VLDL becomes more dense with cholesterol and transitions to an IDL. When the cholesterol content becomes greater than the triglyceride content, the IDL transitions to an LDL.	Transport cholesterol to the cells of the body. LDLs are recognized by an LDL receptor on the cell surface and taken up by the cells via endocytosis.	Triglycerides = 8% Phospholipids = 20% Cholesterol/CE = 50% Protein = 22%
High-density lipoproteins (HDL)	Synthesized in the liver and released into the blood. The HDL then moves through the system picking up apoproteins and free cholesterol. HDL transport their cholesterol back to the liver.	Transport cholesterol from tissues back to the liver.	Triglycerides = 3% Phospholipids = 30% Cholesterol/CE = 17% Protein = 50%

Note: Triglyceride is another name for triacylglycerols.

strenuously after eating a large meal (especially a high-fat meal), the amount of energy obtained from blood lipoproteins is generally small (Turcotte et al. 1995). If one exercises after an overnight fast, the contribution of lipoprotein triacylglycerols is still minimal, since in healthy individuals no chylomicrons would be present and VLDLs would be low.

Oxidation of Fatty Acids

Fatty acids released from adipose cells must go through a series of steps before they can be oxidized for energy within the muscle mitochondria. The steps are outlined next and are illustrated in figure 3.4 (p. 81). A more detailed description of this metabolic process can be found in Achten and Jeukendrup 2004; Jeukendrup 2002; Jeukendrup and colleagues 1998a-b; and Winder 1998.

1. Fatty acids are attached to albumin for transport in the plasma to the muscle. Fatty acid binding proteins (FABP) within muscle cell membranes transport FAs across the membranes and into the cytoplasm of muscle cells.

2. Once FAs are in the cytoplasm of a muscle cell, they can either be re-esterified and stored as intracellular triacylglycerol or be activated for transport into the mitochondria. Fatty acids are transported through the cytoplasm bound to a **cytoplasmic fatty acid binding protein.**

3. If an FA is to be used for β-oxidation, it must first be activated by the enzyme **acyl-CoA synthetase.** This activation occurs outside the mitochondria.

4. The activated FA must then be transported across the mitochondrial inner membrane by **carnitine palmitoyl transferase I (CPT 1)** and **carnitine palmitoyl transferase II (CPT 2),** which work in unison to accomplish this task. First, the CPT 1 located on the outer surface of the mitochondrial membrane converts the fatty acyl-CoA to **acylcarnitine** for transport. Then, on the inner mitochondrial membrane side, CPT 2 reconverts the acylcarnitine back to fatty acyl-CoA for β-oxidation (Winder 1998).

Figure 3.9 describes the process in detail. As the rate-limiting enzyme in this process, CPT 1 regulates the amount of FA entering the mitochondria for oxidation. Malonyl-CoA, which is a potent inhibitor of CPT 1, is elevated when glucose availability is high (Winder 1998). Carnitine is synthesized in the body from two amino acids, lysine and methionine; the synthesis requires the essential nutrients vitamin C, niacin, iron, and vitamin B_6. In addition, we may obtain small amounts of carnitine from animal and dairy foods. Carnitine is considered conditionally essential because healthy individuals can synthesize the amount required in the body; however, under certain clinical conditions, the need may exceed the body's ability to synthesize the compound. In healthy individuals, supplemental carnitine does not improve fat oxidation since the body makes adequate carnitine (see Chapter 6 for more information on carnitine and weight loss). See the review by Foster (2004) for a complete overview of carnitine metabolism in humans.

5. Fatty acyl-CoA undergoes β-oxidation in the mitochondria via a cyclic degradative pathway, with two-carbon units cleaved from the

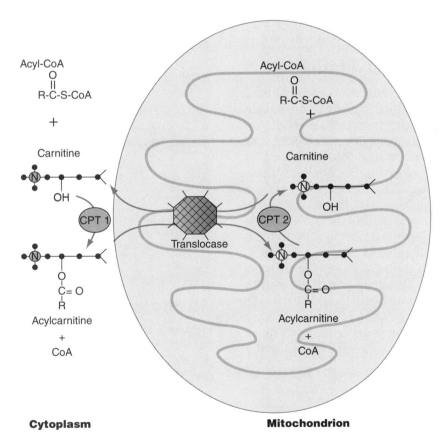

Cytoplasm　　　　　　　　　　**Mitochondrion**

Figure 3.9　The carnitine and fatty acid transport system. R = carbon backbone of fatty acid. CPT 1 = carnitine palmitoyl transferase 1. CPT 2 = carnitine palmitoyl transferase 2.

carboxyl end of the FA in the form of **acetyl-CoA.** Each time the FA goes through the cycle it loses a two-carbon unit, until there are only four carbons remaining. At this point, the four-carbon unit is degraded to produce two acetyl-CoA units. Each rotation of the cycle produces one unit each of acetyl-CoA, flavin adenine dinucleotide ($FADH_2$), and nicotinamide adenine dinucleotide (NADH). The acetyl-CoA units can then enter the TCA cycle for the production of energy (adenosine triphosphate [ATP]). If the acetyl-CoA is completely reduced to oxygen and water in the TCA cycle, 12 ATPs are produced for each unit of acetyl-CoA. The $FADH_2$ and NADH enter the electron transport cycle for further ATP production—each $FADH_2$ unit produces two ATPs, while each NADH yields three ATPs. The total production of ATP from the complete oxidation of one 16-carbon FA yields 129 ATPs (two ATPs are used up in this pathway) (Champe et al. 2008). Oxidation of fat produces three times the energy of an equal amount of glucose. Figure 3.10 shows the β-oxidation process in detail.

Regulation of Fat Oxidation

Since muscle and liver glycogen stores are limited and depletion of these stores contributes to fatigue during exercise, maximization of fat oxidation during exercise might help prevent fatigue and improve exercise performance. Reducing body fat stores may also be appealing for health, fitness, or aesthetic reasons. Even though most people have relatively large fat stores, the ability to oxidize these stores during exercise is limited. While the exact reasons for this limited ability to burn fat have not been identified, researchers working in the area of fat metabolism during exercise (Jeukendrup 2002; Jeukendrup et al. 1998b; Spriet 2002) have outlined a number of factors that might contribute. There may be limitations in the ability to efficiently execute the steps of fat lipolysis or transport at any number of levels, including the following:

- Lipolysis and mobilization of FAs from the adipose tissue

- Transport of FAs to the muscles and within the muscle by transport proteins

- Uptake of FAs across the muscle membrane, either from plasma or from the triacylglycerol in lipoproteins

- Lipolysis and mobilization of FAs from the intramuscular triacylglycerol pools

- Regulation of FA movement across the mitochondrial membranes

If any of these steps are inhibited or limited, the ability to deliver fat to muscle cells for oxidation may be reduced. In addition, a number of factors regulate FA transport and oxidation within the cell (Jeukendrup 2002; Jeukendrup et al. 1998b; Spriet 2002). Glucose availability appears to be a strong regulator of fat oxidation within the cell, with high glucose availability decreasing oxidation of long-chain FAs by inhibiting their transport into the mitochondria (Wolfe 1998). Glucose availability

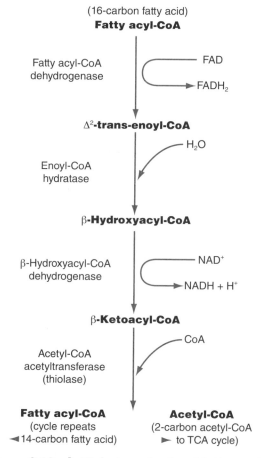

Figure 3.10 Initial steps in β-oxidation using palmitic acid, a 16-carbon fatty acid, as an example. Each turn of the cycle yields one acetyl-CoA unit and shortens the fatty acid by two carbons. The newly formed acetyl-CoA can then go to the tricarboxylic acid (TCA) cycle for further metabolism, while the shorter fatty acid repeats through the cycle. When the fatty acid has been shortened to four carbons, the final turn of the cycle produces two acetyl-CoA units.

Adapted, by permission, from P.C. Champe, R.A. Harvey, and D.R. Ferrier, 2008, *Lippincott's illustrated reviews: Biochemistry*, 4th ed. (Philadelphia, PA: Lippincott, Williams, and Wilkins), 192.

and oxidation appear to be closely coupled (i.e., if glucose is available, it is oxidized). The same is not true of fat since FA availability is generally much higher than required for oxidation. Plasma FFA concentrations during exercise greatly exceed the level needed to meet the fat oxidation capacity of the muscle. Research suggests that FA oxidation rates within the muscle cell during exercise may be controlled by a number of the factors listed earlier (Spriet 2002) and by the availability of glucose, not by the availability of FAs via lipolysis (Carlson et al. 1991; Coyle et al. 1997; Wolfe 1998).

ENHANCEMENT OF FAT OXIDATION

What can a person do to increase burning of fat? Can a supplement like carnitine or a drug like caffeine really increase the burning of fat? A multitude of products are marketed with claims that they increase fat metabolism. Since such products are a multimillion-dollar business in the United States, it is important to understand the science behind fat metabolism. Are these products legitimate or a waste of money? This section addresses training strategies, dietary changes, and ergogenic products thought to improve or enhance the ability to burn fat. Because of wide interest in this topic, a number of reviews have addressed in greater detail the issues we discuss in the next few paragraphs (Brouns and van der Vusse 1998; Hawley et al. 1998; Jeukendrup and Aldred 2004; Kiens and Helge 1998; Lambert et al. 1997; Sherman and Leenders 1995).

Exercise Training

Exercise training enables a person to work harder (higher oxygen uptake) while deriving more energy from fat (both plasma FFAs and intramuscular triacylglycerol) and less from carbohydrate (blood glucose and glycogen) (figure 3.11). A number of researchers have reported the specific physiological and metabolic adaptations that occur with training (Achten and Jeukendrup 2004; Brouns and van der Vusse 1998; Jeukendrup and Aldred 2004; Saltin and Åstrand 1993), which are as follows:

1. Increased numbers of mitochondria and increased activity of enzymes within the mitochondria—including increased concentration of enzymes for the TCA cycle, FA oxidation, and the electron transport system.

2. Increased fatty acyl-CoA synthesis in muscle, plus increased levels of LPL, lipase, carni-

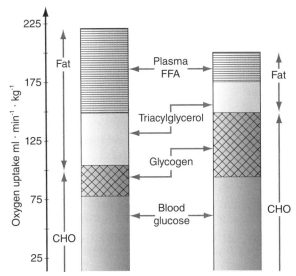

Figure 3.11 The estimated contribution of various substrates to energy metabolism during exercise when the limb is trained or untrained. There is a greater dependence on plasma free fatty acids (FFAs) and triacylglycerol in the trained limb and less reliance on carbohydrate (CHO).

Reproduced with permission of American Society for Nutrition, from *Journal of Clinical Nutrition,* "Free fatty acids and exercise," B. Saltin and P.O. Åstrand, 57: 752S-758S, 1993.

tine, and carnitine transferase—all of which favor improved availability and transport of FAs to the mitochondria for β-oxidation.

3. Increased triacylglycerol storage and oxidation within muscle—more fat is stored closer to the site of oxidation, improving the availability of fat for oxidation during exercise.

4. Increased FFA uptake by the muscle. Exercise increases capillary density of muscle, which in turn improves blood flow and the exchange of FFAs and oxygen; exercise also increases transport of FAs through the sarcolemma. Figure 3.12 (p. 90) illustrates this improvement in FFA uptake, showing that the trained person has a higher FFA uptake compared to the untrained.

5. Alterations in the mobilization of FFAs from the adipose tissue. Exercise may increase the delivery of FFAs from the fat cell to the blood due to increased blood flow in the adipose tissue.

6. Improved cardiovascular respiratory system that enhances oxygen delivery to the muscle for fat oxidation.

Taken collectively, the adaptations listed enhance the body's ability to oxidize fat as a fuel, improve intramuscular fat storage, and increase fat flux (Achten and Jeukendrup 2004; Brouns and van der Vusse 1998; Saltin and Åstrand 1993). Because exercise improves the ability to oxidize fat, it makes sense that the level of exercise intensity required for maximum fat oxidation would vary between trained and untrained individuals. Based on work by Achten and colleagues (2002) and others, the maximal level of fat oxidation occurs at ~64 ± 4% $\dot{V}O_2$max (see figure 3.13). Achten and Jeukendrup (2004) also report that for exercise-trained individuals, maximum rates of fat oxidation occur at exercise intensities between 59% and 65% of $\dot{V}O_2$max, while for untrained individuals the level is 47% to 52% of $\dot{V}O_2$max. Thus, becoming a more trained person means that your maximum fat-oxidizing capabilities occur at a higher intensity of exercise than for a more sedentary individual. This has an advantage for both weight maintenance and weight loss because the trained individual, who can optimally burn fat at a higher $\dot{V}O_2$max, will burn more calories than the sedentary individual in a given amount of time spent exercising. Finally, exercise training also spares endogenous carbohydrate stores that may be needed for prolonged, high-intensity events (see chapter 2), so you can work harder longer.

Exercise training is the best intervention one can recommend to improve a person's ability to burn fat. Unfortunately, many people do not want to put the time and energy into becoming more fit. They are looking for a pill or a potion to improve their fat-burning ability. They want the quick fix! Unfortunately, no legitimate quick fixes are available in the marketplace (but lots of illegitimate ones). This will become evident as you read the rest of this chapter.

High-Fat Diets and Fat Infusions

Both fat and carbohydrate are important energy substrates during exercise. During moderate exercise (60-75% $\dot{V}O_2$max) of long duration (>90 min), however, fat becomes the primary energy substrate as carbohydrate stores are depleted. This depletion of the body's carbohydrate stores is usually manifested by a decrease in blood glucose over time and a depletion of muscle and liver glycogen stores. Depletion of these stores increases reliance on liver gluconeogenesis to provide the glucose necessary to sustain exercise. (See review of the gluconeogenesis pathway in chapter 2.) Ingestion of exogenous carbohydrate

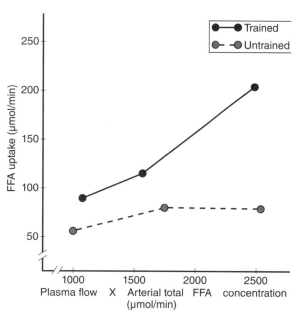

Figure 3.12 Uptake of free fatty acids (FFAs) by the contracting muscle in relation to the amount of FFAs offered to the limb. At a higher inflow of FFAs, the trained individual can utilize a larger fraction of the FFAs available.

Reproduced with permission of American Society for Nutrition, from *Journal of Clinical Nutrition,* "Free fatty acids and exercise," B. Saltin and P.O. Åstrand, 57: 752S-758S, 1993.

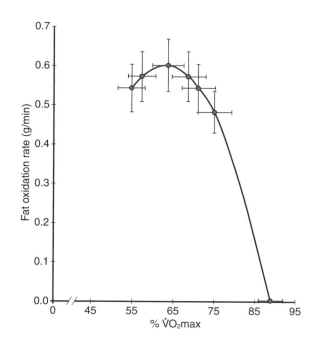

Figure 3.13 Fat oxidation rates versus exercise intensity expressed as percentage of $\dot{V}O_2$max; *N* = 11 subjects; values are mean ± SEM (standard error of the mean).

Reprinted from J. Achten, M. Gleeson, and A.E. Jeukendrup, 2002, "The relationship between maximal fat oxidation and exercise intensity," *Medicine and Science in Sport and Exercise* 34: 92-97.

can delay fatigue but cannot prevent it (Coyle et al. 1986). But when carbohydrate is consumed during exercise, a shift in substrate utilization occurs—glucose feeding suppresses fat lipolysis, mobilization, and oxidation during exercise, thereby reducing the proportion of energy coming from fat. Because the body has limited carbohydrate stores, researchers have examined ways to increase FA availability through diet in an attempt to increase FA oxidation during exercise. If this could be done, then glycogen utilization might be reduced and more fat used as a fuel source during exercise, which could delay fatigue and improve performance (Hawley 2002). Consuming a short-term high-fat diet increases FFA levels in the plasma during rest; subsequently, during exercise, more FAs are taken up by the muscles than if a person has been following a high-carbohydrate diet (Jeukendrup and Saris 1998). Moreover, long-term fat consumption may induce skeletal muscle adaptations that increase the body's ability to oxidize fat as a fuel (Kiens and Helge 1998). Finally, researchers have examined the effect of fat infusions (Intralipid) during exercise to determine if additional fat availability decreases muscle glycogen utilization compared to that in control trials (Odland et al. 1998; Vukovich et al. 1993).

Because of the factors just mentioned, a number of researchers have hypothesized that high-fat diets, either short- or long-term, would increase the availability of fat for oxidation and the ability to oxidize fat during exercise. This in turn would cause the body to become less reliant on carbohydrate for energy, thus sparing muscle glycogen and eventually improving exercise performance. Based on a large body of evidence, the body appears to adapt to the lower carbohydrate availability by becoming a better fat oxidizer (Achten and Jeukendrup 2004; Hawley 2002; Hawley et al. 1998; Jeukendrup and Saris 1998; Sherman and Leenders 1995). If these hypotheses are true, high-fat diets would improve exercise performance by sparing carbohydrate and improving fat oxidation. Researchers have carefully examined these issues, which have been reviewed in detail (Achten and Jeukendrup 2004; Burke and Hawley 2002; Hawley 2002; Helge 2002; Jeukendrup and Aldred 2004). However, the research has produced mixed results due to a number of factors, including differences in experimental designs, training status of the subjects, methods of measuring exercise performance, the percentage of energy derived from fat, and the length of time the high-fat diet was fed (Helge et al. 1998). In general, it appears that researchers agree that high-fat diets can

increase FA oxidation and spare muscle but do not improve performance (Achten and Jeukendrup 2004; Hawley 2002; Burke and Hawley 2002; Burke et al. 2002). For a more retailed review of the impact of high-fat diets on metabolism and exercise performance, see the reviews by Achten and Jeukendrup (2004), Burke and Hawley (2002), Hawley (2002), Helge (2002), and Spriet (2002).

In general, the diets used by researchers examining effects of high-fat meals or diets on glycogen utilization and fat oxidation during exercise can be grouped roughly as follows:

- A single high-fat meal before exercise
- Short-term high-fat diets (three to five days) before exercise
- Moderate-term high-fat diets (one to four weeks) before exercise
- Long-term high-fat diets (more than seven weeks) before exercise
- High-fat diet (either short- or long-term) followed by one or two days of a high-carbohydrate intake

Studies on the effect of high-fat meals (~60-75% of energy) 4 h before endurance exercise (90-120 min) show no differences in exercise performance or work production compared to findings for high-carbohydrate meals (58-87% of energy) (Burke and Hawley 2002). The effect of a high-fat meal on substrate utilization during exercise appears more variable. However, the general consensus is that a short-term high-fat diet (five or six days; 60-70% energy) followed by one or two days of a high-carbohydrate diet (70-80% energy) increases fat oxidation rates and spares muscle glycogen during submaximal exercise compared to high-carbohydrate diets (Burke and Hawley 2002). For example, Okano and colleagues (1998) observed a significantly lower respiratory exchange ratio during exercise when a high-fat meal was fed versus a high-carbohydrate meal. This lower respiratory exchange ratio suggests that a high-fat meal prior to exercise increases fat oxidation during exercise. In studies that used high-fat diets but showed no effect on substrate utilization, dietary fat content was typically lower (55-60% of energy) and no exercise was performed during the diet period (Achten and Jeukendrup 2004). Thus, the research protocol used can dramatically affect the results.

It also appears that two to four weeks of high-fat meals do not negatively affect exercise performance compared to high-carbohydrate diets but do not improve performance either (Burke and Hawley 2002; Helge 2002). For example, Lambert and colleagues (1994) fed five endurance cyclists either a high-fat (76% of energy) or a high-carbohydrate diet (74% of energy) for two weeks in random order separated by two weeks of a normal diet. After each treatment period, the athletes performed three exercise tests in the following order:

1. Wingate test—to test muscle power
2. High-intensity exercise exhaustion test—cycling to exhaustion at 85% of peak power (90% $\dot{V}O_2$max)
3. Moderate-intensity exercise exhaustion test—cycling to exhaustion at 60% of $\dot{V}O_2$max

The results showed that diet had no effect on muscle power output or on the high-intensity exercise exhaustion test. Muscle glycogen utilization during exercise was similar for the two diets during the high-intensity exercise test even though glycogen levels were significantly lower after the high-fat diet (68 mmol/kg/wet mass) compared to the high-carbohydrate diet (121 mmol/kg/wet mass). However, exercise time to exhaustion after moderate-intensity exercise was significantly longer after the high-fat diet (80 min) compared to the high-carbohydrate diet (43 min). This longer endurance time was attributed to a lower respiratory exchange ratio (RER, 0.87) while athletes were on the high-fat diet compared to the high-carbohydrate diet (0.92).

More recent studies addressing the effect of four to five weeks of a high-fat diet on endurance time show mixed results, which may be a consequence of the level of fat fed. Venkatraman and Pendergast (1998) reported improved time to exhaustion in runners fed a moderate-fat diet (32% of energy) compared to a low-fat diet (17% of energy), but no difference between the moderate-fat and the high-fat diet (41% of energy). Unfortunately, the diets were not randomly assigned, and there was no washout period between the diets. Thus, it is difficult to know if there was a carryover effect from one diet to the next. In addition, the level of fat fed in this study was significantly lower than in the 60% to 70% fat diets typically fed in other studies. This makes it difficult to compare these results to those of other high-fat feeding research and emphasizes the importance of standardization of diet with other research studies and the importance of randomization of the diets. Helge

and colleagues (1998) reported no difference in endurance performance in untrained males going through a four-week training period and consuming either a four-week high-fat (62% of energy) or a high-carbohydrate (65% of energy) diet. Time to exhaustion was similar between the groups; however, the high-fat group did have a lower RER during exercise compared both to their own baseline values and to values for the high-carbohydrate group. These results are supported by a recent study by Vogt and colleagues (2003), who fed either a low-fat diet (17% of energy from fat) or a high-fat diet (53% of energy from fat) and found no differences in half-marathon running times or a 20 min all-out time trial. There were no differences between groups for glycogen or oxidative capacity. However, the high-fat diet did produce more intramyocellular lipid and a lower RER. Thus, it appears that feeding a high-fat diet for a short period of time does affect fat metabolism but does not significantly improve performance.

What about the effects of long-term fat feeding? Helge (2002) has carefully reviewed the research in this area and concluded that adoption of a high-fat diet over a number of weeks (two to seven weeks) does not improve endurance performance. One of the first studies done in this area was performed by Helge and colleagues (1996). They fed untrained men either a high-carbohydrate (n = 10, 65% of energy) or a high-fat (n = 10, 62% of energy) diet for seven weeks. All subjects went through endurance training three to four times per week for the duration of the study. At the end of the study, those receiving the high-carbohydrate diet significantly improved exercise endurance time from ~35 min at baseline to 102 min (191% improvement), while the high-fat group improved to only 65 min (85% improvement). Figure 3.14 compares the effect of moderate- and long-term fat feeding on exercise time to exhaustion. Long-term fat feeding appears not to benefit exercise performance.

To summarize current research, high-fat meals before exercise have no effect on performance, while short-term high-fat diets (three to five days) decrease or have no effect on exercise performance compared to high-carbohydrate diets. When high-fat diets are fed for two to four weeks, allowing individuals to adapt metabolically to the diet, the effect on performance is similar to that seen with a high-carbohydrate diet. In other words, high-fat and high-carbohydrate diets produced the same results. However, when high-fat diets are fed for longer periods (seven weeks) and compared to

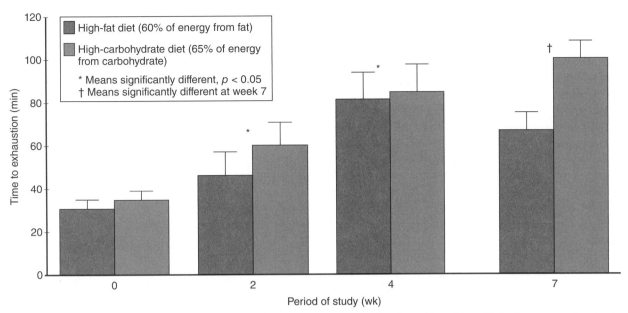

Figure 3.14 Endurance performance to exhaustion measured at baseline (time 0) before exercise training and after two, four, and seven weeks of a high-fat diet compared to a high-carbohydrate diet. Mean values were significantly different from those at week 0 for both diets (*$p < 0.05$). Mean value for the high-carbohydrate diet was significantly different from that for the high-fat diet at week 7 (†$p < 0.05$). Data obtained using Krogh bicycle ergonometer.

Reprinted from B. Kiens and J.W. Helge, 1998, "Effect of high-fat diets on exercise performance," *Proceeding of the Nutritional Society* 57: 73-75. Reprinted with the permission of Cambridge University Press.

high-carbohydrate diets, endurance performance is better on the high-carbohydrate diets (Helge et al. 1996; Kiens and Helge 1998; Helge 2002). At the present time there appears to be no advantage to feeding high-fat diets to athletes—especially the levels of fat fed in experimental studies (~60-70% of energy from fat). These levels of fat are generally not acceptable to most active individuals, can cause gastrointestinal distress, and are not practical. In addition, diets this high in fat are not recommended for good long-term health. Fat infusions during exercise decrease glycogen use but are of no practical value to the active individual, and they are illegal in athletic competition (Hawley 2002; Sherman and Leenders 1995). In summary, based on the limited data available, extremely high-fat diets seem impractical and are not recommended for athletes or active individuals.

Long-Chain Triacylglycerols

In some endurance events (e.g., ultramarathons or triathlons), athletes eat food while competing. In general, the ingestion of **long-chain triacylglycerols (LCTs)**, or triglycerides, during exercise events lasting less than 4 h is not recommended.

Long-chain triacylglycerols comprise three LCFAs and a glycerol backbone. Because LCTs slow gastric emptying, they stay in the gastrointestinal tract longer and enter the blood more slowly than other sources of energy typically used during exercise. Note also that since they are insoluble in water, LCFAs must enter the general circulation via a chylomicron—a much slower process than carbohydrate digestion. Dietary carbohydrate is more readily digested and absorbed, thus, making it more available for energy during exercise than LCTs. The fats transported in chylomicrons are not major contributors of energy to the body during exercise but are thought to contribute to the replenishment of intramuscular fat after exercise is over (Jeukendrup and Saris 1998).

In summary, LCT consumption is generally not recommended during intense exercise lasting less than 4 h (Jeukendrup and Aldred 2004). If the activity is long lasting (e.g., an ultramarathon, a multiday exercise event, or even an all-day hike), foods with LCT are appropriate and even recommended. Even during these types of events, however, the level of fat consumed should usually be low, with the majority of energy coming from carbohydrate.

Medium-Chain Triacylglycerols

Since fat digestion is generally slower than that of carbohydrate, fat stays in the gastrointestinal tract longer before it enters circulation—thus decreasing the immediate availability of exogenous fat as an energy source during exercise. **Medium-chain triacylglycerols (MCTs)** are an exception to this rule since they are digested differently from typical dietary fats. Medium-chain triacylglycerols comprise three MCFAs and a glycerol backbone; however, because MCFAs are only 6 to 12 carbons long, their smaller size alters the way they are digested, transported, and utilized for energy within the body (Jones and Kubow, 2006; Jeukendrup and Aldred 2004). They rapidly exit the stomach into the small intestine. They are digested into MCFAs, which are absorbed across the mucosal membrane almost as rapidly as glucose. Compared with LCFAs, MCFAs are more soluble in water, require less pancreatic lipase and bile salts for digestion, and diffuse rapidly through the unstirred water layer of the gut. Once inside the gut mucosal cells, they do not require resynthesis into triacylglycerols and incorporation into chylomicrons for transport into the blood, as LCFAs do. Medium-chain triacylglycerols enter the portal vein bound to albumin and are transported to the liver as rapidly as glucose. They enter systemic circulation and are available for metabolism 250 times more quickly than LCFAs (Linscheer and Vergroesen 1994). They are not stored in adipose tissue but are oxidized rapidly for energy by the cells, especially in the liver. Within muscle cells, MCFAs are not dependent on carnitine for transport into the mitochondria (Spriet 2002). Finally, MCFAs are metabolized within the muscle about as rapidly as glucose, and preferentially over LCFAs.

These unique characteristics of MCTs and MCFAs have led researchers to suggest that MCTs could be a valuable source of energy during exercise, especially during extreme endurance events (Ivy et al. 1980; Goedecke et al. 2005). It has also been suggested that MCTs may have a glycogen-sparing effect since they are rapidly metabolized for energy (Horowitz et al. 2000) and that they might reduce the need for carbohydrate, which would spare glycogen. In turn, sparing glycogen may help reduce fatigue and thus might be able to improve exercise performance (Horowitz et al. 2000; Vistisen et al. 2003).

A large body of research over the last 15 to 20 years has examined the effect of MCTs on exercise performance, glycogen sparing, and substrate utilization during exercise. One of the first exercise studies done using MCT was by Ivy and colleagues (1980), who studied 10 well-trained male volunteers during 1 h of exercise at 70% $\dot{V}O_2$max under four randomly assigned double-blind conditions:

1. Control (subjects exercised after an overnight fast)
2. MCT (30 g) mixed with cereal and 240 mL (~1 cup) of nonfat milk (total of 621 kcal) fed 1 h before exercise
3. LCT (30 g) mixed with cereal and 240 mL (~1 cup) of nonfat milk (total of 609 kcal) fed 1 h before exercise
4. Cereal only (no added fat) and 240 mL (~1 cup) of nonfat milk (354 kcal, primarily carbohydrate) fed 1 h before exercise

There were no differences in rate of perceived exertion among the four trials. The addition of MCT did not significantly increase the plasma FA levels or the level of fat oxidation during exercise compared to the other treatments. All three experimental meals resulted in approximately 132 g of carbohydrate and 36 g of fat being used for energy, while the control trial utilized 111 g of carbohydrate and 45 g of fat. These authors concluded that MCT in combination with carbohydrate was not a viable energy source during exercise, since all treatments (except the control) utilized the same amounts of fat and carbohydrate. The authors also reported that during preliminary trials, feeding either 50 or 60 g of MCT caused gastrointestinal distress in 100% of their subjects, while 30 g caused distress in only 10% of the subjects. A subsequent study by Decombaz and colleagues (1983) showed similar results. In this study, 12 men consumed either 25 g MCT or 50 g carbohydrate 1 h before exercise and then exercised for 1 h at 60% $\dot{V}O_2$max. The MCT did not spare muscle glycogen use but did account for 10% of total energy expenditure; however, the MCT did not appear to offer any advantages over carbohydrate. These data have been supported by a more recent study by Horowitz and colleagues (2000), who examined the impact of preexercise MCT ingestion (~25 g; 1 h before exercise with a carbohydrate meal [~50 g]) on muscle glycogen sparing during exercise (30 min at 84% maximal O_2 uptake) and found no effect in seven well-trained male cyclists. In this study, the change in muscle glycogen was measured by biopsies taken from the vastus lateralis before and after exercise and calculations of glycogen oxidation using stable isotopes. Thus the addition of MCT to a preexercise carbohydrate meal did not reduce muscle glycogen oxidation during a high-intensity exercise session.

Researchers have also examined the effect of feeding MCT *during* exercise as part of a fluid replacement beverage. Massicotte and colleagues (1992) examined the effect of water, MCT (25 g), or glucose (57 g) ingested during exercise in six healthy young men exercising for 2 h at 65% $\dot{V}O_2$max. The energy provided by MCT and glucose was similar. During exercise, MCTs and carbohydrate were oxidized for energy at similar rates but represented only 7% and 8.5% of total energy expenditure, respectively. Neither the exogenous MCT nor glucose reduced the amount of endogenous carbohydrate utilized. Subsequently Jeukendrup and colleagues (1995, 1996) have reported similar findings. In these experiments, subjects consumed either MCT (~29 g), carbohydrate only, or carbohydrate + MCT during 3 h of cycling at 57% $\dot{V}O_2$max. Results showed that some MCT was oxidized for energy during exercise, but the contribution to total energy expenditure was small (3-7%). Similarly to what was seen in early studies, MCT did not spare muscle glycogen. Even when muscle glycogen levels were low prior to exercise, MCT contributions to total energy expenditure did not improve and remained at ~8% in the 1996 study. Although MCT can be used as a fuel source during exercise, the amount of MCT tolerated in relation to gastrointestinal distress is limited. Feeding higher amounts is therefore not feasible.

The effect of MCT on actual exercise performance has been studied only recently. Van Zyl and colleagues (1996) had six endurance-trained cyclists exercise on three different occasions for 2 h at 60% peak VO_2, then perform a 40 km time trial. Subjects received one of three treatments in random order: 10% glucose solution (100 g/L), 4.3% MCT solution (43 g/L), or 4.3% MCT + 10% glucose solution. Replacing glucose with MCT significantly slowed the time trials by 5.3 min, but combining MCT and glucose in the same drink significantly improved the time trials by 1.7 min compared to glucose alone. The authors did not measure muscle glycogen. Jeukendrup and colleagues (1998d) repeated this study using seven well-trained cyclists, who again exercised for 2 h at 60% $\dot{V}O_2$max and then performed a time trial; however, the time trial consisted of the maximum amount of work that could be done in a 15 min period. Subjects ingested one of four treatments:

1. A 10% carbohydrate solution (170 g glucose)
2. A 10% carbohydrate solution with 5% MCT added (170 g glucose + 85 g MCT)
3. A 5% MCT solution (85 g MCT)
4. A placebo containing artificially colored and flavored water

The authors compared the total amount of work done (in watts [W]) in the various time trials. When subjects consumed the glucose-only beverage (314 ± 19 W) or the glucose + MCT beverage (314 ± 13 W), their performance was similar to that with the placebo (312 ± 18 W). The MCT-only treatment (263 ± 22 W) decreased performance by 17% to 18% compared to the placebo and the other two treatments. The MCT did not affect total carbohydrate or protein utilization during exercise, nor did it alter the amount of exogenous or endogenous carbohydrate used. In other words, MCT use did not spare muscle glycogen. The authors reported that the amount of MCT used in this study did result in some gastrointestinal distress: Two subjects vomited after the MCT trial, and three complained of diarrhea. Belching and bloating were reported with all the treatments except the placebo. The most common complaint was gastrointestinal cramps, which occurred significantly more often when MCT was used. These two studies were similar in that neither found the use of MCT by itself to be beneficial to performance; only the Van Zyl study showed a significant improvement in performance when MCT was combined with carbohydrate. Unfortunately, Van Zyl and colleagues (1996) did not report data on how the subjects responded to the MCT; any benefit of MCT is negated if it causes gastrointestinal distress.

Finally, researchers have examined the impact of MCT before exercise (1 h) and during exercise when MCT is added to a sport beverage (Goedecke et al. 2005; Thorburn et al. 2006). Goedecke and colleagues (2005) fed 32 g of MCT or 75 g of carbohydrate before exercise and then had their ultra-endurance cyclists ingest either a carbohydrate solution (10%) or 4.3% MCT + carbohydrate every 20 min during exercise. Exercise lasted for 270 min at a constant load (50% peak power output), interspersed with four sprints at 60 min intervals followed by a time trial. The researchers found that the athletes were slower when they consumed MCT, and half the subjects reported gastrointestinal distress. Thorburn and colleagues (2006) also examined MCT prior to exercise testing and during exercise. Prior to exercise testing they had a two-week adaptation period in which athletes were fed various levels of fat and carbohydrate. During the actual exercise test they also fed either an MCT or a carbohydrate solution. The two-week feeding period prior to exercise testing was used to see if athletes adapted to MCT, thus reducing the gastrointestinal distress typically seen with feeding of MCT. The results support those already discussed. Athletes experienced gastrointestinal distress during exercise testing (3 h at 50% peak power followed by 10 sprints at maximum intensity) and actually did worse on the MCT trials, in which performance was reduced by 10%. The authors concluded that prefeeding MCT for two weeks helped reduce the gastrointestinal distress experienced by the athletes, but the sprint times were still impaired even though the MCT was better tolerated.

In summary, the use of MCT as a fuel source during exercise has been carefully studied in relation to exercise performance, which usually involves some type of time trial event after an exercise bout lasting 60 to 180 min, and during endurance exercise lasting 60 min or longer (Berning 1996; Brouns and van der Vusse 1998; Goedecke et al. 2005; Horowitz et al. 2000; Jeukendrup and Aldred 2004; Jeukendrup et al. 1998; Thorburn et al. 2006; Vistisen et al. 2003). Although MCTs do contribute to total energy availability during exercise, the contribution to total energy expenditure appears small, ~7% to 8%. In addition, MCTs do not appear to significantly spare muscle glycogen or significantly decrease the amount of endogenous or exogenous carbohydrate used to warrant their ingestion during exercise. Total fat oxidation generally remains the same when MCTs are consumed either before or during exercise, even when glycogen levels are low prior to exercise. This suggests that MCFAs are competing with LCFAs for oxidation during exercise; hence, MCTs may be sparing endogenous fat stores (Brouns and van der Vusse 1998). It may also explain why glycogen is not spared when MCTs are fed either before or during exercise. Feeding higher amounts of MCTs might contribute to a greater proportion of total energy expenditure during exercise, but gastrointestinal distress prevents ingestion of higher doses. Although MCTs empty rapidly from the stomach and MCFAs can be quickly digested, transported, and utilized by the body for energy, use of MCTs as a fuel source during exercise appears limited due to gastrointestinal side effects. Based on the

data available, MCT ingestion either before or during exercise does not appear to spare muscle glycogen or improve exercise performance. A final note: MCTs are very expensive!

Caffeine

Caffeine is one of the most widely used drugs in the world and has long been touted as an ergogenic substance that increases exercise performance and promotes fat burning. Effective January 2008, caffeine was removed from the list of prohibited substances by the World Anti-Doping Agency (WADA 2007). In the United States, the National Collegiate Athletic Association (NCAA) still lists caffeine in the banned-drug class for 2008-2009 with an upper limit of 15 µg/mL for urine (www.ncaa.org). This allowable level of urinary caffeine is very liberal, and most athletes would have to consume caffeine in tablet or suppository form to reach this level (Spriet 1995; Graham 2001). Competitive athletes usually use caffeine for its ability to enhance performance. For most active individuals and recreational athletes, caffeine consumption is little more than a daily habit in the form of coffee, tea, cola, or chocolate—the idea that caffeine might improve exercise performance being a "fringe benefit." For people interested in weight loss, drug companies frequently add caffeine to over-the-counter weight loss products to speed up metabolism and increase metabolic rate. Unfortunately, many such products combine caffeine with other central nervous system stimulants such as ephedrine (ephedra, ma huang) or synephrine (Citrus aurantium, zhi shi, bitter orange)—products that can have serious side effects and should be avoided.

There are three major hypotheses for the ergogenic effect of caffeine during exercise, as outlined next (Graham and Spriet 1996; Spriet 1995; Graham 2001). Various review articles have addressed each of these hypotheses in detail (Clarkson 1993; Dodd et al. 1993; Doherty and Smith 2004; Graham et al. 1994; Graham and Spriet 1996; Kalmar and Cafarelli 2004; Spriet 1995; Graham 2001). To summarize:

1. Caffeine may directly affect the central nervous system and alter one's perception of effort, or it may directly effect neural activation of muscle. See Kalmar and Cafarelli (2004) for a complete review of this hypothesis.

2. Caffeine may directly affect skeletal muscle by altering key enzymes or systems that

regulate carbohydrate breakdown within cells.

3. Caffeine may alter metabolic factors that enhance exercise metabolism and substrate availability, such as increased fat oxidation and decreased carbohydrate utilization. Early in the 1980s it was hypothesized that caffeine directly increases circulating concentrations of epinephrine, which increases mobilization of FFAs from the fat or muscle cells. The increased availability of FFAs increases muscle cell oxidation of fat and improves exercise performance. After nearly 25 years of research, this hypothesis appears to lack support in the research literature (Graham 2001).

It appears that moderate doses of caffeine (3-9 mg/kg body weight) at least 1 h before exercise can enhance performance for well-trained elite or recreational athletes in endurance exercise in controlled research settings. Figure 3.15 shows the results from tests with well-trained recreational runners given caffeine (3, 6, or 9 mg/kg body weight) or a placebo (no caffeine) and asked to run to exhaustion at 85% $\dot{V}O_2$max (Graham and Spriet 1995). A recent meta-analysis by Doherty and Smith (2004) examining the effects of caffeine ingestion on exercise testing showed that caffeine can improve exercise testing outcomes (e.g., exercise tests done in the research laboratory) by 12.3% compared to placebo, with the greatest improvements in endurance exercise versus either graded or short-term exercise tests. When the authors examined the type of exercise protocols used, they found that time-to-exhaustion protocols showed the greatest improvement compared to either graded or nonexhaustion exercise protocols. In the 40 double-blind studies included in this meta-analysis, researchers used pure caffeine (3-13 mg/kg; median = 6 mg/kg) that was administered ~60 min before exercise, not caffeine-containing beverages such as coffee, tea, or cola. The metabolic effects of coffee may be different from those of pure caffeine since there are components in coffee that appear to moderate the effects of caffeine (Graham et al. 1998). The recreational athlete who drinks a cup of coffee and then goes out for a 10K run may not see the performance effects demonstrated in the research laboratory, where a specific level of pure caffeine is fed per kilogram body weight at a set time before exercise begins. Many factors affect both exercise performance and the physiological response to

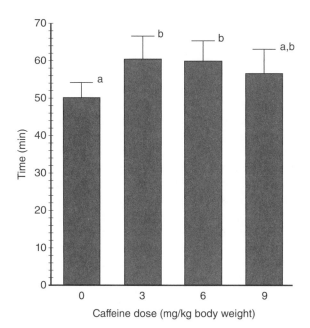

Figure 3.15 Effects of caffeine on exercise time to exhaustion. Data are means for exercise duration after placebo (0 mg/kg) or 3, 6, or 9 mg/kg caffeine. Data for histogram bars with the same letter are not significantly different ($p < 0.05$). The 0 and 3 mg/kg trials were significantly different despite their exhibiting no differences in plasma epinephrine. And the 0 and 9 mg/kg times were not significantly different, although these trials had quite different plasma epinephrine data.

Reprinted from T.E. Graham and L.L. Spriet, 1995, "Metabolic, catecholamine, and exercise performance responses to various doses of caffeine," *Journal of Applied Physiology* 78: 867-874. Used with permission.

caffeine during exercise, including a person's typical or habitual caffeine intake. The metabolic and performance responses of a habitual caffeine user may be very different from those of a nonuser (Bell and McLellan 2002; Graham 2001).

No one physiological mechanism for improved endurance performance with caffeine has been identified. Although about half of the research studies show an increase in plasma FFA concentration early in exercise compared to placebo treatments (Mougious et al. 2003), there is no clear research showing that increased plasma FFAs result in increased fat oxidation during exercise and subsequent muscle glycogen sparing (Graham 2001). Caffeine indirectly affects muscle and adipose tissue by increasing plasma catecholamines, which in turn bind to the β-receptors of the cell membranes, increasing cAMP activity and lipolysis (Hawley et al. 1998). Stimulation of lipolysis is already high during exercise, however, and any caffeine-induced elevation of FFAs comes on top of already high plasma FFA concentrations. This may explain why the effects of caffeine on lipid oxidation are observed only in the initial stages of exercise, when lipolysis and fat oxidation are increasing, and not after 30 min when fat oxidation is high (Hawley et al. 1998). Thus, the performance-enhancing effect of caffeine is most likely related to its effect on the central nervous system rather than to significant effects on fat oxidation and glycogen sparing (Bell et al. 1998; Doherty and Smith 2005; Spriet 1996; Graham 2001).

This suggestion is supported by data from Graham and Spriet (1995) (figure 3.15), who found that a low dose of caffeine (3 mg/kg body weight) was enough to enhance exercise performance but not enough to stimulate the metabolic effects typically attributed to increased fat oxidation. At this level of caffeine, they saw no increase in plasma catecholamines, lipolysis, or plasma FFAs, all of which would have to occur if fat oxidation were enhanced and were the cause for improved performance. Finally, the central nervous system hypothesis for the impact of caffeine on exercise performance is supported by a recent meta-analysis by Doherty and Smith (2005), who examined 21 double-blind, placebo-controlled, laboratory-based studies in which a single oral dose of caffeine (range = 4-10 mg/kg) was given ~60 min prior to exercise. They found that caffeine ingestion reduced rate of perceived exertion during exercise by 5.6% and improved exercise performance by 11.2% compared to values in placebo trials.

In summary, caffeine appears to enhance exercise performance and decrease rate of perceived exertion, and appears to increase fat oxidation at rest, but it does not increase fat oxidation after the first few minutes of exercise. According to recent reviews on caffeine and exercise, use of caffeine as a significant "fat burner" is not substantiated by the research literature (Graham 2001). Exercise is a much greater stimulant of fat oxidation than caffeine supplementation. Yet even the hint of improved fat oxidation leads many consumers to increase caffeine intake. Note, however, that high doses of caffeine can have significant side effects, especially in individuals who are not habitual users: It increases blood pressure at rest and during exercise (Daniels et al. 1998; Kaminsky et al. 1998), and high doses can cause dizziness, headache, insomnia, increased heart rate, and gastrointestinal distress.

Carnitine

Carnitine is marketed as a "fat burner" to sedentary people and athletes. Advertisements claim that carnitine can do everything from decreasing body fat to preventing fatigue. Unlike caffeine, carnitine is an essential substance made by the body and is obtained from the diet in meat products. It is required for the transport of FAs into the mitochondria for β-oxidation (discussed earlier in this chapter). However, in healthy individuals, the body is capable of making adequate amounts of carnitine for FA transport. Although oral L-carnitine supplements increase plasma L-carnitine concentrations, uptake by the muscles remains unchanged (Brouns and van der Vusse 1998; Brass 2000, 2004). Chapter 16 presents more detailed information about carnitine, its role in fat metabolism, and the effect of L-carnitine supplementation on fat loss. To date there is no consistent and convincing evidence that L-carnitine supplementation enhances fat oxidation or improves exercise performance in healthy people (Colombani et al. 1996; Trappe et al. 1994; Brass 2000). Recent research (Karlic and Lohniner 2004) has focused on the impact of carnitine on the immune response and the effect that carnitine may have on the prevention of cellular damage and recovery from exercise stress. The data in this area are too new to allow one to draw a conclusion about the benefit of carnitine supplements in athletes. Data do support the clinical use of L-carnitine supplements in the treatment of cardiovascular disease (Ferrari et al. 2004).

DIETARY FAT RECOMMENDATIONS FOR OPTIMAL PERFORMANCE AND HEALTH

As you read in chapter 1, it is frequently recommended that athletes consume diets containing 45% to 65% of energy from carbohydrate; but this is only part of the story. Active individuals also need adequate fat and protein. But what is the appropriate amount of fat? While we need adequate fat to meet the essential FA requirements, we can meet this need with a few grams per day of flaxseed or fish oil. We also need fat as an energy source and to make our diets palatable. Finally, we want a dietary fat intake that promotes good health and prevents chronic disease. Although the optimal fat and carbohydrate intake for the prevention of chronic disease is still being debated in the research literature, we can give the following general guidelines to active people and athletes. These recommendations should be modified according to an individual's food preferences, training program, energy needs, and health status.

- Carbohydrate should be 45% to 65% of energy intake. For diets very high in energy (>4000-5000 kcal/day), a lower carbohydrate intake (% of energy) provides adequate carbohydrate for glycogen replacement. During times of intense training or competition, carbohydrate intake can be increased, depending on individual needs. People should be encouraged to eat whole grains, fruits, vegetables, low-fat dairy products, and meats. Beans and legumes should be included whenever possible to increase fiber intake. On the day and in the hours before competition, athletes may want to eat low-fiber foods to reduce the feeling of fullness. Simple sugars should be used in moderation, representing <10% of total energy intake—except during high training periods, or for individuals who need additional energy for weight maintenance and who are in good health.

- Fat should be 20% to 35% of energy intake, with <10% of energy from saturated fats and the remaining fat coming from monounsaturated (e.g., olive, canola oil) and polyunsaturated fats (e.g., canola, soy, fish, or corn oil). Athletes who prefer lower-fat diets should take care to ensure that they consume adequate essential FAs. People accustomed to high-fat diets can replace whole-fat foods with fat-modified foods, obtaining additional energy from increased use of unprocessed carbohydrates or protein. People who need to reduce body fat should recognize that reduced-fat or fat-modified foods can be energy dense and should be used in moderation.

- Athletes and active people with chronic disease risk factors should modify fat and carbohydrate intake (both type and amount), based, if possible, on their health risk profiles and blood lipid and blood glucose profiles. For active people with family histories of diabetes, hypertension, or cardiovascular disease, more specific dietary recommendations can be made based on blood lipid and glucose profiles or on the degree of hypertension. These individuals may want to consume diets lower in saturated fats and

higher in whole grains, fruits, and vegetables. In people with abnormal blood lipids or glucose levels, high simple sugar intakes or very low-fat diets (which are usually high in carbohydrate) may lower LDL-cholesterol concentrations, but also increase blood triacylglycerols and lower HDL-cholesterol concentrations. The end result may be a blood lipid profile that does *not* improve their overall risk level! It is advisable that people with such conditions monitor their metabolic responses to any diet.

- People with hypertension may want to consider the DASH (Dietary Approaches to Stop Hypertension) diet outlined on p. 100, or diet recommendations of the American Heart Association (Step 1 or 2 diet) or of the American Diabetes Association. For example, the DASH diet has been demonstrated in research settings to decrease hypertension in both normal and hypertensive individuals. It reduced blood pressure by an average of 5.5 mmHg (systolic) and 3.0 mmHg (diastolic) in 459 adults with systolic blood pressure <160 mmHg and diastolic pressures of 80 to 95 mmHg. It worked even better for individuals with high blood pressure: The systolic fell on average 11.4 mmHg, and the diastolic fell 5.5 mmHg. Since this diet contains ~27% of its energy from fat (depending on the food choices made), it should also improve blood lipid profiles in most individuals. Although the diet shown provides only ~2000 kcal/day, it can be modified to provide additional calories, based on total energy expenditure, without changing the overall meal plan. The diet provides adequate carbohydrate (55-60% of energy) for most recreational or fitness athletes, but may need to be increased for elite athletes unless their energy consumption is already high. Although the absolute amount of carbohydrate provided by this diet is ~300 to 320 g/day, this absolute value will increase as energy intake increases. In addition, protein intake is more than adequate at ~100 g/day, depending on the food selected. Finally, since the DASH diet provides only 2000 kcal/day, it may be a good dietary guide for the athletic woman who wants to lose weight or for older active women who want to maintain weight. Energy intake would need to be increased for most male and female athletes in training, since they need more than 2000 kcal/day.

The Dietary Approaches to Stop Hypertension (DASH) Diet Eating Plan

The number of servings shown here is based on a 2000 kcal/day diet. Additional servings for different energy intake needs follow the same basic eating plan at the 2000 kcal/day diet.

Food group	Daily servings	1 serving equals	Examples and notes	Significance of each food group to the DASH eating plan
Grains and grain products	7-8	1 slice bread, 1/2 cup dry cereal* 1/2 cup cooked rice, pasta, or cereal	Whole wheat breads, English muffin, bagels, grits, oatmeal, pita bread, crackers, unsalted pretzels/popcorn	Major sources of energy and fiber
Vegetables	4-5	1 cup raw leafy vegetable 1/2 cup cooked vegetable 6 oz vegetable juice	Tomatoes, potatoes, carrots, peas, squash, broccoli, turnip greens, sweet potatoes, collards, kale, spinach, beans, artichokes	Rich sources of potassium, magnesium, and fiber
Fruits	4-5	6 oz fruit juice, 1 medium fruit 1/4 cup dried fruit; 1/2 cup fresh, frozen, or canned fruit	Apricots, bananas, dates, grapes, oranges, orange juice, grapefruit, grapefruit juice, mangoes, melons, peaches, pineapples, prunes, raisins, strawberries, tangerines	Important sources of potassium, magnesium, and fiber
Low-fat or nonfat dairy foods	2-3	8 oz milk 1 cup yogurt 1.5 oz cheese	Nonfat or 1% milk, nonfat or low-fat buttermilk, nonfat or low-fat yogurt, part nonfat mozzarella cheese, nonfat cheese	Major sources of protein and calcium
Meats, poultry, fish	2 or less	3 oz cooked meats, poultry, or fish	Select only lean; trim away visible fats; broil, roast, or boil instead of frying; remove skin from poultry	Rich sources of protein and magnesium
Nuts, seeds, and dry beans	4-5 servings per week or 1/2 serving per day	1.5 oz or 1/3 cup dried beans 2 tbsp seeds 1/2 cup cooked legumes	Almonds, filberts, mixed nuts, peanuts, walnuts, sunflower seeds, kidney beans, lentils	Rich sources of energy, magnesium, potassium, protein, and fiber
Fats and oils**	2-3	1 tsp soft margarine 1 tbsp low-fat mayonnaise 2 tbsp light salad dressing	Soft margarine, low-fat mayonnaise, light salad dressing, vegetable oil (such as olive, corn, canola, or safflower)	DASH has >27% of energy as fat, including that in or added to foods
Sweets	5 per week	1 tbsp sugar, 1 tbsp jelly or jam, 1/2 oz jelly beans 8 oz lemonade	Maple syrup, sugar, jelly, jam, fruit-flavored gelatin, jelly beans, hard candy, fruit punch, sorbet, ices	Sweets should be low in fat

*Equals 1/2 to 1-1/4 cup, depending on cereal type. Check the product's nutrition label.

**Fat content changes serving counts for fat and oils: For example, 1 tbsp of regular salad dressing equals 1 serving; 1 tbsp of a low-fat dressing equals 1/2 serving; 1 tbsp of a fat-free dressing equals 0 servings.

The basic DASH eating plan can be modified to fit different energy intake needs, as shown next. The table that follows presents a sample one-day menu for a 2000 kcal diet.

Servings per day	1600 kcal	2100 kcal	2600 kcal	3100 kcal
Grains	6.1	7.7	10.4	12.5
Fruits	3.9	5.2	5.3	6.2
Vegetables	3.6	4.4	5.2	5.8
Low-fat dairy	2.4	2.7	3.2	3.7
Meats, poultry, fish	1.4	1.6	2.0	2.3
Nuts	0.4	0.7	0.7	0.8
Fats	1.8	2.5	3.2	4.1

Sample DASH Menu

Item	Amount	Servings
Breakfast		
Orange juice	6 oz	1 fruit
1% low-fat milk	8 oz	1 dairy
Corn Flakes (with 1 tsp sugar)	1 cup	2 grain
Banana	1 medium	1 fruit
Whole wheat bread (with 1 tbsp jelly)	1 slice	1 grain
Soft margarine	1 tsp	1 fat
Lunch		
Chicken salad	3/4 cup	1 poultry
Pita bread	1/2 slice, large	1 grain
Raw vegetable medley:		1 vegetable
Carrot and celery sticks	3-4 sticks each	
Radishes	2	
Loose-leaf lettuce	2 leaves	
Part nonfat mozzarella cheese	1.5 slice (1.5 oz)	1 dairy
1% low-fat milk	8 oz	1 dairy
Fruit cocktail in light syrup	1/2 cup	1 fruit
Dinner		
Herbed baked cod	3 oz	1 fish
Scallion rice	1 cup	2 grains
Steamed broccoli	1/2 cup	1 vegetable
Stewed tomatoes	1/2 cup	1 vegetable
Spinach salad:		1 vegetable
Raw spinach	1/2 cup	
Cherry tomatoes	2	
Cucumber	2 slices	
Light Italian salad dressing	1 tbsp	1/2 fat
Whole wheat dinner roll	1 small	1 grain
Soft margarine	1 tsp	1 fat
Melon balls	1/2 cup	1 fruit
Snack		
Dried apricots	1 oz (1/4 cup)	1 fruit
Mini pretzels	1 oz (3/4 cup)	1 grain
Mixed nuts	1.5 oz (1/3 cup)	1 nuts
Diet ginger ale	12 oz	—

From S.G. Sheps et al., 1997, National Heart Lung and Blood Institute, National Institutes of Health, Bethesda, MD.

As discussed in chapter 2, making carbohydrate recommendations based on grams of carbohydrate per kilogram body weight is probably the best approach when it comes to determining individual athletes' carbohydrate needs. Table 3.4 provides different protein, fat, and carbohydrate recommendations based on diets that contain 55% to 65% of energy coming from carbohydrate. Once you have selected the ideal carbohydrate recommendations for a particular person, you can use this table to make recommendations for protein and fat. The amount of fat consumed in a diet containing 60% of its energy from carbohydrate varies dramatically with the total number of calories consumed. A 176 lb (80 kg) male athlete consuming 5000 kcal/day with 60% of the energy coming from carbohydrate would consume 750 g (3000 kcal) of carbohydrate and 139 g of fat (1250 kcal). This is equivalent to ~9.5 g of carbohydrate per kilogram body weight, which more than exceeds the amount of carbohydrate needed to replace glycogen at a maximum rate, and 1.7 g of fat per kilogram body weight. For this person, a diet with only 55% of its energy from carbohydrate would still provide 688 g of carbohydrate (8.5 g of carbohydrate per kilogram body weight) and 30% of its energy from fat (167 g fat). (See table 3.4 for the complete compositions of these two diets.) For many male athletes, this level of carbohydrate and fat intake would be more realistic and achievable than a diet obtaining 65% of its energy from carbohydrate—yet it would still easily replace muscle glycogen during heavy training periods.

Thus, making carbohydrate and fat recommendations based solely on percentage of energy coming from carbohydrate may not be realistic or even necessary for most individuals with high energy intakes. This is especially true for athletes who are resistant to dietary changes and those who prefer diets higher in fat. For many athletic

Table 3.4 Examples of High- and Moderate-Carbohydrate Diets of Different Energy Levels for Male and Female Athletes

Energy (kcal/day)	Male (80 kg or 176 lb) % of energy from carbohydrate									Female (55 kg or 121 lb) % of energy from carbohydrate								
	5000			4000			3000			3500			2500			2000		
Carbohydrate																		
(% of energy)	70	60	55	70	60	55	70	60	55	70	60	55	70	60	55	70	60	55
g/day	875	750	688	700	600	550	525	450	413	613	525	481	548	375	344	350	300	275
g/kg BW	10.9	9.4	8.6	8.8	7.5	6.9	6.6	5.6	5.2	11.1	9.5	8.8	8.0	6.8	6.3	6.4	5.5	5.0
g/lb BW	5.0	4.3	3.9	4.0	3.4	3.1	3.0	2.6	2.3	5.1	4.3	2.7	4.5	3.1	2.8	2.9	2.5	2.3
Protein																		
(% of energy)	12	15	15	12	15	15	12	15	15	12	15	15	12	15	15	12	15	15
g/day	150	188	188	120	150	150	90	113	113	105	131	131	75	94	94	60	75	75
g/kg BW	1.9	2.4	2.4	1.5	1.9	1.9	1.1	1.4	1.4	1.9	2.4	2.4	1.4	1.7	1.7	1.1	1.4	1.4
g/lb BW	0.9	1.1	1.1	0.7	0.9	0.9	0.5	0.6	0.6	0.9	1.1	1.1	0.6	0.8	0.8	0.5	0.6	0.6
Fat																		
(% of energy)	18	25	30	18	25	30	18	25	30	18	25	30	18	25	30	18	25	30
g/day	100	139	167	80	111	133	60	83	100	70	97	117	50	69	83	40	56	67
g/kg BW	1.3	1.7	2.1	1.0	1.4	1.7	0.8	1.0	1.3	1.7	1.8	2.1	0.9	1.3	1.5	0.7	1.0	1.2
g/lb BW	0.6	0.8	0.9	0.5	0.6	0.8	0.3	0.5	0.6	1.7	0.6	1.0	0.4	0.6	0.7	0.3	0.5	0.6

BW = body weight.

women, who may consume only 2000 to 2500 kcal/day, it is almost impossible to consume the 500 to 600 g of carbohydrate per day frequently recommended for adequate glycogen replacement in men. A diet this high in carbohydrate would not allow for adequate fat or protein. For example, a 121 lb (55 kg) woman who consumed 6 to 7 g carbohydrate per kilogram body weight would need 330 to 385 g of carbohydrate per day. This is equivalent to 1320 to 1550 kcal from carbohydrate or 60% to 70% of energy coming from carbohydrate based on a 2000 kcal/day diet. For this individual the total carbohydrate intake (g/day) is below the 500 to 600 g/day recommendation for men, but the percentage of energy from carbohydrate is at or above the recommended level. This diet would have to be low in fat (18-25% of energy from fat). A more realistic goal might be 60% to 65% of energy from carbohydrate (300-325 g carbohydrate per day) and 25% of energy from fat (similar to the DASH diet shown on p. 100). This diet would still provide adequate protein (1.4 g/kg based on a 121 lb [55 kg] woman). This level of fat intake is achievable without too many restrictions and is acceptable to most active women. It is also prudent for long-term health and weight maintenance.

CHAPTER IN REVIEW

Fat is an important component in the diets of active people. During weeks and months of heavy exercise training, it is recommended that the diet provide 60% to 65% of its energy from carbohydrate, plus adequate amounts of fat (20-35% of energy) and protein, depending on body size and dietary preferences. Fat should not be eliminated from the diet. Athletes or active individuals who limit fat intake to <15% of energy intake need to make sure that they obtain adequate levels of essential fatty acids

and meet the needs for protein and energy. For active individuals who are dieting for weight loss, a lower-fat diet might be recommended (20-25% of energy from fat). Simple sugars should not be used to replace fat in the diet; the emphasis should rather be on whole grains, fruits, and vegetables, plus low-fat meat and dairy products (see the general DASH diet food selection on p. 100). Beans and legumes should be included whenever possible. This type of diet ensures that adequate fiber and micronutrients are consumed along with adequate protein, fat, and carbohydrate. People concerned about body weight should exercise caution when buying low-fat or reduced-fat foods. Products labeled reduced-fat are not necessarily low in calories. It is best to use low-fat versions of whole-fat foods, which provide the same micronutrients, protein, and carbohydrate composition as the full-fat food but are lower in fat and energy (kilocalories and fat per serving). People with risk factors for chronic disease may need to manipulate their dietary intakes based on their disease risk factors and their level of activity. A registered dietitian can help make more specific dietary recommendations in these cases. Finally, it is prudent for all athletes and active people to reduce saturated fat to less than 10% of energy intake in order to help reduce the risk of developing chronic disease.

Although a number of products are marketed to athletes to "improve fat oxidation," no scientific data support the claims of significantly improved fat oxidation. Exercise training is the only method clearly documented in the research literature to improve fat oxidation—a trained individual is a better fat oxidizer than an untrained individual. Exercise training also improves blood lipid and blood glucose profiles and reduces blood pressure, thus reducing the risk of cardiovascular disease, hypertension, and diabetes.

Key Concepts

1. Explain the functions, classifications, and dietary sources of fat.

Dietary fat is a primary source of energy, provides the essential fatty acids and fat-soluble vitamins, and adds flavor and palatability to foods. Fat is part of the structural component of cell membranes and tissues and is the means by which the body stores extra energy. Dietary fats can be classified by their chain length, their level of saturation, their shape, or by the food processing methods applied to the fat (e.g., hydrogenation). Dietary fat is found primarily in the form of triacylglycerols (triglycerides), which contain saturated, monounsaturated, or polyunsaturated fatty acids. Foods with an obviously high concentration of fat, such as butter, oils, and margarine, are called visible fats. Prepared foods that are high in fat, such as cookies, cakes, and desserts, are called invisible fats. Animal foods (meats, dairy, eggs) are generally much higher in fat than plant foods (fruits, vegetables, grains).

2. Compare and contrast the current fat intake of active and inactive individuals.

The body appears to have an unlimited ability to store fat in adipose tissue. In general, active people have lower body fat stores than sedentary people, and women have higher body fat levels than men. Typical fat intake for the general population is ~34% of energy intake, which represents a decrease over the last 30 years from 45% of energy. However, absolute total fat intake (g/day) has increased slightly over the last 5 to 10 years due to an increase in total energy intake. Reported fat intakes of active individuals vary dramatically depending on the sport and gender, with athletes in endurance sports or those who are dieting usually reporting lower fat intakes (<35% of energy from fat).

3. Understand fat metabolism during exercise and the sources of this fat.

Exercise is a strong stimulator of fat lipolysis due to the dramatic increase in blood catecholamines that occurs with exercise. The amount of fat lipolysis, mobilization, and oxidation that occurs during exercise depends on one or more of the following factors: fitness level; the type, intensity, and duration of the exercise; availability of fat reserves in the muscle; the ability to mobilize and transport fatty acids to the muscles; the composition of the meal prior to exercise; and the availability of carbohydrate. Fat mobilized for energy during exercise comes from adipose tissue, intramuscular fat, or fat consumed in the meal before exercise. Fatty acid breakdown, mobilization, and transport from the adipose tissue to the muscle cell employ a number of metabolic pathways and transport proteins. Intramuscular fatty acids can be more readily used as an energy source by the exercising muscle (compared with those from adipose tissue) since no blood transport is required. Regulation of fat oxidation depends primarily on one's ability to mobilize fatty acids from the adipose tissue and to transport these fatty acids to the muscle for uptake, and on the mobilization of fatty acids from intramuscular fats.

4. Identify factors that can enhance or inhibit fat oxidation during exercise.

Increasing one's level of fitness is the primary factor that appears to enhance fat oxidation during exercise. Exercise training increases the body's ability to oxidize fat (1) by increasing the mitochondrial content of the muscle and increasing the activities of various enzymes involved in fat oxidation and mobilization; (2) by increasing fatty acid uptake by the muscle; (3) by enhancing mobilization of fatty acids from adipose tissue; and (4) by improving the cardiovascular respiratory system, which augments oxygen delivery to the muscle. Other factors—for example, high-fat diets (~60-75% of energy from fat), long-chain fatty acids, medium-chain triacylglycerol, caffeine, and carnitine—have been examined as to their ability to improve fat oxidation during exercise. In general, none of these factors appreciably improves fat oxidation during exercise.

5. Discuss the current dietary fat recommendations for active individuals.

Fat intakes of 20% to 35% of energy are generally recommended for active individuals, while extremely low-fat diets (<15% of energy) appear to offer no health or performance benefit. Fat recommendations for individual athletes should be based on the individual's health, current dietary intake, sport, body weight and composition goals, and food preferences.

Key Terms

α-linolenic acid 70

acetyl-CoA 88

acylcarnitine 87

acyl-CoA synthetase 86

carnitine palmitoyl transferase I (CPT 1) 87

carnitine palmitoyl transferase II (CPT 2) 87

chylomicron 85

cis fatty acid 70

cytoplasmic fatty acid binding protein 86

docosahexaenoic acid (DHA) 71

eicosapentaenoic acid (EPA) 71

epinephrine 80

essential fatty acid 70

fatty acid (FA) 72

fatty acid binding protein (FABP) 82

fatty acid translocase (FAT/CD36) 82

free fatty acid (FFA) 80

glycerol 72

hormone-sensitive lipase (HSL) 80

hydrogenation 70

insulin 83

invisible fat 74

linoleic acid 70

lipolysis 80

lipoprotein 85

lipoprotein lipase (LPL) 85

long-chain fatty acid (LCFA) 73

long-chain triacylglycerol (LCT) 93

medium-chain fatty acid (MCFA) 73

medium-chain triacylglycerol (MCT) 94

monoglyceride lipase (MGL) 82

monounsaturated 73

polyunsaturated 73

re-esterification 82

saturated 73

short-chain fatty acid (SCFA) 73

trans fatty acid 70

triacylglycerol (triglyceride) 80

very low-density lipoprotein (VLDL) 85

visible fat 74

Additional Information

Jeukendrup AE, Aldred S. Fat supplementation, health, and endurance performance. Nutrition 2004;20(7-8):678-688.

> Gives an overview of the role of various fats in athletic performance. Reviews long-chain triglycerides, fish oil, conjugated linoleic acid, and medium-chain triglycerides.

Kalmar JM, Cafarelli E. Caffeine: a valuable tool to study central fatigue in humans? Exerc Sport Sci Rev 2004;32(4):143-147.

> Carefully outlines the mechanism for caffeine's ergogenic effect on exercise performance, with specific attention to the central effects hypothesis.

Spriet LL. Regulation of skeletal muscle fat oxidation during exercise in humans. Med Sci Sports Exerc 2002;34(9):1477-1484.

> Excellent overview of the role of carbohydrate and fat as energy substrate during aerobic exercise. Provides in-depth diagrams of the regulation of adipose tissue lypolysis during exercise, energy production in the skeletal muscle, and fat transport and uptake.

National Heart Lung and Blood Institute. The Dietary Approaches to Stop Hypertension—Sodium Study (DASH-Sodium). www.nhlbi.nih.gov/resources/deca/descriptions/dashs.htm.

> This Web page gives an overview of the DASH research study, including methods and results. You can find more about the DASH eating plan at this Web page: www.nhlbi.nih.gov/hbp/prevent/h_eating/h_eating.htm.

References

Achten J, Gleeson M, Jeukendrup AE. Determination of the exercise intensity that elicits maximal fat oxidation. Med Sci Sports Exerc Jan 2002;34(1):92-97.

Achten J, Jeukendrup AE. Optimizing fat oxidation through exercise and diet. Nutrition Jul-Aug 2004;20(7-8):716-727.

Austria JA, Richard MN, Chahine MN, Edel AL, Malcolmson LJ, Dupasquier CMA, Pierce GN. Bioavailability of alpha-linolenic acid in subjects after ingestion of three different forms of flaxseed. J Am Coll Nutr 2008;27(2):214-221.

Beals KA, Manore MM. Nutritional status of female athletes with subclinical eating disorders. J Am Diet Assoc 1998;98:419-425.

Bell DG, Jacobs I, Zamecnik J. Effects of caffeine, ephedrine and their combination on time to exhaustion during high-intensity exercise. Eur J Appl Physiol 1998;77:427-433.

Bell DG, McLellan TM. Exercise endurance 1, 2, and 6 h after caffeine ingestion in caffeine users and nonusers. J Appl Physiol 2002;93(4):1227-1234.

Berning JR. The role of medium-chain triglycerides in exercise. Int J Sport Nutr 1996;6:121-133.

Brass EP. Supplemental carnitine and exercise. Am J Clin Nutr 2000;72(2) suppl:618S-623S.

Brass EP. Carnitine and sports medicine: use or abuse? Ann NY Acad Sci 2004;1033:67-78.

Briefel RR, Johnson CL. Secular trend in dietary intake in the United States. Ann Rev Nutr 2004;24:401-431.

Brouns F, van der Vusse GJ. Utilization of lipids during exercise in human subjects: metabolic and dietary constraints. Br J Nutr 1998;79:117-128.

Burke L. Nutrition for recovery after training and competition. In: Burke L, Deakin V eds. Clinical sports nutrition, 3rd ed. Sydney: McGraw-Hill, 2006;415-453.

Burke LM, Hawley JA. Effects of short-term fat adaptation on metabolism and performance of prolonged exercise. Med Sci Sports Exerc 2002;34(9):1492-1498.

Burke LM, Hawley JA, Angus DJ, Cox RG, Clark SA, Cummings NK, Desbrow B, Hargreaves M. Adaptations to short-term high-fat diet persist during exercise despite high carbohydrate availability. Med Sci Sports Exerc 2002;34(1):83-91.

Callaway CW. The role of fat-modified foods in the American diet. Nutr Today 1998;33(4):156-163.

Calorie Control Council (CCC). National consumer survey. Most popular reduced-fat products. Why people used reduced fat products. Atlanta: CCC, 2006. www.caloriecontrol.org. Accessed Dec 2006.

Carlson MG, Snead WL, Hill JO, Nurjhan N, Campbell PJ. Glucose regulation of lipid metabolism in humans. Am J Physiol 1991;261(24):E815-E820.

Champe PC, Harvey RA, Ferrier DR. Lippincott's illustrated reviews: biochemistry, 4th ed. Philadelphia: Lippincott, 2008;173-200.

Chanmugam P, Guthrie JF, Cecilio S, Morton JF, Basiotis PP, Anand R. Did fat intake in the United States really decline between 1989-1991 and 1994-1996? J Am Diet Assoc 2003;103(7):867-872.

Clarkson PM. Nutritional ergogenic aids: caffeine. Int J Sport Nutr 1993;3:103-111.

Colombani P, Wenk C, Kunz I et al. Effects of L-carnitine supplementation on physical performance and energy metabolism of endurance-trained athletes: a double-blind crossover field study. Eur J Appl Physiol 1996;73:434-439.

Cortright RN, Muoio DM, Dohm GL. Skeletal muscle lipid metabolism: a frontier for new insights into fuel homeostasis. J Nutr Biochem 1997;8:228-245.

Coyle EF, Coggan AR, Hemmert MK, Ivy JL. Muscle glycogen utilization during prolonged strenuous exercise when fed carbohydrate. J Appl Physiol 1986;61(1):165-172.

Coyle EF, Jeukendrup AE, Wagenmakers AJM, Saris WHM. Fatty acid oxidation is directly regulated by carbohydrate metabolism during exercise. Am J Physiol 1997;273(36):E268-E275.

Daniels JW, Mole PA, Shaffrath JD, Stebbins CL. Effects of caffeine on blood pressure, heart rate, and forearm blood flow during dynamic leg exercise. J Appl Physiol 1998;85(1):154-159.

Decombaz J, Arnaud MJ, Milon H et al. Energy metabolism of medium-chain triglycerides versus carbohydrates during exercise. Eur J Appl Physiol 1983;52:9-14.

Dodd SL, Herb RA, Powers SK. Caffeine and endurance performance: an update. Sports Med 1993;15:14-23.

Doherty M, Smith PM. Effects of caffeine ingestion on exercise testing: a meta-analysis. Int J Sport Nutr Exerc Metab 2004;14(6):626-646.

Doherty M, Smith PM. Effects of caffeine ingestion on rating of perceived exertion during and after exercise: a meta-analysis. Scand J Med Sci Sports 2005;15(2):69-78.

Dreon DM, Fernstrom HA, Williams PT, Krauss RM. A very-low-fat diet is not associated with improved lipoprotein profiles in men with a predominance of large, low-density lipoproteins. Am J Clin Nutr 1999;69:411-418.

Dyck DJ, Peters SJ, Glatz J et al. Functional differences in lipid metabolism in resting skeletal muscle of various fiber types. Am J Physiol 1997;272(35):E340-E351.

Ferrari R, Merli E, Cicchitelli G, Mele D, Fucili A, Ceconi C. Therapeutic effects of L-carnitine and propionyl-L-carnitine on cardiovascular diseases: a review. Ann NY Acad Sci 2004;1033:79-91.

FDA Register P99-27. FDA proposes new rules for trans fatty acids in nutrition labeling, nutrient content claims, and health claims. Washington, DC: HHS News. www.fda.gov/bbs/topics/NEWS/NEW00698.html. Accessed Dec 2006.

Fogelholm M, Koskinen R, Laakso J, Rankinen T, Ruokonen I. Gradual and rapid weight loss: effects on nutrition and performance in male athletes. Med Sci Sports Exerc 1993;25(3):371-377.

Fogelholm M, Rehunen S, Gref C et al. Dietary intake and thiamin, iron, and zinc status in elite Nordic skiers during different training periods. Int J Sport Nutr 1992;2:351-365.

Food Processor SQL (software program), Version 10.0. ESHA Research, Salem, OR.

Foster DW. The role of the carnitine system in human metabolism. Ann NY Acad Sci 2004;1033:1-16.

Goedecke JH, Clark VR, Noakes TD, Lambert EV. The effects of medium-chain triacylglycerol and carbohydrate ingestion on ultra-endurance exercise performance. Int J Sport Nutr Exerc Metab 2005;15(1):15-27.

Graham TE. Caffeine and exercise: metabolism, endurance and performance. Sports Med 2001;31(11):785-807.

Graham TE, Hibbert E, Sathasivam P. Metabolic and exercise endurance effects of coffee and caffeine ingestion. J Appl Physiol 1998;85(3):883-889.

Graham TE, Rusch JWE, van Soeren MH. Caffeine and exercise: metabolism and performance. Can J Appl Physiol 1994;19:111-138.

Graham TE, Spriet LL. Metabolic, catecholamine, and exercise performance responses to various doses of caffeine. J Appl Physiol 1995;78(3):867-874.

Graham TE, Spriet LL. Caffeine and exercise performance. In: Sports science exchange. Barrington, IL: Gatorade Sports Science Institute, 1996;9:1-6.

Hawley JA. Effect of increased fat availability on metabolism and exercise capacity. Med Sci Sports Exerc 2002;34(9):1485-1491.

Hawley JA, Brouns F, Jeukendrup A. Strategies to enhance fat utilization during exercise. Sports Med 1998;25:241-267.

Hawley JA, Dennis SC, Lindsay FH, Noakes TD. Nutritional practices of athletes: are they sub-optimal? J Sports Sci 1995;13:S75-S87.

Heird WC, Lapilone A. The role of essential fatty acids in development. Ann Rev Nutr 2005;25:549-571.

Helge JW. Long-term fat diet adaptation effects on performance, training capacity, and fat utilization. Med Sci Sports Exerc 2002;34(9):1499-1504.

Helge JW, Richter EA, Kiens B. Interaction of training and diet on metabolism and endurance during exercise in man. J Physiol 1996;492(1):293-306.

Helge JW, Wulff B, Kiens B. Impact of a fat-rich diet on endurance in man: role of the dietary period. Med Sci Sports Exerc 1998;30(3):456-461.

Horowitz JF, Mora-Rodriguez R, Byerlye LO, Coyle EF. Lipolytic suppression following carbohydrate ingestion limits fat oxidation during exercise. Am J Physiol 1997;273(36):E768-E775.

Horowitz JF, Mora-Rodriguez R, Byerlye LO, Coyle EF. Pre-exercise medium-chain triglyceride ingestion does not alter muscle glycogen use during exercise. J Appl Physiol 2000;88(1):219-225.

Hurley BF, Nemeth PM, Martin WH, Hagberg JM, Dalsky GP, Holloszy JO. Muscle triglyceride utilization during exercise: effect of training. J Appl Physiol 1986;60(2):562-567.

Institute of Medicine (IOM), Food and Nutrition Board. Dietary reference intakes for energy, carbohydrate, fiber, fat, fatty acids, cholesterol, protein, and amino acids (macronutrients). Washington, DC: National Academies Press, 2005.

Ivy JL, Costill DL, Fink WJ, Maglischo E. Contribution of medium and long chain triglyceride intake to energy metabolism during prolonged exercise. Int J Sports Med 1980;1:15-20.

Jeukendrup AE. Regulation of fat metabolism in skeletal muscle. Ann NY Acad Sci 2002;967:217-235.

Jeukendrup AE, Aldred S. Fat supplementation, health and endurance performance. Nutrition 2004;20(7-8):678-688.

Jeukendrup AE, Saris WHM. Fat as a fuel during exercise. In: Berning JR, Steen SN eds. Nutrition for sport and exercise. Gaithersburg, MD: Aspen, 1998;59-75.

Jeukendrup AE, Saris WHM, Brouns F, Halliday D, Wagenmakers AJM. Effects of carbohydrate (CHO) and fat supplementation on CHO metabolism during prolonged exercise. Metabolism 1996;45(7):915-921.

Jeukendrup AE, Saris WHM, Schrauwen P, Brouns F, Wagenmakers AJM. Metabolic availability of medium-chain triglycerides co-ingested with carbohydrate during prolonged exercise. J Appl Physiol 1995;79(3):756-762.

Jeukendrup AE, Saris WHM, Wagenmakers AJM. Fat metabolism during exercise: a review—part I. Int J Sports Med 1998a;19(4):231-244.

Jeukendrup AE, Saris WHM, Wagenmakers AJM. Fat metabolism during exercise: a review—part II. Regulation of metabolism and the effects of training. Int J Sports Med 1998b;19(5):293-302.

Jeukendrup AE, Saris WHM, Wagenmakers AJM. Fat metabolism during exercise: a review—part III. Effects of nutritional interventions. Int J Sports Med 1998c;19(6):371-379.

Jeukendrup AE, Thielen JJHC, Wagenmakers AJM, Brouns F, Saris WHM. Effect of medium-chain triacylglycerol and carbohydrate ingestion during exercise on substrate utilization and subsequent cycling performance. Am J Clin Nutr 1998d;67:397-404.

Jones PJH, Kubow S. Lipids, sterols, and their metabolites In: Shils ME, Shike M, Ross AC, Caballero B, Cousins RJ eds. Modern nutrition in health and disease. Philadelphia: Lea & Febiger, 2006;92-135.

Kalmar JM, Cafarelli E. Caffeine: a valuable tool to study central fatigue in humans? Exerc Sport Sci Rev 2004;32(4):143-147.

Kaminsky LA, Martin CA, Whaley MH. Caffeine consumption habits do not influence the exercise blood pressure response following caffeine ingestion. J Sports Med Phys Fit 1998;38:53-58.

Karlic H, Lohninger A. Supplementation of L-carnitine in athletes: Does it make sense? Nutrition. 2004;20:7-9-715.

Kiens B, Essen-Gustavsson B, Christensen NJ, Saltin B. Skeletal muscle substrate utilization during submaximal exercise in man: effect of endurance training. J Physiol 1993;469:459-578.

Kiens B, Helge JW. Effect of high-fat diets on exercise performance. Proc Nutr Soc 1998;57:73-75.

Lambert EV, Hawley JA, Goedecke J, Noakes TD, Dennis SC. Nutritional strategies for promoting fat utilization and delaying the onset of fatigue during prolonged exercise. J Sports Sci 1997;15:315-324.

Lambert EV, Speechly DP, Dennis SC, Noakes TD. Enhanced endurance in trained cyclists during moderate intensity exercise following 2 weeks adaptation to a high-fat diet. Eur J Appl Physiol 1994;69:287-293.

Lichtenstein AH, Van Horn L. Very low-fat diets. Circulation 1998;98:935-939.

Massicotte D, Peronnet F, Brisson GR, Hillaire-Marcel C. Oxidation of exogenous medium chain free fatty acids during prolonged exercise: comparison with glucose. J Appl Physiol 1992;73(4):1334-1339.

Moss J. Labeling of trans fatty acid content in food, regulations and limits—the FDA view. Atheroscler Suppl 2006;7(2):57-59.

Mougious V, Ring S, Petridou A, Nikolaidis MG. Duration of coffee- and exercise-induced changes in the fatty acid profile of human serum. J Appl Physiol 2003;94(2):476-484.

Odland LM, Heigenhauser GJF, Wong D, Hollidge-Horvat MG, Spriet LL. Effects of increased fat availability on fat-carbohydrate interaction during prolonged exercise in men. Am J Physiol 1998;274(43):R894-R904.

Okano G, Sato Y, Murata Y. Effect of elevated blood FFAs levels on endurance performance after a single fat meal ingestion. Med Sci Sports Exerc 1998;30(5):763-768.

Onywera VO, Kiplamai FK, Tuitoek PJ, Boit MK, Pitslidis YP. Food and macronutrient intake of elite Kenyan distance runners. Inter J Sport Nutr Exerc Metab 2004;14(6):709-719.

Oscai LB, Essig DA, Palmer WK. Lipase regulation of muscle triacylglycerol hydrolysis. J Appl Physiol 1990;69(5):1571-1577.

Pathways of Nutritional Biochemistry. Carnitine and fatty acid synthesis. J Nutr Biochem 1991;2:381.

Romijn JA, Coyle EF, Sidossis LS et al. Regulation of endogenous fat and carbohydrate metabolism in relation to exercise intensity. Am J Physiol 1993;265(28):E380-E391.

Saltin B, Åstrand PO. Free fatty acids and exercise. Am J Clin Nutr 1993;57(suppl):752S-758S.

Saris WHM, van Erp-Baart MA, Brouns F, Westerterp KR, ten Hoor F. Study of food intake and energy expenditure during extreme sustained exercise: the Tour de France. Int J Sports Med 1989;10(suppl 1):S26-S31.

Sheps SG, Black HR, Cohen JD et al. The sixth report of the Joint National Committee on Prevention, Detection, Evaluation, and Treatment of High Blood Pressure. Arch Intern Med 1997;157(24):2413-2446.

Sherman WM, Leenders N. Fat loading: the next magic bullet? Int J Sport Nutr 1995;5:S1-S12.

Sigman-Grant M. Can you have your low-fat cake and eat it too? The role of fat-modified products. J Am Diet Assoc 1997;97(suppl): S76-81.

Spriet LL. Caffeine and performance. Int J Sport Nutr 1995;5:S84-S99.

Spriet LL. Regulation of skeletal muscle fat oxidation during exercise in humans. Med Sci Sports Exerc 2002;34(9):1477-1484.

Thompson J, Manore MM, Vaughan L. The science of nutrition. San Francisco: Benjamin Cummings, 2008.

Thorburn MS, Vistisen B, Thorp RM et al. Attenuated gastric distress but no benefit to performance with adaptation to octanoate-rich esterified oils in well-trained male cyclists. J Appl Physiol Dec 2006;101(6):1733-1743.

Trappe SW, Costill DL, Goodpasture B, Vukovich VD, Fink WJ. The effects of L-carnitine supplementation on performance during interval swimming. Int J Sports Med 1994;15:181-185.

Turcotte LP, Richter EA, Kiens B. Lipid metabolism during exercise. In: Hargreaves M ed. Exercise metabolism. Champaign, IL: Human Kinetics, 1995;99-130.

U.S. Department of Agriculture Center for Nutrition Policy and Promotion. Is total fat consumption really decreasing? Nutrition Insights 1995, vol. 5. Reprinted in Nutr Today 1998;33:171-172.

U.S. Department of Agriculture and Department of Health and Human Services. Dietary guidelines for Americans, 2005. http://www.health.gov/DietaryGuidelines/

Van Zyl CG, Lambert EV, Hawley JA, Noakes TD, Dennis SC. Effects of medium-chain triglyceride ingestion on fuel metabolism and cycling performance. J Appl Physiol 1996(6);80:2217-2225.

Venkatraman JT, Pendergast D. Effects of the level of dietary fat intake and endurance exercise on plasma cytokines in runners. Med Sci Sports Exerc 1998;30(8):1198-1204.

Vistisen B, Nybo L, Xu X, Hoy CE, Kiens B. Minor amounts of plasma medium-chain fatty acids and no improvement time trial performance after consuming lipids. J Appl Physiol 2003;95(6):2434-2443.

Vogt M, Puntschart A, Howald H, Meuller B, Mannhart C, Gfeller-Tuescher L, Mullis P, Hoppeler H. Effects of dietary fat on muscle substrates, metabolism and performance in athletes. Med Sci Sports Exerc 2003;35(6):952-960.

Vukovich MD, Costill DL, Hickey MS, Trappe SW, Cole KJ, Fink WJ. Effect of fat emulsion infusion and fat feeding on muscle glycogen utilization during cycling exercise. J Appl Physiol 1993;75(4):1513-1518.

Westerterp-Plantenga MS. Fat intake and energy-balance effects. Physiol Behav Dec 30 2004;83(4):579-585.

Whalen J, Rust C. Innovative dietary sources of n-3 fatty acids. Ann Rev Nutr 2006;26:75-103.

Wijendran V, Hayes KC. Dietary n-6 and n-3 fatty acid balance and cardiovascular disease. Ann Rev Nutr 2004;24:597-615.

Winder WW. Malonyl CoA—regulator of fatty acid oxidation in muscle during exercise. In: Holloszy J ed. Exerc Sport Sci Rev. Baltimore: Williams & Wilkins, 1998;117-132.

Wolfe RR. Metabolic interactions between glucose and fatty acids in humans. Am J Clin Nutr 1998;67(suppl):519S-526S.

Wolfe RR, Klein S, Carraro F, Weber JM. Role of triglyceride-fatty acid cycle in controlling fat metabolism in humans during and after exercise. Am J Physiol 1990;258(21):E382-E389.

World Anti-Doping Agency (WADA). The World Anti-Doping code. The 2008 prohibited list. International standard. Sep 22, 2007. www.wada-ama.org/rtecontent/document/2008_List_En.pdf. Accessed Aug 2008.

CHAPTER 4

Protein and Exercise

Chapter Objectives

After reading this chapter you should be able to

- describe the functions and classifications of proteins,
- list and describe the primary methods of assessing protein status,
- discuss dietary sources of protein,
- discuss the metabolism of protein during and postexercise, and
- describe the dietary protein recommendations for active individuals.

The role of protein, a required macronutrient, in sport nutrition has been controversial. Before the 20th century, diets of athletes were typically high in protein because protein was considered the primary energy source for exercise. In addition, many cultures believed that consuming the muscle of an animal resulted in a direct transfer of that animal's strength and prowess to the athlete.

However, the primary energy sources fueling exercise are carbohydrate and fat, not protein. Rather, as an essential nutrient, protein has a critical role in the health and performance of athletes. Widespread confusion exists among many exercise professionals and the lay public regarding both the role that protein plays during exercise and the protein needs of active people. The following are some questions frequently posed concerning protein and exercise:

- Do athletes and active people need more protein than sedentary people?
- Do strength athletes have a high protein requirement?
- Can a vegetarian diet provide adequate protein for athletes?
- Are risks associated with high protein intakes or protein supplementation?

This chapter reviews the roles of protein in relation to exercise and addresses these questions. Protein metabolism during exercise is an active area of scientific inquiry. Some of the confusion can be clarified, but more research is needed. Finally, the chapter provides dietary protein recommendations for active people.

FUNCTIONS AND CLASSIFICATIONS

Protein is a nutrient that is critical to both the structure and function of the body. It is more appropriate to use the term "proteins" than "protein," as there are a multitude of proteins in the human body. The three-dimensional shape and sequence of amino acids determine the functional role of any particular protein within the body. Proteins have many exercise-related functions, including the following:

- Proteins serve as building materials for bone, ligaments, tendons, muscles, and organs.
- They serve as enzymes that facilitate reactions associated with energy production and fuel utilization, as well as the building and repair of body tissues, especially muscle.
- They serve as hormones that are involved with energy metabolism (e.g., insulin, glucagon, epinephrine).
- They maintain fluid and electrolyte balance (e.g., blood albumin plays a significant role in maintaining colloidal pressure within blood vessels).
- They assist with the maintenance of acid–base balance.
- Transport proteins carry a number of substances such as micronutrients, drugs, and oxygen within the body (e.g., hemoglobin transports oxygen from the lungs to the working muscle; transferrin transports minerals such as iron; albumin transports micronutrients and drugs) and move nutrients into the cells.
- Proteins can provide energy during and following exercise, particularly in situations of low carbohydrate and energy status.

Protein is unique among the energy nutrients (fat, carbohydrate, protein, and alcohol), since it contains nitrogen (N). Proteins, both in the diet and in the body, are made up of **amino acids** that contain at least one nitrogen amine group. When body proteins are broken down, the amino acids can be oxidized for energy to CO_2 and water; the nitrogen group is eliminated in the urine, primarily as urea. The same is true when extra dietary protein is consumed: The amino acids are oxidized for energy, with the extra nitrogen eliminated as urea. The body does not store extra protein the way it stores dietary carbohydrate as glycogen and extra energy or dietary fat as body fat.

The amino acids found in dietary protein are typically classified as essential or nonessential (see "Classification of Common Amino Acids"), although the essentiality of an amino acid may depend on one's age, genetic makeup, or health status. **Essential**, or **indispensable, amino acids** must be consumed in the diet, while the body can synthesize the **nonessential**, or **dispensable, amino acids**. All amino acids are important for good health, growth, and the maintenance and repair of tissue. "Classification of Common Amino Acids" lists two amino acids as **conditionally essential amino acids** since requirements for them change when synthesis becomes limited or when the diet provides inadequate amounts of precursors (Matthews et al. 2006). For example, the body makes tyrosine from the essential amino acid phenylalanine and makes cysteine from the essential amino acid methionine. If the diet is low in phenylalanine or methionine, the body may not synthesize adequate amounts of these two amino acids, and their essentiality in the diet increases. "Classification of Common Amino Acids" also lists special amino acids that are commonly found in the body, such as 3-methylhistidine, a modification of histidine after the latter is incorporated into muscle. The role of 3-methylhistidine in protein status is discussed later in this chapter.

The current Recommended Dietary Allowance (RDA) for protein, estimated for sedentary healthy adults, is 0.8 g/kg body weight (Institute of Medicine 2005). This value is estimated to meet the daily protein needs of most healthy adults; the unique needs of active adults were not included in this estimation.

In 2005 the Institute of Medicine (IOM) published Dietary Reference Intakes (DRIs) for specific nutrients, including protein (IOM 2005). The DRIs are a set of reference values that include the RDA for protein, which ranges from approximately 0.8 to 1.5 g/kg (or about 0.3 to 0.7 g/lb) depending on age. The DRIs are based on the concept that there is a range of protein intakes for optimal protein utilization. Because exercise increases oxygen

Classification of Common Amino Acids

Essential (Indispensable) Amino Acids

Isoleucine

Leucine

Lysine

Methionine

Phenylalanine

Threonine

Tryptophan

Valine

Histidine*

Nonessential (Dispensable) Amino Acids

Alanine

Arginine

Aspartic acid

Asparagine

Glutamic acid

Glutamine

Glycine

Proline

Serine

Conditionally Essential Amino Acids

Cysteine

Tyrosine

Some Special Amino Acids

Alloisoleucine

Citrulline

Homocysteine

Hydroxylysine

Hydroxyproline

3-Methyhistidine

Ornithine

*The essentiality for histidine has been shown only for infants, but small amounts are also needed for adults.

Adapted, by permission, from D.E. Matthews, 2006, Proteins and Amino Acids. In *Modern nutrition in health and disease*, 10th ed., edited by M.E. Shils et al. (Philadelphia, PA: Lippincott Williams and Wilkins), 26.

transport, fuel utilization, and energy needs and can stimulate tissue growth and repair, there is ongoing speculation that the current RDA may not be adequate for active people. Before discussing the specific protein needs of athletes and active people, we review the assessment techniques used to measure protein status.

METHODS OF ASSESSING PROTEIN STATUS

There are a variety of ways to assess protein status, and each method has its limitations. These methods have been useful in expanding our knowledge of the roles of proteins in exercise. Many of the protein assessment methods are time-consuming and invasive and require sophisticated laboratory equipment. The challenges of these procedures have limited our ability to assess the protein status of large numbers of active people. Furthermore, the information gathered from a traditional method such as nitrogen balance provides a more general perspective regarding protein use by the body, while a contemporary method that employs amino acids to trace protein metabolism can be used to characterize specific aspects of protein use not only by the body, but also by tissues of interest (i.e., skeletal muscle).

Nitrogen Balance

Nitrogen balance involves assessing the relationship between dietary protein intake, which contains ~16% nitrogen, and nitrogen lost from the body. When protein (or nitrogen) intake is greater than the amount lost by the body, one is said to be in **positive nitrogen balance,** or positive nitrogen status. This state is considered to be anabolic and occurs during growth and development, weight gain, pregnancy, lactation, and times of muscle healing or recovery from injury. When protein (or nitrogen) intake is less than the amount excreted, one is in a state of **negative nitrogen balance** or catabolism. This state occurs with weight loss, illness, burns, or injury. When protein (or nitrogen) intake is equal to the amount excreted, one is in nitrogen balance. A state of nitrogen balance typically occurs in healthy adults during times of weight maintenance.

One must consider a number of variables when assessing nitrogen balance. The following are some of the key nitrogen sources that must be estimated or measured in order to determine nitrogen balance in an individual:

- Dietary nitrogen intake (assessed by calculating total protein intake [g/day divided by 6.25] or by directly measuring nitrogen in food)
- Total urinary nitrogen (primarily nitrogen from urea [86-90% of total urinary nitrogen], creatinine [4.5%], ammonia [2.8%], uric acid [1.7%], and other N-containing compounds [5.0%])
- Total fecal nitrogen (primarily nitrogen from undigested proteins, sloughed-off cells, and bacteria within the gut)
- Dermal and other miscellaneous nitrogen losses (primarily nitrogen in exfoliated cells and nitrogen lost in blood, sweat, nails, hair, and semen)

Total urinary nitrogen and fecal nitrogen are directly measured using the **Kjeldahl technique** (Gibson 2005). The Kjeldahl technique uses sulfuric acid to digest the material, a strong base to liberate the nitrogen as ammonia, and a colorimetric assay or titration to determine the nitrogen content. Due to the labor and time required to use this technique, total urinary and fecal nitrogen content is rarely measured outside of a research setting. Instead, urinary urea nitrogen is used to estimate total urinary nitrogen since 85% to 90% of total urinary nitrogen is accounted for by urinary urea nitrogen (Gibson 2005). The use of urinary urea nitrogen to estimate total urinary nitrogen is controversial, and researchers disagree about the extent to which the errors associated with this estimation are clinically significant. This simple method of calculating nitrogen balance using urinary urea nitrogen is sometimes referred to as **crude nitrogen balance** (see "Equations Used to Calculate Nitrogen Balance").

The nitrogen balance procedure is challenging to the volunteer being assessed as well as to the researcher. The volunteer must be willing to perform multiple 24 h urine and fecal collections. The dietary protein intake is best measured if the volunteer follows a standardized diet—which means that all the food he or she eats must be measured before consumption, and duplicate meals must be

Highlight

Equations Used to Calculate Nitrogen Balance

Two equations can be used to calculate nitrogen balance (Gibson 2005). The first estimates total urinary and fecal nitrogen losses. The second estimates nitrogen balance using urinary urea nitrogen and adds a constant value as a single estimate of both total fecal and dermal nitrogen losses.

Equation 1

Nitrogen balance = I − (U − Ue) + (F − Fe) + S

where I = (protein intake in grams) / 6.25 (this gives an estimate of nitrogen intake); U = total urinary nitrogen; Ue = endogenous urinary nitrogen; F = fecal nitrogen; Fe = endogenous fecal nitrogen losses; S = dermal nitrogen losses (nitrogen lost in sweat and sloughed-off skin cells).

Endogenous urinary and fecal nitrogen losses refer to the nitrogen that is excreted in urine or feces on a protein-free diet; although this nitrogen is "lost," these losses within the body are not typically quantified.

Equation 2

Nitrogen balance = (Protein intake in grams / 6.25 − (Urinary urea nitrogen [in grams] + 4*)

*The value 4 is derived by estimating 2 g/day of N lost in feces and from the skin and another 2 g/day from other miscellaneous loses of N in the urine and from the body.

To further simplify the estimation of nitrogen balance, a constant value of 2 g is generally used to account for fecal and dermal losses; an additional 2 g approximates the nonurea nitrogen components of urine and other miscellaneous nitrogen losses (blood, nails, hair, semen) (MacKenzie et al. 1985). This method is sometimes called crude nitrogen balance.

Advantages and Limitations of Methods Used to Estimate Protein Status

Method	Advantages	Limitations
Nitrogen balance	• Relatively accurate measure of protein status • Cost-effective means of monitoring clinical patients if crude nitrogen balance is used	• Time-consuming • Laborious • Subject compliance must be very good • Assesses only net nitrogen status
Tracer methodology	• Can estimate how protein synthesis, oxidation, and degradation contribute to overall protein status • Relatively noninvasive	• Expensive • Requires specialized gas chromatograph-mass spectrometry equipment • Labeled amino acid may not respond in the same manner to exercise as nonlabeled amino acids • Assumptions about certain metabolic issues may not hold true during exercise
3-Methylhistidine	• Noninvasive • Inexpensive • Can be measured in a standard clinical laboratory	• Metabolism of contractile proteins in gut and skin can confound results • Does not indicate protein synthesis, degradation, or oxidation

prepared and analyzed for their nitrogen content. It is imperative that the participant eat only the foods prescribed and that body weight be stable throughout the testing period. Compliance of the participant plays a major role in the accuracy of estimating nitrogen balance. The advantages and limitations of the nitrogen balance method and other methods used to estimate protein status are listed on this page. Although these limitations exist with the nitrogen balance method, nitrogen balance data can be used as a basis for measuring change in response to a diet or exercise intervention and can provide insight regarding the body's use of protein.

Tracer Methodology

A second method of estimating protein status uses labeled exogenous **isotopic tracers** to model protein turnover. Labeled amino acids, specifically ^{13}C, ^{14}C, and ^{15}N, are administered orally or intravenously to "trace" or "follow" the metabolism of their naturally occurring or nonlabeled counterparts. The procedures vary depending on what aspect of protein turnover is being modeled (i.e., whole body vs. individual tissues), but generally involve determining the enrichment or specific activity (ratio of labeled to nonlabeled) of the tracer in body fluids, tissues, and excretion products such as urine and expired air. Figure 4.1 illustrates the single-pool model of whole-body protein metabolism measured with a labeled amino acid tracer (Matthews et al. 2006). The amino acid tracer enters the free amino acid pool, for which amino acids are derived from dietary protein intake, protein breakdown within the body, and the synthesis of nonessential amino acids. The labeled amino acid leaves the free amino acid pool via protein synthesis (i.e., incorporation into body proteins) or amino acid oxidation. Oxidation results in the production of urea, ammonia (NH_3), and CO_2.

This method provides an estimate of amino acid or protein turnover, which is composed of both protein synthesis and protein breakdown. The method is commonly used to estimate the rate at which the labeled amino acid is incorporated into body tissues as an indicator of protein synthesis. See the reports of Wolfe and colleagues (1984) and Matthews and colleagues (2006) for detailed description of tracer methodology. The primary advantage of the tracer method over nitrogen balance is that the former reflects the metabolic fate of an individual amino acid, thereby providing estimates of protein synthesis, oxidation, and degradation. It is important to note, however,

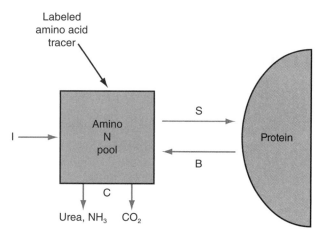

Figure 4.1 Single-pool model of whole-body protein metabolism measured with a labeled amino acid tracer. The amino acid enters the free pool from dietary intake (I) or as amino acid released from protein breakdown (B); it leaves the free pool via amino acid oxidation (C) to urea, ammonia (NH_3), and CO_2 or when used in protein synthesis (S).

Adapted, by permission, from D.E. Matthews, 2006, Proteins and Amino Acids. In *Modern nutrition in health and disease*, 10th ed., edited by, M.E. Shils et al. (Philadelphia, PA: Lippincott Williams & Wilkins), 39.

that the turnover of a single amino acid does not necessarily represent the turnover of all amino acids. Therefore, a number of amino acids have been employed as isotopic tracers in efforts to characterize whole-body protein turnover as well as protein utilization by specific tissues, such as skeletal muscle.

3-Methylhistidine Excretion

Protein status and metabolism, especially in the muscle, can also be estimated by measuring **3-methylhistidine** (3-MH) (also known as N-methylhistidine) in the urine. Most 3-MH, which is formed by the methylation of histidine after it is incorporated into contractile proteins, is found in muscle tissue. Since the body cannot recycle 3-MH from degraded contractile proteins (i.e., muscle tissue), 3-MH is excreted in the urine (Matthews et al. 2006). An increased level of 3-MH in the urine may indicate increased breakdown of the contractile proteins actin and myosin. Since dietary meat confounds the measurement of 3-MH, subjects must follow a controlled diet when this method is employed for assessment of skeletal muscle protein breakdown.

The excretion of 3-MH is expressed as a ratio to creatinine excretion in order to adjust for changes in renal clearance and to correct for individual differences in muscle mass. This method is controversial, the primary objection being that 3-MH is not specific to skeletal muscle breakdown (there are small amounts of contractile proteins in the gut and skin), and that the turnover of these other tissues can contribute significantly to the total 3-MH excreted in the urine (Matthews et al. 2006). Despite this limitation, many researchers value this method as a noninvasive, relatively simple, and inexpensive indicator of protein breakdown.

DIETARY SOURCES OF PROTEIN

Protein is abundant in the American diet and in the diets of other developed countries. While meat and dairy products contain high levels of protein, a significant amount of our dietary protein comes from cereals, grains, nuts, and legumes. Even many fruits (e.g., apricots, blueberries, and apples) and vegetables (e.g., asparagus and green beans) contain small amounts of protein. **Protein quality** is determined by both the amino acid content and the **digestibility** of the protein (IOM 2005). Proteins derived from plant foods are approximately 85% digestible; those in a mixed diet of meat products and refined grains are approximately 95% digestible. Based on these differences in digestibility, it is recommended that people who eat no flesh or dairy products consume 10% more protein daily (or 0.9 g/kg body weight per day compared to the current adult RDA of 0.8 g/kg). This qualification is also based on the protein quality, or "completeness" of the dietary protein.

The term **complete protein** typically refers to proteins that contain all the essential amino acids when consumed at the recommended level of protein intake (Messina and Messina 1996). Complete proteins are considered high-quality proteins. While plant proteins have been generally classified as **incomplete protein,** and perhaps of lesser quality than animal proteins, all of the amino acids appear in plant proteins, but in lower amounts as compared to meat. Thus, one needs to eat more of a plant protein source in order to obtain adequate amino acids. In some cases one must consume more than one source of plant protein in order to obtain all the amino acids. Grains tend to lack lysine, for example, and legumes tend to lack methionine. **Mutual supplementation** involves consuming plant protein sources with complementary amino acid combinations (such as soybeans and rice, wheat bread and peanut butter, pinto beans and corn tortillas) at each meal to obtain sufficient amounts of all essential amino acids from the diet. Studies of adults have shown that it is not really necessary to consume these foods together at the same meal, as the endogenous protein levels in the gut are maintained between meals and can be used for protein synthesis at subsequent meals (Messina and Messina 1996). These findings highlight the importance of consuming high-protein sources throughout the day if one follows a vegetarian diet.

A separate protein requirement does not exist for vegetarians, and the RDA for protein for non-vegetarian adults of 0.8 g/kg body weight is considered sufficient for vegetarians consuming complementary mixtures of plant proteins (IOM 2005). Protein recommendations are also expressed as a percentage of total energy. The acceptable macronutrient distribution range (AMDR) for protein is 10% to 35% (IOM 2005). Contrary to the belief of many, most people in the United States easily meet their protein needs. Active people at risk for inadequate protein intakes are generally those who are not consuming adequate energy.

Table 4.1 reviews the protein content of common foods consumed in the United States. Clearly, individuals who eat a varied diet and consume adequate energy on a regular basis can easily meet the RDA for protein. An example: Doug weighs 180 lb (81.8 kg) and briskly walks 10 miles (16 km) every week. Assuming that his requirement matches the RDA, Doug needs 0.8 g of protein per kilogram body weight, or 65.4 g of protein per day. If he consumes 2/3 cup of oatmeal with 1/2 cup nonfat milk for breakfast and 4 oz (115 g) chicken breast with no skin and 8 fl oz (240 mL) of nonfat milk for lunch, his protein intake from these foods alone is approximately 53 g, or 80% of the RDA—and his energy intake is only 417 kcal! Since Doug typically consumes 2500 to 2800 kcal/day to maintain his body weight, he easily meets his protein needs by eating other foods.

Vegetarians are also quite able to meet their daily protein needs. Messina and Messina (1996) reviewed numerous studies of vegetarians and reported that protein intakes ranged between 12% and 14% and between 10% and 12% of the total energy consumed by lacto-ovo vegetarians and vegans, respectively. Beans, nuts, soy, eggs, and dairy products are excellent protein sources that can be eaten by **lacto-ovo vegetarians** (who eat eggs and dairy products), while people consuming **vegan** diets (no animal products of any kind) can obtain adequate protein from beans, nuts, soy, and other plant sources. It is important that vegetarians consume a wide variety of foods; some may need supplements of micronutrients such as vitamin B_{12}, iron, and zinc. However, both sedentary and physically active vegetarians are capable of meeting their daily protein needs without requiring supplementation if they eat a variety of foods and meet their energy needs.

A common question is, "Don't athletes need more protein?" We discuss this topic in detail later in this chapter. The quick answer is yes. The protein needs of both strength and endurance athletes can be approximately 1.5 to 2.0 times higher than the present adult RDA (Lemon 1998), with the exact amount dependent on a number of factors, including intensity and duration of exercise (Tarnopolsky 2004).

Protein Intake of the General U.S. Population

Large epidemiological surveys have estimated the dietary intake of the U.S. population. The National Health and Nutrition Examination Survey (NHANES 1999-2000) analyzed the energy and macronutrient intakes of persons 2 months of age and older (Wright et al. 2004). The average protein intake of men over age 20 years was 15.5% of total energy and for women was 15.1%. The mean protein intake for men was ~98 g/day and for women ~71 g/day. Table 4.2 lists the protein intakes of the total population of adult men and women surveyed across age groups. The survey did not provide data on intake per unit of body weight.

Another large survey examining the protein intake of Americans was the randomized primary prevention trial (MRFIT, Multiple Risk Factor Intervention Trial) conducted in the United States from 1973 through 1982. The nutrient intake of 12,847 men ages 35 to 57 years was determined prior to intervention (Tillotson et al. 1997). The average protein intake of this population was 16.4% of total energy intake (~99 g protein per day). The participants reported consuming 24% of their energy from meat and 11% from dairy products. Average energy intake was reported to be approximately 2420 kcal/day. Follow-up data from the NHANES I survey showed similar findings, with the average protein intake of 2580 men and 4567 women reported as 16.6% and 17.0% of total energy intake, respectively (Kant et al. 1995).

Table 4.1   Protein Content of Foods Commonly Consumed in the United States

Food	Serving size	Protein (g)
Beef		
Ground, lean, baked (16% fat)	3.5 oz	24.3
Corned beef, brisket, cooked	3.5 oz	18.3
Prime rib, broiled (1/2 in. trim)	3.5 oz	20.9
Top sirloin, broiled (1/4 in. trim)	3.5 oz	27.4
Poultry		
Chicken breast, broiled, no skin	3.0 oz	25.3
Chicken thigh, BBQ, with skin	2.2 oz	14.5
Chicken drumstick, BBQ, with skin	2.5 oz	15.8
Turkey breast meat, roasted, Louis Rich	3.5 oz	19.9
Turkey dark meat, roasted, no skin	3.5 oz	28.7
Seafood		
Cod, steamed	3.5 oz	22.1
Salmon, Chinook, baked	3.5 oz	25.5
Shrimp, steamed	3.5 oz	20.8
Oysters, boiled	3.5 oz	18.6
Tuna, water packed, drained	3.5 oz	29.4
Dairy		
Whole milk (3.3% fat)	8 fl. oz	8.0
1% milk	8 fl. oz	8.0
Nonfat milk	8 fl. oz	8.4
Low-fat yogurt	8 fl. oz	12.9
American cheese, processed	1 oz	6.5
Swiss cheese	1 oz	6.4
Cottage cheese, low fat 2%	1 cup	31.0
Nuts and beans		
Peanuts, dry roasted	1 oz	6.7
Peanut butter, creamy	2 tbsp	8.2
Almonds, blanched	1 oz	6.0
Beans, refried	1/2 cup	6.9
Kidney beans, red	1/2 cup	9.3
Grains and cereals		
Oatmeal, quick, cooked	1 cup	6.1
Malt-O-Meal, cooked	1 cup	3.6
Cheerios	1 1/4 cup	4.3
Frosted Flakes	3/4 cup	1.1
Grape-Nuts	1/4 cup	3.4
Rye bread	1 slice	2.7
Whole wheat bread	1 slice	2.7
Cheez-It crackers	12 crackers	1.2
Triscuit crackers	3 crackers	1.1
Vegetables and fruits		
Banana	1 medium	1.2
Apple, raw with skin	1 medium	0.3
Orange, raw, navel	1 medium	1.3
Asparagus, boiled	1/2 cup (6 spears)	2.3
Green snap beans, canned	1/2 cup	0.8
Broccoli, raw, chopped	1/2 cup	1.3
Mushrooms, raw, pieces	1/2 cup	0.7

Values from Food Processor 7.21, ESHA Research, Salem, OR.

The results of these large epidemiological surveys show that the U.S. population reports eating 16% to 17% of total energy intake as protein. The reported energy intakes from these studies range from approximately 1800 to over 3000 kcal/day for men and from approximately 1400 to 2000 kcal/day for women. Based on these energy intake values, the reported protein intakes are more than adequate to meet the current adult RDA.

Table 4.2 Protein Intake by Sex and Age (NHANES 1999-2000)

Sex and age	Mean intake (g/day)	Energy intake (% of total)
Males		
20-39 years	105	14.9
40-59 years	102	15.8
60-74 years	85	16.1
Females		
20-39 years	74	14.6
40-59 years	69	15.2
60-74 years	65	16.2

Values from "Trends in intake of energy and macronutrients-United States, 1971-2000," *MMWR*, Feb 6, 2004, Vol. 53(4). Available: http://www.cdc.gov/mmwr/PDF/wk/mm5304.pdf

Protein Intake of Active People

Many athletes, particularly those participating in strength- and bodybuilding-related activities, are concerned with meeting their protein needs. This concern has led many athletes to consume large amounts of protein and amino acid supplements to ensure adequate protein intakes. Are athletes and active people eating enough protein? Are supplements needed?

Numerous scientific studies have analyzed the protein intake of athletes. Table 4.3 summarizes data from several representative reports. On average, the reported protein intakes are well above the adult RDA, and many even exceed recommended levels for athletes (see "Dietary Protein Recommendations for Active Individuals" later in this chapter). However, some athletes are at risk for low protein intakes—including female gymnasts, distance runners, figure skaters, and dieting wrestlers. These athletes sometimes compromise their protein intakes by consistently consuming too little energy. Athletes who are unable to consume sufficient energy and therefore sufficient protein due to time constraints, for example, may benefit from protein supplementation. However, the supplement should not be a routine meal replacement, but rather a supplement in the true

Table 4.3 Self-Reported Protein Intakes of Athletes

Reference	Sport type	Sex	Protein intake (g/kg body weight)	Protein intake (% total kcal)
Burke et al. 1991	Triathlon	M	2.0	13
	Marathon	M	2.0	14.5
	Football	M	1.5	15
	Weightlifting	M	1.9	18
Peters and Goetzsche 1997	Ultradistance running	M	1.4	16.7
Keith et al. 1996	Bodybuilding	M	2.7	22.5
Niekamp and Baer 1995	Distance running	M	1.6	12.8
Bolster et al. 2005	Distance running	M	1.7	17.1
Kleiner et al. 1994	Bodybuilding	M	3.1	37.7
Rico-Sanz et al. 1998	Soccer	M	2.2	14.4
Kleiner et al. 1994	Bodybuilding	F	2.7	35.8
Peters and Goetzsche 1997	Ultradistance running	F	1.2	15.1
Felder et al. 1998	Surfing	F	1.5	17
Wiita and Stombaugh 1996	Distance running	F	1.1	14.1
Walberg-Rankin et al. 1993	Bodybuilding	F	1.9[a]	22.6[a]

[a] Average value over five time periods.

sense in that it provides additional energy and protein to assist the athlete in meeting his or her total daily nutrient requirements. The concept of protein or nutritional supplementation is considered with specific regard to nutrient timing in the chapter highlight on p. 121.

METABOLISM OF PROTEIN DURING AND AFTER EXERCISE

Dietary protein is digested into small peptides (single amino acids linked together) and single amino acids. These peptides and amino acids are absorbed by various transport mechanisms in the gut mucosal cells, where peptides are further digested to single amino acids. The single amino acids are then transported to the liver via the portal vein. The liver regulates the release of amino acids into the **free amino acid pool** located in the blood and tissues (see figure 4.2). Small amounts of undigested protein may be lost in the feces. The amino acids in the free amino acid pool are either metabolized for energy or synthesized into new body tissues or other nitrogen-containing compounds. Using the assessment techniques described earlier in this chapter (e.g., nitrogen balance and isotopic tracers), researchers can determine the fate of dietary proteins and individual amino acids during and after exercise.

Protein turnover in the body is dynamic, since amino acids are continuously exchanged between body proteins and free amino acid pools and proteins are always being synthesized and degraded. When a person is in energy and protein balance, there will be no significant change in the size of the total protein pool at the end of a day. However, throughout the course of the day there is a diurnal cycling of proteins, in which gains and losses occur with feeding and fasting (figure 4.3).

Many factors can influence protein metabolism during and following exercise—including exercise intensity, carbohydrate availability, type of exercise, energy intake, gender, training level, and age. The following sections review what we know about how the type of exercise, intensity of exercise, and training status affect protein metabolism. See the work of Lemon (1998, 1995), Tarnopolsky (2004), and Phillips and colleagues (2004) for more detailed reviews of these factors and their relationship with protein metabolism.

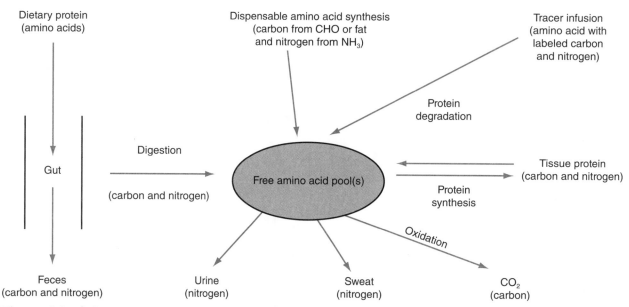

Figure 4.2 Schematic representation of protein kinetics. Shown are the movement and ultimate fate of both carbon and nitrogen from amino acids. All amino acids pass through the free amino acid pool; although only a small percentage of the body's amino acids are found there at any time (the vast majority are in tissue proteins), the importance of the free amino acid pool is indicated by its large size and central location. Nitrogen balance (status) studies assess net nitrogen retention (intake minus excretion), while metabolic tracer studies assess the component processes of protein kinetics (oxidation, synthesis, and degradation/breakdown).

Reprinted, by permission, from P.W. Lemon, 1998, "Effects of exercise on dietary protein requirements," *International Journal in Sport Nutrition* 8: 426-447.

Type of Activity and Protein Metabolism

Resistance and endurance exercise rely on different energy systems for fuel. Resistance training relies primarily on the phosphagen system (stored adenosine triphosphate [ATP] and creatine phosphate) and anaerobic glycolysis to provide ATP for use during exercise. Fatty acids and amino acids are not typical sources of fuel for resistance exercise. On the other hand, endurance exercise, particularly of submaximal intensity, allows for greater oxygen availability, thereby using aerobic mechanisms for ATP production. During endurance exercise, fuel sources can include stored energy (carbohydrate, fat, and to a lesser extent protein). Despite these differences in fuel utilization and the fact that protein is not typically a major energy source in endurance exercise, a single session of either resistance or endurance exercise can influence protein metabolism.

Given that the phenotypical outcomes of routine training between the two modes of exercise differ (strength training leads to increased muscle size and strength while endurance training results in enhanced aerobic capacity), it can be presumed that each type of exercise will uniquely influence protein metabolism.

Resistance Exercise

Changes in muscle size are ultimately the result of alterations in rates of protein synthesis, breakdown, or both. For muscle to grow, rates of synthesis must exceed those of breakdown. Resistance exercise provides the stimulus for muscle growth since training of this type typically results in an increase in muscle protein synthesis postexercise (Phillips et al. 1997; Biolo et al. 1995; Chesley et al. 1992). This increase in synthesis can last for up to 48 h following a resistance training session (Phillips et al. 1997; Phillips 2004). The increase in synthetic rates will also be associated with increased rates of protein breakdown (Phillips et al. 1997; Phillips 2004) unless dietary amino acids are provided, highlighting the importance of nutrient intake following resistance exercise if muscle gain is desired (figure 4.4).

It is a common belief that strength athletes require significantly higher protein intakes than sedentary individuals or endurance athletes. Nitrogen balance studies suggest that strength athletes do require higher protein intakes to maintain nitrogen balance (Tarnopolsky et al. 1992; Lemon et al. 1992; Walberg et al. 1988). Figure 4.5 illustrates the responses of novice bodybuilders to one month of strength training at two levels of dietary protein. On the lower protein intake (0.99

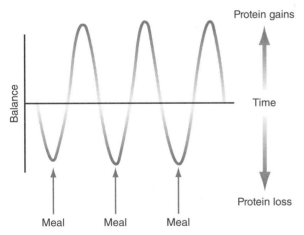

Figure 4.3 A diurnal pattern of feeding and fasting occurs throughout the day, with fasting resulting in protein losses that are restored upon feeding. When persons are in energy and protein balance, the end result is that there are no appreciable gains or losses in protein.

Adapted from *Journal of American College of Nutrition,* vol. 24, "Dietary protein to support anabolism with resistance exercise in young men," pgs. 134S-139S, Copyright 2004, with permission from Elsevier.

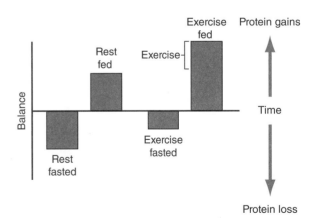

Figure 4.4 Resistance exercise attenuates the negative net balance associated with fasting. However, not until a protein-containing meal is fed does protein balance become positive. Exercise has an additive effect to resistance exercise in promoting positive balance with regard to muscle protein.

Adapted from S.M. Phillips, J.W. Hartman, and S.B. Wilkinson, 2004, "Dietary protein to support anabolism with resistance exercise in young men," *Journal of American College of Nutrition* 24: 134S-139S.

g/kg per day), all but one subject were in negative nitrogen balance. At the higher intake (2.62 g/kg per day), all subjects achieved positive nitrogen balance. Regression analysis indicated that nitrogen balance occurred at a protein intake of 1.43 g/kg per day, while the recommended allowance (requirement + Standard Deviation [SD]) for these strength athletes is 1.6 to 1.7 g/kg per day. Other evidence shows that no further increase in protein synthesis occurs at protein intakes higher than 2.0 g/kg per day (Fern et al. 1991). Lemon (1995) theorized that strength athletes need more protein in order to accelerate the rate of muscle protein synthesis, to decrease the rate of protein breakdown during and following strength training, or both. A recent review by Phillips (2004) suggested that strength athletes need ~1.33 g/kg per day of protein based on nitrogen balance studies.

Gene expression, which refers to the process by which DNA is converted into the structure and functions of a cell (i.e., proteins), can be broken down into two major processes. **Transcription** refers to the process in which DNA is transcribed to mRNA, and **translation** refers to the process in which mRNA is translated into proteins. Over the last decade sport nutrition research has begun to focus on mechanisms at the molecular level that can explain the adaptations that occur in response to exercise. In particular, resistance exercise has

proven to be a stimulus for increasing protein synthesis by increasing rates of translation (Bolster et al. 2003). Amino acids, particularly leucine, are also important in influencing translation (Anthony et al. 2000). Bolster and colleagues (2004) and Kimball and colleagues (2002) provide more comprehensive review of resistance exercise, amino acids, and their molecular regulation.

Endurance Exercise

Studies of the effects of endurance exercise on protein metabolism indicate that moderate- to high-intensity endurance exercise stimulates the oxidation of leucine (Babij et al. 1983; Evans et al. 1983; Hagg et al. 1982). Moreover, blood urea concentrations increase during endurance exercise, resulting in increased urinary urea excretion following exercise. These findings suggest that protein oxidation increases during endurance exercise—and that protein needs of endurance athletes are probably higher than the current RDA. Additional protein may also be required to repair any muscle damage caused by intense endurance training (Lemon 1995; Phillips 2004; Tarnopolsky 2004). Nitrogen balance studies suggest that the dietary protein intake necessary to support nitrogen balance in endurance athletes ranges from 1.2 to 1.4 g/kg per day (Brouns et al. 1989; Friedman and Lemon 1989; Meredith et al. 1989; Gaine et

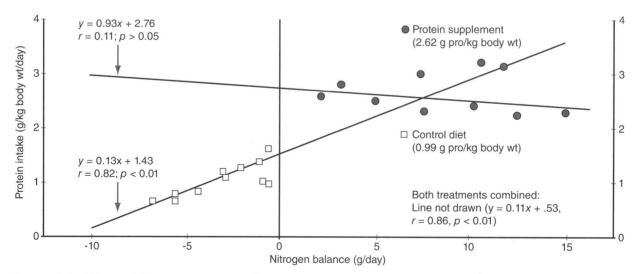

Figure 4.5 Effect of dietary protein intake on nitrogen balance (status). The strong linear relationship between these two variables is lost at high protein intakes (2.62 g/kg per day); based on the lower protein intake (0.99 g/kg per day), the protein requirement (i.e., protein intake at which nitrogen balance occurs at the y-intercept) is 1.43 g/kg per day (200-212% of the current RDA).

Reprinted from P.W. Lemon et al., 1992, "Protein requirements and muscle mass/strength changes during intensive training in novice bodybuilders," *Journal of Applied Physiology* 73: 767-775. Used with permission.

Nutrient Timing: A New Concept

In 2004, Drs. John Ivy and Robert Portman published *Nutrient Timing* , a book that contains innovative concepts (the Nutrient Timing System) designed to help strength training individuals optimize muscle growth and minimize muscle damage. The aim of the book is to shift emphasis in nutritional practices from solely *what* you eat to include *when* you eat. The authors used their expertise in the areas of exercise physiology, performance, recovery, and sport supplementation to compile research in support of the Nutrient Timing System.

The key principle behind the book's claims is that muscle is uniquely sensitive to particular nutrients during its 24 h growth cycle and that improved muscle growth, strength, and power can occur if the right combination of nutrients is delivered to the muscles at the right time. The Nutrient Timing System divides the 24 h growth cycle into three major phases: (1) the energy phase, (2) the anabolic phase, and (3) the growth phase.

Phase 1: The Energy Phase

The energy phase is the workout itself, with the following Nutrient Timing System goals.

Increase Nutrient Delivery to Muscles and Spare Muscle Glycogen

- Providing carbohydrate during exercise will spare glycogen and increase muscular endurance.
- Providing a small amount of protein during or before exercise will spare muscle by decreasing the demand for amino acid release from muscle (particularly the branched-chain amino acids).

Limit Immune System Suppression

- Providing carbohydrate during exercise helps maintain immune function.
- Carbohydrate consumption during exercise also attenuates rise in cortisol (a catabolic hormone).

Minimize Muscle Damage

- Providing carbohydrate during exercise attenuates rise in cortisol and the inflammatory response.
- Providing antioxidants (vitamins C and E) during exercise may be beneficial.

Set the Nutritional Stage for a Faster Recovery Following Your Workout

- Provision of carbohydrate and protein during exercise minimizes glycogen usage, immune system suppression, and muscle damage, thereby allowing for faster recovery.
- The protein ingested during exercise can set the stage for an increase in protein synthesis postexercise.

Phase 2: The Anabolic Phase

The anabolic phase is the 45 min period postexercise, which has the following Nutrient Timing System goals.

Shift Metabolic Machinery From a Catabolic State to an Anabolic State

- Carbohydrate and protein (3:1 to 4:1 ratio) consumption postexercise stimulates insulin (anabolic hormone).
- Carbohydrate and protein intake following exercise blunts cortisol release.

Speed the Elimination of Metabolic Wastes (i.e., Lactic Acid) by Increasing Muscle Blood Flow

- Increased insulin increases blood flow.
- Nitric oxide (synthesized from the amino acid arginine) can increase blood flow.

(continued)

Replenish Muscle Glycogen Stores

- Immediate carbohydrate ingestion postexercise is most effective in replenishing glycogen.
- Evidence indicates that the addition of protein to carbohydrate aids in replenishment.

Initiate Tissue Repair and Set the Stage for Muscle Growth

- Protein consumption postexercise is critical in maximizing synthetic response to resistance exercise.
- The addition of carbohydrate provides further stimulation of insulin release, thereby further increasing synthetic rates.

Reduce Muscle Damage and Bolster the Immune System

- Consuming a protein and carbohydrate postexercise may reduce soreness, infections, and joint problems.
- The restoration of glutamine (an amino acid important in immune function) that occurs following consumption of protein and carbohydrate postexercise may contribute to enhanced immunity.

Phase 3: The Growth Phase

The growth phase is the 18 to 24 h period when the majority of muscle and strength gains occur. This phase is divided into two segments: (1) the rapid segment (1 to 5 h postexercise) and (2) the sustained segment (5 h postexercise until your next workout).

Nutrient Timing System Goals for the Rapid Segment

Maintain Insulin Sensitivity

- Carbohydrate and protein consumed during the anabolic phase and during the rapid segment maintain muscle's anabolic activity for up to 3 to 4 h after the anabolic phase.
- Carbohydrate and protein consumed during the anabolic phase and during the rapid segment, maintain muscle's anabolic sensitivity for up to 3 to 4 h after the anabolic phase.

Maintain Anabolic State

- Small feedings of carbohydrate and protein every 1 to 2 h postexercise maintain elevated rates of protein synthesis.
- Glycogen replenishment occurs with frequent consumption of carbohydrate and protein.

Nutrient Timing System Goals for the Sustained Segment

Maintain Positive Nitrogen Balance and Stimulate Protein Synthesis

- It is important to consume enough protein throughout training to meet your needs (see protein recommendations section).
- Consuming adequate protein helps to maintain nitrogen balance and ensure that amino acids are available to sustain protein synthesis and reduce protein breakdown.

Promote Protein Turnover and Muscle Development

- Maintain elevated blood levels of amino acids by regularly consuming protein-containing meals and snacks throughout the day.
- Consume adequate energy from carbohydrate and fat to ensure amino acids are not used as fuel source.

Adapted from J. Ivy and R. Portman, 2004, *Nutrient timing* (Laguna Beach, CA: Basic Health Publications, Inc.).

al. 2006). See table 4.4 for an overview of protein intakes required to achieve nitrogen balance.

Protein contributes to energy production during and after exercise in the following ways:

- Amino acids can become substrates for gluconeogenesis to prevent hypoglycemia.
- Amino acids can be converted to Krebs cycle intermediates and contribute to acetyl-CoA oxidation (see figure 4.6).
- Amino acids can be oxidized directly in the muscles for energy.

Endurance exercise affects not only whole-body protein turnover but also skeletal muscle protein turnover. A limited number of studies have examined human skeletal muscle protein turnover in response to endurance exercise. Research in humans has shown that walking (Sheffield-Moore et al. 2004; Carraro et al. 1990) and swimming (Tipton et al. 1996) exercise stimulate mixed muscle protein synthesis in the recovery period. The effects of endurance exercise on muscle protein breakdown in humans have not been studied using direct measurements. Similar to research on resistance training, studies addressing the effects of nutrient intake after endurance exercise highlight the importance of eating immediately after a

Table 4.4 Protein Levels Required for Nitrogen Balance

Endurance exercise	Sex	$\dot{V}O_2$max (mL · kg^{-1} · min^{-1})	Protein (g/kg per day)
Meredith et al. 1989	Males	55 (older) 55 (young)	0.94
Tarnopolsky et al. 1988	Males	76	1.6
Friedman and Lemon 1989	Males	65	1.49
Gaine et al. 2006	Males	71	1.2

Resistance exercise	Sex	Training status	Protein (g/kg per day)
Tarnopolsky et al. 1992	Males	Trained	1.41
Tarnopolsky et al. 1988	Males	Trained	1.2
Lemon et al. 1992	Males	Untrained	1.4-1.5

workout. In one study, consuming a protein–carbohydrate supplement immediately postexercise, but not 3 h postexercise, resulted in positive muscle protein balance and a more positive whole-body protein balance (Levenhagen et al. 2001).

Effect of Exercise Intensity on Protein Metabolism

Babij and colleagues (1983) found that oxidation of leucine increased linearly with exercise intensity (figure 4.7)—indicating that the body increases its use of amino acids during endurance exercise and that high-intensity exercise results in greater oxidation of amino acids. And if endurance athletes are increasing their oxidation of amino acids, they clearly need to increase their intake of protein.

The mechanism responsible for this increase in leucine oxidation appears to be an increase in the activity of **branched-chain lactoacid dehydrogenase,** which is the rate-limiting enzyme in the oxidation of the BCAAs (branched-chain amino acids—leucine, isoleucine, and valine) (Kasperek and Snider 1987). Exercise performed at less than 55% to 60% $\dot{V}O_2$max does not appear to stimulate amino acid oxidation (Todd et al. 1984; Butterfield and Calloway 1984).

Energy and Carbohydrate Availability

The link between energy availability and protein utilization has been recognized for over 50 years. When energy intake is not sufficient, there is an increase in the use of protein for energy-yielding functions rather than for the more preferred functional and structural roles of protein (Calloway and Spector 1954). Since carbohydrate is one of the primary fuel sources for endurance exercise, carbohydrate or glycogen availability has been shown to be directly related to protein utilization during exercise. When carbohydrate stores are limiting (i.e., glycogen depletion), there is an increase in the oxidation of amino acids for fuel during exercise. This scenario can occur in persons whose training diet is insufficient to replenish glycogen used during glycogen-depleting exercise of high intensities and long duration.

Gender Effects on Protein Metabolism

The majority of studies regarding exercise and protein utilization have involved the use of male

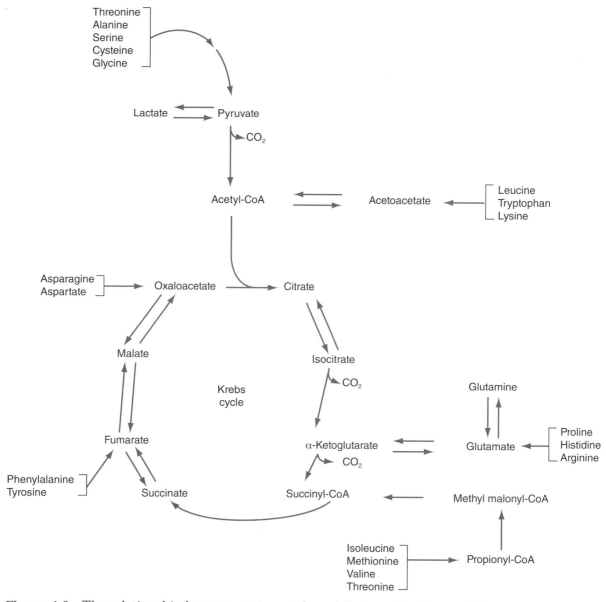

Figure 4.6 The relationship between amino acids and Krebs cycle intermediates.

Adapted, by permission, from P.C. Champe, R.A. Harvey, and D.R. Ferrier, 2008, *Lippincott's illustrated reviews: Biochemistry,* 4th ed. (Philadelphia, PA: Lippincott Williams & Wilkins), 269.

subjects. However, there is evidence of gender differences in protein utilization in response to exercise. It has been shown that females rely to a greater extent on fat for fuel during exercise while oxidizing fewer amino acids and excreting less nitrogen than males (Tarnopolsky 2004; Tarnopolsky et al. 1990; Phillips et al. 1993). Further exploration into gender differences in protein metabolism for resistance and endurance exercise, as well as the mechanisms responsible for these differences, is needed.

Changes in Protein Metabolism Resulting From Training Adaptations

Although many studies show that protein turnover (and therefore protein requirements) increases with exercise, Butterfield (1987) has cautioned that the body may adapt to exercise training over time, with protein needs returning to baseline levels. Butterfield (1987) suggested that the tran-

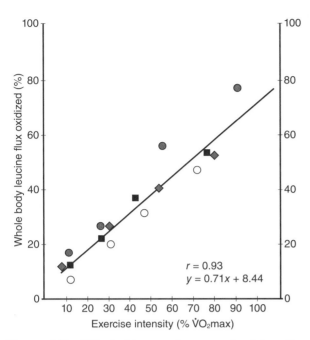

Figure 4.7 Effect of increasing exercise intensity on oxidation of the amino acid leucine. As the intensity of endurance exercise increases, there is a nearly linear increase in amino acid oxidation.

Adapted from P. Babij, S.M. Matthews, and M.J. Rennie, 1983, "Changes in blood ammonia, lactate and amino acids in relation to workload during bicycle ergometer exercise in man," *European Journal of Applied Physiology and Occupational Physiology* 50: 405-411.

sient change in protein metabolism occurs for 12 to 14 days after the initiation of training, and that protein metabolism returns to baseline levels after three to four weeks of training. Figure 4.9 shows that individuals initiating a cycling program experienced a negative nitrogen balance with the initiation of training, but that nitrogen balance was restored after 20 days of training with no change in dietary protein intake (Gontzea et al. 1975). A number of studies support these observations, having demonstrated that endurance exercise training results in a "more efficient" handling of protein by the body, with improvements in nitrogen balance and decreases in leucine oxidation noted following training (Butterfield and Calloway 1984; Gaine et al. 2005).

That said, the concept of accommodation versus adaptation, put forth by Young and colleagues, must be considered (Young et al. 1989). **Accommodation** refers to the achievement of nitrogen balance resulting from a downregulation of physiological processes in order to retain nitrogen, whereas **adaptation** refers to a level of protein intake that is sufficient to promote synthesis of enzymes, growth

of capillaries, and support immune function necessary for the beneficial adaptations to endurance training to occur. Therefore, the improvements in protein utilization in response to endurance exercise that occur without changes in protein intake may be an accommodation response, and a greater protein intake may be more beneficial to optimize endurance training adaptations.

DIETARY PROTEIN RECOMMENDATIONS FOR ACTIVE INDIVIDUALS

The following recommendations are based on many of the aforementioned studies of protein metabolism during and following exercise:

- People who regularly engage in endurance activities need dietary protein intake of 0.55 to 0.64 g/lb body weight per day (1.2-1.4 g/kg body weight per day, or 1.5 to 1.75 times the current adult RDA).

- People who regularly engage in strength exercise need dietary protein intake of 0.73 to 0.77 g/lb body weight per day (1.6-1.7 g/kg body weight per day, or 2.0 to 2.1 times the current adult RDA).

Since protein turnover is an energy-requiring process, optimal use of dietary protein by the body requires that the energy needs of the individual be met. Increasing protein intake while energy intake is adequate and constant does not improve nitrogen balance or protein utilization (Calloway and Spector 1954). Consumption of protein in excess of what is needed for maintenance, synthesis, or repair of proteins is of little benefit to the body, as this leads to an increase in the oxidation of protein as a fuel source (Bolster et al. 2005). As a result, energy balance, or the consumption of adequate calories to meet those expended, is important to protein metabolism so that amino acids are spared for protein synthetic processes and not oxidized to assist in meeting energy needs. Since exercise training contributes to energy expenditure, participation in routine exercise programs challenges this relationship. Attention to energy intake is therefore of particular importance with regard to training-specific nutritional strategies focused on optimal protein utilization.

Many nutrition professionals are concerned that the high protein intakes of some athletes can have adverse effects (Lemon 1998), including

Amino Acid Supplementation and Central Fatigue Hypothesis

The **central fatigue hypothesis (CFH)** was first proposed by Newsholme and coworkers in 1987 as a possible mechanism contributing to the onset of fatigue during endurance exercise. In brief, there are two causes of fatigue resulting from prolonged aerobic exercise: peripheral fatigue and central fatigue. **Peripheral fatigue** is the failure of the individual to maintain the expected power or force needed to continue the exercise bout due to changes in the peripheral environment, including the depletion of fuel sources to the muscle (low blood glucose or reduced muscle glycogen, for example) or an increase in lactate. In contrast, **central fatigue** is associated with specific alterations in the function of the central nervous system that are not explained by peripheral markers of fatigue (Gleeson 2005). The CFH is based on the premise that an increase in serotonin levels in the brain during exercise results in the perception of fatigue. The relation between protein, or amino acids in particular, to the onset of central fatigue is illustrated in figure 4.8.

The critical endpoint is the production of the neurotransmitter serotonin (5-hydroxytryptamine, 5-HT) in the brain. Tryptophan, an essential amino acid, is the precursor to serotonin. Tryptophan circulates in the blood either bound to albumin or as free tryptophan. Transport of tryptophan into the brain is dependent on the concentration of free tryptophan in the blood and the ability of free tryptophan to compete successfully with the **branched-chain amino acids** or **BCAA** (leucine, isoleucine, valine) for transport into the brain. Therefore, the ratio of free tryptophan to the BCAA in the blood can hypothetically affect the amount of serotonin produced in the brain, thereby influencing an individual's perception of fatigue (Newsholme and Blomstrand 2006). Since free fatty acids (FFAs) compete more effectively than tryptophan for albumin, an increase in circulating FFAs increases the amount of free tryptophan.

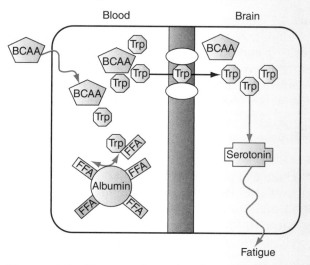

The CFH is based on the notion that the typical substrate profile associated with

Figure 4.8 Proposed mechanism for central fatigue.

submaximal exercise of prolonged duration sets the stage for central fatigue by increasing the transport of free tryptophan to the brain and increasing serotonin production. The following are the changes that occur in circulating levels of BCAA, FFAs, and free tryptophan during exercise to predispose an endurance athlete to central fatigue:

- An increase in the uptake of BCAA by muscle for energy
- An increase in blood FFAs as they are mobilized to fuel the muscles
- An increase in circulating free tryptophan since FFAs are binding to albumin
- An increase in the ratio of free tryptophan to BCAA
- An increase in brain tryptophan levels as tryptophan more effectively competes for transport across the blood–brain barrier
- Increased production of serotonin due to increased tryptophan and the perception of fatigue

Given the basis for the CFH, it may seem logical to supplement with protein, or more specifically the BCAA, to prevent the onset of central fatigue during endurance exercise. Theoretically, an increase in the BCAA should decrease the free tryptophan:BCAA ratio, thereby limiting free tryptophan entry into the brain (Gleeson 2005; Newsholme and Blomstrand 2006). Unfortunately, there is no scientific evidence to date to support the benefit of such supplementation practices to the athlete or to athletic performance. More research is needed to determine whether or not consumption of BCAA-rich proteins or individual BCAA supplementation prior to or during endurance exercise can prevent the onset of central fatigue.

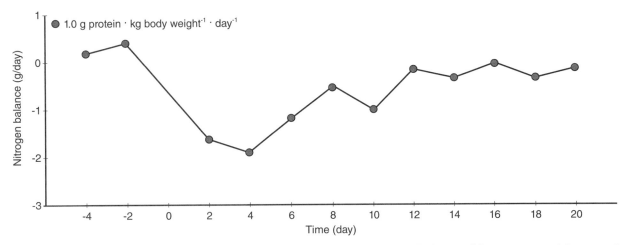

Figure 4.9 Effect of several weeks of endurance training on nitrogen balance. Men consumed 1 g protein per kilogram body weight per day for 12 days before and 20 days after initiation of a cycling program. Note that nitrogen balance is no longer negative (or restored) by day 12.

This article was published in *Nutrition Reports International,* Vol 11, I. Gontzea, P. Sutzescu, and S. Dumitrache, "The influence of adaptation to physical effort on nitrogen balance in man," pgs. 231-236, Copyright Elsevier 1975.

- renal damage,
- increased urinary calcium excretion,
- increased serum lipoprotein levels and higher risk for heart disease,
- dehydration, and
- possible toxicity from large doses of individual amino acids.

Some of these adverse effects appear only in certain populations. High-protein diets are dangerous for people with kidney or liver disease, for example, but have not been shown to cause damage in healthy individuals (Martin et al. 2006). Protein consumption increases the excretion of urinary calcium, but its impact on the retention of calcium is debatable (IOM 1997). Urinary calcium loss appears to occur only in people who obtain their additional protein from purified protein supplements (vs. from foods, which also contain phosphorus). Dehydration may occur as a result of increased water loss from additional nitrogen excretion that occurs with higher protein intakes; therefore athletes consuming higher-protein diets should be attentive to fluid intake (Martin et al. 2006). Athletes and active people should assess

their current protein intake to determine if an increase is warranted. Although no one should exceed the recommendations listed previously, there is no evidence to suggest that protein intake of 1.2 to 2.0 times the RDA is hazardous for basically healthy people (Martin et al. 2005).

CHAPTER IN REVIEW

This chapter has reviewed the important role of protein in supporting exercise and ensuring adequate recovery from exercise. Studies of nitrogen balance and metabolic tracers show that strength athletes and endurance athletes need more protein than most people—but only about 1.2 to 2.0 times the current adult RDA, which is lower than the protein level many athletes already consume and within the AMDR for protein. By consuming adequate energy and a varied diet, most athletes—including vegetarians—can obtain adequate dietary protein without the need for supplements. People following higher-protein diets should drink extra fluids to avoid becoming dehydrated; people at risk for heart or kidney disease or for bone loss should avoid excessive protein.

Key Concepts

1. Describe the functions and classifications of proteins.

Proteins serve as critical components of building materials for bone, ligaments, tendons, muscles, and organs. Proteins are also enzymes and hormones; they assist with maintaining fluid and acid–base balance; and they are an important energy source during and following exercise. Amino acids are classified as essential or nonessential; both classes are critical for health, growth, and maintenance and repair of tissue.

2. List and describe the primary methods of assessing protein status.

The three primary assessment methods are nitrogen balance, isotopic tracers, and 3-methylhistidine excretion. Each method has advantages and limitations. While nitrogen balance gives a good indication of whole-body nitrogen balance, it cannot estimate protein synthesis, oxidation, or degradation. Tracer methods can estimate these variables, but these methods are expensive and do not necessarily reflect the activity of all amino acids. The 3-methylhistidine method indicates degradation levels of contractile proteins but is confounded by dietary meat intake and by excretion of contractile proteins from the gut and skin.

3. Discuss dietary sources of protein.

Protein is abundant in the U.S. diet, with meat and dairy products containing high amounts of protein. Adequate protein can also be obtained in the vegetarian diet: Cereals, grains, nuts, and legumes contain significant amounts of protein, and mutual supplementation can be used to obtain complete protein. The U.S. population generally consumes adequate dietary protein, but athletes with low energy intakes are vulnerable to inadequate protein intakes.

4. Discuss the metabolism of protein during and postexercise.

Protein plays many roles during and after exercise. Amino acids are used as substrates for gluconeogenesis and as Krebs cycle intermediates; they also are used for energy in the muscle and for building and repair of tissues following exercise. Protein utilization is affected by exercise intensity and duration, training level, energy intake, and carbohydrate availability. Debate continues as to the protein needs of active people. Although rigorous training can temporarily cause a negative nitrogen balance, nitrogen balance can be restored once the body has adapted to the training.

5. Describe the dietary protein recommendations for active individuals.

The protein intake for people regularly participating in endurance activities should be about 0.55 to 0.64 g/lb per day (or 1.2-1.4 g/kg per day, 1.5-1.75 times the current adult RDA). The protein intake of people regularly engaging in strength exercise should be about 0.73 to 0.77 g/lb per day (or 1.6-1.7 g/kg per day, 2.0-2.1 times the current adult RDA).

Key Terms

3-methylhistidine 114

accommodation 125

adaptation 125

amino acid 110

branched-chain amino acid
  (BCAA) 126

branched-chain lactoacid dehydrogenase 123

central fatigue 126

central fatigue hypothesis (CFH) 126

complete protein 114

conditionally essential amino acid 110

Additional Information

Burke L, Deakin V. Clinical sports nutrition, 3rd ed. Sydney, Australia: McGraw-Hill, 2006.

> This is an edited reference book for sport nutrition professionals, sports medicine practitioners, coaches, trainers, and students of sport nutrition or sport science. Topics include exercise physiology and metabolism, assessment of nutritional status in athletes, energy and macronutrient requirements of athletes, weight loss and making weight in athletes, disordered eating, and micronutrient needs. The book also covers special topics such as the female athlete triad, the aging athlete, athletes with special needs, and supplements.

Burke L. Practical sports nutrition. Champaign, IL: Human Kinetics, 2007.

> This book provides information that is applied, practical, and useful to the health professional working with athletes in a number of different sports—road cycling, swimming, sprinting, long-distance running, and many others. Each chapter offers a comprehensive review of competition, training, physique and physiology, lifestyle and culture, dietary surveys, sport foods and supplements—all tailored to the specific sport. Also included are discussions of issues and challenges arising in each sport, with useful examples of how to successfully tackle sport-specific problems.

Dunford M. ed. Sports nutrition: a practice manual for professionals, 4th ed.United States: American Dietetic Association, 2005.

> This manual was written by the Sports, Cardiovascular and Wellness Nutritionists (SCAN) dietetics practice group (DPG) of the American Dietetic Association. The manual is designed to deliver the essential information that health and fitness professionals need in order to work with athletes of all ages and proficiency levels. Topics are presented in four sections: "Sports Nutrition Basics," "Screening and Assessment," "Sports Nutrition Across the Life Cycle," and "Sport Specific Guidelines." The "At-A-Glance" feature provides sport-specific information for 18 sports.

Protein and protein hydrolysates in sports nutrition (suppl). Int J Sport Nutr Exerc Metab 2007;17:S1-S117.

> This supplement to the journal comprises a series of papers by researchers in exercise science and protein metabolism that provide an overview of various aspects of the application of protein and protein hydrolysates in sport nutrition. Two articles from this supplement are highlighted here, but other topics include protein digestion and absorption, use of amino acids by the brain, protein requirements for active individuals, the interaction of protein and carbohydrate, and the role of protein and protein hydrolysates in improving postexercise recovery. In particular, see (1) van Loon LJ, Kies AK, Saris WH, "Protein and protein hydrolysates in sports nutrition," S1-S4, and (2) van Loon LJ, "Application of protein or protein hydrolysates to improve postexercise recovery," S103-S116.

References

Anthony JC, Anthony TG, Kimball SR, Vary TC, Jefferson LS. Orally administered leucine stimulates protein synthesis in skeletal muscle of postabsorptive rats in association with increased eIF4F formation. J Nutr 2000;130:139-145.

Babij P, Matthews SM, Rennie MJ. Changes in blood ammonia, lactate and amino acids in relation to workload during bicycle ergometer exercise in man. Eur J Appl Physiol Occup Physiol 1983;50:405-411.

Biolo G, Maggi SP, Williams BD, Tipton KD, Wolfe RR. Increased rates of muscle protein turnover and amino acid transport after resistance exercise in humans. Am J Physiol 1995;268:E514-E520.

Bolster DR, Jefferson LS, Kimball SR. Regulation of protein synthesis associated with skeletal muscle hypertrophy by insulin-, amino acid- and exercise-induced signalling. Proc Nutr Soc 2004;63:351-356.

Bolster DR, Kubica N, Crozier SJ et al. Immediate response of mammalian target of rapamycin (mTOR)-mediated signalling following acute resistance exercise in rat skeletal muscle. J Physiol 2003;553:213-220.

Bolster DR, Pikosky MA, Gaine PC et al. Dietary protein intake impacts human skeletal muscle protein fractional synthetic rates after endurance exercise. Am J Physiol Endocrinol Metab 2005;289:E678-E683.

Brouns F, Saris WH, Stroecken J et al. Eating, drinking, and cycling. A controlled Tour de France simulation study, part II. Effect of diet manipulation. Int J Sports Med 1989;10 suppl 1:S41-S48.

Burke LM, Gollan RA, Read RSD. Dietary intakes and food use of groups of elite Australian male athletes. Int J Sport Nutr 1991;1:378-394.

Butterfield GE. Whole-body protein utilization in humans. Med Sci Sports Exerc 1987;19:S157-S165.

Butterfield GE, Calloway DH. Physical activity improves protein utilization in young men. Br J Nutr 1984;51:171-184.

Calloway DH, Spector H. Nitrogen balance as related to caloric and protein intake in active young men. Am J Clin Nutr 1954;2:405-412.

Carraro F, Stuart CA, Hartl WH, Rosenblatt J, Wolfe RR. Effect of exercise and recovery on muscle protein synthesis in human subjects. Am J Physiol 1990;259:E470-E476.

Champe PC, Harvey RA, Ferrier DR. Lippincott's illustrated reviews: biochemistry, 4th ed. Philadelphia: Lippincott Williams & Wilkins, 2008.

Chesley A, MacDougall JD, Tarnopolsky MA, Atkinson SA, Smith K. Changes in human muscle protein synthesis after resistance exercise. J Appl Physiol 1992;73:1383-1388.

Evans WJ, Fisher EC, Hoerr RA, Young VR. Protein metabolism and endurance exercise. Phys Sportsmed 1983;63-72.

Felder JM, Burke LM, Lowdon BJ, Cameron-Smith D, Collier GR. Nutritional practices of elite female surfers during training and competition. Int J Sport Nutr 1998;8:36-48.

Fern EB, Bielinski RN, Schutz Y. Effects of exaggerated amino acid and protein supply in man. Experientia 1991;47:168-172.

Friedman JE, Lemon PW. Effect of chronic endurance exercise on retention of dietary protein. Int J Sports Med 1989;10:118-123.

Gaine PC, Pikosky MA, Martin WF, Bolster DR, Maresh CM, Rodriguez NR. Level of dietary protein impacts whole body protein turnover in trained males at rest. Metabolism Apr 2006;55(4):501-507.

Gaine PC, Viesselman CT, Pikosky MA et al. Aerobic exercise training decreases leucine oxidation at rest in healthy adults. J Nutr 2005;135:1088-1092.

Gibson RS. Principles of nutritional assessment, 2nd ed. New York: Oxford University Press, 2005.

Gleeson M. Interrelationship between physical activity and branched-chain amino acids. J Nutr 2005;135:1591S-1595S.

Gontzea I, Sutzescu P, Dumitrache S. The influence of adaptation to physical effort on nitrogen balance in man. Nutr Rep Int 1975;11:231-236.

Hagg SA, Morse EL, Adibi SA. Effect of exercise on rates of oxidation, turnover, and plasma clearance of leucine in human subjects. Am J Physiol 1982;242:E407-E410.

Institute of Medicine (IOM), Food and Nutrition Board, National Academy of Sciences. Dietary reference intakes. Calcium, phosphorus, magnesium, vitamin D, and fluoride. Washington, DC: National Academy Press, 1997.

Institute of Medicine (IOM), Food and Nutrition Board, National Academy of Sciences. Dietary reference intakes for energy, carbohydrate, fiber, fat, fatty acids, cholesterol, protein, and amino acids. Washington, DC: National Academies Press, 2005.

Ivy JL, Portman R. Nutrient timing. North Bergen, NJ: Basic Health, 2004.

Kant AK, Graubard BI, Schatzkin A, Ballard-Barbash R. Proportion of energy intake from fat and subsequent weight change in the NHANES I epidemiologic follow-up study. Am J Clin Nutr 1995;61:11-17.

Kasperek GJ, Snider RD. Effect of exercise intensity and starvation on activation of branched-chain keto acid dehydrogenase by exercise. Am J Physiol 1987;252:E33-E37.

Keith RE, Stone MH, Carson RE, Lefavi RG, Fleck SJ. Nutritional status and lipid profiles of trained steroid-using bodybuilders. Int J Sport Nutr 1996;6:247-254.

Kimball SR, Farrell PA, Jefferson LS. Invited review: Role of insulin in translational control of protein synthesis in skeletal muscle by amino acids or exercise. J Appl Physiol 2002;93:1168-1180.

Kleiner SM, Bazzarre TL, Ainsworth BE. Nutritional status of nationally ranked elite body-builders. Int J Sport Nutr 1994;4:54-69.

Lemon PW. Effects of exercise on dietary protein requirements. Int J Sport Nutr 1998;8:426-447.

Lemon PWR. Do athletes need more dietary protein and amino acids? Int J Sport Nutr 1995;5:S39-S61.

Lemon PW, Tarnopolsky MA, MacDougall JD, Atkinson SA. Protein requirements and muscle mass/strength changes during intensive training in novice bodybuilders. J Appl Physiol 1992;73:767-775.

Levenhagen DK, Gresham JD, Carlson MG, Maron DJ, Borel MJ, Flakoll PJ. Postexercise nutrient intake timing in humans is critical to recovery of leg glucose and protein homeostasis. Am J Physiol Endocrinol Metab 2001;280:E982-E993.

Martin WF, Armstrong LE, Rodriguez NR. Dietary protein intake and renal function. Nutr Metab (Lond) 2005;2:25.

Martin WF, Cerundolo LH, Pikosky MA et al. Effects of dietary protein intake on indices of hydration. J Am Diet Assoc 2006;106:587-589.

Matthews DE. Proteins and amino acids. In: Shils ME, Shike M, Ross AC, Caballero B, Cousins RJ eds. Modern nutrition in health and disease, 10th ed. Philadelphia: Lippincott Williams & Wilkins, 2006;23-61.

MacKenzie TA, Clark NG, Bistrian BR, Flatt JP, Hallowell EM, Blackburn GL. A simple method for estimating nitrogen balance in hospitalized patients; a review and supporting data for a previously proposed technique. J Am Coll Nutr 1985;4:575-581.

Meredith CN, Zackin MJ, Frontera WR, Evans WJ. Dietary protein requirements and body protein metabolism in endurance-trained men. J Appl Physiol 1989;66:2850-2856.

Messina M, Messina V. The dietitian's guide to vegetarian diets. Gaithersburg, MD: Aspen, 1996.

Newsholme EA, Acworth IN, Blomstrand E. Amino acids, brain neurotransmitters and a functional link between muscle and brain that is important in sustained exercise, 1st ed. Montrouge, France: Eurotext, 1987.

Newsholme EA, Blomstrand E. Branched-chain amino acids and central fatigue. J Nutr 2006;136:274S-276S.

Niekamp RA, Baer JT. In-season dietary adequacy of trained male cross-country runners. Int J Sport Nutr 1995;5:45-55.

Peters EM, Goetzsche JM. Dietary practices of South African ultradistance runners. Int J Sport Nutr 1997;7:80-103.

Phillips SM. Protein requirements and supplementation in strength sports. Nutrition Jul-Aug 2004;20(7-8):689-695.

Phillips SM, Atkinson SA, Tarnopolsky MA, MacDougall JD. Gender differences in leucine kinetics and nitrogen balance in endurance athletes. J Appl Physiol 1993;75:2134-2141.

Phillips SM, Hartman JW, Wilkinson SB. Dietary protein to support anabolism with resistance exercise in young men. J Am Coll Nutr 2004;24:134S-139S.

Phillips SM, Tipton KD, Aarsland A, Wolf SE, Wolfe RR. Mixed muscle protein synthesis and breakdown after resistance exercise in humans. Am J Physiol 1997;273:E99-E107.

Rico-Sanz J, Frontera WR, Molé PA, Rivera MA, Rivera-Brown A, Meredith CN. Dietary and performance assessment of elite soccer players during a period of intense training. Int J Sport Nutr 1998;8:230-240.

Sheffield-Moore M, Yeckel CW, Volpi E et al. Postexercise protein metabolism in older and younger men following moderate-intensity aerobic exercise. Am J Physiol Endocrinol Metab 2004;287:E513-E522.

Tarnopolsky LJ, MacDougall JD, Atkinson SA, Tarnopolsky MA, Sutton JR. Gender differences in substrate for endurance exercise. J Appl Physiol 1990;68:302-308.

Tarnopolsky M. Protein requirements for endurance athletes. Nutrition Jul-Aug 2004;20(7-8):662-668.

Tarnopolsky MA, Atkinson SA, MacDougall JD, Chesley A, Phillips S, Schwarz HP. Evaluation of protein requirements for trained strength athletes. J Appl Physiol 1992;73:1986-1995.

Tarnopolsky MA, MacDougall JD, Atkinson SA. Influence of protein intake and training status on nitrogen balance and lean body mass. J Appl Physiol 1988;64:187-193.

Tillotson JL, Bartsch GE, Gorder D, Grandits GA, Stamler J. Food group and nutrient intakes at baseline in the Multiple Risk Factor Intervention Trial. Am J Clin Nutr 1997;65:228S-257S.

Tipton KD, Ferrando AA, Williams BD, Wolfe RR. Muscle protein metabolism in female swimmers after a combination of resistance and endurance exercise. J Appl Physiol 1996;81:2034-2038.

Todd KS, Butterfield GE, Calloway DH. Nitrogen balance in men with adequate and deficient energy intake at three levels of work. J Nutr 1984;114:2107-2118.

Walberg JL, Leidy MK, Sturgill DJ, Hinkle DE, Ritchey SJ, Sebolt DR. Macronutrient content of a hypoenergy diet affects nitrogen retention and muscle function in weight lifters. Int J Sports Med 1988;9:261-266.

Walberg-Rankin J, Eckstein Edmonds C, Gwazdauskas FC. Diet and weight changes of female bodybuilders before and after competition. Int J Sport Nutr 1993;3:87-102.

Wiita BG, Stombaugh IA. Nutrition knowledge, eating practices, and health of adolescent female runners: a 3-year longitudinal study. Int J Sport Nutr 1996;6:414-25.

Wolfe R, Wolfe MH, Nadel ER, Shaw JHF. Isotopic determination of amino acid-urea interactions in exercise in humans. J Appl Physiol 1984;221-229.

Wright JD, Kennedy-Stephenson J, Wang CY, McDowell MA, Johnson CL. National Center for Health Statistics, CDC. Trends in intake of energy and macronutrients-United States, 1971-2000. MMWR Feb 2004;6:80-82.

Young VR, Bier DM, Pellett PL. A theoretical basis for increasing current estimates of the amino acid requirements in adult man, with experimental support. Am J Clin Nutr 1989;50:80-92.

CHAPTER 5

Energy and Nutrient Balance

Chapter Objectives

After reading this chapter you should be able to

- explain the energy and nutrient balance equations,
- understand the concept of nutrient balance and the contributions of carbohydrate, protein, fat, and alcohol to energy balance,
- identify the various components of energy expenditure, how they are measured, and the contribution of energy expenditure to the energy balance equation, and
- understand the role of energy intake in the energy balance equation.

Most individuals maintain a stable body weight over time. Think about your own body weight—how much has it fluctuated over the last year? Over the last five years? Unless you diet frequently or have dramatically changed your activity level, your body weight has probably been relatively stable. What factors play a role in weight stability? How can our bodies maintain body weight within such a narrow range, especially when we pay little attention to the amount of energy we consume or expend each day? This chapter addresses these questions. First we present the energy balance equations and discuss the concept of energy and macronutrient balance. To understand energy balance and why a person gains, loses, or maintains weight, you must know the factors that influence energy intake and expenditure.

ENERGY AND MACRONUTRIENT BALANCE EQUATIONS

The classic energy balance equation states that if energy intake (total kilocalories consumed) equals energy expenditure (total kilocalories expended), then weight is maintained. However, this equation does not allow for changes in body composition and energy stores, nor does it help us understand the many factors associated with weight change, especially weight gain. We now know that maintenance of body weight and body composition over time requires not only that energy intake equal energy expenditure—but also that intakes of protein, carbohydrate, fat, and alcohol equal their oxidation rates. People who meet these criteria are in **energy balance** and will maintain their weight and body composition. A number of factors affect these components of energy balance. Some of them may be further modified by socioeconomic, physiological, and psychological influences (Flatt 1993). These factors, which are listed next, vary among individuals in their importance and influence.

- Genetic makeup
- Dietary intake and habits
- Physical activity and activities of daily living
- Environmental conditions
- Lifestyle

Maintenance of body weight and composition depends on how these factors influence the energy balance principles presented in the sidebar on this page.

The equations given are both dynamic and time dependent, allowing for the effect of changing energy stores on energy expenditure over time. Swinburn and Ravussin (1993) illustrate this point with the following example. What would happen if you consumed an extra chocolate chip cookie (~100 kcal each) every day for 40 years? The amount of extra energy would equal 1.5 million kcal. If we assume that there are ~3500 kcal/lb (7700 kcal/kg) of adipose tissue, your weight gain would be about 417 lb (190 kg) over this 40-year period. Yet this clearly does not happen. If you really ate these extra kilocalories every day for 40 years, you would probably gain only about 6 lb (2.7 kg). After a short period of positive energy balance, the extra kilocalories would cause you to gain weight (both fat and lean tissues), and your larger body size would increase energy expenditure sufficiently to balance the extra kilocalories consumed. Of course, the amount of weight you gain will depend on the number of extra kilocalories you eat, the composition of those kilocalories (i.e., the amount of fat, carbohydrate, protein, or alcohol), and your energy expenditure. Thus, weight gain can result from an initial positive energy balance, but also can eventually restore energy balance (see "Example of Weight Stability").

MACRONUTRIENT BALANCE

Alterations of energy intake or expenditure are just one part of the energy balance picture. Changes in the type and amount of macronutrients con-

---

Energy and Nutrient Balance Equations Required for Long-Term Weight Maintenance

1. Energy Balance

Rate of energy input (Dietary energy + Stored energy) = Rate of energy expenditure.

2. Nutrient Balance

Rate of protein intake = Rate of protein oxidation.

Rate of fat intake = Rate of fat oxidation.

Rate of carbohydrate intake = Rate of carbohydrate oxidation.

Rate of alcohol intake = Rate of alcohol oxidation.

Example of Weight Stability

To illustrate how weight stable we appear to be, here is an example from research done in Germany in 1902 (as reported by Keesey 1980). A researcher reported being weight stable while ingesting 1766 kcal/day for one year. The next year he increased his energy intake to 2199 kcal/day, and then to 2403 kcal/day for the third year. Thus, he consumed nearly 160,000 more kilocalories in the second year than the first, and approximately 230,000 more kilocalories in the third year compared to year 1. The researcher's weight changed little over this time (he reported gaining only several pounds), although energy intake increased 26%.

sumed (protein, fat, carbohydrate, alcohol) and the oxidation of these nutrients within the body must also be considered. In fact, it is difficult to separate these two factors when explaining energy balance. Under normal physiological conditions, carbohydrate, protein, and alcohol are not easily converted to body fat (Swinburn and Ravussin 1993; Flatt 2001); increases in the intake of nonfat nutrients stimulate their oxidation rates proportionally. Fat is different. Increased fat intake does *not* immediately stimulate fat oxidation, increasing the probability that dietary fat will be stored as adipose tissue (Saris and Tarnopolsky 2003; Westerterp 1993). The type of food consumed therefore plays a major role in the amount of energy consumed and expended each day (Acheson et al. 1984; Swinburn and Ravussin 1993). In addition, degree of fatness, metabolic conditions such as diabetes, level of fitness, and fat mass may alter how the body oxidizes macronutrients. The following section reviews each of these nutrients and the roles they play in energy balance.

Carbohydrate Balance

Carbohydrate balance is precisely regulated by the body (Acheson, Schultz et al. 1988; Flatt 1988; Jebb et al. 1996; Saris 2003). Ingestion of carbohydrate stimulates both glycogen storage and glucose oxidation and inhibits fat oxidation. The degree to which the body stores carbohydrate as glycogen may also affect carbohydrate and energy balance. For example, Eckel and colleagues (2006) recently demonstrated that people who are able to increase glycogen storage with increased carbohydrate ingestion are more resistant to weight gain. One way to increase your ability to store glycogen is to become more physically fit. Glucose not stored as glycogen is thought to be oxidized directly in almost equal balance to that consumed (Flatt et

al. 1985; Flatt 2001). Conversion of excess dietary carbohydrate and protein to triacylglycerides (de novo lipogenesis) apparently does not occur to a significant extent in normal-weight people except in nonphysiological conditions (Hellerstein et al. 1991; Saris 2003): Only when very large amounts of carbohydrate are consumed over several consecutive days, *and* dietary energy is in excess of need (~30-50% or more) (McDevitt et al. 2001), does the body appear to convert the excess carbohydrate to fat in the form of triacylglyceride (Acheson, Schutz et al. 1982; McDevitt et al. 2001).

Researchers have also examined whether the type of carbohydrate consumed during periods of overfeeding matters in the conversion of carbohydrate to fat. McDevitt and colleagues (2001) found that there was no difference in de novo lipogenesis when lean and obese women were overfed a diet with 50% sucrose or glucose over a 96 h period. As figure 5.1 illustrates, consumption of carbohydrate promotes the oxidation of carbohydrate—and any excess energy stored appears to come directly from dietary fat made available by inhibition of fat oxidation. For example, Jebb and colleagues (1996) overfed three lean men for 12 days and measured changes in energy expenditure and changes in protein, fat, and carbohydrate oxidation in a metabolic chamber (figure 5.2). The diet provided 15% of its energy as protein, 35% as fat, and 50% as carbohydrate, while energy intake was 33% higher than required to maintain energy balance. Carbohydrate and protein oxidation matched intake, while fat oxidation was not sensitive to fat intake. The subjects consumed 150 g of fat per day but oxidized only 59 g. The result was a 6.5 lb (2.9 kg) weight gain during the 12-day period. The researchers verified the inability of fat oxidation to match dietary fat intake when they underfed three lean men for 12 days using the same mixed diet. Energy intake was 67% less than required

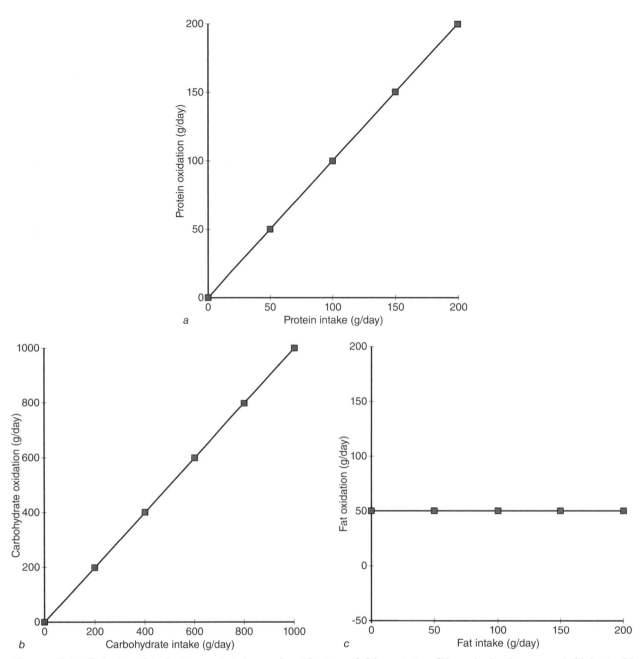

Figure 5.1 Relationship between intake and oxidation of *(a)* protein, *(b)* carbohydrate, and *(c)* fat in 21 weight-stable men (*n* = 11) and women (*n* = 10) after seven days of consuming a diet that contained 62% of energy from carbohydrate and 26% of energy from fat.

Reprinted, by permission, from C.D. Thomas et al., 1992, "Nutrient balance and energy expenditure during ad libitum feeding of high-fat and high-carbohydrate diets in humans," *American Journal of Clinical Nutrition* 55: 934-942.

to maintain energy balance. Again, carbohydrate and protein oxidation matched dietary intakes, but fat did not. The subjects consumed 20 g of fat but oxidized 59 g. The subjects lost on average 7 lb (3.2 kg) in 12 days. Changes in fat balance explained 74% of the energy imbalance during the overfeeding period and 84% of the imbalance during the underfeeding period.

The metabolic consequences of the preferential storage of dietary fat are significant. The energy required to digest, absorb, and convert carbohydrate energy to adenosine triphosphate (ATP) is greater than that lost in converting dietary fat to ATP—leaving only about 75% to 80% of the carbohydrate energy available for work, whereas 90% to 94% of the fat energy is available (Flatt 2001) (see

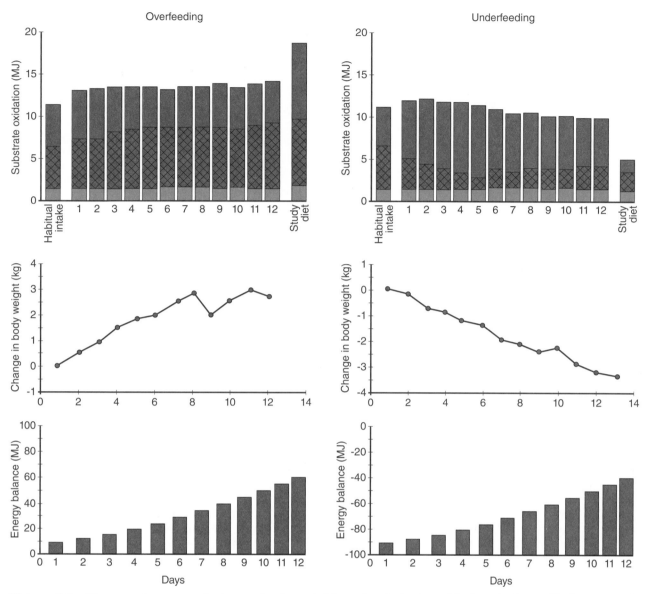

Figure 5.2 Changes in energy balance, body weight, and substrate oxidation during a 12-day period of overfeeding or underfeeding. Overfeeding consisted of a mixed diet (15% of energy from protein, 35% from fat, 50% from carbohydrate) that was 33% higher in energy than required to maintain energy balance. Underfeeding consisted of the same mixed diet, which was 67% lower in energy than required to maintain energy balance. Top graphs show changes in energy expenditure with over- and underfeeding and the contributions from separate macronutrients. Gray bar = protein; hatched bar = carbohydrate; blue bar = fat. To convert MJ (megajoules) to kilocalories: MJ × 1000 / 4.184 = kcal.

Reprinted, by permission, from S.A. Jebb et al., 1996, "Changes in macronutrient balance during over- and underfeeding assessed by 12-d continuous whole-body calorimetry," *American Journal of Clinical Nutrition* 64: 259-266.

table 5.1). Thus, when dietary fat is stored as adipose tissue, it may represent a greater relative fuel reservoir than had previously been considered.

The body's glycogen storage capacity is limited to 1.1 to 1.8 lb (~500-800 g) in the liver and skeletal muscle combined, a capacity much smaller than that for protein or fat. Exercise training can increase the storage capacity, but even then it

cannot be enlarged much past ~4.4 lb (2 kg). Glycogen storage fluctuates greatly in response to feeding and exercise: Feeding increases and exercise decreases glycogen stores. Conversely, becoming physically fit increases one's ability to store glycogen, making this carbohydrate unavailable for conversion to fat. Flatt (1988, 2001) proposed that a carbohydrate "appetite" drives people to

Table 5.1 Calculated Cost of Nutrient Thermogenesis and Energy Stored in Humans and the Net ATP Yields

Nutrient	Storage form	Thermogenesis[a]	Cost of nutrient storage[b]	ATP yields (% of total energy)[d]
Glucose	Glycogen (liver)	6-8%	5-10%	75%
	Glycogen (muscle)	–	5-10%	
	Fat (adipose)	–	24-28%[c]	
Fat	Fat (adipose)	2-3%	4-7%	90%
Protein	Protein	25-40%	25-40%	60%

[a] In percent of the energy content of the infused nutrient.
[b] In percent of the energy content of the stored nutrient.
[c] In humans under normal physiological conditions, little de novo synthesis of triglycerides (fat) occurs from excess protein or carbohydrate.
[d] Net ATP yields after ATP required for transport, activation, recycling, regeneration, and excretion of the substrate being oxidized is accounted for.

Adapted from E. Jequier, 1992, Regulation of thermogenesis and nutrient metabolism in the human: relevance for obesity. In *Obesity,* edited by P. Bjorntorp ad B.N. Brodoff (Philadelphia, PA: Lippincott, Williams, and Wilkins), 130-135; J.P. Flatt, 1978, The biochemistry of energy expenditure. In *Recent advances in obesity research II,* edited by G. Bray (London: John Libby), 211-228; J.P. Flatt, 2001, "Macronutrient composition and food selection," *Obesity Research* 9(4): 256S-262S.

replenish glycogen stores and that satiety occurs when this replenishment is complete. Researchers at Laval University in Quebec (Tremblay et al. 1991) have shown that people on a high-fat diet (i.e., a diet low in carbohydrate) may overconsume energy to satisfy the drive for carbohydrate. The overconsumption results in a positive energy balance, which can increase amounts of adipose tissue. Some researchers feel that this approach is too simplistic and that control of carbohydrate appetite may result from relative rates of breakdown and synthesis (flux) of both carbohydrate and fat (Friedman and Tordoff 1986). Other investigators have been unable to show such a drive for maintenance of carbohydrate stores. Stubbs and colleagues (1993) found that men given diets of varying carbohydrate content did not change energy intake on the day after being fed a diet providing either 3% of energy from carbohydrate (depletion diet) or 47% (control diet). However, the study lasted only one day, and the diet provided during the control phase may have been sufficient to replenish any glycogen stores used by these inactive individuals over the one day of testing. These investigators also found that carbohydrate oxidation decreased with the lower carbohydrate intake and increased with the higher carbohydrate intake.

Protein Balance

The concept of protein or nitrogen balance (see chapter 4) is essential to the discussion of energy balance. The body adjusts to a wide range of protein intakes by altering the oxidation rate of dietary protein. After anabolic needs are met, the carbon skeletons of any excess amino acids are diverted into the energy substrate pool where they are used for energy production. The adequacy of total energy intake, and carbohydrate intake in particular, appears to dramatically affect this process. Inadequate intakes of either energy or carbohydrate result in negative protein balance and may adversely affect the balances of individual amino acids (Krempf et al. 1993). Conversely, excess intake of either energy or carbohydrate will spare protein, which is then available to support brief periods of protein accumulation until the protein pool is expanded to a new balance point. At this point, the degradation of endogenous protein matches the available exogenous protein. Excess protein consumed or protein made available through protein sparing may contribute indirectly to fat storage by sparing dietary fat, as seen with the consumption of excess carbohydrate energy. However, excess dietary protein is not made directly into triacylglycerides (or triglycerides) and stored as fat.

Fat Balance

Fat balance is not as precisely regulated as protein and carbohydrate balance. Figure 5.1 shows that as fat intake increases, fat oxidation does not increase proportionately. In marked contrast to carbohydrate stores, body adipose tissue stores are large, and most evidence shows that the acute intake of fat has little influence on fat oxidation

(Thomas et al. 1992; Westerterp-Plantenga 2003). Because most research shows that fat intake does not directly promote fat oxidation, it is now commonly accepted that excess energy eaten as dietary fat is stored as triacylglyceride in adipose tissue, with little energy being consumed in the storage process. How quickly one's fat oxidation adapts to match fat intake may depend on a number of factors, including level of obesity or one's propensity to gain weight (Flatt 2001).

Over the long term, a positive fat balance due to excess energy intake leads to a progressive increase in total body fat stores in an attempt to achieve energy balance. These expanded stores also increase the free fatty acid (FFA) concentrations in the blood. This increase in circulation of FFAs may slightly increase fat oxidation and probably promotes recycling. Thus, the larger adipose tissue mass promotes increased fat oxidation. When the new rate of fat oxidation equals the rate of fat intake, a person again achieves fat balance (and hence energy balance)—but at a significantly higher body weight (figure 5.3).

If increasing fat stores allows fat oxidation to match fat intake, then obesity may be viewed as a compensatory mechanism to reestablish energy balance at a new steady state in response to the chronic ingestion of excess energy (Flatt 2001). For example, Astrup and colleagues (1994) found a higher rate of fat oxidation in obese women (40%) as compared to nonobese women (36%) after adjusting for their percentage of energy from dietary fat, age, and 24 h energy balance. Percentage of fat oxidation also increased with fat mass—the higher the fat mass, the greater an individual's fat oxidation rate. Schutz and colleagues (1992) reported that an excess fat intake of 20 g/day (180 kcal/day) would lead to an increase in body fat of 22 lb (10 kg) before fat balance would be achieved with a corresponding increase in fat oxidation. Thus, in susceptible sedentary individuals, the expansion of fat stores is a prerequisite to increase fat oxidation to match a high percentage of dietary fat energy. Schutz and colleagues (1992) found a decrease in fat oxidation in obese women losing weight.

Alcohol Balance

Alcohol is a "priority fuel," which means that alcohol oxidation rises quickly after its ingestion until all of it is cleared from the body. Alcohol suppresses the oxidation of fat and to a lesser degree that of protein and carbohydrate (Shelmet et al. 1988; Suter 2005). Alcohol is not converted

to triacylglycerides and stored as fat, nor can it contribute to the formation of muscle or liver glycogen. It may, however, indirectly divert fat to storage by providing an alternative and preferred energy source for the body (Sonko et al. 1994; Suter 2005). Thus, at ~7 kcal/g, alcohol can contribute significantly to total daily energy intake; individuals who consume alcohol may have to reduce their consumption of energy from other dietary components to maintain energy balance.

Alcohol can contribute to changes in energy balance in other ways besides adding additional energy to the diet. Although alcohol adds kilocalories to the meal in which it is consumed, there appears to be minimal reduction of food intake to compensate for the extra energy consumed in alcohol (Yoemans et al. 2003). This means that you may consume more kilocalories at a meal that includes alcohol. In fact, alcohol may actually stimulate appetite and increase the number of kilocalories consumed in a meal from food. Other ways in which alcohol may affect energy balance are by decreasing fatty acid oxidation and altering neurochemical and peripheral systems that help regulate energy balance (Yoemans et al. 2003). Thus, it is important to ask about alcohol consumption when addressing the issue of energy balance with an individual. See the review by Suter (2005) for a complete overview of the impact of alcohol on weight gain and obesity.

ENERGY EXPENDITURE

Energy expenditure is one side of the energy balance equation. Any alteration in energy expenditure can result in weight gain or loss if energy intake and composition are held constant. In this section, we review the various components of energy expenditure and how these components are measured; we also discuss how being physically active can influence these components. Because direct assessment of energy expenditure is difficult, we present methods for predicting energy expenditure based on age, gender, and anthropometric measurements.

Components of Energy Expenditure

The components of total daily energy expenditure are generally divided into three main categories: (1) **resting metabolic rate (RMR), basal metabolic rate (BMR),** or **resting energy expenditure (REE)** (see "What Are the Differences Between

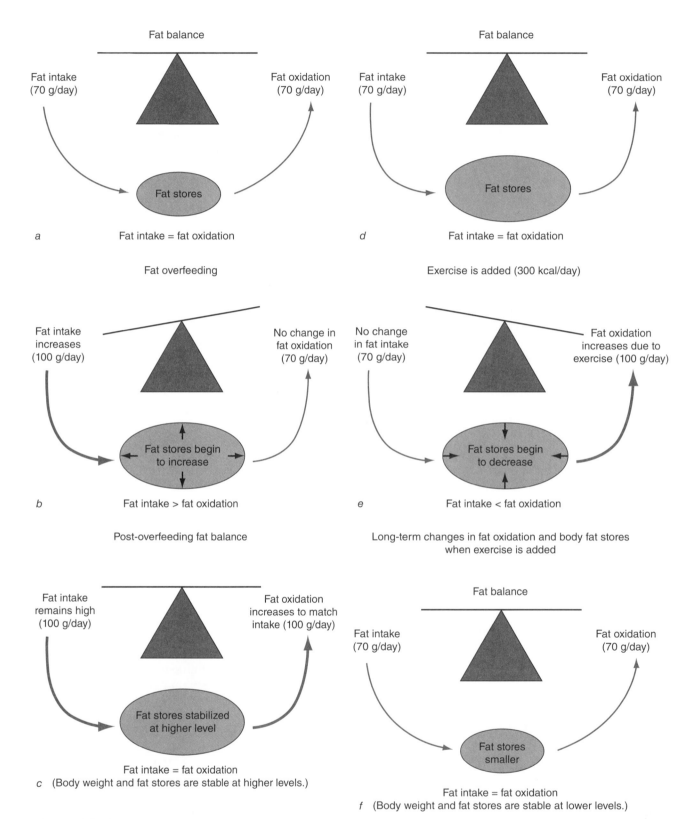

Figure 5.3 Schematic illustration of the proposed long-term adaptations in fat oxidation and body fat storage induced by *(a* through *c)* excess dietary fat over a prolonged period and *(d* through *f)* exercise.

Highlight

What are the Differences Between RMR, BMR, REE, and SMR?

In the research literature, the terms RMR, BMR, and REE are often used interchangeably; you may also see references to **sleeping metabolic rate (SMR)**. If BMR is used, it usually means that the measurements are taken after the subject has stayed overnight in a metabolic chamber or a research ward and has not eaten in the last 12 h. If RMR or REE is used, it usually means that the subject slept at home and drove or was driven to the research lab for testing. Resting metabolic rate and BMR usually differ by less than 10%. If SMR is reported, it means that the subject slept in a metabolic chamber and technicians measured the metabolic rate during sleep (usually the period of fewest movements). The SMR is usually 5% to 10% lower than the BMR. Read the research methods carefully so that you know which technique was used for data collection. In general, BMR may better represent the energy required at rest because the subject does not have to get up, dress, and drive to a research site. However, some researchers now report that BMR and RMR are similar *if* strict research protocols are followed during data collection (Bullough and Melby 1993; Thompson et al. 1995; Turley et al. 1993).

RMR, BMR, REE, and SMR?"); (2) thermic effect of food; and (3) energy expended in physical activity and activities of daily living, or as it is frequently called, the thermic effect of activity. The RMR is the energy required to maintain the systems of the body and to regulate body temperature at rest. Resting metabolic rate is measured in the morning after an overnight fast (12 h) while the individual is resting in a bed. The person must be comfortable and free from stress, medications, or any other stimulation that would increase metabolic activity. The room where RMR is measured should be quiet, temperature controlled, and free of distractions. The RMR accounts for approximately 60% to 80% of total daily energy expenditure in most sedentary healthy adults (Levine 2005; Ravussin et al. 1986; Ravussin and Bogardus 1989). In active individuals this percentage varies greatly—it is not unusual for some athletes to expend 1000 to 2000 kcal/day just in sport-related activities. When Thompson and colleagues (1993) determined energy balance in 24 elite male endurance athletes over three to seven days, they found that RMR represented only 38% to 47% of total daily energy expenditure. Beidleman and colleagues (1995) reported similar figures for active women. During days of repetitive heavy competition, such as ultramarathons, RMR may represent <20% of total energy expenditure (Rontoyannis et al. 1989).

The **thermic effect of food (TEF)** represents the increase in energy expenditure above RMR that results from the consumption of food and beverage throughout the day. Although TEF is frequently used interchangeably with the thermic effect of a meal, the terms are not synonymous. The **thermic effect of a meal (TEM)** represents the increase in metabolic rate above RMR after a meal has been eaten. It is easier to measure TEM than TEF because of the difficulties in trying to assess the cumulative energy cost of all foods consumed within a day. Most research literature on the energy costs of active individuals presents TEM unless the researchers are able to use a metabolic chamber. Figure 5.4 (p. 142) illustrates the TEM concept by showing the increase in metabolic rate above RMR over a 3 h period on two different occasions in male triathletes fed a meal containing approximately 750 kcal.

The TEF includes the energy cost of food digestion, absorption, transport, metabolism, and storage within the body. The TEF usually accounts for approximately 6% to 10% of total daily energy expenditure, but can vary from 4% to 15% (Hollis and Mattes 2005) depending on the total number of kilocalories in a meal, types of foods consumed, and the degree of obesity. The TEF has two general components: obligatory and facultative thermogenesis. **Obligatory thermogenesis** is the energy cost associated with digestion, absorption, and transport of nutrients and with the synthesis of protein, fat (triacylglycerides), and carbohydrate (glycogen). Approximately 50% to 75% of the TEF can be attributed to the obligatory component (Flatt 1992). Research has shown that

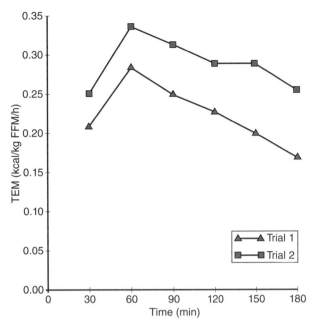

Figure 5.4 Thermic effect of a meal (TEM) on two different occasions in male triathletes consuming 12 kcal/kg of fat-free mass (FFM) (~750 kcal). The TEM was calculated as the difference between resting metabolic rate (RMR) and the thermic response to the test meal. The liquid meal provided 60% of energy from carbohydrate, 25% of energy from fat, and 15% of energy from protein.

Adapted from J. Thompson, M.M. Manore, and J.S. Skinner, 1993, "Resting metabolic rate and thermic effect of a meal in low- and adequate-energy intake male endurance athletes," *International Journal of Sport and Nutrition* 3: 194-206.

the measured TEF is higher than the theoretical cost of nutrient digestion, absorption, and storage (Acheson et al. 1984). The energy expended above obligatory thermogenesis is termed **facultative thermogenesis** and is due primarily to sympathetic nervous system activity. For example, after ingestion of a meal or after the infusion of glucose, plasma levels of norepinephrine increase. If medication blocks this release of norepinephrine, the TEF of food declines (Acheson et al. 1984). Thus, the TEF is a combination of the energy required to digest and metabolize the food we eat and the energy expended due to sympathetic nervous system activity brought about by seeing, smelling, and eating food.

The **thermic effect of activity (TEA)** is the most variable component of energy expenditure. It includes the energy cost of daily activities above RMR and TEF, such as purposeful activities of daily living (making dinner, dressing, cleaning house) or planned exercise events (running, weight train-

ing, walking). It also includes the energy cost of involuntary muscular activity such as shivering, fidgeting, and maintenance of posture. This type of movement is called **spontaneous physical activity (SPA)** or **nonexercise activity thermogenesis (NEAT)** (Levine et al. 1999; Ravussin and Swinburn 1993). Nonexercise activity thermogenesis is defined as the energy expended for everything we do that is not sleeping, eating, or sport or exercise types of activities. Levine (2004; Levine et al. 2001) has popularized this term to separate it from the movement we do each day that is not programmed physical activity, such as working at a desk, walking to have lunch, or standing to greet someone. He has suggested that NEAT may help explain why some people are obese and others are not (Levine et al. 2005). Levine and his colleagues (2005) compared the NEAT in 10 mildly obese and 10 lean sedentary individuals and found that obese individuals were seated 2 h/day longer than lean individuals and that lean individuals were standing or ambulating 2.5 h/day more than obese individuals. This difference in NEAT accounted for a difference of 350 ± 65 kcal/day (Levine et al. 2005; Ravussin 2005) (see figure 5.5). Thus, this component of TEA may help explain why some people gain weight and others do not. The TEA may be only 10% to 15% of total daily energy expenditure in sedentary persons but may be as high as 50% in active people, especially those who do some type of movement in their job.

The addition of RMR, TEF, and TEA should account for 100% of total energy expenditure (figure 5.6). A number of factors can increase energy expenditure above normal baseline levels (e.g., cold, fear, stress, and various medications). The thermic effect of these factors is frequently referred to as **adaptive thermogenesis (AT)**. Adaptive thermogenesis represents a temporary increase in thermogenesis that may last for hours or even days, depending on the duration and magnitude of the stimulus (e.g., a serious physical injury, the stress associated with an upcoming event, going to a higher altitude, or the use of certain medications) (table 5.2 p. 144).

Biological Factors That Influence Resting Metabolic Rate

A variety of factors can influence RMR for a given individual on any given day. Table 5.2 briefly outlines these factors, which one should consider when measuring or predicting an individual's RMR. This section reviews the most common

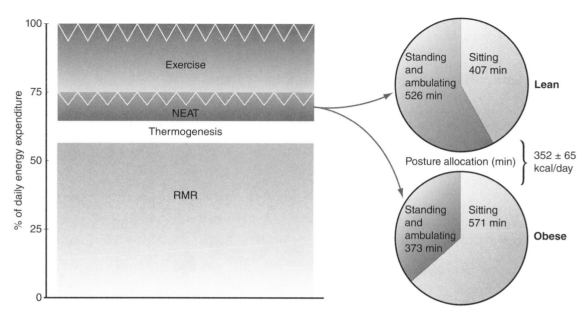

Figure 5.5 Contributions of nonexercise activity thermogenesis (NEAT) and differences in NEAT between sedentary lean and obese individuals.

From E. Ravussin, 2005, "A NEAT way to control weight?" *Science* 307(Jan 28): 530-531. Reprinted with permission from AAAS.

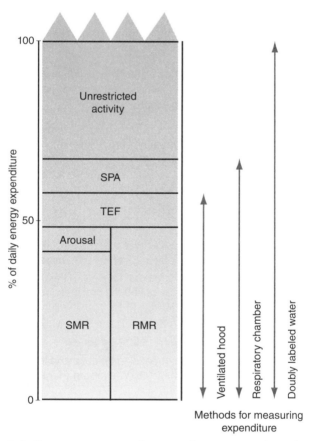

Methods for measuring expenditure

Figure 5.6 Components of daily energy expenditure in humans and methods of measurement. Daily energy expenditure can be divided into three major components: the resting metabolic rate (RMR) (sum of the sleeping metabolic rate [SMR] and the energy cost of arousal), which usually represents 50% to 70% of daily energy expenditure; the thermic effect of food (TEF), which represents ~6% to 10% of daily energy expenditure; and the energy cost of physical activity and movement (sum of spontaneous physical activity [SPA] and unrestricted or voluntary physical activity, including nonexercise activity thermogenesis [NEAT]), which represents 20% to 40% of daily energy expenditure.

Adapted from E. Ravussin and B.A. Swinburn, 1993, Energy metabolism. In *Obesity: Theory and therapy,* edited by J.A. Stunkard and T.A. Wadden (New York: Raven Press Ltd.) 97-123; J.A. Levine, 2004, "Non-exercise activity thermogenesis (NEAT)," *Nutrition Reviews* 62(7): S82-S97.

Table 5.2 Factors That Influence Resting Metabolic Rate (RMR)

Factor	Effect on RMR
Body size Weight Fat-free mass (FFM) Fat mass (FM)	↑RMR with ↑weight ↑RMR with ↑FFM ↑RMR with ↑FM (Bray and Atkinson 1977)
Age	↓<1-2% per decade between second and seventh decades (Keys et al. 1973)
Gender	↑RMR in males versus females (Ferraro et al. 1992)
Impact of genetics	RMR shows familial relationship (Bouchard et al. 1989; Bogardus et al. 1986)
Ethnicity	↓RMR in African Americans ~10%
Physical activity Fitness level (trained vs. untrained) Acute exercise (excess postexercise oxygen consumption)	Variable responses dependent on duration, intensity, and type of training Variable responses dependent on intensity and duration of exercise
Physiological factors Body temperature Severe dieting or starvation Feasting or overeating Illness, catabolic conditions, injury Menstrual cycle (variable responses reported) Growth, pregnancy	12%↑ RMR with each 1° C↑ body temperature ↓RMR (Weinsier et al. 2000) ↑RMR ↑RMR RMR↑ in luteal phase (100-300 kcal/day) versus follicular phase (Ferraro et al. 1992; Bisbee et al. 1989; Solomon et al. 1982) ↑RMR with ↑body weight
Hormonal and drug influences Thyroid hormones ↑Catecholamines ↑Cortisol ↑Growth hormone Alcohol Smoking; nicotine Caffeine (coffee, tea, cola, pills) Nicotine + caffeine	↓RMR if thyroid hormones are below normal levels; ↑RMR if thyroid hormones are abnormally high ↑RMR ↑RMR ↑RMR ↑RMR (Klesges et al. 1994) Four cigarettes ↑RMR by 3% over 3 h (Collins et al. 1994); gum containing 1 mg or 2 mg nicotine ↑ by 3.7% and 4.9%, respectively (Jessen et al. 2003) Single dose of 100 mg oral caffeine ↑RMR by 3-4% over 150 min (Dulloo et al. 1989); a single dose of 200 mg oral caffeine ↑RMR by 5-8% (Collins et al. 1994); 4 mg/kg dose ↑RMR by 13-15% by 30 min (Yoshida et al. 1994) ↑RMR by 7.9%, 6.3%, 8.5%, and 9.8% when the following doses of nicotine (mg)/caffeine (mg) were given: 1/50, 2/50, 1/100, and 2/100 (Jessen et al. 2003)
Other substances: spices and tea (capsaicin, black pepper, green tea)	↑RMR is variable depending on dose and level of active substances that influence thermogenesis (Westerterp-Plantenga et al. 2006)

influences on RMR and discusses how they may be altered in active individuals.

Effects of Age, Gender, and Body Size on Resting Metabolic Rate

It is well documented that RMR is influenced by age, gender, and body size, including fat-free mass (FFM) and fat mass. Three of these variables (FFM, age, and gender) generally explain about 80% of

the variability in RMR (Bogardus et al. 1986). Since FFM, which includes organs and muscles, is very metabolically active tissue, any change in FFM dramatically influences RMR. Figure 5.7 shows the strong linear relationship between FFM and RMR. This relationship appears to hold for all individuals regardless of sex or race. In general, men have larger RMRs than women simply because they usually weigh more and have more FFM, but other factors may contribute to the male–female differ-

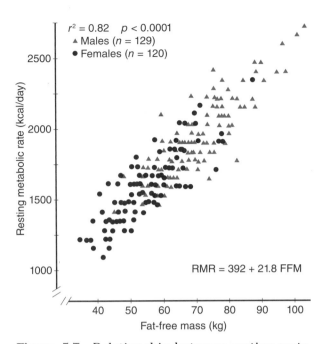

$r^2 = 0.82 \quad p < 0.0001$
▲ Males (n = 129)
● Females (n = 120)

RMR = 392 + 21.8 FFM

Figure 5.7 Relationship between resting metabolic rate (RMR) and fat-free mass (FFM).

Reprinted, by permission, from E. Ravussin and C. Bogardus, 1989, "Relationship of genetics, age and physical fitness to daily energy expenditure and fuel utilization," *American Journal of Clinical Nutrition* 49: 968-975.

ences (Blanc et al. 2004). Ferraro and colleagues (1992) found lower RMRs in women than in men (~100 kcal/day less) even after controlling for differences in FFM, fat mass, and age. Conversely, Blanc and colleagues (2004) found no differences in RMR between elderly men and women (70-79 years) after controlling for FFM. The differences in these two studies may be due to the age of the participants, since the Blanc study used sedentary subjects in their eighth decade of life.

Age also influences RMR, which declines ~1% to 2% per decade from the second through the seventh decade of life (Keys et al. 1987). Part of the decrease is attributed to the decline in FFM that frequently occurs with aging, especially as people lead more sedentary lifestyles. Yet not all the decline in RMR that occurs with aging is attributed to decreases in FFM. A study by Vaughan and colleagues (1991) showed a small but significant negative impact of age on metabolic rate independent of FFM, fat mass, and gender. These researchers used a metabolic chamber to measure metabolic rates of 39 elderly and 64 young men and women. After adjusting for differences in FFM, fat mass, and gender, they found significantly lower BMRs (~100 kcal/day) in the elderly versus the younger

subjects. Although the exact effect of age on RMR has not yet been determined, it seems clear that the decrease in RMR with age will be minimized for people who stay physically active throughout their lives.

Effect of Genetics on Resting Metabolic Rate

It is now known that RMR has a genetic component: Individuals within families tend to have similar RMRs. After measuring RMR in 130 nondiabetic adult southwestern American Indians from 54 families (figure 5.8 p. 146), Bogardus and colleagues (1986) found that family membership explained 11% of the variability in RMR ($p < 0.0001$). In studies of twins and parent–child pairs, Bouchard and colleagues (1989) reported that heritability explained approximately 40% of the variability in RMR after adjustments were made for age, gender, and FFM. Finally, recent research documents lower RMR in African American women after controlling for lean tissue, aerobic fitness level, weight, percentage of body fat, and age (Hunter et al. 2000). This lower RMR was attributed to a low volume of metabolically active organ tissue. Thus, it appears that a number of genetic factors can influence RMR, which can secondarily affect body weight.

Effect of Body Temperature on Resting Metabolic Rate

Although we know that RMR increases as body temperature increases above normal, for example in febrile diseases (see table 5.2), until recently it was not known whether a relationship existed between RMR and body temperature within normal temperature ranges. After adjusting for differences in body size, body composition, and age, Rising and colleagues (1992) found a strong positive correlation ($r = 0.80$; $p < 0.0001$) between metabolic rate and body temperature within the range of 95.0° to 97.7° F (35.0-36.5° C). The question remains: Are lower body temperatures inherited, thus predisposing one to a lower RMR and an increased risk for obesity?

Effect of Reproductive Hormones on Resting Metabolic Rate

Researchers have examined the fluctuations in RMR over the phases of the menstrual cycle. Some studies show that RMR values are lowest during the follicular phase of the cycle and highest during the luteal phase (Bisbee et al. 1989;

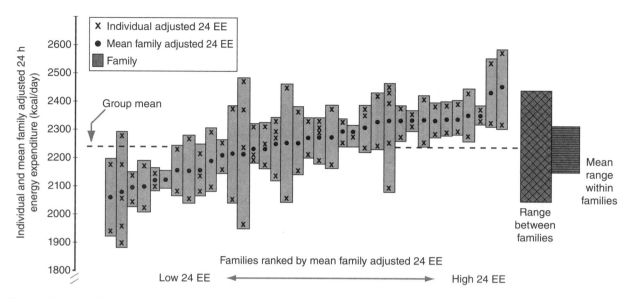

Figure 5.8 Individual and mean family 24 h energy expenditure (24 EE) adjusted for fat-free mass, fat mass, age, and sex. Intrafamily correlation coefficient was 0.26. Families are ranked according to adjusted resting metabolic rate (RMR). The range of mean family adjusted RMR and the mean range within families are depicted by the hatched bars on the right.

Solomon et al. 1982). Figure 5.9 illustrates this change in RMR by measuring sleep metabolic rate (SMR), a component of RMR over the menstrual cycle. The difference in RMR between these two phases is estimated to be approximately 100 to 300 kcal/day; however, adaptations in energy intake appear to mimic the changes in RMR. Barr and colleagues (1995) reported that women consume approximately 300 kcal/day more during the luteal phase of the menstrual cycle (end of the cycle) as compared with the follicular phase (beginning of the cycle). Thus, the increased energy expenditure, due to a higher RMR during the luteal phase, is compensated for by an increase in energy intake during this period. Conversely, Weststrate (1993) showed no effect of menstrual cycle on RMR, and Piers and coworkers (1995) showed no effect of menstrual cycle phase on RMR or energy intake.

Recently, Day and colleagues (2005) examined changes in RMR in 14 premenopausal women before and after suppression of progesterone and estrogen using pharmacological methods in the midluteal phase of the menstrual cycle. Using this method, researchers were able to determine the change in RMR when these reproductive hormones were suppressed, as you would see in amenorrhea or menopause, compared to that in a normal menstrual cycle. They found that suppression of estrogen and progesterone significantly

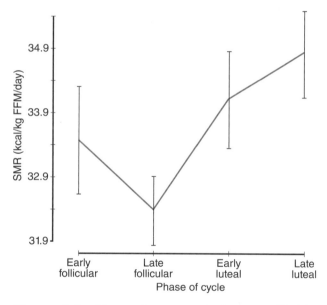

Figure 5.9 Mean sleep metabolic rate (SMR) (kcal/kg of Fat Free Mass [FFM] per day) at four phases of the menstrual cycle.

decreased RMR by 71 kcal/day ($P = 0.002$). Thus, phase of the menstrual cycle should be recorded when RMR or energy intake is measured in premenopausal females. Ideally, if repeated measures of energy intake or RMR are being recorded, they should be taken at the same time during the menstrual cycle. These data are supported by research indicating that RMR was significantly lower in female athletes with menstrual dysfunction (nine periods within the last 12 months) compared to athletes with normal menstrual function (~111 kcal/day lower; $P < 0.02$) (Lebenstedt et al. 1999). If a female is amenorrheic (not menstruating) or postmenopausal, these fluctuations in RMR do not occur. In postmenopausal women, this lower RMR may contribute to weight gain (Day et al. 2005).

Effect of Exercise or Physical Activity on Resting Metabolic Rate

Exercise can affect energy expenditure both directly and indirectly. Metabolism increases during exercise, directly increasing the amount of energy expended. Exercise can also increase energy expenditure indirectly by increasing the amount of FFM, which in turn elevates RMR. Researchers have asked the following questions:

1. Within the general population, do aerobically trained people have higher RMRs than untrained individuals?

2. For a given individual, does becoming more aerobically trained increase RMR?

3. Does metabolic rate stay elevated for a time after exercise is over?

Does Aerobic Training Increase Resting Metabolic Rates?

Researchers have addressed this question by comparing the RMRs of aerobically trained and untrained people while trying to match for FFM. We know that FFM accounts for the majority of variability in RMR between individuals, and we often assume that trained individuals would have more FFM than untrained. Thus, by matching individuals for FFM, we can eliminate this confounding variable to see if exercise-trained individuals have a higher RMR. Figure 5.10 summarizes some of the current studies in this area. Results have been mixed. For example, Poehlman and colleagues (1990) found that active men had RMRs significantly (~5%) higher than those of untrained men of similar size and FFM, but Broeder and colleagues (1992) found no significant difference in RMR between active and inactive men—mean RMR was only 3.4% higher in the trained group. As yet there is no consensus in this area of research

(see "Why Is the Research Literature Inconsistent Regarding the Effect of Exercise on Metabolism?" on p. 150).

As figure 5.10 demonstrates, researchers have reported a wide range of differences in RMR (~3-16%). The discrepancies in these data may be due to a number of factors, including the subjects' levels of fitness, types of training program, methods used for measuring RMR, and levels of **energy flux** (a factor that includes kilocalories expended in exercise compared with kilocalories consumed each day, and also the amount of time between exercise sessions). Concerning the last point, RMR values may be influenced by acute changes in exercise energy expenditure or energy intake or both. Bullough and colleagues (1995), for example, found that athletes' RMRs measured after three days of high-intensity exercise (90 min of cycling at 75% $\dot{V}O_2$max) were significantly higher than when measured after three days of no exercise. During each of these periods, the

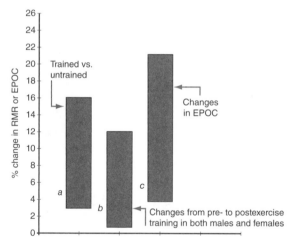

Figure 5.10 Effect of exercise on resting metabolic rate (RMR) and excess postexercise oxygen consumption (EPOC). *(a)* Effect of exercise on RMR in young trained and untrained men. *(b)* Effect of exercise training on posttraining RMR in previously untrained men and women. *(c)* Effect of exercise and exercise intensity on changes in EPOC. In each case, bar represents range of changes reported in the literature. See appendixes C.3 through C.5 for the research literature used to make this graph.

Adapted from R.C. Bullough et al., 1995, "Interaction of acute changes in exercise energy expenditure and energy intake on resting metabolic rate," *American Journal of Clinical Nutrition* 61: 473-481.

amount of energy fed matched energy expenditure. The authors also compared the RMRs of the trained group with those of an untrained control group and found no differences between groups if the trained group was measured after three days of no exercise. However, there were significant differences (~16%) between the trained and untrained groups when RMR was measured in the trained group after three days of high-intensity exercise. The researchers also found that if energy intake was low on high-exercise days, RMR was not elevated as compared to RMR on high-exercise days when energy intake was adequate (see figure 5.11).

Another factor that influences RMR is the timing of the RMR measurement related to physical activity, eating, and the use of stimulants such as caffeine and nicotine. Herring and colleagues (1992) examined RMR 15, 39, 63, and 87 h after the last exercise bout in nine long-distance female runners. By 39 h postexercise, RMR had declined by 8%. This lower RMR was maintained up to 87 h postexercise. Thus, if RMR is measured within 24 h of the last exercise bout, it may be higher than if measured 35 to 48 h afterward. However, since most active people exercise five to seven days per week, there is rarely a time when no exercise occurs for a 48 h period. In fact, many athletes actually train twice a day, so they rarely have even a 24 h period in which they do not exercise. Timing of the meal around exercise can also alter RMR. Haugen and colleagues (2003) found that RMR was significantly higher (~100 kcal/day) if measured in the afternoon after a 4 h fast than when measured in the morning after a 12 h fast. The same was true if RMR was measured in the afternoon after subjects had fasted 4 h, abstained from caffeine, and had no exercise versus in the morning after a 12 h fast, with exercise and caffeine controlled. In this study, RMR was ~100 kcal/

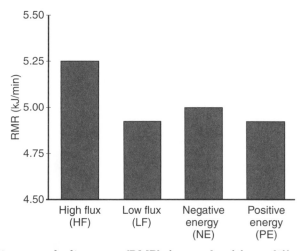

Figure 5.11 Average resting metabolic rates (RMR) for each of four different energy balance or flux conditions in eight highly trained men (mean ± SEM). High flux was significantly different from all other conditions ($P < 0.05$). Trained male athletes were used for the following four conditions:

- High flux (HF): Subjects were in a state of high energy flux, exercising at 75% $\dot{V}O_2$max for 90 min on each of three days while consuming a controlled diet adequate to maintain energy balance. High-flux turnover is characterized by high energy intake and exercise energy expenditure.

- Low flux (LF): Subjects were in a state of low energy flux, abstaining from exercise for three days while consuming a controlled diet adequate to maintain energy balance.

- Negative energy (NE) balance: Subjects were in NE balance, exercising at 75% $\dot{V}O_2$max for 90 min on each of three days while consuming the controlled diet designed to maintain energy balance during LF.

- Positive energy (PE) balance: Subjects were in PE balance, abstaining from exercise for two days while consuming the controlled diet designed to maintain energy balance during HF.

PE = High energy intake and high energy expenditure

Adapted, by permission, from R.C. Bullough et al., 1995, "Interaction of acute changes in exercise energy expenditure and energy intake on resting metabolic rate," *American Journal of Clinical Nutrition* 61: 473-481.

day higher in the afternoon setting compared to the morning setting. Thus, it is important to control the environment in which RMR is measured in order to ensure that one has measured a true RMR. Choosing the exact time to measure RMR postexercise in active individuals can be difficult! See the review by Levine (2005) for a detailed description of how the various components of energy expenditure should be measured.

For a Given Individual, Does Becoming More Aerobically Trained Increase Resting Metabolic Rate?

Researchers have examined pre- and posttraining RMRs in sedentary individuals who participated in exercise training programs (see figure 5.10*b*). Published data on change in RMR with exercise training range from <1% to 12%. For example, Wilmore and colleagues (1998) saw no change in RMR in 74 men and women (17-63 years) who participated in a 20-week endurance training program (cycle exercise) that increased $\dot{V}O_2$max by 17.9%. But Poehlman and Danforth (1991) reported an 11.8% increase in RMR in 19 older subjects (64 ± 1.6 years) participating in an eight-week endurance training program (cycle exercise). Again, the

mixed results presumably depend on a number of variables such as age, gender, level of obesity, type of training program used, and levels of fitness achieved. Although there appears to be no consensus in this area, we do know that becoming more physically active can increase or preserve FFM. This increased activity may in turn help to stabilize or increase RMR.

Does Metabolic Rate Stay Elevated After Exercise Is Over?

It is now well documented that oxygen consumption remains elevated for a short time after exercise has stopped (Gaesser and Brooks 1984; Osterberg and Melby 2000). During this cool-down period, heart rate and metabolic processes usually return to normal within a short time. How quickly the return to homeostasis occurs depends on a number of factors including level of training, age, environmental conditions, and intensity and duration of the exercise. Can exercise significantly increase oxygen consumption after exercise (the term generally used is **excess postexercise oxygen consumption** or **EPOC**)? Figure 5.12 illustrates the change in EPOC with different exercise intensities and durations in 10 trained male triathletes.

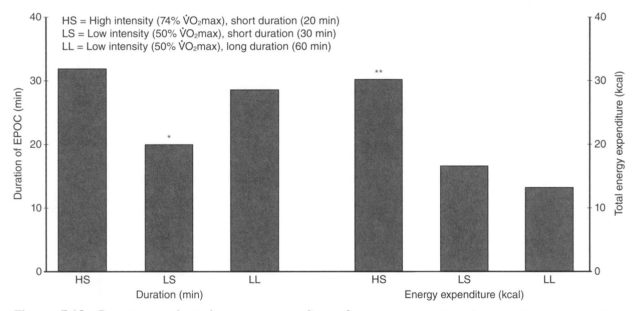

HS = High intensity (74% $\dot{V}O_2$max), short duration (20 min)
LS = Low intensity (50% $\dot{V}O_2$max), short duration (30 min)
LL = Low intensity (50% $\dot{V}O_2$max), long duration (60 min)

Figure 5.12 Duration and total energy expenditure for excess postexercise oxygen consumption (EPOC) in 10 trained male triathletes performing three cycle ergometer exercises. *Significantly different ($p < 0.05$) from HS and LL for duration. **Significantly different ($p < 0.05$) from LS and LL for energy expenditure.

Adapted, by permission, from D.A. Sedlock, J.A. Fissinger, and C.L. Melby, 1989, "Effect of exercise intensity and duration on post-exercise energy expenditure," *Medicine and Science in Sports and Exercise* 21: 662-666.

In this study, EPOC appears to be greater after high-intensity exercise, although the duration is short (20 min).

For how long and to what magnitude does EPOC increase after an exercise bout? Does a strenuous exercise session on one day significantly increase oxygen consumption on subsequent days? Figure 5.10 gives the range of changes in EPOC (~4-21%) reported in the research literature. It appears that to produce a significant increase in EPOC, exercise intensity must be high or the duration of exercise must be long. A normal exercise bout of 30 to 60 min of moderate intensity (50-65% $\dot{V}O_2$max) does not appear to significantly elevate EPOC for any appreciable length of time after the exercise ends—oxygen levels usually return to normal within 1 h. However, if exercise is of high intensity or of long duration, EPOC appears to be elevated for hours after exercise. In some cases, oxygen consumption is even elevated on subsequent days after strenuous exercise.

The type of exercise performed (aerobic vs. strength training) may also influence EPOC. Most research examining the effect of exercise on EPOC uses aerobic activity as the mode of exercise. However, Melby and colleagues (1993) observed a significant EPOC in trained males lifting weights for 90 min. On the morning after the exercise session, oxygen consumption was elevated by 5% to 10% over baseline levels. This same study was repeated in women with the same results. After 100 min of resistance exercise, EPOC was elevated by 4.2% the morning after the exercise compared to the morning after no exercise had occurred (Osterberg and Melby 2000). Thus, although it is well documented that O_2 consumption is elevated after exercise, the magnitude and duration of the elevation appear to depend on the intensity and duration of the exercise bout as well as the type of exercise.

Factors That Influence the Thermic Effect of Food

A number of factors can influence how our bodies respond metabolically when we consume food. Some of these factors are associated with physiological characteristics such as genetic background, age, level of physical fitness, sensitivity to insulin, or level of obesity. Other factors are associated with the meal, such as its size, composition, palatability, and timing.

Effect of Food Composition and Meal Size on the Thermic Effect of Food

The TEF can last for several hours after a meal and depends on the size of the meal consumed (number of kilocalories) and its composition (percentage of kilocalories from protein, fat, carbohydrate, alcohol) (Stock 1999). In general, the thermic effect of a mixed diet is about 6% to 10% of total daily energy intake; however, the total TEF also depends on the macronutrient composition of the diet. For example, the thermogenic effect of glucose is 5% to 10%, while the thermic effect of fat is 3% to 5% and that of protein is

---

Highlight

Why Is the Research Literature Inconsistent Regarding the Effect of Exercise on Metabolism?

A variety of factors may contribute to the inconsistency of published data on the effect of exercise on metabolism (especially on RMR):

- Some experiments used only a small number of subjects, and in some there was great variability in the subjects' characteristics (level of training, FFM, body size, age, diet behaviors).
- The time of the RMR measurements after the last exercise bout has not been standardized.
- Methods for measuring oxygen consumption vary (no repeated measures, no standardization of protocol), making comparisons between studies difficult.
- There often is variability in repeated measurements on the same individual due to prior dietary practices, exercise patterns, or other uncontrolled variables.
- Experimental subjects have variable levels of training (minutes exercised per week) and fitness (level of $\dot{V}O_2$max).

20% to 30% (Flatt 1992, 2001). The lower thermic responses for carbohydrate and fat are due to the lower energy requirement to store carbohydrate as glycogen and fat as triacylglycerides, as compared to the energy-expensive synthesis of proteins from amino acids. Because of the higher thermic effect of protein, it may play an important role in regulating food intake, by influencing satiety, and body weight (Westerterp-Plantenga 2003). The TEF also depends on how the body uses the energy it consumes: Is the body going to use the food for immediate energy, or will the energy be stored? If the energy will be stored, in what form will it be stored?

Table 5.1 reviews the energy costs of storing various macronutrients. For example, the amount of energy required to store dietary carbohydrate as glycogen is much lower than when dietary carbohydrate is converted to endogenous fat and stored. In general, converting dietary carbohydrate or protein to stored fat requires more energy than converting dietary fat to stored fat. In weight-stable, normal-weight people who consume a mixed diet, however, synthesis of fat from carbohydrate appears to be negligible. Under normal physiological conditions, excess protein and carbohydrate consumed are preferentially used for energy, while fat is stored. Diets higher in fat generally have a lower TEF than diets that contain more carbohydrate or protein—and a meal higher in kilocalories will have a higher TEF compared to a low-kilocalorie meal, which has fewer kilocalories and less food to be digested, transported, and stored. For example, the TEF of a person who consumes 3000 kcal/day would be 180 to 300 kcal/day, while someone consuming only 1500 kcal/day would have a TEF of 90 to 150 kcal/day. The total TEF for a day does not appear to be influenced by meal size or number, only the total number of kilocalories consumed. (Belko and Barbieri 1987). Thus, the TEF depends on the number of kilocalories consumed during the day and the composition of those kilocalories.

In the research laboratory, it is time-consuming to measure TEF and TEM; and these parameters are the least reproducible components of energy expenditure. Of the two measures, the TEM is more frequently used to measure metabolic response to food because it is more reproducible and also because the procedure is less expensive than measuring TEF in a metabolic chamber (Tataranni et al. 1995). The TEM represents the metabolic response to a single meal (usually over a 6 h period), while the TEF represents the metabolic response to all the food consumed during the day. As mentioned earlier, these terms are frequently used interchangeably in the research literature, so you need to look carefully at the methods to determine what was being measured. To determine the reproducibility of these measurements, one can measure an individual's day-to-day variability for TEM as well as the variability among individuals. Houde-Nadeau and colleagues (1993) reported the within-subject coefficient of variation for TEM to be 10.7%, while the between-subject variability was twice as high at 24%. These investigators measured TEM in four men and four women on three different occasions for 6 h. The subjects ate a standardized meal of 792 kcal (44% carbohydrate, 16% protein, 40% fat). The measured TEM was 7% after 6 h; but since the increased energy expenditure due to the meal had not returned to baseline, the total TEM was actually higher. This study showed no significant difference between men and women for TEM when values were expressed as kilocalories per hour. However, when the values were expressed as a percentage of RMR, the response was 10.7% for the women and 5% for the men after 6 h.

Effect of Exercise on the Thermic Effect of Food

The effect of acute exercise on TEF appears to depend on a number of factors, including the level of obesity, the timing of the meal and of the exercise session, the intensity and duration of the exercise, and the level of fitness. Segal and colleagues (1992) reported that exercise before a meal had no significant effect on TEM in lean subjects but increased TEM in obese subjects by 40%. However, the absolute increase in total kilocalories was small (10-15 kcal over 3 h). Few current data are available on the effect of exercise before and after a meal in exercise-trained subjects. Nichols and colleagues (1988) reported that in trained swimmers (both men and women), 45 min of swimming significantly increased the metabolic response to a meal by 18 kcals when the meal was fed before exercise, compared with feeding only the meal with no exercise (20.2 kcal/h). However, a difference of 18 kcal over the 4 h measurement period and the long-term significance of this difference is probably small, especially considering the high variability in the TEM measurement between individuals. More recently, Denzer and Young (2003) examined the impact of a single bout of resistance exercise on the TEF (660 kcal) for 2 h after exercise in both men and women. They found that exercise significantly increased TEF, but the difference was only 16 kcal (67 kJ/2 h) compared to no exercise. Again, the impact this energy difference would have on energy balance may be small and would depend on the frequency of eating immediately after a resistance exercise bout.

Measurement of Total Daily Energy Expenditure

Total daily energy expenditure or its components can be measured in the laboratory or can be estimated with prediction equations. We will discuss the most commonly used laboratory techniques as well as prediction equations that can be used to estimate energy expenditure when laboratory facilities are not available.

Calorimetry

Energy expenditure in humans can be assessed by either direct or indirect calorimetry. **Direct calorimetry** measures the amount of heat given off by the body through radiation, convection, and evaporation. Since neither oxygen nor carbon dioxide is stored in the body under normal physiological conditions, **indirect calorimetry** estimates the heat released through oxidative processes by measuring rates of oxygen consumption and carbon dioxide production. Under basal conditions, the two methods give identical results; but due to cyclical changes in body temperature throughout the day, direct calorimetry cannot be used to assess heat production for periods less than 24 h (Jequier and Shultz 1983). Direct calorimetry uses an airtight calorimetric chamber; the heat produced by the body warms the water surrounding the chamber (figure 5.13). Research-

ers calculate the amount of energy expended from the recorded changes in water temperature. This method is very expensive and is not currently used. Indirect calorimetry is much less expensive and is the method of choice for many researchers. Indirect calorimetry uses either a metabolic chamber or a mask, hood, or mouthpiece in which gases are collected and analyzed for a specified period of time.

Indirect calorimetry assumes that one can estimate metabolic rate by measuring the rate of transformation of chemical energy into heat. It involves measuring the oxygen consumed, the carbon dioxide produced, and, if possible, the amount of urinary nitrogen excreted (to provide an estimate of protein oxidation). The amounts of oxygen and carbon dioxide exchanged in the lungs closely represent the use and release of these substances by the body tissues.

Indirect calorimetry measures the amounts of oxygen consumed and carbon dioxide produced during various activities in order to estimate the amount of energy being expended during those activities. The ratio between the volume of carbon dioxide produced and the volume of oxygen consumed (VCO_2:VO_2), termed the nonprotein **respiratory quotient (RQ),** represents the ratio between oxidation of carbohydrates and lipids (see the following discussion of respiratory exchange ratio). Various published formulas permit estimation of total energy expenditure, using data on the amount of each energy substrate oxidized and the amounts of oxygen consumed and carbon dioxide produced. Appendix C.1 provides some of the most frequently used formulas. Figure 5.14 shows the equipment used in indirect calorimetry.

Highlight

What Is a Calorie?

A calorie (small "c") is defined as a unit of energy that is equivalent to 4.184 absolute joules or J. A joule is a designated measure of heat that is equivalent to the energy required to raise the temperature of 1 pound of water 1° F. Since a calorie is a fraction of a joule, it is the heat generated to raise the temperature of 1 gram of water 1° C. In the United States and in the popular press, the term calorie is actually referring to a kilocalorie or 1000 calories (small "c"). Thus, 1 food calorie (small "c") is equal to 1 kcal, or the amount of energy required to raise 1 kilogram of water from 15° to 16° C. As mentioned earlier, we use the term kilocalorie (kcal) through this book, which is equivalent to the term "calorie" typically used on food labels, in the popular press, and when people are referring to the energy content of food.

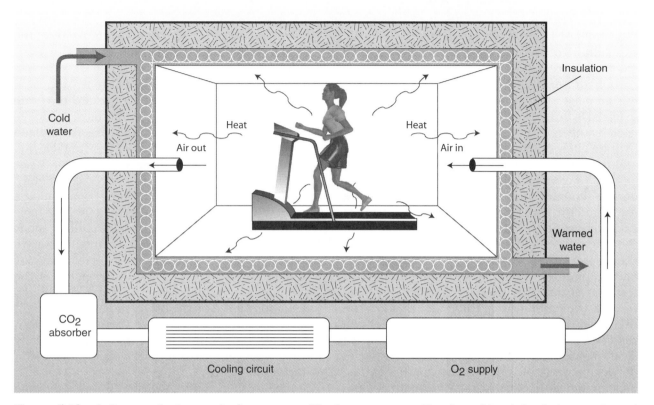

Figure 5.13 A direct calorimeter for human use. The heat generated by the subject's body is transferred to the air and walls of the chamber (through conduction, convection, and evaporation). This heat, produced by the subject, is then measured via recording of the temperature change in the air and water flowing through and around the chamber, respectively. The heat change is a measure of the subject's metabolic rate.

Reprinted, by permission, from J. H. Wilmore, D.L. Costill, and W.L. Kenney, 2008, *Physiology of sport and exercise,* 4th ed. (Champaign, IL: Human Kinetics), 101.

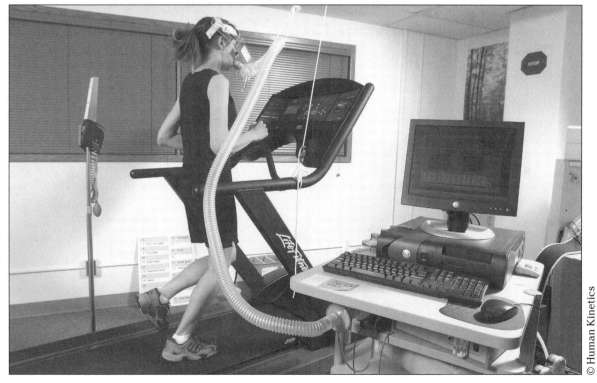

Figure 5.14 Indirect calorimetry.

Consuming 1 L of oxygen typically results in the expenditure of approximately 4.81 kcal if the fuels oxidized represent a mixture of protein, fat, and carbohydrate.

One must also know the types of foods being oxidized in order to estimate the amount of energy used by the body because fat, protein, and carbohydrate differ dramatically in their energy content and in their content of carbon and oxygen. The amount of oxygen used during exercise depends on the types of fuels being burned and can be estimated through calculation of the **respiratory exchange ratio (RER)**. This ratio is calculated in the same way as RQ. As mentioned in "What Is the Difference Between Respiratory Quotient (RQ) and Respiratory Exchange Ratio (RER)?", the two terms are frequently used interchangeably even though their definitions differ. True RQ is the exchange of oxygen and carbon dioxide at the *cellular level,* but since this parameter cannot be easily measured, RER is used to represent the ratio between carbon dioxide and oxygen that can be measured from expired gases using indirect calorimetry. The assumption is that RER adequately represents what is occurring metabolically at the cellular level under steady-state conditions.

The RER indicates the types of fuels being oxidized for energy at any particular time. Values for RER range from 1.0 to 0.7, with pure carbohydrate having a value of 1.0 and pure fat having a value of 0.7. When a molecule of glucose is oxidized completely, equal amounts of oxygen and carbon dioxide are used and released—thus the RQ or RER for glucose is 1.0. If fat is oxidized completely, the RQ or RER is 0.7. Most people consuming a mixed diet of protein, fat, and carbohydrate have an RER value between 0.82 and 0.87. During times of high exercise intensity, RER will move closer to 1.0; during times of fasting or low energy intake, RER will be closer to 0.7. Thus, RER depends on the composition of the foods consumed, the energy demands placed on the body, and whether weight is being maintained. Yet there are times when RER does not reflect what is occurring metabolically (e.g., hyperventilation can artificially elevate RER during exercise).

Finally, the energy available to the body from the combustion of the food that we consume is not

Highlight

What Is the Difference Between Respiratory Quotient (RQ) and Respiratory Exchange Ratio (RER)?

As the ratio between CO_2 produced and O_2 consumed (VCO_2:VO_2), RQ is an indication of the types of fuels being burned for energy at the cellular level. Since we cannot easily measure what is occurring at the cellular level, we measure RER. The RER is also calculated, using indirect calorimetry, as the ratio between CO_2 production and O_2 from expired gases (it thus represents the CO_2 released and the O_2 retained in lung tissue). Because RQ and RER are calculated using the same equation, the terms are often used interchangeably. However, it is appropriate to use RQ only when calculations are made to estimate cellular metabolism. When expired gases are measured and used to estimate fuel utilization, the term RER should be used. Nutrition research literature more frequently uses the term RQ, while exercise scientists tend to use the term RER. Here is an example of glucose oxidation and the resulting RER value:

$$6\ O_2 + C_6H_{12}O_6 \rightarrow 6\ CO_2 + 6\ H_2O + 38\ ATP.$$

Thus, the RER = 6 CO_2 / 6 O_2 = 1.

Here is an example of fat oxidation and the resulting RER, using a theoretical triacylglycerol containing two molecules of stearic acid and one of palmitic acid:

$$C_{55}H_{106}O_6 + 76.5\ O_2 \rightarrow 55\ CO_2 + 53\ H_2O.$$

Thus, the RER = 55 CO_2 / 76.5 O_2 = 0.719.

identical to the energy liberated when that same food is burned in a bomb calorimeter (e.g., burned until totally combusted) outside of the body in a furnace (Buchholz and Schoeller 2004) (see table 5.3). Thus, the energy available to the body when food is consumed is called metabolizable energy and will vary from the energy content obtained when food is burned outside the body. In addition, the amount of metabolizable energy available from a particular meal or diet will depend on the composition of the diet, especially the amount of protein or fiber in the diet (Buchholz and Schoeller 2004). Thus, the actual amount of food energy available to the body from each macronutrient has been estimated compared to the heat of combustion. These values are given in table 5.3 along with the level of variability associated with each macronutrient.

Doubly Labeled Water

Because calorimetry requires that a subject be confined to a laboratory setting or a metabolic chamber, it is difficult to measure a person's free-living or habitual activity. Several field methods for determining energy expenditure have been tested, ranging from factorial methods (described later in this chapter) to heart rate monitors, accelerometers, and pedometers. Unfortunately, these methods have disadvantages that frequently make them unacceptable for use with certain groups, or they can be too time-consuming to use with large populations (Schoeller and Racette 1990). Recently the **doubly labeled water (DLW)** technique has

been validated as a field method for determining total daily energy expenditure (figure 5.6).

The DLW ($^2H_2{}^{18}O$) method has become a valuable tool for determining free-living energy expenditures. This method was first developed for use in animals but eventually was applied to humans (Schoeller et al. 1986). The DLW method is a form of indirect calorimetry based on the differential elimination of ^2H (deuterium) and ^{18}O from body water following a dose of water labeled with these two stable isotopes. The deuterium is eliminated as water, while the ^{18}O is eliminated as both water and carbon dioxide. The difference between the two elimination rates is a measure of carbon dioxide production (Coward and Cole 1991; Prentice et al. 1991). The method differs from traditional indirect calorimetry in that it measures only CO_2 production and not oxygen (O_2) consumption. One advantage to the method is that it can measure energy expenditure in free-living subjects for three days to three weeks and requires only periodic collection of urine for measurement of the isotope elimination rates. Another advantage is that it is free of bias, and subjects can engage in normal daily activities without the interruption of writing down activities or wearing a heart rate monitor. The DLW method has been validated and is used to measure energy expenditure in a number of populations, including athletes (Sjodin et al. 1994; Westerterp et al. 1986), lean (Seale et al. 1993) and obese individuals (Prentice et al. 1986; Ravussin et al. 1991), and children (Kaskoun et al. 1994). It has become a valuable tool for validating

Table 5.3 Available Energy When Food Is Burned in a Bomb Calorimeter Versus That Available When a Mixed Diet Is Fed[1]

Macronutrient	Heat of combustion (kcal/g) from bomb calorimeter	Coefficient of availability (%)	Available energy (kcal/g total nutrients) for the body
Protein	5.65	92	4.0[2]
Fat	9.40	95	8.9[3]
Carbohydrate	4.10	97	4.0

[1] Represents the amount of energy (kcal/g) generated from a mixed meal when it is burned in a bomb calorimeter versus the amount of energy (kcal/g total nutrient) available to the body when that same meal is consumed. Fiber in food is not completely digested by the body so cannot yield the same amount of energy as when it is burned in a bomb calorimeter.

[2] Corrected for unoxidized material in the urine, that is, (5.65 kcal/g × 0.923) – 1.25 kcal/g. An additional correction is made for protein. For each g of N in the urine, there is unoxidized matter to yield an average of 1.25 kcal/g. This value is subtracted from the heat of combustion of protein. This correction factor is based on original research by Atwater, Rubner, and Bryant and is described by Buchholz and Schoeller (2004).

[3] The energy availability of fat is typically rounded to 9 kcal/g.

Reprinted, by permission, from A.C. Buchholz and D.A. Schoeller, 2004, "Is a calorie a calorie?" *American Journal of Clinical Nutrition* 79(suppl): 899S-906S.

other less expensive field methods of measuring energy expenditure, such as pedometers, heart rate monitors, motion sensors, and uniaxial and triaxial accelerometers (Schoeller and Racette 1990; Ainslie et al. 2003). The major disadvantages of the technique are as follows:

1. It is too expensive for large population-based studies.

2. Specialized expertise is required for the analysis of the isotope concentration in body fluids by mass spectrometry.

3. It has a five times greater potential error on the energy expenditure calculation because it uses only the caloric equivalent of carbon dioxide and not the caloric equivalent of oxygen (Jequier et al. 1987).

4. Its experimental variability can be high (5-8.5%), both when the technique is repeated in the same individual and when it is repeated between individuals (Goran et al. 1994; Ainslie et al. 2003).

Predicting Energy Expenditure

How can we estimate or predict total energy expenditure outside the laboratory setting? As mentioned earlier, total energy expenditure comprises RMR, TEF, and TEA. One of the most common ways to estimate total energy expenditure is to first estimate RMR using a prediction equation and then multiply RMR by an appropriate activity factor. This is called the factorial method. A number of RMR prediction equations have been developed using populations differing in age, gender, level of obesity, and activity level. In general, it is best to use the RMR prediction equation most representative of the population with whom you are working. For example, if you want to predict the RMR of young active women, employ an equation developed with that population. "Equations for Estimating Resting Metabolic Rate (RMR) in Healthy Individuals" lists some of the commonly used RMR prediction equations and the populations from which they were developed. Most of these RMR prediction equations were developed using sedentary individuals. In an effort to determine which of the RMR prediction equations works best for active individuals, Thompson and Manore (1996) compared actual RMR values measured in the laboratory with RMR values predicted by equations listed in "Equations for Estimating Resting Metabolic Rate (RMR) in Healthy Individuals." They found that for both active men and women, the Cunningham equation

best predicted RMR; the Harris-Benedict equation was the next best predictor. Figure 5.15 shows how closely these equations predicted RMR in a group of endurance-trained men and women. Because the Cunningham equation requires the measurement of lean body mass (LBM), the Harris-Benedict equation is easier to use when LBM cannot be directly measured. However, in less active populations, the equation of Mifflin and colleagues (1990) has been shown to be the best predictor of RMR.

Factorial Methods for Predicting Total Daily Energy Expenditure Once a value for RMR has been obtained either by estimation or by direct measurement, **total daily energy expenditure (TDEE)** can be estimated by a variety of factorial methods that differ in labor intensiveness and in the level of respondent burden. Appendix C.2 describes these methods in detail. The easiest methods multiply RMR by an appropriate **activity factor (AF)** to estimate TDEE. This factor may be as low as 10% to 20% of RMR for a bedridden person and as high as >100% for a very active individual. Although many laboratories establish unique activity factors for their particular research setting, factors of 1.3 to 1.6 are commonly used with sedentary people or for those doing only light activity. One activity factor can be applied to the whole day, or a weighted activity factor can be determined. This activity factor is then multiplied by the RMR to provide a TDEE value in kilocalories per day. For example, if an individual has an RMR of 1500 kcal/day and an activity factor of 1.3, then the daily energy expenditure will be 30% above RMR or 1950 kcal/day (1500 × 1.3 = 1950 kcal/day).

A third method estimates a **general activity factor (GAF)** and a **specific activity factor (SAF)**. The GAF represents energy expended for everyday activities like walking about, driving, watching TV, and going to class (table 5.4); SAF is activity expended in planned or purposeful activity like running, swimming, cycling, or weight training for a designated amount of time at a specific level of intensity. The GAF is calculated as indicated earlier; to obtain SAF, the amount of time spent in a specific activity is multiplied by the energy required for that activity in kilocalories per kilogram body weight per minute (see appendix E.3 for tables giving these values). The GAF and SAF are then added together to get the total amount of energy expended per day in activity. This value is added to the estimated RMR value to give a subtotal for energy expenditure; an additional 6% to 10% is then added to this value to represent

Equations for Estimating Resting Metabolic Rate (RMR) in Healthy Individuals

Harris-Benedict (1919)[a]

Males: RMR = 66.47 + 13.75 (wt) + 5 (ht) − 6.76 (age).

Females: RMR = 655.1 + 9.56 (wt) + 1.85 (ht) − 4.68 (age).

Owen and Colleagues (1986)[b]

Active females: RMR = 50.4 + 21.1 (wt).

Inactive females: RMR = 795 + 7.18 (wt).

Owen and Colleagues (1987)[c]

Males: RMR = 290 + 22.3 (LBM).

Males: RMR = 879 +10.2 (wt).

Mifflin and Colleagues (1990)[d]

RMR = 9.99 (wt) + 6.25 (ht) − 4.92 (age) + 166 (sex; male = 1, female = 0) − 161.

Cunningham (1980)[e]

RMR = 500 + 22 (LBM).

World Health Organization (1985)[f]

Sex	Age range (years)	Equation to derive RMR in kcal/day
Males	0-3	$(60.9 \times wt) - 54$
	3-10	$(22.7 \times wt) + 495$
	10-18	$(17.5 \times wt) + 651$
	18-30	$(15.3 \times wt) + 679$
	30-60	$(11.6 \times wt) + 879$
	60	$(13.5 \times wt) + 487$
Females	0-3	$(61.0 \times wt) - 51$
	3-10	$(22.5 \times wt) + 499$
	10-18	$(12.2 \times wt) + 746$
	18-30	$(14.7 \times wt) + 496$
	30-60	$(8.7 \times wt) + 829$
	>60	$(10.5 \times wt) + 596$

[a] The Harris-Benedict equation was published in 1919, based on 136 men and (mean age 27 ± 9 years; mean weight 64 ± 10 kg) 103 women (mean age 331 ± 14 years; mean weight 56.5 ± 11.5 kg) (n = 239 subjects). The subjects included some trained male athletes. The investigators derived different equations for men and women and included weight, height, and age as variables. Researchers frequently report that the Harris-Benedict equation overpredicts RMR by >15%.

[b] Owen and colleagues' (1986) equation was developed using 44 lean and obese women; eight of the women were trained athletes (ages 18-65 years; 48-143 kg). None of the women were menstruating during the study, and all reported having been weight stable for at least one month.

[c] Owen and colleagues' (1987) equation was developed using 60 lean and obese men (ages 18-82 years; weight range 60-171 kg). All had been weight stable for at least one month. No athletes were included in this study.

[d] Mifflin and colleagues (1990) used 498 healthy lean and obese subjects (247 females and 251 males), aged 18 to 78 years; weight ranged from 46 to 120 kg for the women and from 58 to 143 kg for the men. No mention was made of the physical activity level of the subjects.

[e] Cunningham (1980) used 223 subjects (120 males and 103 females) from the 1919 Harris and Benedict database. Cunningham eliminated 16 males who had been identified as trained athletes. In this study, LBM accounted for 70% of the variability of BMR. The age variable did not account for much of the variability because the age range of the group was narrow. Lean body mass had not been determined for the Harris-Benedict equation, so Cunningham estimated LBM based on body mass (kg) and age.

[f] The World Health Organization (1985) derived these equations from BMR data: wt = weight (kg); ht = height (cm); age = age (years); and LBM = lean body mass (kg).

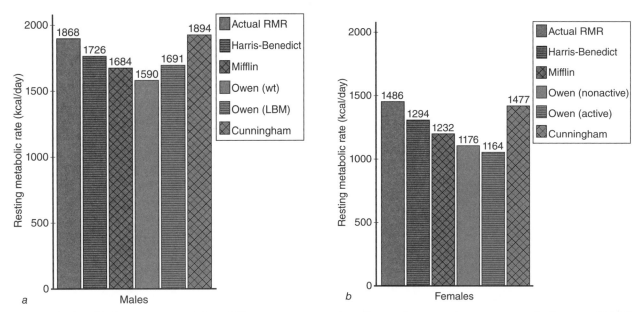

Figure 5.15 *(a)* Comparison of five different equations for the prediction of resting metabolic rate (RMR) in endurance-trained men compared to actual measured RMR. *(b)* Comparison of five different equations (see "Equations for Estimating Resting Metabolic Rate (RMR) in Healthy Individuals") for the prediction of RMR in endurance-trained women compared to actual measured RMR. LBM = lean body mass.

Reprinted from *Journal of the American Dietetic Association,* Vol 96, J.L. Thompson and M.M. Manore, "Predicted and measured resting metabolic rate of male and female endurance athletes," pgs. 30-34. Copyright 1996, with permission from Elsevier.

TEF. The final number represents the total energy expended in a day or TDEE (see appendix C.2 for an example). This method is relatively easy to use with active individuals who follow specific training or exercise programs and who already keep training logs.

A final method of estimating total energy expenditure is to record all activities over a 24 h period, then calculate (using energy expenditure tables) the total energy expended in each of these activities (kilocalories per kilogram body weight per minute). The kilocalories expended in the various activities are then added together to represent the total amount of energy expended for that day (appendix C.2). Many computer programs allow you to calculate energy expenditure in this way. See appendix E.2 for a sample 24 h energy expenditure form. Regardless of which method is used, keep in mind that all values are estimates. The accuracy of these values depends on how carefully activity is recorded and on the accuracy of the database that was used to generate the energy estimates.

Dietary Reference Intakes Method for Estimating Energy Requirements Recently the Institute of Medicine (IOM) developed prediction equations for estimated energy requirements (EER) as part of the Dietary Reference Intakes (DRIs) for energy and macronutrients based on cross-sectional DLW data acquired from individual investigators. These investigators had collected the data on a number of persons with a range of ages and activity levels but within normal body size (body mass index [BMI] = 18.5-25 kg/m^2) (IOM 2005). It is suggested that this method replace the factorial methods, which may underestimate energy needs (IOM 2005). Thus the Dietary Reference Committee for Energy and Macronutrients felt that the DLW method would provide a more accurate estimate of EER for most individuals. In calculating EER, age, weight, and height are used in the equation along with a physical activity coefficient (PA). The PA is determined from the physical activity level (PAL) of the individual, where PA = TDEE / BEE (basal energy expenditure). An average of 60 min of daily moderate-intensity physical activity (e.g., walking/jogging at 3-4 mph [4.8-6.4 km/h]) or shorter periods of more vigorous exertion (e.g., jogging for 30 min at 5.5 mph [~9 km/h]) were associated with a normal BMI and therefore were recommended for normal-weight individuals. The amount of physical activity the DRI committee used to represent

Table 5.4   Approximate Energy Expenditure for Various Activities in Relation to Resting Needs for Males and Females of Average Size

Activity category[a]	Representative values for activity factor per unit of time of activity	kcal/min
Resting Sleeping, reclining	RMR × 1.0	1-1.2
Very light Seated and standing activities, painting trades, driving, laboratory work, typing, sewing, ironing, cooking, playing cards, playing a musical instrument	RMR × 1.5	Up to 2.5
Light Walking on a level surface at 2.5 or 3 mph, garage work, electrical trades, carpentry, restaurant trades, house cleaning, child care, golf, sailing, table tennis	RMR × 2.5	2.5-4.9
Moderate Walking 3.5 to 4 mph, weeding and hoeing, carrying a load, cycling, skiing, tennis, dancing	RMR × 5.0	5.0-7.4
Heavy Walking with a load uphill, tree felling, heavy manual digging, basketball, climbing, football, soccer	RMR × 7.0	7.5-12.0

[a] When reported as multiples of basal needs, the expenditures of males and females are similar.

an "active" lifestyle, corresponding to a PAL >1.6. (See "Estimated Energy Requirements" p. 160.)

The DRIs are provided for general healthy populations; therefore, a recommended level of physical activity for weight loss for an obese individual was not determined by the DRI committee. In addition, the DRI committee made a distinction between physical activity and exercise, viewing the latter as more vigorous and required for improvement in physical fitness. For the DLW data collected and used to calculate the EER prediction equations, the average PAL was 1.75, which is equivalent to walking 5 to 7 miles/day (8-11 km) at 3 to 4 mph. Knowing these comparisons helps one to determine how to estimate an individual's PAL and to decide what "activity" category the person should be placed in. In addition, a complete list of various physical activities and their associated PAL values are provided by the DRI committee (see IOM 2005).

To use the EER method, first determine the PAL (see "Estimated Energy Requirements" p. 160) and the PA associated with PAL. Once you know the PA, you can use the equations provided to determine the EER for men and women 19 years and older. An example of calculating the EER of an active individual is also given. Although this method is faster than the factorial method, it does not allow for the calculation of TDEE in highly active individuals, since the highest PA may not be reflective of the level of activity engaged in by elite athletes or very active recreational athletes. Thus, the energy needs of highly active individuals may still need to be estimated using the factorial method. The IOM also has EER equations for children (IOM 2005).

ENERGY INTAKE

Since energy intake is one side of the energy balance equation, knowing total energy intake gives some indication of total energy expenditure if body weight is stable. Collection and assessment of dietary intake is the most frequently used procedure for monitoring energy and nutrient intakes in active individuals. The goal is to achieve the most accurate possible description of a person's typical food intake, then to use that information (1) to assess mean energy and nutrient intakes, (2) to make recommendations for changing or improving food habits, (3) to determine the need for micronutrient supplements, or (4) to help the person achieve his or her dietary or weight goal or both.

Estimated Energy Requirements (EER) Equations for Men and Women Ages 19 Years and Older[1-3]

EER for Men Ages 19 and Older

$$EER = 662 - (9.53 \times age\ [years]) + PA \times (15.91 \times weight\ [kg] + 539.6 \times height\ [m])$$

where PA is the physical activity coefficient:

PA = 1.00 if PAL is estimated to be ≥1.0 and <1.4 (sedentary).

PA = 1.11 if PAL is estimated to be ≥1.4 and <1.6 (low active).

PA = 1.25 if PAL is estimated to be ≥1.6 and <1.9 (active).

PA = 1.48 if PAL is estimated to be ≥1.9 and <2.5 (very active).

Example: A male long-distance runner (23 years, 179 cm, 80 kg) is a graduate student who trains 2 h/day. When he is not training, he is relatively sedentary and spends his time walking to class, sitting in class, studying, and working at the computer. If we used the highest PAL value (very active = 1.9-2.5) to represent his activity level, which corresponds to a PA of 1.48, his EER would be as follows:

$$EER = 662 - (9.53 \times 23\ years) + 1.48 \times (15.91 \times 80\ kg + 539.6 \times 1.79\ m).$$
$$EER = 662 - (219) + 1.48 \times (1273 + 966).$$
$$EER = 3756\ kcal/day.$$

Note: Based on the factorial methods given in appendix C.2 for this same individual, the TDEE was calculated as 5153 kcal/day with the combined method (method 3) and 5129 kcal/day with the specific activity factor method (method 4). Thus, the DRI method underestimates the energy demand of this athlete because the EER equation and the estimated PA values are not based on data from individuals with exceptionally high levels of physical activity.

EER for Women Ages 19 and Older

$$EER = 354 - (6.91 \times age\ [years]) + PA \times (9.36 \times weight\ [kg] + 726 \times height\ [m])$$

where PA is the physical activity coefficient:

PA = 1.00 if PAL is estimated to be ≥1.0 and <1.4 (sedentary).

PA = 1.12 if PAL is estimated to be ≥1.4 and <1.6 (low active).

PA = 1.27 if PAL is estimated to be ≥1.6 and <1.9 (active).

PA = 1.45 if PAL is estimated to be ≥1.9 and <2.5 (very active).

Example: An active woman (41 years, 163 cm, 64.4 kg) exercises ~7.5 h/week in both aerobic activities and weight training. Estimated PAL is considered "active" with a PAL between 1.6 and 1.9 a PA of 1.27.

$$EER = 354 - (6.91 \times 41\ years) + PA \times (9.36 \times 64.4\ kg + 726 \times 1.63\ m).$$
$$EER = 354 - (283) + 1.27 \times (603 + 1183).$$
$$EER = 2339\ kcal/day.$$

Note: Based on the factorial methods given in appendix C.2 for this same individual, the TDEE was calculated as 2208 kcal/day with activity factor method 1 and 2415 kcal/day with activity factor method 2.

[1] Individual doubly labeled water (DLW) data were not used in the estimates to make these equations if the PAL value was <1.0 or greater than 2.5. Cross-sectional data from DLW were used to define a recommended level of physical activity, based on the physical activity level (PAL) associated with a normal body mass index (BMI) range of 18.5 to 25 kg/m². An "active" lifestyle is recommended for all normal-weight individuals and corresponds to a PAL of 1.6 or greater. This would include an average of 60 min of daily moderate-intensity physical activity (e.g., walking/jogging at 3-4 mph [4.8-6.4 km/h]) or shorter periods of more vigorous exertion (e.g., jogging for 30 min at 5.5 mph [~9 km/h]).

[2] Source: Institute of Medicine (IOM), Food and Nutrition Board, 2005, *Dietary reference intakes for energy, carbohydrate, fiber, fat, fatty acids, cholesterol, protein, and amino acids* (Washington, DC: National Academy Press), 184-185.

[3] To convert pounds to kilograms: pounds / 2.2 = kg; to convert inches to meters: inches × 2.54 / 100 = m.

Collecting dietary data is only part of the assessment process. The data then must be analyzed using a computerized nutrient analysis program, with the results compared to nutrient standards or goals. Energy intakes must be compared to estimated energy expenditure values. To avoid introducing additional error into the process of dietary assessment, care should be taken in choosing and using a computerized nutrient analysis program; the program should allow you to enter additional food data, such as specific sport foods or supplements, that may not be in the database.

Once diet data are analyzed, results are usually compared to some type of dietary standard. Although a variety of standards are available, the most commonly used standards are the DRIs, which include the Recommended Dietary Allowances (RDAs) (IOM 1997, 1998, 2001, 2005); *Dietary Guidelines for Americans* (U.S. Department of Agriculture 2005); and MyPyramid—"Steps to a Healthier You" (U.S. Department of Agriculture 2005) (all discussed in chapter 1). Additional recommendations for nutrient intakes are frequently made for active individuals, especially female athletes (see chapter 15).

CHAPTER IN REVIEW

This chapter has discussed the components that determine energy balance—both energy input (dietary energy plus the contribution of energy stores within the body) and energy expenditure. We have covered how the various components of energy expenditure can be measured. For any one individual, the factors that influence energy balance may be numerous, including gender, age, family history, dietary choices, level of daily activity, and stress level. If a person wishes to permanently change body size, then one or more of the components of energy balance must be altered over an extended period of time. The following chapter presents methods for doing this.

◆

Key Concepts

1. **Explain the energy and nutrient balance equations.**

   Energy balance, or long-term weight maintenance, requires that the amount and composition of energy input (both from dietary sources and from stored energy in the body) equal energy expended. It also requires that the oxidation of protein, fat, and carbohydrate equal the proportion in which they are consumed within the diet. Thus, energy balance depends not only on the balance between energy intake and energy expenditure but also on the oxidation rate of the energy consumed (carbohydrate, protein, fat, and alcohol).

2. **Understand the concept of nutrient balance and the contributions of carbohydrate, protein, fat, and alcohol to energy balance.**

   Nutrient balance means that oxidation rates of dietary protein, fat, carbohydrate, and alcohol are equal to their intake. Oxidation of protein and carbohydrate closely match their dietary intake—as protein or carbohydrate intake increases, so does its oxidation within the body. Fat oxidation is less sensitive to change in dietary fat intake: An excess of dietary fat results in increased fat storage. Since in humans there is little synthesis of endogenous fat from excess dietary carbohydrate or protein, increased intakes of these nutrients increase their oxidation rates, resulting in dietary fat being stored in adipose tissue. Alcohol is a priority fuel that undergoes rapid oxidation while suppressing the oxidation of other substrates, especially fat.

3. **Identify the various components of energy expenditure, how they are measured, and the contribution of energy expenditure to the energy balance equation.**

   Total daily energy expenditure includes RMR, TEF, TEA (daily activities, exercise, SPA, NEAT, and AT). Of these factors, TEA can vary the most and is most susceptible to lifestyle changes, while TEF is the most difficult to measure and has a greater degree of variability. A variety of factors can influence RMR. Some are fixed and cannot be changed (e.g., age, gender, genetics), while others may be influenced by lifestyle (e.g., level of fitness and FFM). Energy expenditure needs are generally estimated in the laboratory using indirect calorimetry and 24 h activity logs or estimated using prediction equations such as the DRI predication equations.

4. Understand the role of energy intake in the energy balance equation.

Total daily energy intake is one side of the energy balance equation. If a person is in energy balance, energy intake equals energy expenditure. Knowing total energy intake provides some indication of total energy expenditure if weight is stable. It is difficult and time-consuming to record accurate total daily energy intakes that represent typical dietary patterns.

Key Terms

activity factor (AF) 156
adaptive thermogenesis (AT) 142
basal metabolic rate (BMR) 139
direct calorimetry 152
doubly labeled water (DLW) 155
energy balance 134
energy flux 147
excess postexercise oxygen consumption (EPOC) 149
facultative thermogenesis 142
general activity factor (GAF) 156
indirect calorimetry 152
nonexercise activity thermogenesis (NEAT) 142

obligatory thermogenesis 141
respiratory exchange ratio (RER) 154
respiratory quotient (RQ) 152
resting energy expenditure (REE) 139
resting metabolic rate (RMR) 139
sleeping metabolic rate (SMR) 141
specific activity factor (SAF) 156
spontaneous physical activity (SPA) 142
thermic effect of activity (TEA) 142
thermic effect of a meal (TEM) 141
thermic effect of food (TEF) 141
total daily energy expenditure (TDEE) 156

Additional Information

Buchholz AC, Schoeller DA. Is a calorie a calorie? Am J Clin Nutr 2004;79(suppl):899S-906S.

This review paper evaluates the data and potential mechanisms for increases in weight loss in subjects consuming diets high in protein, low in carbohydrate, or both. Does a calorie from protein differ from a calorie of carbohydrate?

Institute of Medicine (IOM), Food and Nutrition Board. Dietary reference intakes for energy, carbohydrate, fiber, fat, fatty acids, cholesterol, protein, and amino acids. Washington, DC: National Academy Press, 2005.

This is the source for DRIs for energy and the macronutrients, providing a complete review of the literature and presenting the data and rationale for the new DRIs for protein, fat, and carbohydrate and the bases for the new energy expenditure tables.

Levine JA. Non-exercise activity thermogenesis (NEAT). Nutr Rev 2004;62(7):S82-S97.

A complete review of the role of NEAT in regulating body weight, including methods for measurement, variability of NEAT, and how changes in energy balance affect NEAT.

Suter PM. Is alcohol consumption a risk factor for weight gain and obesity? Crit Rev Clin Lab Sci 2005;43(3):197-227.

A complete review of how the body metabolizes alcohol, including the various metabolic pathways and the effects of alcohol on energy and substrate balance. The role of alcohol in fat distribution and the research on the relationship between alcohol intake and body weight are also reviewed.

References

Acheson KJ, Schutz Y, Bessard T, Ravussin E, Jequier E, Flatte JP. Glycogen storage capacity and de novo lipogenesis during massive carbohdyrate overfeeding in man. Am J Clin Nutr 1988;48:240-247.

Acheson KJ, Ravussin E, Wahren J, Jequier E. Thermic effect of glucose in man. Obligatory and facultative thermogenesis. J Clin Invest 1984;74(5):1572-1580.

Ainslie PN, Reilly T, Westerterp KR. Estimating human energy expenditure: a review of techniques with particular reference to doubly labelled water. Sports Med 2003;33(9):683-698.

Astrup A, Buemann B, Western P, Toubro S, Raben A, Christensen NJ. Obesity as an adaptation to a high-fat diet: evidence from a cross-sectional study. Am J Clin Nutr 1994;59:350-355.

Barr SI, Janelle KC, Prior JC. Energy intakes are higher during the luteal phase of ovulatory menstrual cycles. Am J Clin Nutr 1995;61:39-43.

Beidleman BA, Pahl JL, De Souza MJ. Energy balance in female distance runners. Am J Clin Nutr 1995;61:303-311.

Belko AZ, Barbieri TF. Effect of meal size and frequency on the thermic effect of food. Nutr Res 1987;7:237-242.

Bisbee JT, James WPT, Shaw MA. Changes in energy expenditure during the menstrual cycle. Br J Nutr 1989;61:187-199.

Blanc S, Schoeller DA, Bauer D, Danielson ME, Tylasvsky F, Simonsick EM, Harris TB, Kritchevsky SB, Everhart JE. Energy requirements in the eighth decade of life. Am J Clin Nutr 2004;79:303-310.

Bogardus C, Lillioja S, Ravussin E et al. Familial dependence of the resting metabolic rate. N Engl J Med 1986;315:96-100.

Bouchard C, Tremblay A, Nadeau A et al. Genetic effect in resting and exercise metabolic rates. Metabolism 1989;38:364-470.

Bray GA, Atkinson RL. Factors affecting basal metabolic rate. Prog Food Nutr Sci 1977;2(8):395-403.

Broeder CE, Burrhus KA, Svanevik LS, Wilmore JH. The effect of aerobic fitness on resting metabolic rate. Am J Clin Nutr 1992;55:795-801.

Buchholz AC, Schoeller DA. Is a calorie a calorie? Am J Clin Nutr 2004;79(suppl):899S-906S.

Bullough RC, Gillette CA, Harris MA, Melby CL. Interaction of acute changes in exercise energy expenditure and energy intake on resting metabolic rate. Am J Clin Nutr 1995;61:473-481.

Bullough RC, Melby CL. Effect of inpatient versus outpatient measurement protocol on resting metabolic rate and respiratory exchange ratio. Ann Nutr Metab 1993;27:24-32.

Butterfield G, Tremblay A. Physical activity and nutrition in the context of fitness and health. In: Bouchard C, Shephard RJ, Stevens S eds. Physical activity, fitness and health. International proceedings and consensus statement. Champaign, IL: Human Kinetics, 1994;257-269.

Collins LC, Cornelius MF, Vogel RL, Walker JF, Stamford BA. Effect of caffeine and/or cigarette smoking on resting energy expenditure. Int J Obesity 1994;18:551-556.

Coward WA, Cole TJ. The doubly labeled water method for the measurement of energy expenditure in humans: risks and benefits. In: Whitehead RG, Prentice A eds. New techniques in nutritional research. New York: Academic Press, 1991;139-176.

Cunningham JJ. A reanalysis of the factors influencing basal metabolic rate in normal adults. Am J Clin Nutr Nov 1980;33(11):2372-2374.

Day DS, Gozansky WS, Van Pelt RE, Schwartz RS, Kohrt WM. Sex hormone suppression reduces resting energy expenditure and β-adrenergic support of resting energy expenditure. J Clin Endocrinol Metab 2005;90:3312-3317.

Denzer CM, Young JC. The effect of resistance exercise on the thermic effect of food. Int J Sport Nutr Exerc Metab 2003;13:396-402.

Dulloo AG, Geissler CA, Horton T, Collins A, Miller DS. Normal caffeine consumption: influence on thermogenesis and daily energy expenditure in lean and post-obese human volunteers. Am J Clin Nutr 1989;49:44-50.

Eckel RH, Hernandez TL, Bell M L, Weil KM, Shepard TY, Grunwald GK, Sharp TA, Francis CC, Hill JO. Carbohydrate balance predicts weight and fat gain in adults. Am J Clin Nutr 2006;83:803-808.

Ferraro R, Lillioja S, Fontvieille AM, Rising R, Bogardus C, Ravussin E. Lower sedentary metabolic rate in women compared to men. J Clin Invest 1992;90:780-784.

Flatt JP. The biochemistry of energy expenditure. In: Bray G ed. Recent advances in obesity research II. London: John Libbey, 1978;211-228.

Flatt JP. Importance of nutrient balance in body weight regulation. Diabetes Metab Rev 1988;4(6):571-581.

Flatt JP. The biochemistry of energy expenditure. In: Bjornthrop P, Brodoff BN eds. Obesity. New York: Lippincott, 1992;100-116.

Flatt JP. Dietary fat, carbohydrate balance, and weight maintenance. Ann NY Acad Sci 1993;683:122-140.

Flatt JP. Macronutrient composition and food selection. Obesity Res 2001;9(4):256S-262S.

Flatt JP, Ravussin E, Acheson KJ, Jequier E. Effects of dietary fat on postprandial substrate oxidation and on carbohydrate and fat balance. J Clin Invest 1985;76:1019-1024.

Friedman MI, Tordoff MG. Fatty acid oxidation and glucose utilization interact to control food intake in rats. Am J Physiol 1986;251(20):R840-R845.

Gaesser GA, Brooks GA. Metabolic bases of excess post-exercise oxygen consumption: a review. Med Sci Sports Exerc 1984;16(1):29-43.

Goran MI, Poehlman ET, Danforth E. Experimental reliability of the doubly labeled water technique. Am J Physiol 1994;266:E510-E515.

Harris JA, Benedict FG. A biometric study of basal metabolism in man. Carnegie Inst Wash pub. no. 279. Philadelphia: Lippincott, 1919;227.

Haugen HA, Melanson EL, Tran ZV, Kearney JT, Hill JO. Variability of measured resting metabolic rate. Am J Clin Nutr 2003;78:1141-1144.

Hellerstein MK, Christiansen M, Kaempfer S. Measurement of de novo hepatic lipogenesis in humans using stable isotopes. J Clin Invest 1991;87:1841-1852.

Herring JL, Mole PA, Meredith CN, Stern JS. Effect of suspending exercise training on resting metabolic rate in women. Med Sci Sports Exerc 1992;24(1):59-65.

Hollis JH, Mattes RD. Are all calories created equal? Emerging issues in weight management. Curr Diabetes Rep 2005;5:374-378.

Houde-Nadeau M, de Jonge L, Garrel DR. Thermogenic response to food: intra-individual variability and measurement reliability. J Am Coll Nutr 1993;12(5):511-516.

Hunter GR, Weinsier RL, Darnel BE, Zuckerman PA, Goran MI. Racial difference in energy expenditure and aerobic fitness in premenopausal women. Am J Clin Nutr 2000;71:500-506.

Institute of Medicine (IOM), Food and Nutrition Board. Recommended dietary allowances, 10th ed. National Research Council. Washington, DC: National Academy Press, 1989.

Institute of Medicine (IOM), Food and Nutrition Board. Dietary reference intakes for calcium, phosphorus, magnesium, vitamin D, and fluoride. Washington, DC: National Academy Press, 1997.

Institute of Medicine (IOM), Food and Nutrition Board. Dietary reference intakes for thiamin, riboflavin, niacin, vitamin B-6, folate, vitamin B-12, pantothenic acid, biotin, and choline. Washington, DC: National Academy Press, 1998.

Institute of Medicine (IOM), Food and Nutrition Board. Dietary reference intakes for vitamin A, vitamin K, arsenic, boron, chromium, copper, iodione, iron, manganese, molybdenum, nickel, silicon, vanadium, and zinc. Washington, DC: National Academy Press, 2001.

Institute of Medicine (IOM), Food and Nutrition Board. Dietary reference intakes for energy, carbohydrate, fiber, fat, fatty acids, cholesterol, protein, and amino acids. Washington, DC: National Academy Press, 2005.

Jebb SA, Prentice AM, Goldberg GR, Murgatroyd PR, Black AE, Coward WA. Changes in macronutrient balance during over- and underfeeding assessed by 12-d continuous whole-body calorimetry. Am J Clin Nutr 1996;64:259-266.

Jequier E. Regulation of thermogenesis and nutrient metabolism in the human: relevance for obesity. In: Bjorntorp P, Brodoff BN eds. Obesity. Philadelphia: Lippincott, 1992;130-135.

Jequier E, Acheson K, Schultz Y. Assessment of energy expenditure and fuel utilization in man. Ann Rev Nutr 1987;7187-7208.

Jequier E, Shultz Y. Long-term measurement of energy expenditure in humans using a respiration chamber. Am J Clin Nutr 1983;38:989-998.

Jessen AB, Toubro S, Astrup A. Effect of chewing gum containing nicotine and caffeine on energy expenditure and substrate utilization in men. J Am Clin Nutr 2003;77:1442-1447.

Kaskoun MC, Johnson RK, Goran MI. Comparison of energy intake by semiquantitative food-frequency questionnaire with total energy expenditure by the doubly labeled water method in young children. Am J Clin Nutr 1994;60:43-47.

Keesey RE. The set-point analysis of the regulation of body weight. In: Stunkard AJ ed. Obesity. Philadelphia: Saunders, 1980;144-165.

Keys A, Taylor HL, Grande F. Basal metabolism and age of adult man. Metabolism 1973;22(4):579-587.

Klesges RC, Mealer CZ, Klesges LM. Effects of alcohol intake on resting energy expenditure in young women social drinkers. Am J Clin Nutr Apr 1994;59(4):805-809.

Krempf M, Hoerr RA, Pelletier VA, Marks LA, Gleason R, Young VR. An isotopic study of the effect of dietary carbohydrate on the metabolic fate of dietary leucine and phenylalanine. Am J Clin Nutr 1993;57:161-169.

Lebenstedt M, Platte P, Pirke K. Reduced resting metabolic rate in athletes with menstrual disorders. Med Sci Sports Exerc 1999;31(9):1240-1256.

Levine JA. Non-exercise activity thermogenesis (NEAT). Nutr Rev 2004;62(7):S82-S97.

Levine JA. Measurement of energy expenditure. Public Health Nutr 2005;87(7A):1123-1132.

Levine JA, Eberhardt NL, Jensen MD. Role of non-exercise activity thermogenesis in resistance to fat gain in humans. Science 1999;283(Jan 8):212-214.

Levine JA, Lanningham-Foster LM, McCrady SK, Krizan AC, Olson LR, Kane PH, Jensen MD, Clark MM. Interindividual variation in posture allocation: Possible role in human obesity. Science 2005;307(Jan 28):584-589.

Levine J, Melanson EL, Westerterp KR, Hill JO. Measurement of the components of nonexercise activity thermogenesis. Am J Physiol Endocrinol Metab 2001;281:E670-E675.

McDevitt RM, Bott SJ, Haring M, Coward WA, Bluck LJ, Prentice AM. De novo lipogenesis during controlled overfeeding with sucrose or glucose in lean and obese women. Am J Clin Nutr 2001;74:737-746.

Melby C, Scholl C, Edwards G, Bullough R. Effect of acute resistance exercise on post-exercise energy expenditure and resting metabolic rate. J Appl Physiol 1993;75(4):1847-1853.

Mifflin MD, St. Jeor ST, Hill LA, Scott BJ, Daugherty SA, Koh YO. A new predictive equation for resting energy expenditure in healthy individuals. Am J Clin Nutr 1990;51:241-247.

Nichols J, Ross S, Patterson P. Thermic effect of food at rest and following swim exercise in trained college men and women. Ann Nutr Metab 1988;32:215-219.

Osterberg KL, Melby CL. Effect of acute resistance exercise on postexercise oxygen consumption and resting metabolic rate in young women. Int J Sport Nutr Exerc Metab 2000;10:71-81.

Owen OE, Holup JL, D'Alessio DA et al. A reappraisal of the caloric requirements of men. Am J Clin Nutr 1987;46:875-885.

Owen OE, Kavle E, Owen RS et al. A reappraisal of caloric requirements in healthy women. Am J Clin Nutr 1986;44:1-19.

Piers LS, Diggavi SN, Rijskamp J, van Raaij JMA, Shetty PS, Hautvast JGAJ. Resting metabolic rate and thermic effect of a meal in the follicular and luteal phases of the menstrual cycle in well-nourished Indian women. Am J Clin Nutr 1995;61:296-302.

Poehlman ET, Danforth E Jr. Endurance training increases metabolic rate and norepinephrine appearance rate in older individuals. Am J Physiol Aug 1991;261(2)Pt 1:E233-239.

Poehlman ET, McAuliffe TL, Van Houten DR, Danforth E. Influence of age and endurance training on metabolic rate and hormones in healthy men. Am J Physiol 1990;259(22):E66-E72.

Prentice AM, Black AE, Coward WA et al. High levels of energy expenditure in obese women. Br Med J 1986;292:983-987.

Prentice AM, Diaz EO, Murgatroyd PR, Goldberg GR, Sonko BJ, Black AE, Coward WA. Doubly labeled water measurements and calorimetry in practice. In: Whitehead RG, Prentice A eds. New techniques in nutritional research. New York: Academic Press, 1991;177-207.

Ravussin E. A NEAT way to control weight? Science 2005;307(Jan 28):530-531.

Ravussin E, Bogardus C. Relationship of genetics, age and physical fitness to daily energy expenditure and fuel utilization. Am J Clin Nutr 1989;49:968-975.

Ravussin E, Harper IT, Rising R, Bogardus C. Energy expenditure by doubly labeled water: validation in lean and obese subjects. Am J Physiol 1991;261:E402-E409.

Ravussin E, Lillioja S, Anderson TE, Christin L, Bogardus C. Determinants of 24-hour energy expenditure in man: methods and results using a respiratory chamber. J Clin Invest 1986;78:1568-1578.

Ravussin E, Swinburn BA. Energy metabolism. In: Stunkard JA, Wadden TA eds. Obesity: theory and therapy. New York: Raven Press, 1993;97-123.

Rising R, Keys A, Ravussin E, Bogardus C. Concomitant inter-individual variation in body temperature and metabolic rate. Am J Physiol 1992;263(26):E730-E734.

Rontoyannis GP, Skoulis T, Pavlou KN. Energy balance in ultramarathon running. Am J Clin Nutr 1989;49:976-979.

Saris WHM. Sugars, energy metabolism and body weight control. Am J Clin Nutr 2003;78(suppl):850S-857S.

Saris WHM, Tarnopolsky MA. Controlling food intake and energy balance: which macronutrient should we select? Curr Opin Clin Nutr Metab Care 2003;6:609-613.

Schoeller DA, Racette SB. A review of field techniques for the assessment of energy expenditure. J Nutr 1990;120:1492-1495.

Schoeller DA, Ravussin E, Schutz Y, Acheson KJ, Baertschi P, Jequier E. Energy expenditure by doubly labeled water: validation in humans and proposed calculation. Am J Physiol May 1986;250(5)Pt 2:R823-830.

Schutz Y, Tremblay A, Weinsier RL, Nelson KM. Role of fat oxidation in the long-term stabilization of body weight in obese women. Am J Clin Nutr 1992;55:670-674.

Seale JL, Conway JM, Canary JJ. Seven-day validation of doubly labeled water method using indirect room calorimetry. J Appl Physiol 1993;74(1):402-409.

Sedlock DA, Fissinger JA, Melby CL. Effect of exercise intensity and duration on post-exercise energy expenditure. Med Sci Sports Exerc 1989;21(6):662-666.

Segal KR, Chun A, Coronel P, Valdez V. Effects of exercise mode and intensity on postprandial thermogenesis in lean and obese men. J Appl Physiol 1992;72(5):1754-1763.

Shelmet JJ, Reichard GA, Skutches CL, Hoeldtke RD, Owen OE, Boden G. Ethanol causes acute inhibition of carbohydrate,

fat, and protein oxidation and insulin resistance. J Clin Invest 1988;81:1137-1145.

Sjodin AM, Andersson AB, Hogberg JM, Westerterp KR. Energy balance in cross-country skiers: a study using doubly labeled water. Med Sci Sports Exerc 1994;26(6):720-724.

Solomon SJ, Kurzer MS, Calloway DH. Menstrual cycle and basal metabolic rate in women. Am J Clin Nutr 1982;36:611-666.

Sonko BJ, Prentice AM, Murgatroyd PR, Goldberg GR, van de Ven MLHM, Coward WA. Effect of alcohol on postmeal fat storage. Am J Clin Nutr 1994;59:619-625.

Stock MJ. Gluttony and thermogenesis revisited. Int J Obesity 1999;23:1105-1117.

Stubbs RJ, Murgatroyd PR, Goldberg GR, Prentice AM. Carbohydrate balance and the regulation of day-to-day food intake in humans. Am J Clin Nutr 1993;57:897-903.

Suter PM. Is alcohol consumption a risk factor for weight gain and obesity? Crit Rev Clin Lab Sci 2005;43(3):197-227.

Swinburn B, Ravussin E. Energy balance or fat balance? Am J Clin Nutr 1993;57(suppl):766S-771S.

Tataranni PA, Larson DE, Snitker S, Ravussin E. Thermic effect of food in humans: methods and results from use of a respiratory chamber. Am J Clin Nutr 1995;61:1013-1019.

Thomas CD, Peters JC, Reed WG, Abumrad NN, Sun M, Hill JO. Nutrient balance and energy expenditure during ad libitum feeding of high-fat and high-carbohydrate diets in humans. Am J Clin Nutr 1992;55:934-942.

Thompson JL, Manore MM. Predicted and measured resting metabolic rate of male and female endurance athletes. J Am Diet Assoc 1996;96(1):30-34.

Thompson J, Manore MM, Skinner JS. Resting metabolic rate and thermic effect of a meal in low- and adequate-energy intake male endurance athletes. Int J Sport Nutr 1993;3:194-206.

Thompson JL, Manore MM, Skinner JS, Ravussin E, Spraul M. Daily energy expenditure in male endurance athletes with differing energy intakes. Med Sci Sports Exerc 1995;27(3):347-354.

Tremblay A, Lavallee N, Almeras N, Allard L, Despres JP, Bouchard C. Nutritional determinants of the increase in energy intake associated with a high-fat diet. Am J Clin Nutr 1991;53:1134-1137.

Turley KR, McBride PJ, Wilmore JH. Resting metabolic rate measured after subjects spent the night at home vs at a clinic. Am J Clin Nutr 1993;58:141-144.

U.S. Department of Agriculture (USDA). MyPyramid—steps to a healthier you. Washington, DC: Human Nutrition Information Service, 2005.

U.S. Department of Agriculture (USDA) and U.S. Department of Health and Human Services (USDHHS). Dietary guidelines for Americans 2005: key recommendations for the general population. http://www.health.gov/dietaryguidelines/dga2005/recommendations.htm Accessed January 2009.

Vaughan L, Zurlo F, Ravussin E. Aging and energy expenditure. Am J Clin Nutr 1991;53:821-825.

Weinsier RL, Nagy TR, Hunter GR, Darnell BE, Hensrud DD, Weiss HL. Do adaptive changes in metabolic rate favor weight regain in weight-reduced individuals? An examination of the set-point theory. Am J Cin Nutr 2000;72:1088-1094.

Westerterp KR. Food quotient, respiratory quotient, and energy balance. Am J Clin Nutr 1993;57(suppl):759S-765S.

Westerterp KR, Sarris WHM, van Es M, ten Hoor F. Use of doubly labeled water technique in humans during heavy sustained exercise. J Appl Physiol 1986;61(6):2162-2167.

Westerterp-Plantenga M. The significance of protein in food intake and body weight regulation. Curr Opin Clin Nutr Metab Care 2003;6:635-638.

Westerterp-Plantenga M, Diepvens K, Joosen AMCP, Berube-Parent S, Tremblay A. Metabolic effects of spices, tea, and caffeine. Physiol Behav 2006;89:85-91.

Weststrate JA. Resting metabolic rate and diet induced thermogenesis: a methodological reappraisal. Am J Clin Nutr 1993;58:592-601.

Wilmore JH, Stanforth PR, Hudspeth LA et al. Alterations in resting metabolic rate as a consequence of 20 wk of endurance training: the HERITAGE Family Study. Am J Clin Nutr 1998;68:66-71.

World Health Organization. Energy and protein requirements. Report of a Joint FAO/WHO/UNU Expert Committee. Technical report series 724. Geneva: World Health Organization, 1985;206. (This equation was reprinted in the 1989 National Research Council book on RDAs.)

Yoemans MR, Caton S, Hetherington MM. Alcohol and food intake. Curr Opin Clin Nutr Metab Care 2003;6:639-644.

Yoshida T, Sakane N, Umekawa T, Kondo M. Relationship between basal metabolic rate, thermogenic response to caffeine, and body weight loss following combined low calorie and exercise treatment in obese women. Int J Obesity 1994;18:345-350.

CHAPTER 6

Achieving Healthy Body Weight

Chapter Objectives

After reading this chapter you should be able to

- discuss the role of diet and exercise in achieving healthy body weight,
- describe the recommendations for maintaining a healthy body weight,
- discuss the weight concerns of athletes, and
- define the recommendations for weight gain.

Katie is a soccer player faced with the challenge of losing body weight in order to regain her competitive edge. She recently gained 20 lb (9.1 kg) during her recovery from knee surgery. Her body fat has increased from 17% to 27%, and she knows that in order to compete at her best, she needs to lose body fat and weight and gain fat-free mass (FFM). While her physician and family recommend that she achieve this weight loss slowly, Katie feels pressure to lose the weight quickly, using whatever means possible. She feels that the more quickly she can lose the weight, the sooner she can rejoin the team and feel better about herself.

The need or desire to lose weight is common among competitive athletes; however, it is also common among many recreational athletes and sedentary individuals who wish to alter their physical appearance. Individuals throughout the United States appear to be obsessed with body weight and an aesthetically pleasing body shape. It has been estimated that at any one time, at least 29% to 33% of the U.S. population are dieting (Calorie Control Council 2007). Ironically, it appears that many individuals who are dieting are either underweight or of normal weight. The Behavioral Risk Factor Surveillance System survey done by the Centers for Disease Control and Prevention (CDC) showed that in adults age 18 to 24 years, 20% of normal-weight individuals were dieting in 2003, while 45% to 67% of overweight and obese individuals were dieting (McCracken et al. 2007). While weight loss would be recommended in Katie's case, many people are inappropriately concerned with weight loss. Why do people who are normal weight or underweight diet for weight loss? Many feel that they are still not thin enough in relation to society's standards or the image they wish to portray. Unfortunately, concerns with body weight are not limited to adults. Research has shown that U.S. girls as young as 12 to 14 years of age express concerns about body weight and actually restrict energy intake (National Adolescent Student Health Survey 1989). These data were supported in a recent study that followed the dieting behaviors of ~15,000 children between the ages of 9 and 15 years over a four-year period (Field et al. 2003). Researchers found that when the study started, ~30% of girls and 16% of boys were dieting to either maintain or lose weight. Even more distressing is the number of young adolescents who use smoking to control their weight. Data from the National Health and Nutrition Examination Survey (NHANES) III study showed that 23% of normal-weight adolescent girls used smoking to lose weight (Strauss and Mir 2001). These data emphasize that preoccupation with body weight and shape can begin at a young age.

With the widespread anxiety in our society about weight, one might guess that the prevalence of obesity is on the decline. On the contrary, the U.S. population is becoming more obese, with an estimated 66% of adults either overweight or obese (CDC 2007; Ogden et al. 2006). A paradox exists: Those who need to lose weight are not dieting, but those who do not need to lose weight are dieting. Why aren't overweight people dieting? There are probably many answers to this question. One answer is that people have tried numerous diets, have been unsuccessful, and are unwilling to try again. One characteristic of individuals who are unsuccessful at weight maintenance is a past dieting history, with more frequent dieting associated with higher weight gain after the diet is over (Pasman et al. 1999). A major focus of obesity research today is how to help people keep the weight off once the diet is over (Ball et al. 2002+; Donnelly et al. 2004; Hill et al. 2005).

Being overweight (or incorrectly viewing oneself as overweight) is very stressful. Overweight individuals are often portrayed as lazy, stupid, and unsuccessful and are targets of ridicule. The media constantly suggest that the only way to be desirable and adorable is to be thin and perfectly proportioned. Defining optimal body weights and educating people about healthy ways to achieve and maintain optimal body weight appear to be critical to the emotional and physical health of athletes and other members of our society.

ROLE OF DIET AND EXERCISE IN ACHIEVING A HEALTHY BODY WEIGHT

What is a healthy or optimal body weight? How do you determine your optimal body weight? Although identifying an optimal or healthy weight is very difficult because no charts or tables provide the answer, the following criteria are frequently used to help determine healthy body weight:

- Weight that can be maintained without constant dieting or restraining food intake
- Weight at which health risks are minimized and good health is promoted
- Weight that promotes good eating habits
- Weight that allows one to participate in some type of physical activity
- Weight that can be accepted by the individual
- Weight that allows optimal performance in the sport of one's choice
- Weight that takes into consideration one's genetic makeup and family history of body weight and body shape
- Weight appropriate for one's age and level of physical development

Thus, optimal body weight should promote good health and be "reasonable" in terms of whether or not it can be achieved and maintained. If people are constantly dieting or are repeatedly gaining and losing weight, they may be trying to achieve or maintain an unrealistic or "in your dreams" body weight.

Conversely, there are many sports that require a low body weight. Athletes involved in such sports may find that they are lighter during specific phases of their training and competition. For example, a ski jumper, wrestler, or cyclist will be lighter during the competitive phase and gain weight during the off-season since it is unrealistic to maintain a low body weight throughout the entire year. While it is important for athletes to achieve and maintain a healthy body weight throughout the year, some athletes target body weights that are difficult to maintain postcompetition. It is important for these athletes to regain some weight during the off-season.

Determination of Body Size, Percentage of Body Fat, and Fat Distribution

There are a variety of methods for determining body size, percentage of body fat, and body fat distribution. All are used to some extent to determine whether or not a person is at risk for developing health problems related to being overfat. In addition, change in body size is often used to determine whether a weight loss program has been successful. Although weight loss should not be the only criterion for success, it is often a major component measured in any weight loss effort.

Body Mass Index

One way of expressing body size is to use the body mass index. The **body mass index (BMI)** is defined as a ratio of weight (in kilograms) to the square of height (in meters squared), that is, kg/m^2. To estimate BMI using pounds and inches, multiply $(lb/in.^2) \times 703$. **Overweight** is defined as a BMI between 25 and 29.9 kg/m^2, and **obesity** is defined as a BMI ≥30 (National Heart, Lung and Blood Institute [NHLBI] 1998). Although BMI is relatively easy and inexpensive to measure, it has some major disadvantages. It gives no information about a person's percentage of body fat, fat distribution, or amount of FFM; and it does not account for differences in frame size, age, activity level, or gender. For example, a male bodybuilder who weighs 210 lb (95.3 kg), has a height of 68 in. (1.72 m), and has 6% to 8% body fat would have a BMI of 32 kg/m^2. According to our previous definition, this individual would be considered obese from his BMI value, although his actual body fat percentage is very low. This person is very active, moreover, and his risk for chronic diseases is low. "The Relationship Between Weight and Body Mass Index" (p. 170) demonstrates how changes in body weight affect BMI. Finally, remember that clinical judgment needs to be used when one is interpreting BMI, since a number of situations can influence accuracy, such as edema, high muscularity, muscle wasting, and short stature (NHLBI 2000).

The National Heart, Lung and Blood Institute of the National Institutes of Health (NIH) has developed a risk assessment table for use with BMI and waist circumference measurements (shown as table 6.1). This table helps classify individuals based on both their BMI and body fat distribution. For example, an individual with a small waist and a BMI of 28 kg/m^2 would be classified as having increased risk. However, if this same person had a large waist circumference, he or she would be classified as high risk. It is important to remember that this table has limited application to people who have disproportionately greater FFM for a given height (weightlifters, bodybuilders, football and basketball players).

Percentage Body Fat

Most determinations of body fat percentage involve estimating the ratio of body fat to FFM. Chapter 7 describes the techniques in detail. While knowing an individual's body fat is useful in both clinical and sport settings, it does not give an indication of the distribution of body fat and FFM, or of whether the body fat is present predominantly subcutaneously or within the tissues. Please refer to chapter 7 for more details regarding body composition assessments.

Body Fat Distribution

Body fat distribution is assessed to determine where body fat deposits are located. The body shape of people with upper body fat is referred to as android or "apple shaped." The body shape of people with body fat located in the lower part of the body (buttocks, hips, and thigh regions) is referred to as gynoid or "pear-shaped." It has been hypothesized that upper body or abdominal obesity increases the risk for elevated blood lipids, glucose, and insulin—changes that may eventually lead to cardiovascular disease (CVD), diabetes, and hypertension (Klein et al. 2007). Others argue that total body obesity is just as good a predictor of CVD as measurements of abdominal obesity (Reaven 2007). In general, men tend to have a higher incidence of upper body obesity while women have a higher incidence of lower body obesity. Body fat distribution may be one of the factors that contribute to the higher incidence of CVD in men than in premenopausal women.

Body fat distribution is usually determined through measurement of the **waist circumference** or measurement of the ratio of abdominal visceral fat (the fat around the internal organs) to subcutaneous fat (fat located directly under the skin) using **computed tomography (CT)** or **magnetic resonance imaging (MRI)** (Klein et al. 2007). The waist circumference is a simple and inexpensive field measurement for determining body fat distribution; however, it cannot distinguish between visceral and subcutaneous fat. Visceral abdominal fat is more closely associated

The Relationship Between Weight and Body Mass Index

Body mass index (BMI) is one of the most frequently reported measures of body size in the research literature. To better understand the concept of BMI and how it changes as weight changes, do the following exercise using your own weight and height. First, determine your own BMI (using English measures, calculate weight/height^2 using the units ($[\text{lb/in.}^2] \times 703$); then calculate how your BMI will change as you repeatedly add 10 lb (4.5 kg) to your weight. Keep adding 10 lb (4.5 kg) until you have reached a BMI of 40 kg/m^2. If you started with a BMI >20 kg/m^2, subtract 10 lb (4.5 kg) from your current weight until you have reached a BMI of less than 20 kg/m^2. Now, using table 6.1, determine your health risk classification based upon the ranges of BMI you calculated. The following example is given for a woman who is 60 in. (1.52 m) tall and weighs 110 lb (50 kg).

Weight (lb)	Weight (kg)	BMI (kg/m²)	Health risk classification
100	45.5	19.6	—
110	50.0	21.5	—
120	54.5	23.5	—
130	59.0	25.4	Increased or high
140	63.6	27.4	Increased or high
150	68.2	29.4	Increased or high
160	72.7	31.3	High or very high
170	77.3	33.3	High or very high
180	81.8	35.2	Very high
190	86.4	37.2	Very high
200	90.9	39.1	Very high
210	95.5	41.0	Extremely high

Table 6.1 **Classification of Overweight and Obesity by Body Mass Index (BMI), Waist Circumference, and Associated Disease Risk**

	BMI (kg/m²)	Obesity class	Disease risk* relative to normal weight and waist circumference	
			Men ≤102 cm (≤40 in.) Women ≤88 cm (≤35 in.)	Men >102 cm (>40 in.) Women >88 cm (>35 in.)
Underweight	<18.5		—	—
Normal⁺	18.5-24.9		—	—
Overweight	25.0-29.9		Increased	High
Obesity	30.0-34.9	I	High	Very high
	35.0-39.9	II	Very high	Very high
Extreme obesity	≥40	III	Extremely high	Extremely high

* Disease risk for type 2 diabetes, hypertension, and cardiovascular disease. ⁺Increased waist circumference can be a marker for increased risk even in persons of normal weight.

Reprinted from National Heart, Lung and Blood Institute, 1998, "Clinical guidelines on the identification, evaluation, and treatment of overweight and obesity in adults," *The evidence report* (Washington, DC: National Institutes of Health, U.S. Dept. of Health and Human Services).

with increased risk of disease than subcutaneous fat. Figure 6.1 represents CT scans of two different individuals—a young man with a lower amount of abdominal visceral fat and a middle-aged man with a higher amount of intra-abdominal visceral fat. Because determining body fat distribution using CT scans is expensive and is predominantly done for research purposes, the waist circumference is the more frequently used technique.

The waist circumference is fairly easy to measure, but specific measurement guidelines need to be followed. Unfortunately, in the past, measurement sites have not been standardized, making comparisons between research studies difficult. The NHLBI recommends the following method as a standard (see figure 6.2):

1. To measure waist circumference, locate the upper hip bone and the top of the right iliac crest. Place a measuring tape in a horizontal plane around the abdomen at the level of the iliac crest.

2. Before reading the tape measure, ensure that the tape is snug but does not compress the skin and is parallel to the floor. The measurement is made at the end of a normal expiration.

All measurements should be done with a flexible tape and recorded in centimeters. Increased health risks are associated with a waist circumference of >102 cm (40 in.) for men and >88 cm (35 in.) for women (see table 6.1). For a more detailed

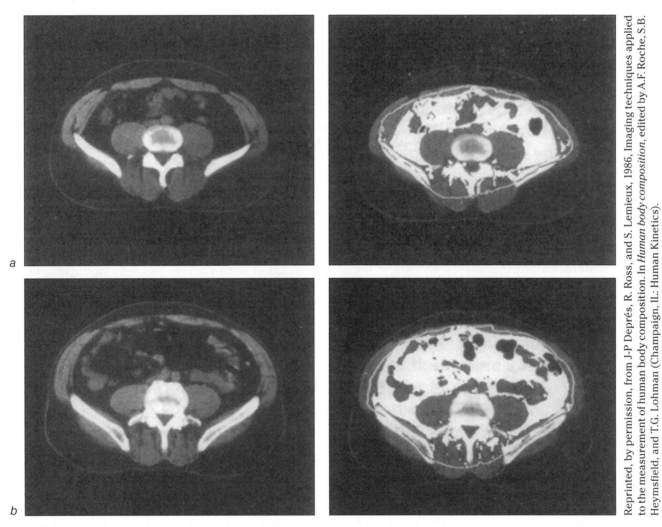

Reprinted, by permission, from J-P Després, R. Ross, and S. Lemieux, 1986, Imaging techniques applied to the measurement of human body composition. In *Human body composition*, edited by A.F. Roche, S.B. Heymsfield, and T.G. Lohman (Champaign, IL: Human Kinetics).

Figure 6.1 Cross-sectional images of the abdomen obtained by computed tomography (CT) at L4-L5 in (*a*) a young man with excess intra-abdominal visceral fat and (*b*) a middle-aged man matched for total body fat mass (19.8 kg). The visceral adipose tissue area (96 cm^2 for the young man and 155 cm^2 for the middle-aged man), which is delineated by a line within the muscle wall surrounding the abdominal cavity, is highlighted in the images on the right.

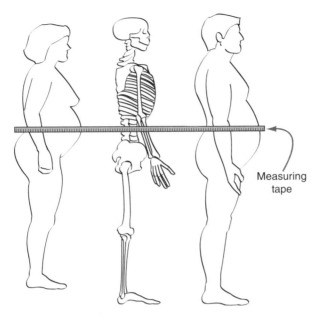

Measuring
tape

Figure 6.2 Measuring tape position for waist (abdominal) circumference measurement in adults.

Reprinted from NHLBI, NIH, 2002, "The practical guide: Identification, evalution, and treatment of overweight and obesity in adults," NIH Publication No. 02-4084, January, pg. 9.

discussion of the issues surrounding the measurement of waist circumference, see Klein and colleagues 2007.

As table 6.1 indicates, once waist circumference increases above 102 cm (>40 in.) for men and above 88 cm (>35 in.) for women, risks increase for hypertension, heart disease, and diabetes. Thus, if a person has a BMI of 28 kg/m^2 and increased abdominal fat (waist circumference above the cutoff), his or her relative risk for disease is higher than for someone with the same BMI but a smaller waist. This general risk assessment assumes that other disease risk factors are similar. Body mass index is highly positively correlated with waist circumference, so as one increases, so does the other (Reaven 2007; Ford et al. 2003).

The exact mechanism linking higher levels of body fat, especially abdominal visceral body fat, with increased risk for chronic disease has been the focus of extensive research (Eckel et al. 2005; Grundy 2006; Rader 2007; Reaven 2007). Reaven (1994) was one of the early researchers examining the relationship between high abdominal fat and increased blood insulin, glucose, and lipid levels. Adipose tissue, especially visceral fat, leads to an increased breakdown and release of non-esterified free fatty acids (NEFAs). These can overload the muscle, liver, and β-cells of the pancreas with lipid

and are considered a major contributor to insulin resistance (Grundy 2006; Eckel et al. 2005). This increase in NEFAs also leads to hyperlipidemia. Visceral fat is located close to the body's internal organs, from which venous blood drains directly into the portal vein, which in turn flows to the liver. High levels of NEFAs in the portal vein result in high levels of NEFAs entering the liver, which provides substrate for triglyceride synthesis and increased very low-density lipoprotein (VLDL) production by the liver. These high levels of NEFAs also alter insulin-mediated signaling in the body, including the liver, muscle, and adipose tissue, leading to hyperinsulinemia and abnormal glucose control (Eckel et al. 2005). Hyperinsulinemia can also increase sodium retention by the kidneys, which can contribute to higher risk of hypertension. In addition, increased VLDL production by the liver can lead to elevated blood levels of VLDL-cholesterol and low-density lipoprotein (LDL)-cholesterol, which are both risk factors for CVD. Figure 6.3 is a schematic diagram of this proposed mechanism linking high visceral body fat with increased disease risk.

Obesity, especially abdominal obesity, is highly correlated with abnormal biochemical profiles (high blood lipids, insulin, and glucose) as compared to lower body obesity, which is often considered relatively "benign" (Klein et al. 2007). It is not, however, truly benign: Lower body obesity can also contribute to increased NEFAs, stress the weight-bearing joints, contribute to varicose veins and osteoarthritis, and discourage participation in regular physical activity due to the discomfort associated with carrying excess body weight. For reviews on the relationship between body fat and disease risk see the reviews by Eckel and colleagues (2005), Grundy (2006), Reaven (2007), and Rader (2007).

Health Problems Associated With Obesity

Uncomplicated obesity is seldom fatal; once body size (or BMI) reaches a certain critical point, however, mortality increases. The J-shaped curve in figure 6.4 shows the relationship between BMI and mortality: Mortality increases as BMI increases above 25 kg/m^2, with the sharpest risk associated with a BMI >30 kg/m^2. From this curve, one would also conclude that the risk of mortality increases at a BMI <20 kg/m^2.

Yet there are some problems with the data used to generate the curve in figure 6.4. First, women

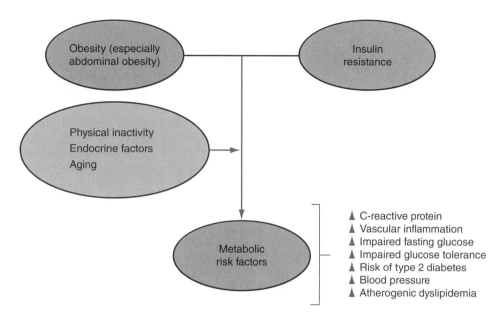

Figure 6.3 A proposed mechanism linking high visceral body fat with increased disease risk.

Reprinted by permission from Macmillan Publishers Ltd: *Nature Reviews,* S.M. Grundy, "Drug therapy of the metabolic syndrome: minimizing the emerging crisis of polypharmacy," 5: 295-309. Copyright 2006.

have a different curve than men; women have a lower mortality risk than men at similar weights. This difference may be related to a number of factors, including fat distribution, hormonal differences, self-care behaviors, or disease treatment. Second, individuals who may have had low body weights (and BMI) due to illness or cigarette smoking were not eliminated from the analyses. If these data are eliminated from the analyses, the curve of the relationship between BMI and risk of mortality changes, with no increased risk of mortality observed at a lower BMI. In a 14-year epidemiological study of more than 1 million men and women, Calle and colleagues (1999) found that white men and women in all age groups had a higher risk of death from all causes—but especially CVD and cancer—as their BMI increased. The lowest death rates occurred at a BMI of about 24 kg/m² for men and 23 kg/m² for women. Mortality risks for black men and women, however, were not strongly associated with BMI. A study of nurses in the United States showed that the BMI associated with the lowest risk of mortality was less than 20 kg/m², which represents body weights at least 15% less than the U.S. average for women similar in age to those studied (Manson et al. 1995). These data suggest that the lowest mortality is associated with very low BMI values. However, this is an area of controversy, as others argue that higher BMI values are associated with increased mortality

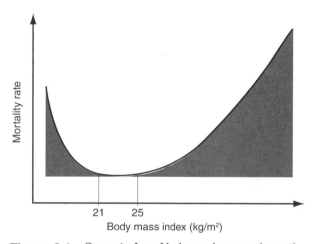

Figure 6.4 Generic J- or U-shaped curve describing the relationship of body mass index (BMI) to mortality.

Reprinted from T.B. Van Itallie, 1992, Body weight, morbidity, and longevity. In *Obesity,* edited by B. Bjorntorp and B.N. Brodoff (Philadelphia, PA: Lippincott, Williams, and Wilkins).

only in individuals who lead a sedentary lifestyle *and* consume a high-fat, low-fiber diet (Gaesser 1999). For a detailed discussion of whether people can be at low risk for chronic disease if they are fit and fat, see reviews by Willett and colleagues (1999) and LaMonte and Blair (2006).

Obesity may play a role in morbidity by either causing or exacerbating certain diseases. Figure 6.5 illustrates how obesity may exacerbate an existing health problem (Bray 1992). An individual with a BMI of 37 kg/m² has twice the risk of all-cause mortality as someone with a BMI of 23 kg/m². Results from the NHANES II (Van Itallie 1985) showed a 2.9 times greater risk of developing diabetes in obese as compared to nonobese people. Thus, obesity may increase the risk of developing certain diseases as well as increase the risk of dying from obesity-related diseases. Note that health risks related to obesity are also risks associated with a sedentary lifestyle. It can

be quite difficult to separate the health effects of excess body fat from those of inactivity. In fact, Wei and colleagues (1997) showed that regular exercise improved the lipid profiles of men, and the improvement was similar for overweight and normal-weight men. Lee and colleagues (1999) also found that unfit lean men had a significantly higher risk of all-cause and CVD mortality than fit obese men. A number of health disorders thought to be caused or exacerbated by obesity (Saltzman 2006) are listed on this page.

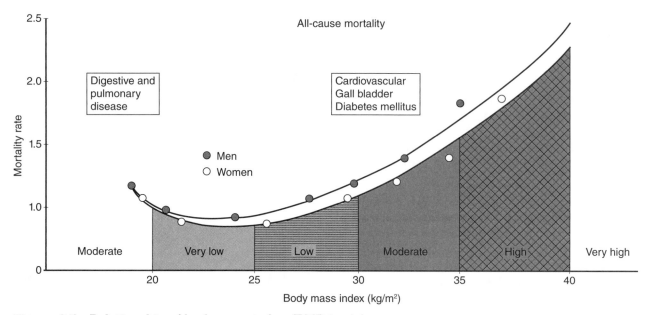

Figure 6.5 Relationship of body mass index (BMI) to risk.
Reprinted, by permission, from G.A. Bray, 1992, "Pathophysiology of obesity," *American Journal of Clinical Nutrition* 55: 488S-494S.

Health Effects of Obesity

Cardiovascular	**Pulmonary**	**Endocrine**	**Genitourinary**	**Musculoskeletal**
Coronary heart disease	Asthma	Type 2 diabetes	Urinary incontinence	Osteoarthritis
Stroke	Obstructive sleep apnea	Dyslipidemia	Proteinuria	Back pain
Congestive heart failure	Pulmonary embolus	Metabolic syndrome	**Cancer**	Gout
Cardiomyopathy	Obesity hypoventilation syndrome	Infertility	Breast	**Neurological and Sensory**
Left ventricular hypertrophy		**Gastrointestinal**	Colon	Pseudotumor cerebri
Sudden death		Gastroesophageal reflux	Endometrium	Macular degeneration
Deep vein thrombosis		Gallstones	Esophagus	
		Nonalcoholic fatty liver disease	Gastric cardia	
			Gallbladder	

Reprinted from E. Saltzman, 2006, Obesity as a health issue. In *Present knowledge in nutrition,* 9th ed, Vol II, edited by B.A. Bowman and R.M. Russell (Washington, DC: ILSI Press), 640.

WEIGHT LOSS INTERVENTIONS

Over the last 30 years, numerous approaches have been used for weight loss. Highly trained athletes and individuals participating in regular physical activity possess the greatest potential for combining energy restriction with physical activity when appropriate. It is important for any person attempting to lose weight to include regular physical activity in his or her weight loss program. The primary goal of a weight loss program is to improve health by lowering body fat while maintaining or increasing the proportion of FFM or muscle tissue. If FFM can be increased or maintained during weight loss, it is easier to sustain resting metabolic rate (RMR) and the reduced level of body fat. Preserving FFM is also important to increase muscle strength and the ability to perform physical activity and activities of daily living. Since many people not currently involved in regular physical activity are attempting to lose weight using only energy restriction, it is important to understand the role that diet in itself plays in the scheme of weight loss.

Before we discuss the various diets used for weight loss, we need to first set the ground rules for weight loss. Here are some basic facts about dieting that are important to remember, regardless of the diet used:

- Kilocalories (kcal) or calories are important! Decreasing energy intake below the level of energy expenditure can reduce body weight. The amount of weight lost for a given energy deficit is difficult to predict for any one person since the energy deficit needed to bring about weight loss appears to be highly individualized. Thus, we cannot expect everyone to respond the same to any given dietary treatment—many people report eating very few kilocalories without experiencing weight loss and feel they are truly "resistant" to weight loss. However, Bray and Gray (1988) have reported that no healthy adult who has ever been studied in a metabolic chamber required less than 1200 kcal/day to maintain body weight. Note also that the lowest-energy diets do not always bring about the best weight loss results. Because severely restricted diets result in loss of FFM and subsequent decrease in RMR, they are rarely successful in producing lasting weight loss.

- Composition of the diet is important. A dieting person needs to know the amount of energy consumed each day and also the percentage of energy coming from carbohydrate, fat, protein, and alcohol. The composition of the diet may affect weight loss differently in different people. Some individuals prefer and do better with a higher-protein diet than with the typical low-fat approach when initiating a diet. The nutrient composition of the diet can also affect weight loss and changes in body composition. Finally, diet composition may be important for weight maintenance; consumption of a moderate-fat diet is significantly associated with long-term successful weight maintenance (Phelan et al. 2006).

- Protein intake is important, especially the ratio of nitrogen (or protein) intake to energy intake. When a low-calorie diet is consumed, a higher nitrogen:kilocalorie ratio is required than is normally recommended in a weight maintenance diet. Higher-quality protein is also required to maintain FFM. Because people on reduced-energy diets use some dietary protein for energy instead of for building and repair of body tissues, a higher intake of protein is necessary to meet their needs. This is especially true for people who exercise while reducing energy intake. In addition, protein may help regulate appetite during phases of energy restriction.

- Frequency of meals is another important factor. It may be better for dieters to consume small meals throughout the day than to eat all of the day's kilocalories in one large meal. Frequent feedings may help improve regulation of blood glucose and insulin, improve nitrogen retention, and increase the ability to maintain self-control. People who become too hungry have a greater tendency to overconsume when food is finally available. Researchers have examined the role of breakfast and meal consistency on weight maintenance, finding that people who maintained weight loss were more likely to eat breakfast daily and had a higher level of physical activity than non-breakfast eaters (Wyatt et al. 2002). However, whether breakfast will help keep the weight off or help one maintain a lower BMI may depend on the type of breakfast consumed (de la Hunty and Ashwell 2007). In addition, Gorin and colleagues (2004) found that meal consistency resulted in smaller weight gains over a one-year period. In this study, participants who reported a consistent diet regimen throughout the week were 1.5 times more likely to maintain their weight within 5 lb (2.3 kg) than those who dieted more strictly on weekdays and had a looser diet regimen on the weekend, on holidays, and during vacations.

All of the commonly used diets can produce weight loss because they restrict energy intake (Freedman et al. 2001). Unfortunately, few promote good eating habits, long-term weight maintenance strategies, physical activity, and good health. Understanding these diets will help you make better weight loss recommendations to your clients and help you evaluate the next fad diet that comes along. In the following sections we briefly discuss the various types of weight loss diets. For complete evidence-based analyses of the research literature regarding the effectiveness of these diets, see the work of Freedman and colleagues (2001) and Bravata and colleagues (2003). Tangney and colleagues (2005) have also reviewed these plans to determine their efficacy in maintenance of weight loss for at least one year.

Starvation Diets

Starvation or fasting is often used as a quick method to lose unwanted pounds. **Starvation diets** are usually defined as those providing <200 kcal/day (Bray and Gray 1988). The primary advantage of a starvation diet is the very rapid weight loss that occurs. However, these diets have a number of serious problems:

- There are major protein losses, including from muscle and organ tissues.
- There are major fluid and electrolyte losses, which can also lead to problems with hypotension and dehydration.
- Malnutrition often develops, including nutrient deficiencies and bone loss—especially if the diet is followed without medical supervision and for an extended period of time.
- Refeeding needs to be done slowly: Accumulation of fat can occur even with the consumption of moderately few kilocalories.
- Long-term success is poor, with individuals usually regaining most or all of the weight lost.
- Resting metabolic rate is blunted, which reduces the number of kilocalories one can consume to maintain body weight.

The severity of these problems depends on how long people are on the diet and whether or not they are exercising while they are consuming little or no food. Starvation dieting is never recommended for weight loss, especially for active individuals.

Very Low-Calorie Diets

Very low-calorie diets (VLCDs) are usually defined as diets providing <800 kcal/day (Tsai and Wadden 2006; NHLBI 1998). These diets have been in existence since the 1930s but did not become popular until the 1970s. Interest in VLCDs as an effective weight loss treatment stemmed from the success of complete starvation in achieving spectacular weight loss. The negative side effects associated with starvation diets, including large losses of lean body tissue (especially from muscles and organs) and even death, made them unpopular with patients and professionals.

The limitations of starvation diets led to the development of the **protein-sparing modified fast (PSMF)** in the early 1970s. The PSMF consisted of a high-protein (usually 1.5 g/kg body weight or ~70 to 100 g protein per day) and low-kilocalorie (200-400 kcal/day) meal plan, with all of the protein and energy coming from lean meat (high-quality protein sources). This diet was modestly successful because it resulted in improved nitrogen balance while still producing rapid weight loss. Very low-calorie diets also can improve many comorbid conditions by decreasing elevated blood pressure, improving blood lipid profiles and glucose tolerance, and improving breathing in individuals with pulmonary problems. In the late 1970s, VLCDs composed of low-quality protein sources (hydrolyzed gelatin and collagen) became extremely popular. By 1977, approximately 98,000 Americans were using liquid-protein VLCDs as their sole source of food for at least one month, and 37,000 Americans were using this type of diet as their sole source of food for two months or more (Van Itallie and Yang 1984). During 1977 and 1978, 58 deaths were reported in obese adults who had recently been on or were currently using these diets. Many of these otherwise healthy people died of cardiac arrhythmias due to catabolism of cardiac tissue during the dietary period (Van Itallie and Yang 1984). A significant positive correlation was found between BMI before initiation of the VLCD and months of survival while on the VLCD. Very low-calorie diets should be supervised by physicians or other qualified health care professionals and are appropriate only for severely overweight people; a limit should be placed on the length of time a person consumes a VLCD.

There is disagreement about whether some carbohydrate should be included in the VLCD. Very low-calorie diets containing little or no carbohydrate are termed **ketogenic diets,** as they stimulate production of ketones to provide an alternative source of energy for the central nervous system. However, increased ketone production can be dangerous if maintained for prolonged periods of time; thus monitoring is important. Very low-calorie diets containing carbohydrates are termed nonketogenic diets. Support for ketogenic VLCDs stems from the fact that these diets produce more rapid weight loss due to increased dieresis and that they suppress insulin levels, which can increase fat utilization and spare protein breakdown (Blackburn et al. 1986). Others argue that inclusion of some carbohydrate (nonketogenic diet) is important to prevent excess fluid and electrolyte losses and the hypotension that may accompany these losses.

Low-Calorie Diets

Low-calorie diets (LCDs) are those that provide 1000 to 1500 kcal/day and may comprise regular foods, specially formulated foods, or a combination of these (NHLBI 1998). These diets typically provide less than 30% of total energy from fat, provide enough carbohydrate to avoid **ketosis** (abnormal increase of ketone bodies—i.e., acetoacetate, acetone, or β-hydroxybutyrate), and usually involve vitamin and mineral supplementation. Commercial programs in this category include those from Weight Watchers, Diet Center, and Jenny Craig. Slim-Fast is an example of a specially formulated over-the-counter food designed as a meal replacement in this type of diet program. Although weight loss on these diets—averaging 1 to 3 lb/week (0.5 to 1.5 kg/week)—is not as rapid as with VLCDs, long-term compliance may be improved, and there are fewer side effects. Low-kilocalorie diets are relatively safe, and healthy obese individuals can initiate them without physician supervision. It is important to investigate the nutritional adequacy of these diets, however, as they can range from low-fat, high-carbohydrate, nutritionally balanced plans to diets void of nutritional value.

Note that the diets just reviewed are too low in energy and carbohydrate for most women and for all men, regardless of activity level. These diets cannot replace the glycogen necessary for engaging in exercise. The diets were designed to help obese or overweight people lose weight and were not intended for use by active individuals or athletes with only small weight loss goals. They are too low in energy for most active individuals engaged in an intense training program who might be trying to maintain lean tissue while losing fat. While many people follow these types of diets, their long-term maintenance of weight loss is very poor unless permanent lifestyle changes are made.

Tsai and Wadden (2006) recently compared VLCDs to LCDs to determine if the rapid weight loss typically achieved with VLCDs can be better maintained than with the more conventional LCD. They found that VLCDs were not any better at producing long-term weight loss than the LCD. Thus, there is no real benefit to following a VLCD versus a LCD if long-term weight loss is the goal. In addition, LCDs are typically less expensive, safer, and easier to adhere to than VLCDs.

Low-Carbohydrate, High-Protein Diets

Diets classified as low-carbohydrate, high-protein diets, also called high-fat, low-carbohydrate diets, are numerous (Freedman et al. 2001). These diets can range from low to moderate energy intakes and are typically packaged under a variety of names and marketing strategies. In general, these diets comprise foods containing ~25% to 30% or more of the energy from protein, <100 g/day from carbohydrate, and the balance from fat (~55-65% of energy) (Freedman et al. 2001). Whether consumers can actually follow these levels of macronutrient intake is still in question, since many consumers view a low-carbohydrate diet as one that restricts bread and grains but lets them eat as many fruits and vegetables as they desire. This "self-described" low-carbohydrate diet approach does not match the carbohydrate recommendations of the Dr. Atkins diet (2003) (<20 g/day in the induction phase; <90 g/day in the maintenance phase). This level of carbohydrate (<100 g/day) should never be recommended for training athletes, especially endurance athletes, because the carbohydrate level is too low to support strenuous exercise, maintain blood glucose levels, and replace muscle glycogen. The Recommended Dietary Allowance (RDA) for carbohydrate is 130 g/day, which is the average minimum amount of glucose utilized by the brain (Institute of Medicine 2005). This level of carbohydrate (130 g/day) is also too low for athletes, but higher than that recommended by the Dr. Atkins diet (2003). Two mechanisms have been proposed to support the use of high-protein types of diets for weight loss (Manore and Thompson, 2008):

- High-protein diets, which are also typically high in fat, are more satiating, making these diets easier to follow than lower protein diets for some individuals. A diet plan that can be followed is more likely to bring about success. In addition, the thermic effect of protein is higher than that for carbohydrate or fat, which means that more energy is expended in the absorption, digestion, and metabolism of protein.

- A lower-carbohydrate diet produces less insulin (or insulin "surges") than is produced with consumption of a high-carbohydrate meal; lower levels of insulin may lead to reduced fat storage and improved glucose regulation.

Over the last 10 years, research on the benefits and risks of low-carbohydrate diets for weight loss and health has exploded, with researchers setting up camp on both sides of the issue (Astrup 2001; Astrup et al. 2002; Crowe 2005; Phinney 2004; Volek et al. 2005; Westman et al. 2007). According to research on whether low-carbohydrate, high-protein (or high-fat) diets result in greater weight loss than energy-equivalent low-fat, high-carbohydrate diets (e.g., conventional diet), people initially lose weight faster on the low-carbohydrate diets, but after 12 months the total weight loss is similar (Foster et al. 2003). An extensive review of this literature, using an evidence-based approach, showed that individuals following these types of diets typically lose weight because energy intake is reduced. However, researchers found no "metabolic" advantage to these diets with respect to losses in body weight or body composition (Freedman et al. 2001). In the end, the majority of weight loss associated with low-carbohydrate diets is related to decreased energy intake (Bravata et al. 2003). Thus as mentioned earlier, in the end, calories count. The major disadvantage of applying a low-carbohydrate diet plan to the lifestyle of an athlete is that this type of diet will result in glycogen depletion, leaving the athlete with limited or no capability to perform high-intensity activities. Another disadvantage is the rapid weight loss due to diuresis, or water loss, as stored carbohydrates are oxidized. While the weight loss goals are achieved, these diets leave one feeling lethargic, short-tempered, dehydrated, and unable to engage in strenuous exercise. Carbohydrate is a critical fuel for athletic performance, and consuming inadequate amounts of carbohydrate hinders the athlete's cognitive ability and the ability to train and perform optimally on a daily basis. These diets can also lead to fluid and electrolyte imbalances.

Another claim regarding low-carbohydrate diets is that they more effectively regulate blood glucose and insulin, which should reduce storage of excess carbohydrate as body fat. Insulin is a strong anabolic hormone that signals the cells to store glucose and fat, and dietary carbohydrate results in the secretion of insulin. The majority of the research on glucose and insulin regulation, weight loss, and responses to various diets has used subjects with obesity, with type 2 diabetes or other glucose regulation problems, or both. People in these groups are not the metabolic peers of highly trained athletes. Healthy athletes and active individuals have good glucose tolerance and insulin sensitivity compared to their healthy sedentary counterparts (Niakaris et al. 2005). The metabolic response of a sedentary obese individual or of someone with type 2 diabetes to a particular dietary regimen can be quite different than that of an active individual fed the same diet. For example, Niakaris and colleagues (2005) compared the glycemic response of healthy lean male sprint runners, endurance runners, and sedentary controls to a 75 g oral glucose tolerance test. They found that the basal plasma insulin and the insulinemic responses to the glucose load were significantly higher in controls than in the athletes ($p < 0.05$, $p < 0.02$, respectively), while there were no differences between endurance and sprint runners. In addition, both groups of athletes were more insulin sensitive than controls, regardless of the measure of insulin sensitivity used ($p < 0.05$). This study demonstrates the positive benefit of physical activity on the ability of the body to metabolize glucose.

High-protein, low-carbohydrate diets for weight loss will always be around because they initially bring success and clinically can be used for treatment of some health conditions. These diets need to be used with care with athletes and active individuals and should not be used during periods of high-intensity training or competition. Finally, low-carbohydrate diets (<90 g/day) typically cannot be maintained for long periods of time by most people; thus their use during weight maintenance is limited (Phelan et al. 2006).

Moderate Energy Restriction Diets

Very low-calorie diets and LCDs can result in substantial weight loss but are also associated with large losses of FFM and decreases in RMR. These changes make long-term weight maintenance very difficult. In addition, these types of diets typically do not take into account body size, gender, food preferences, sport, or level of physical activity. Thus, it is becoming increasingly common to recommend **moderate energy restriction diets** combined with physical activity, both aerobic and resistance training, in an attempt to prevent the loss of metabolically active tissues.

Moderate energy restriction diets do not prespecify a recommended energy level for all individuals. These types of diets produce a specific energy deficit through diet (e.g., energy restriction of –300 kcal/day) or exercise (e.g., –300 kcal/day), or both, to bring about a total energy reduction (e.g., –600 kcal/day). The exact level of energy deficit induced will depend on the individual's current dietary habits and training schedule. For some athletes, increasing energy expenditure may not be possible because they are already exercising at a high level. Thus they produce an energy deficit by decreasing energy intake only, but not to the extent that physical activity is negatively affected.

The goal in these weight loss programs is to achieve a weight loss defined in pounds per week (kilograms per week), or to decrease total body weight by a designated percentage, or both. Energy intake is decreased to a lower level than currently needed to maintain body weight, and expenditure is increased above the current level. For example, a female athlete (current body weight 120 lb or 55 kg) may aim to lose 10 lb (4.5 kg), which also represents 8% of her current body weight. It is assumed that this athlete maintains weight on her current diet while exercising 1 h/day. To achieve a weight loss of ~1 lb/week (~0.45 kg), she should accumulate an energy deficit of 500 kcal/day (~1 lb of fat contains ~3500 kcal). As it is best to target weight and fat loss during the off-season, she may choose to engage in an additional 30 min of exercise (e.g., running for 20 min at a pace of 6.5 min/mile [~275 kcal]) and to eat 225 kcal less on a daily basis. Remember that as weight is lost, the total amount of energy needed to maintain weight decreases because the body is getting smaller. Thus, weight loss will slow as the individual gets closer to the target weight if the same diet and activity plans are maintained.

Using this approach to weight loss, especially fat loss, may work better for active people than a predetermined energy intake such as that provided by a 1200 kcal/day diet. This level of energy intake is too low and will result in a lowering of RMR and a loss of lean tissue, because it is below the RMR requirement of most individuals. An active person cannot replace muscle glycogen when energy intake is this low. Finally, if energy intake is too low, the individual will not be able to adhere to the diet plan and still maintain a training or fitness program.

While weight loss is less rapid with moderate energy restriction diets, as compared to diets employing more severe energy reductions, FFM and RMR do not appear to be compromised. In addition, healthy dietary practices can be stressed with moderate energy restriction, thereby assisting people with long-term maintenance of healthy body weight. Finally, this approach allows people to work toward their fitness or exercise goals as well.

Low Energy-Dense Diets

Not everyone wants to count calories. Is there a diet plan that can help people lose weight by making better food choices without constantly counting calories? Research shows that people can successfully lose weight on diets composed mainly of low-energy-dense foods such as unprocessed carbohydrates (e.g., whole grains, legumes, beans, whole fruits, and vegetables) and lean protein sources (e.g., lean meats, fish, poultry, eggs and egg whites, low-fat dairy). Typically, these diets are low in energy density (kcal/g of food), high in water content, lower in fat, and higher in fiber than the typical low calorie diet. People on a **low-energy-dense diet** self-select to eat less food (e.g., fewer calories per day), yet report feeling satiated (Ello-Martin et al. 2005; Bell and Rolls 2001). These diets are higher than other diet plans in total volume of food consumed because they focus on foods with high water content and bulk. Dr. Barbara Rolls, one of the primary researchers in this area, has called this the "volumetric weight-control plan" (Rolls and Barnett 2000). This approach does not include fluids that contain high energy such as juice drinks or soda but encourages the use of broth-based soup, salads, and whole fruits and vegetables (Mattes 2006; Rolls et al. 2004, 2005; Ledikwe et al. 2006). If low-energy-dense foods are combined with smaller portion sizes, there is an additive effect, which leads to sustained decreases in energy intake (Rolls et al. 2006). Thus, weight loss can occur when individuals are allowed ad libitum consumption of low-energy-dense foods, selecting foods that are nutrient rich, less processed, and lower in fat. These findings are encouraging for people who find it difficult to count calories, as weight loss may be possible without the deprivation and sacrifice associated with more severe dieting.

How can someone lose weight on an ad libitum, unprocessed low-energy-dense diet? First, there is evidence that people eating these diets consume significantly less energy than those consuming an ad libitum higher-fat or higher-energy-dense diet (Duncan et al. 1983; Lissner et al. 1987; Schutz et al. 1989; Tremblay et al. 1989; Bell and Rolls 2001; Ledikwe et al. 2006). The lower energy intake is due to the greater volume of food that is high in fiber and water and lower in fat than an individual's more typical diet, which usually contains more processed foods. The increased bulk leads to feeling fuller after eating, which prevents overeating. In addition, it appears that eating a high-volume diet with less refined carbohydrate causes a person to feel less hungry between meals (Duncan et al. 1983). These diets have a low energy density per gram of food (kcal/g): One can eat large amounts of whole fruits and vegetables while consuming relatively few kilocalories. Note, however, that it is possible to eat a **high-carbohydrate diet** that has a *high* energy density per gram of food (e.g., fat-free cookies, fat-free frozen yogurt or ice cream) and *not* lose weight—you might even gain weight. Such diets comprise highly processed carbohydrate foods, which are energy dense and contain few vitamins and minerals. This point was demonstrated by Bell and Rolls (2001), who found that women consumed 20% less daily energy on a low-energy-dense diet compared to a high-energy-dense diet (~450 kcal less per day), yet ratings of hunger and fullness were similar between diets. Women also ate the least on the low-energy-dense, low-fat diet (25% energy from fat) compared to a diet with either 35% or 45% percent of energy from fat (see figure 6.6).

Reducing dietary fat intake can also change body weight and energy intake (Lissner et al. 1987; Ello-Martin et al. 2007). For example, Lissner and colleagues (1987) fed three different diets varying in fat content (low, moderate, and high fat) to 24 healthy, nonsmoking young university females. Each diet was fed for two weeks, and participants were told to eat as much as they liked of the foods

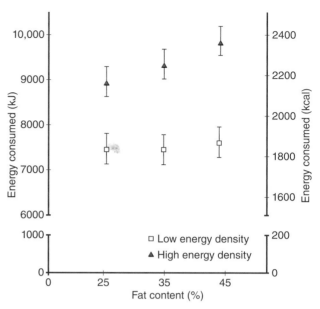

Figure 6.6 Total daily energy consumed with the energy density of the diets manipulated. There was a significant main effect of energy density ($P < 0.0001$) and fat content ($P < 0.02$). Lean and obese women consumed significantly less energy when following the low-energy-dense versus the high-energy-dense diet and less energy in the low-fat (25% of energy from fat) than in the high-fat (45% of energy from fat) diet.

Reprinted, by permission, from E.A. Bell and B.J. Rolls, 2001, "Energy density of foods affects energy intake across multiple levels of fat content in lean and obese women," *American Journal of Clinical Nutrition* 73: 1010-1018.

served. Changes in weight and energy intake are shown in figure 6.7. Compared to participants on the moderate-fat diet, individuals spontaneously ate 11% less energy on the low-fat diet and 15% more energy on the high-fat diet. In addition, there was a significant increase in body weight over a 14-day period on the high-fat diet as compared to the diets relatively low or moderate in fat (Lissner et al. 1987).

Popular or Fad Diets

Fad diets are those that enjoy short-lived success and popularity and are based on a marketing gimmick. Athletes can be particularly vulnerable to fad dieting because of their intense desire to optimize body composition and performance. Celebrities and other well-known persons endorse these diets in an attempt to give them credibility. Justification for these diets is typically based on a scientific or biochemical claim that may be speculative and unproven. Consumers must remember that if the claims associated with the

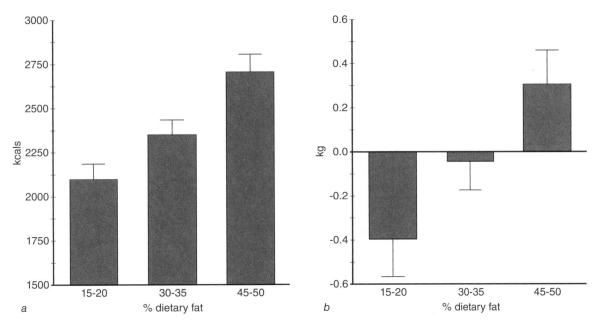

Figure 6.7 *(a)* Mean daily energy intake per 14-day dietary treatment, with the treatments differing in dietary fat intake. Energy intakes were significantly different among diets ($P < 0.0001$). *(b)* Mean changes in body weight over each 14-day treatment period, calculated as day 14 minus day 1. Weight loss was significantly different among diets at $p < 0.001$.

Reprinted, by permission, from L. Lissner et al., 1987, "Dietary fat and the regulation of energy intake in human subjects," *American Journal of Clinical Nutrition* 46: 886-892.

diets were true, there would be no need for people to continue dieting and no need for the next fad diet! For example, if the Dr. Atkins diet, popular in the 1970s, had worked, there would be no need for the "new and improved" Dr. Atkins' New Diet Revolution in the 1990s and 2000s. As mentioned earlier, more modified versions of the Dr. Atkins diet are here to stay but are characterized by less carbohydrate restriction. Because LCDs bring about quick weight loss, they may be used to help people begin or "jump-start" a weight loss regimen.

There will always be a new fad diet in the marketplace, so it is important to understand how to evaluate each new diet and give good dietary advice to your clients. The criteria listed next will help you recognize a potential fad diet or nutrition program. If the diet either you or your clients are considering is associated with one of the following, it is probably just another fad diet:

1. The claim that the diet is new, modern, improved, or recently discovered, with no scientific data available to back up the claim

2. The claim that weight or fat loss will be rapid, usually more than 2 lb (0.9 kg) per week

3. The claim of successful weight loss with no or little physical exercise

4. Inclusion of special foods that are expensive and difficult to find; suggestion that foods should be consumed in a particular order or "combination"; suggestion that consumption of certain "bad" foods should be avoided; or inclusion of "magic" or "miracle" foods that will burn fat

5. Inclusion of a rigid menu that must be followed daily; restriction to a limited list of foods (these diets frequently require adherents to eat the same foods day after day)

6. Inclusion of supplemental meals, foods, or nutrient supplements with the claim that they will cure disease or a variety of ailments

Until we figure out how to solve the obesity problem, the consumer will be bombarded with new weight loss products and programs promising fast weight loss. It is important for nutrition and fitness professionals to educate consumers about the limitations of these products and programs. While some may be physically harmless (albeit expensive), others can cause illness or even death. It is always important to consider the safety and efficacy of any fad diet, including the associated supplements, before recommending it to a client.

Weight Loss Supplements

Weight loss supplements are in the news and on the Web. Just as with fat diets, there is always a new weight loss supplement, with marketers touting its benefits and promising a quick fix. Weight loss and sport nutrition supplements are big business, with over $16.8 billion spent in 2005 (*Nutrition Business Journal* 2006). It appears that the quickest way to get rich is to develop a weight loss supplement and get it to market, regardless of the ethics involved. Currently there is no regulation of the weight loss industry, so the consumer must beware.

This section outlines the types of weight loss supplements on the market, which typically fall into one of four categories depending on their hypothesized mechanism for bringing about weight loss. We briefly review these categories and provide examples of the type of weight loss supplement marketed within each. The next time you see a weight loss supplement advertised, check whether it fits into one of these categories. Remember that many weight loss supplements combine different types of substances into one product, so it is important to read the labels carefully. For a more extensive review of dietary and herbal supplements for weight loss, see the review articles by Dwyer and colleagues (2005), Pittler and colleagues (2005), Pittler and Ernst (2004), Saper and colleagues (2004), and Thomas (2005). You can also search the International Bibliographic Information on Dietary Supplements (IBIBS) database from the NIH Office of Dietary Supplements (http://grande.nal.usda.gov/ibids/index.php) for current published research studies on dietary weight loss supplements and ingredients.

Products Said to Block Absorption of Macronutrients and Energy

The products known as carbohydrate and fat blockers are hypothesized to work by blocking the absorption of energy-containing macronutrients.

- Carbohydrate blockers contain α-amylase inhibitors, proposed to inhibit α-amylase and prevent carbohydrate digestion and absorption. In this way, the energy contained in the starch-based carbohydrate food does not get absorbed, leading to weight loss. To date, no research supports the efficacy of

these products for weight loss (Hollenbeck et al. 1983).

- Fat blockers are designed to decrease the amount of fat and bile absorbed, thus reducing total energy intake. The major ingredient in most fat blockers marketed today is chitosan, a cellulose-type polysaccharide extracted mainly from the exoskeletons of marine crustaceans. The authors of a recent **meta-analysis** (see "What Is a Meta-Analysis?"), reviewing the efficacy of chitosan for weight loss, concluded that the effects were minimal (Mhurchu et al. 2005). Gades and Stern (2005) examined the fat-trapping capacity of chitosan by feeding 12 men and 12 women a control diet for four days, followed by the control diet plus chitosan for another four days. They collected fecal samples from each period to determine the amount of fat trapped by chitosan. They found that with the control diet plus chitosan, fecal fat excretion increased by 1.8 g/day (16 kcal/day) for the men and 0.0 g/day for the women and concluded that the amount of fat trapped by chitosan was clinically insignificant.

Products Said to Boost Metabolism by Acting as Stimulants

Products that fit into the metabolism-boosting category include caffeine, green tea, ephedrine/ephedra (ma huang), guarana, Seville orange (Citrus aurantium), yerba maté, and yohimbe. In general, these products all contain caffeine or ephedra-type stimulants. Frequently they are combined in weight loss products along with diuretics to help reduce body weight.

- Ephedrine alkaloids were banned by the U.S. Food and Drug Administration (FDA) in February 2004 because they were considered to "present unreasonable risk of illness or injury under the conditions of use recommended" (FDA 2004). Although challenged, this ban was upheld by the 10th Circuit U.S. Court of Appeals in 2006 (FDA 2006). At the time of this ruling, a 133,000-page administrative record had been compiled by the FDA, supporting its finding that ephedrine alkaloids and related products posed unreasonable risk of illness to users. A review of several studies showed that ephedra helped with short-term weight loss (~0.9 kg/month) but that it stressed the cardiovascular system

What Is a Meta-Analysis?

Meta-analysis is a research method that combines the results of many studies into an overall result, or "effect," of one or more interventions. This form of research is usually conducted in research areas that are controversial or have yielded copious equivocal findings, or both. For example, meta-analyses have been conducted to determine whether VLDCs are better than conventional LCDs in achieving long-term weight loss (Tsai and Wadden 2006), to determine the effect of diet or diet plus exercise on RMR (Thompson et al. 1996), and to assess the effectiveness of diet or diet plus exercise on amount of weight loss (Curioni and Lourenco 2005; Shaw et al. 2006). Proponents of meta-analytical research claim that it is an accurate, unbiased research process that can combine numerous research findings from a variety of settings to determine treatment effectiveness. Those opposed to meta-analysis believe that it is fraught with bias and is akin to comparing "apples and oranges." Regardless of one's stance on the use of meta-analyses, it is important to remember that a meta-analysis is only as good as the original studies that it includes.

and raised blood pressure (Pittler and Ernst 2004; Thomas 2005). In-depth reviews of ephedra have been published by Abourashed and colleagues (2003), Haller and colleagues (2004), Shekelle and colleagues (2003), and Soni and colleagues (2004).

- Green tea contains caffeine and catechins, which are strong antioxidants and anti-inflammatory compounds. The caffeine and catechins in tea may work together to increase thermogenesis and thus increase energy expenditure (Cabrera et al. 2006). Catechins, which are considered to be among the active ingredients in green tea, may also alter lipid metabolism, which means that this supplement also falls into the category discussed next.

- Guarana and yerba maté contain caffeine, while Seville orange (Citrus aurantium) contains synephrine, which is structurally similar to epinephrine. Yohimbe, a stimulant similar to caffeine and ephedra, is extracted from yohimbe bark. There is no evidence that these products are effective for long-term weight loss (Fugh-Berman and Meyers 2004; Pittler et al. 2005).

Products Said to Change Macronutrient Partitioning and Body Composition

Items that fall into this category are calcium, L-carnitine, chromium picolinate, conjugated linoleic acid, green tea, and pyruvate. These substances are hypothesized to work by changing either fat or carbohydrate metabolism, thus reducing fat storage or increasing fat metabolism or both. Many of these substances have been the focus of a tremendous amount of research, with the jury still out on their efficacy for weight loss or fat loss. Here we briefly review some of these supplements.

- The role that calcium may play in weight control has been extensively researched, with no consensus on the impact of calcium intake on body weight. It has been hypothesized that an increase in calcium intake or dairy consumption is associated with a lower body weight and decreased weight gain. For more in-depth information on this topic, see the reviews by Barr (2003), Heaney (2003), Rajpathak and colleagues (2006), Teegarden (2003), and Zemel (2004).

- L-carnitine is essential for fatty acid metabolism. It has long been hypothesized that if carnitine can be increased in the muscle, fat oxidation will be increased, which could affect body composition and endurance performance. However, in order for carnitine to be effective, it must be taken up by the muscle cell. Currently, there is a lack of evidence that carnitine ingested in supplemental form is taken up by muscle. For a review of the impact of carnitine on exercise performance, see Karlic and Lohninger 2004. There is no evidence that carnitine is an effective weight loss agent (Villani et al. 2000).

- Chromium picolinate is an essential trace metal believed to increase lean muscle mass and promote fat loss while enhancing the effects of insulin. A recent meta-analysis showed small changes in weight (<0.45 lb/week or <0.2 kg/week) with chromium supplementation lasting 6 to 14 weeks (Pittler et al. 2003). Conversely, Vincent (2003) has reviewed the chromium picolinate literature and reports no benefit of supplementation on body composition.

- Conjugated linoleic acid (CLA) is hypothesized to increase lean tissue mass and decrease body fat on the basis of extensive research in animals documenting this phenomenon; however, research in humans has not produced the same results. Two recent meta-analyses have examined the effect of supplementation on fat loss and on weight regain after completion of a weight loss program. A meta-analysis by Whigham and colleagues (2007) showed a small (0.1 lb/week or 0.05 kg/week) but significant change in fat mass with 3.2 g/day of CLA over a 6- to 24-month period. Conversely, a review by Larsen and colleagues (2003) showed no significant difference in either body weight or fat mass regain in CLA users (3.4 g/day for one year) compared to placebo groups. Thus, based on the cost of the supplement and the duration required to see any change in weight, there is little benefit of the supplement for weight loss. Information on the safety of CLA over long periods of use is limited.

- Hydroxycitrate (HCA) is the active ingredient in the rind of the fruit *Garcinia cambogia,* a species native to India. Hydroxycitrate is an inhibitor of ATP-citrate-lyase, the enzyme that cleaves citrate into oxaloacetate and acetyl-CoA for endogenous fat synthesis. Thus, it is hypothesized that HCA can reduce fat synthesis if carbohydrate intake is in excess. Hydroxycitrate is also hypothesized to increase fat oxidation and suppress appetite. At the present time, research does not support increased fat oxidation, appetite suppression, or fat loss with HCA supplementation (Heymsfield et al. 1998; Kovacs et al. 2001; Mattes and Bormann 2000).

Products Said to Suppress Appetite and Increase Satiety

Supplements that fall into this category include soluble fibers such as psyllium, glucomannan and guar gum, and hoodia gordonii, a South African plant used for appetite suppression. Soluble fiber can absorb water within the gut and theoretically increase the sense of satiety, thus lowering caloric intake. Although fiber has definite health benefits, there are no data supporting fiber supplements for weight loss. Pittler and Ernst (2001) reviewed the research literature on guar gum and found no effect of supplementation on body weight. Side effects of guar gum supplementation are primarily flatulence, diarrhea, and gastrointestinal pain and complaints. At the present time, there are no research studies in humans on the effectiveness of hoodia gordonii in suppressing appetite and reducing body weight.

ADDING EXERCISE TO WEIGHT LOSS PROGRAMS

It is well established that diet alone and diet combined with exercise can result in weight loss. Exercise plays a number of important roles in regard to body weight and health. Many active people consume more energy than sedentary obese individuals but maintain a lean physique. Active people also have a healthier BMI and body fat distribution than do sedentary or detrained individuals (Williams and Thompson 2006). Furthermore, an active lifestyle may prevent or minimize the weight gain observed with aging. Among those who are active and overweight, the risk of morbidity and mortality is much lower than it is for sedentary overweight and lean individuals.

Weight loss occurs when energy intake is less than energy expenditure. Exercise alone can be used to increase energy expenditure, resulting in weight loss if energy intake is not increased to compensate for the higher energy expenditure. Table 6.2 lists energy expenditures for various activities. The energy expended for any given activity is usually expressed per kilogram body weight or as a multiple of RMR. Although these energy values are useful as a guide, they may not be exact. A number of errors are inherent in the estimation of energy expenditure (see chapter 14 for detailed discussion). Appendix E.3 provides a more complete table of energy expenditure values.

Exercise-induced weight loss depends on both the total amount of energy expended and the types of fuels used for energy during the activity. Exercising is an ideal way to increase fat oxidation since skeletal muscle readily uses fat for energy. Fat oxidation is also proportionately greater during prolonged exercise of low to moderate intensity as compared to exercise performed at

Table 6.2   Energy Expenditure for Various Physical Activities

Activity	Energy expenditure (kcal · min⁻¹ · kg⁻¹)	Energy expenditure for selected body weights (kcal/min)			
		110 lb (50 kg)	130 lb (59 kg)	150 lb (68 kg)	170 lb (77 kg)
Cycling					
Leisure (5.5 mph)	0.064	3.2	3.8	4.4	4.9
Leisure (9.4 mph)	0.100	5.0	5.9	6.8	7.7
Racing	0.169	8.5	10.0	11.5	13.0
Dancing					
Aerobic (medium)	0.103	5.2	6.1	7.0	7.9
Aerobic (intense)	0.135	6.7	7.9	9.2	10.4
Ballroom	0.051	2.6	3.0	3.5	3.9
Walking (normal pace)					
Asphalt road	0.080	4.0	4.7	5.4	6.2
Fields and hillsides	0.082	4.1	4.8	5.6	6.3
Running (horizontal)					
11 min, 30 s/mile	0.135	6.8	8.0	9.2	10.5
8 min/mile	0.208	10.8	12.5	14.2	16.0
6 min/mile	0.252	13.9	15.6	17.3	19.1
Swimming					
Backstroke	0.169	8.5	10.0	11.5	13.0
Breaststroke	0.162	8.1	9.6	11.0	12.5
Crawl, fast	0.156	7.8	9.2	10.6	12.0
Crawl, slow	0.128	6.4	7.6	8.7	9.9

Adapted, by permission, from B.E. Ainsworth et al., 1993, "Compendium of physical activities: classification by energy costs of human physical activities," *Medicine and Science in Sport and Exercise* 25: 71-80.

a higher intensity (Flatt 1992). Activities causing the greatest energy expenditure are those that are endurance related and use large muscle groups (e.g., running or cross-country skiing) (table 6.2). Remember also that fat oxidation is maximized at activities of low to moderate intensity (figure 6.8). This means that performing activities such as walking, swimming, aerobics, and bicycling at low to moderate intensities increases relative fat oxidation (i.e., the majority of the energy will come from fat) as compared to activities of greater intensity. However, the *total* energy expenditure over a given period of time for low- to moderate-intensity activities is less than that for more intense activities such as running. A critical point to remember is that the *relative* contribution of fat as a fuel is greater during moderate exercise than during intense exercise, when carbohydrate contributes proportionately more energy (figure 6.8). However, it is the *total* energy and nutrient balance over an entire day that determines the absolute amount of fat used as a fuel.

One of the first studies to show the importance of both time and intensity of exercise in weight loss was done by Tremblay and colleagues (1994). Their results indicate that high-intensity intermittent training may result in greater fat loss than moderate-intensity endurance training. The subjects performed either 20 weeks of continuous cycling (four times per week for 30-45 min at 60-85% of maximal heart rate reserve) or 15 weeks of high-intensity intermittent training (19 short- and 16 long-interval workouts, accompanied by 25 sessions of continuous cycling, 30 min each). The high-intensity exercisers showed a significantly greater reduction in skinfold thickness than the endurance exercisers, despite the fact that the energy cost of the high-intensity program was less than half that of the endurance program. One mechanism to explain these findings was the significant increase in muscle **3-hydroxyacyl coenzyme A dehydrogenase (HADH)** enzyme activity with high-intensity training; HADH is a marker of β-oxidation, with increased activity of

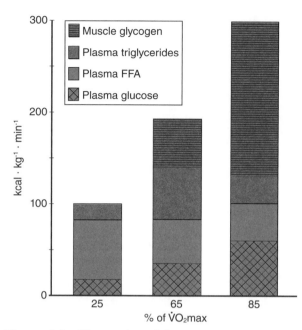

Figure 6.8 Illustration of the crossover from lipid to carbohydrate dependency as exercise intensity increases from mild (25% $\dot{V}O_2$max) to hard (85% $\dot{V}O_2$max). FFA= Free fatty acids.

Reprinted from J.A. Romijn et al. 1993, "Regulation of endogenous fat and carbohydrate metabolism in relation to exercise intensity and duration," *American Journal of Physiology* 265(3) Pt 1: E380-391. Used with permission.

this enzyme indicating an increase in fat oxidation. Other factors that were not measured may also explain these findings, including increased excess postexercise oxygen consumption (EPOC), suppression of food intake, increased metabolic cost of tissue damage related to the high-intensity exercise, or some combination of these.

It is important to emphasize that many people are not physically capable of performing high-intensity exercise due to their low fitness level, age, or health problems. For these people, participation in low- to moderate-intensity endurance-type activities will still be effective for weight loss. Athletes naturally engage in high-intensity activity in training and during competition. Thus, there typically is no need to incorporate high-intensity exercise into a weight loss regimen in this population. In fact, including some lower-intensity activities such as jogging or cycling in the training schedule at specific times of the day (e.g., morning before breakfast, or before or after practice) may be a more feasible and effective approach for weight loss.

Resistance training also plays a critical role in weight loss (Jakicic et al. 2001). It may not significantly increase energy expenditure, and fat is not the predominant fuel source for resistance training—but increasing one's FFM, which is a result of resistance training, increases RMR (Ballor et al. 1988; Broeder et al. 1992; Tremblay et al. 1986). Resistance training can also help reshape the body by toning or adding FFM (or both)—a goal often sought by those who are trying to lose weight.

Effect of Exercise Alone on Weight Loss

Despite the importance of exercise for health and maintenance of lean tissue, most studies do not support the contention that exercise alone results in significant weight loss (Jakicic et al. 2001) unless exercise levels are high (~700 kcal/day) and other energy factors are held constant (Ross et al. 2000). If exercise alone does result in weight loss, the loss is usually small (~0.09 kg/week) for both men and women (Epstein and Wing, 1980; Garrow and Summerbell 1995). Most subjects participating in these studies did not lose as much weight as expected from their increased energy expenditure. Since energy intake was not controlled, presumably either a compensatory increase in energy intake occurred with the increase in energy expenditure, or the subjects decreased the duration or intensity of activities associated with daily living. These changes would result in relatively small perturbations in body weight.

For exercise alone to be effective in weight loss, energy intake must be maintained at a level lower than that of total daily energy expenditure. Exercising women lost significant amounts of weight when their energy intake was held constant at sedentary maintenance levels (Keim et al. 1990). These women lost approximately 1.1 lb/week (0.5 kg/week) when walking on a treadmill six days a week at a level equal to 25% of their energy intake. They lost weight because they were not allowed to compensate for their increased energy expenditure. Note, however, the results of research by Woo and colleagues (1982): Subjects allowed an ad libitum diet did not compensate for the excess energy expended in daily walking and had an average weight loss of 1.8 lb/week (0.8 kg/week). For exercise to assist in maintaining healthy body weight, it is important not only to practice some form of regular exercise training but also to increase activities of daily living. See "Methods for Increasing Total Daily Energy Expenditure" for suggestions on ways to increase daily activity levels (in addition to an organized exercise session).

Highlight

Methods for Increasing Total Daily Energy Expenditure

Here are a few suggestions for increasing total energy expenditure. Please keep in mind that the list is by no means exhaustive.

- Leave your desk frequently at work, and take the stairs between floors.
- Skip the escalators and elevators at the mall or at work, and take the stairs instead.
- Park farther away from your destination (or walk instead).
- Walk to lunch when the weather permits.
- Play with your children, grandchildren, or pets on a regular basis.
- Clean the house a little every day. Not only will you expend energy, but cleaning will not seem like such an overwhelming chore.
- Replace some of your television viewing time with gardening, fixing up your home, or some other active hobby.
- Do stretching and resistance training activities while watching television.
- Take a 10 min walk during your break or lunchtime or after dinner.

Not only can performing these activities help increase total daily energy expenditure, but research shows that they can be just as effective as structured exercise in improving fitness and health (Andersen et al. 1999; Brown et al. 2007; Dunn et al. 1999).

When trying to lose weight, people must not increase energy intake to compensate for the energy expended during exercise. From the information presented in this chapter, it appears that consuming a diet high in less processed carbohydrates (e.g., whole grains, legumes, beans, whole fruits, and vegetables) and lean protein sources while increasing activity should result in weight loss over time. Combining moderate-intensity (or even high-intensity) exercise with a diet high in nutrient-rich carbohydrates, moreover, can promote fat oxidation. Consumption of a diet high in carbohydrate also supports participation in exercise, as it ensures adequate glycogen stores and helps maintain endurance (Bogardus et al. 1981).

Diet and Exercise in Weight Loss and Weight Maintenance

Research data clearly show that energy restriction results in weight loss and that exercise alone without compensatory increases in energy intake can also lead to gradual losses of body weight. It has been suggested throughout this chapter that the most effective regimen for weight loss is com-bining diet with exercise. This section addresses the validity of the following claims for combining energy restriction with exercise:

- Exercise prevents the decrease in RMR seen with dieting.
- Exercise added to dieting increases the amount of weight lost.
- Exercise added to dieting helps preserve FFM.

Does Exercise Prevent the Decrease in RMR Seen With Dieting?

Numerous researchers have attempted to determine the additive effects of exercise and diet on RMR, yet there appears to be no clear understanding of the issue. Some have suggested that exercise can prevent the decrease in RMR observed with dieting (Svendsen et al. 1993; Thompson et al. 1997); others either show no effect of exercise or find that RMR can decline even further when exercise is added to dietary restriction (Donnelly et al. 1991, 1994; Heymsfield et al. 1989; van Dale et al. 1990). A number of factors can contribute to these discrepancies. For example, level of energy restriction, intensity and type of prescribed exercise, duration of the diet and exercise program, and the characteristics of the subjects can all influence the results reported in the literature.

A meta-analysis of the effects that diet alone and diet plus exercise regimens have on RMR reviewed all of the available studies (Thompson et al. 1996). In this analysis, exercise (predominantly endurance exercise) was found to prevent some of the decrease in RMR observed with dieting. However, a number of unique factors in these studies may limit widespread application of this analysis:

- Very few studies were available on men or postmenopausal women.
- The majority of studies prescribed energy intakes less than 800 kcal/day.
- The endurance exercise prescribed in most studies was moderate in intensity (50-70% of $\dot{V}O_2$max).
- Only half of the studies combined strength training with endurance exercise.
- No studies employed only strength training.
- The average duration of the studies was nine weeks.

The results of this meta-analysis suggest that adding moderate-intensity endurance exercise can prevent some of the RMR decrease when obese, premenopausal women diet. A recent review by Stiegler and Cunliffe (2006) examined the role that diet and exercise play in the maintenance of FFM and RMR during weight loss. They found that two key factors are important for maintaining FFM: (1) including strength training in a weight loss program and (2) obtaining adequate protein in the diet to help maintain FFM. Unfortunately, preserving FFM does not always prevent a decline in RMR. Thus, until we know the mechanisms that are important for maintaining both FFM and RMR during periods of weight loss, it is prudent to consume adequate amounts of high-quality protein and include both endurance and strength training exercises.

Does Exercise Increase the Amount of Weight Lost and Help Preserve FFM Over Dieting Alone?

One would assume that adding exercise to dietary restriction would increase the energy deficit and thus lead to greater weight loss. However, the plethora of studies addressing the effectiveness of diet alone or diet plus exercise regimens on weight loss and changes in body composition do not overwhelmingly support this assumption. Although individual studies have not always demonstrated significant differences in body weight between diet and diet plus exercise groups, recent meta-analyses have shown significant differences (Curioni and Lourenco 2005; Shaw et al. 2006). Curioni and Lourenco (2005) compared six randomized clinical trials ranging from 10 to 52 weeks that also followed subjects (n = 265) for one year after the weight loss intervention. They found a 20% greater weight loss in diet plus exercise programs (–13 kg) compared to diet-only programs (–9.9 kg) and a 20% greater sustained weight loss after one year (Curioni and Lourenco 2005). A second meta-analysis (Shaw et al. 2006) showed a small but significant increase in weight loss in diet plus exercise programs (–1.1 kg) compared to diet-only programs. Thus, there appears to be a small but significant positive effect on weight loss and retention of weight loss if physical activity is added to an energy reduction diet.

This lack of greater weight loss with the addition of exercise to a diet program is most likely due to a decrease in the total amount of energy expended over the day, or an increase in energy intake that compensates for the energy expended during exercise, or both. There is evidence that exercisers compensate for their increased energy expended by increasing the time spent sleeping, sitting, and lying down during the day. Dieters, on the other hand, appear to spend more time in sedentary activities because their lack of energy intake makes them feel "more tired." Note that most studies of diet and exercise are done on an "outpatient" basis, which increases the probability that subjects may be consuming more kilocalories per day than prescribed in the diet. These additional kilocalories would explain why most people participating in diet and exercise studies do not lose as much weight as would be predicted from the prescribed energy deficit.

While adding exercise to a diet plan not lead to substantially greater weight loss, it does appear to increase the amount of body fat lost. Endurance exercise not only results in the oxidation of fat; it also increases the potential to sustain FFM in a way not observed with dieting alone (Donnelly et al. 1991; Garrow and Summerbell 1995). Adding exercise to dietary restriction can enhance fat loss and maintain or slow the loss of FFM that consistently occurs with dieting alone. It is important to emphasize that the studies demonstrating significant losses of FFM involved relatively low energy intakes (<1000 kcal/day). Less restrictive diets may have much less impact on loss of FFM. The most critical role that exercise may play is in maintaining weight loss after the diet is over. Experts in the area of weight loss consistently stress the importance of regular exercise to achieve both weight loss and the long-term maintenance of weight loss (Jakicic et al. 2001; Donnelly et al. 2009).

RECOMMENDATIONS FOR MAINTAINING OR GAINING WEIGHT

Not everyone wants to lose weight. Some individuals want to maintain their current weight (e.g. not gain weight), while others want to gain weight, usually lean tissue. The following section discusses successful strategies you can recommend to your clients for weight maintenance throughout the life span. This section also gives specific diet and exercise recommendations for individuals who want to gain weight, specifically lean tissue, in a healthy manner.

Maintaining a Healthy Body Weight

Maintaining a healthy or optimal body weight appears to be linked to successfully addressing three lifestyle issues on a daily basis:

- Consuming a diet low in fat and high in whole and less processed carbohydrate (e.g., high in fruits, vegetables, whole grains, legumes, and beans)
- Participating in regular exercise and leading an active lifestyle
- Making appropriate behavioral modifications related to dietary intake and exercise ("Components of a Behavior Modification Program for Weight Loss or Weight Maintenance" reviews the components of a behavior modification program)

People who are successful at long-term maintenance of weight loss report that incorporating healthy lifestyle modifications into daily life is critical to their success. Moreover, it is essential that people accept the fact that maintenance of healthy body weight is a lifelong process (see "Case Study: Weight Loss in an Overweight Active Woman" p. 190 and "The National Weight Control Registry" p. 191).

Highlight

Components of a Behavior Modification Program for Weight Loss or Weight Maintenance

Berkel and colleagues (2005) reviewed the components of behavioral interventions for obesity. The following is a brief synopsis of the important components of any behavior modification program aimed at weight loss or weight maintenance. Note that these programs address nutrition and exercise, reinforcing the important interactions among diet, exercise, and behavior on weight loss and weight maintenance.

- **Self-monitoring:** Involves completing regular records on amount, location, and circumstances surrounding food intake to assess initial patterns of eating and exercise behavior. Also used to track motivation and document positive changes in behavior.
- **Goal setting:** Involves determining reasonable and achievable goals within the context of one's life. What has to be done daily to achieve this goal? For example, how much energy or how many grams of fat should be consumed daily? How much physical activity in minutes per week should be achieved? A later section of the chapter addresses how to help clients reach their goals.
- **Nutrition:** Requires going beyond just counting calories (kilocalories). Involves understanding the nutrient composition of foods and setting specific dietary goals, such as decreasing energy and fat intake or eating more nutrient-dense foods (e.g., carrots instead of jelly beans). Also includes educating oneself on the importance of healthy eating regardless of energy intake.

(continued)

Components of a Behavior Modification Program   *(continued)*

- **Exercise:** Involves learning how to increase activities of daily living, including the gradual introduction of a regular exercise program into one's lifestyle. Requires committing to a lifetime of physical activity.

- **Stimulus control:** Involves controlling the environment in which one consumes food, such as keeping food out of sight, avoiding the purchase of problematic foods, eating at specific times and places, and breaking habitual eating routines.

- **Problem solving:** Involves identifying potential barriers to carrying out goals and the program that has been set up to reach these goals, selecting possible solutions to these barriers, and learning to implement the solutions.

- **Cognitive reconstruction:** Involves recognizing and improving thoughts and beliefs about one's body, one's life, and chances of success for weight loss and long-term maintenance.

- **Relapse prevention:** Involves realizing that lapses will occur, but learning how one keeps them from turning into relapse. Clients learn to find help in a number of places, for example, to obtain positive support from fellow dieters, family members, and friends. Also involves preventing the undermining of the dieting effort by spouse or family members and avoiding ridicule of efforts by peers.

Highlight

Case Study:
Weight Loss in an Overweight Active Woman

Margaret is 5 ft 5 in. tall (165 cm), is 35 years old, and weighs 160 lb (72.6 kg). Her BMI is 26.7 kg/m², and she recently had her body fat measured at 33%. Margaret was a competitive athlete in college and has remained active. She has always struggled with her weight, which has ranged from 135 lb (62 kg) to 170 lb (77 kg) throughout her adult life. She currently walks/runs an average of 25 miles (40 km)/week and attends a 90 min yoga class once a week. While Margaret considers herself fit, she would like to decrease her body fat since she has had consistently elevated serum LDL-cholesterol levels for the past three years. Her doctor recommended that she lose 15 lb (6.8 kg). Margaret's diet and activity logs show that she requires approximately 2500 kcal/day to maintain her current body weight and activity level. While individuals certainly differ, a universal rule of thumb is that one must have an energy deficit of 3500 kcal in order to lose 1 lb of fat.

Margaret would like to lose her excess body fat rapidly but knows from her previous dieting experiences that she is more likely to maintain weight loss with a more gradual program. She has decided to maintain her current activity level (increasing her activity level exacerbates her chronic lower leg pain), reminding herself that she should perform some sort of physical activity at least four days a week. She has decided to decrease her energy intake by 500 kcal/day, which should result in a weight loss of ~1 lb/week (0.45 kg/week). Her goal is to maximize fat loss and minimize loss of muscle tissue. Margaret feels that this is a realistic goal, as she can skip the chocolate bar she eats every afternoon (220 kcal), give up the two light beers she drinks every night after work (180 kcal), and eat one less piece of toast for breakfast in the morning (100 kcal). In addition, she plans to pay close attention to the amount of saturated fat in her diet, eating less than 10% of her total fat intake as saturated fat in an attempt to lower her LDL-cholesterol levels. By reducing her daily energy intake in this manner, Margaret should reach her weight goal of 145 lb (66 kg) in approximately 15 weeks. It is important for Margaret to remember that as she gets closer to her goal weight, the rate of weight loss will be slower than at the beginning of the program. This response is primarily due to her lower body weight (since she weighs less, the energy deficit will be less than the original 500 kcal/day) and may also be due to the potential reduction in RMR that occurs with dietary restriction and weight loss.

The National Weight Control Registry

In 1994, Drs. Rena Wing, PhD, of Brown Medical School and James Hill, PhD, of the University of Colorado Health Sciences Center founded the National Weight Control Registry (NWCR) (www.nwcr.ws). To date, this project is the largest prospective investigation of long-term successful weight loss maintenance. The goal of the project was to find individuals who had been successful at weight loss and describe the strategies that they used to achieve and maintain weight loss long-term. Currently, the NWCR is tracking over 5000 individuals who have lost significant amounts of weight and kept it off for long periods of time. In order to be part of the registry, people need to be 18 years or older, to have lost at least 30 lb (6.6 kg), and to have maintained this weight loss for at least one year. Once enrolled in the program, individuals are periodically asked to fill out detailed questionnaires about their successful weight loss, current weight maintenance strategies, and other health-related behaviors for the purpose of determining the behavioral and psychological characteristics of weight maintainers, as well as the strategies they use to maintain weight loss. Participants also fill out annual follow-up surveys so that their weight maintenance can be continually tracked. Thus the NWCR is not a randomized controlled study, but rather looks at who has been successful at weight loss and at weight loss maintenance. On average, 80% of the participants are women and 20% are men who have lost 66 lb (30 kg) and kept the weight off for 5.5 years. The average woman is 45 years of age and weighs 145 lb (66 kg), and the average man is 49 years of age and weighs 190 lb (86 kg). Of course, these averages hide the huge diversity of the individuals involved in the study, as well as facts such as the following:

- Weight loss has ranged from 30 to 300 lb (13.6-136 kg).
- Duration of successful weight loss has ranged from 1 to 66 years.
- Some participants have lost the weight rapidly, while others have lost it very slowly—over as many as 14 years.

The following are strategies used by these individuals to lose weight and keep it off. Some of the information has been adapted from a review of the NWCR by Manore (2004).

- **Methods of weight loss.** Almost everyone in the registry has used a combination of diet and exercise to lose the weight, with 45% reporting that they lost the weight on their own and 55% reporting using some type of program. Nearly all of the participants (98%) reported that they modified their food intake in some way to lose weight, while 94% said that they increased their physical activity. The most common form of physical activity reported is walking. Nearly all of the participants have reported that their weight loss has led to significant improvements in energy levels, physical mobility, general mood, self-confidence, and physical health (Klem et al. 1997). Participants (~42%) state that keeping the weight off has not been as difficult as losing it initially (Klem et al. 1997). This is especially true in individuals who have kept the weight off for more than two years (Klem et al. 2000).

- **Strategies for weight maintenance.** Since the initiation of the NWCR, investigators have been analyzing the data to determine successful weight maintenance strategies (Gorin et al. 2004; Hill and Wing 2003; Klem et al. 1997; McGuire et al. 1998; Phelan et al. 2007; Raynor et al. 2006; Shick et al. 1998; Wyatt et al. 2002). In general, most participants report continuing to maintain a low-calorie, low-fat diet and doing high levels of physical activity. The following are some of the specific and most frequently mentioned strategies used by participants who have been successful at maintaining weight loss.

  -*Eating breakfast.* Nearly 80% of participants report eating breakfast every day, with only 4% reporting never eating breakfast. How might eating breakfast contribute to successful weight maintenance? Although there were no differences in total energy intake between frequent breakfast eaters and less frequent breakfast eaters (three times a week or less), breakfast eaters reported being more physically active (Wyatt et al. 2002).

(continued)

The National Weight Control Registry *(continued)*

-*Monitoring energy and fat intake.* A common characteristic of registry participants is that they continue to monitor their energy and fat intake even after the weight loss period is over. On average, participants consume diets with ~24% of energy from fat and have energy intakes lower than average (Shick et al. 1998). As a group, 80% consume diets with <30% of energy from fat, while 35% consume diets with less than 20% of energy from fat. The strategies employed to control food intake include limiting intake of certain high-fat foods, eating less food per meal, counting grams of fat or calories, eating regular meals, and adhering to the same diet regimen throughout the week (Klem et al. 1997; Gorin et al. 2004). Diet consistency across the week appears to help people prevent weight gain (Gorin et al. 2004).

-*Exercising daily.* Being physical active is an important characteristic of registry participants, with 90% reporting that they exercise, on average, about 1 h or more per day. Weekly energy expenditures from physical activity average ~2800 kcal: ~2500 kcal/week for women and 3300 kcal/week for men (Hill and Wing 2003; Klem et al. 1997). The most common forms of physical activity reported are cycling, aerobics, walking, and running (Klem et al. 1997). Comparison of the levels of physical activity between successful weight loss maintainers and people who had always maintained a normal weight showed that the weight loss maintainers spent significantly more time in high-intensity forms of physical activity and spent more minutes per week doing physical activity (Phelan et al. 2007).

- *Engaging in less sedentary activity.* It has long been recognized that sedentary behaviors, especially TV viewing, may contribute to weight gain. Raynor and colleagues (2006) examined the TV viewing of registry participants and found that 62% watched <10 h of TV per week, with 36% reporting that they watched <5 h/week. This level of TV viewing is much lower than the national average of 28 h/week.

-*Monitoring weight.* Nearly 75% of the registry participants weigh themselves at least once a week (Klem et al. 1997). Thus, regularly monitoring weight appears to be a behavior that is important for ensuring that weight regain does not occur.

What we have learned from the participants in the NWCR is that good nutrition, physical activity, and self-monitoring are important for keeping the weight off once it has been lost. Individuals who are successful at weight loss and the maintenance of weight loss appear to employ similar strategies. They eat breakfast, exercise regularly, monitor their diet for both energy and fat intake, participate in less TV watching, and weigh themselves regularly.

Gaining Weight

Weight gain is also a concern for many athletes. The ideal would be to achieve maximal gains in lean tissue and minimal gains in fat tissue. It may be unrealistic, however, to expect to gain exclusively lean tissue on a weight gain program. The key to gaining weight is to consume more energy than one expends. Consuming a diet higher in nutrient-dense carbohydrates and lower in fat, yet still high in kilocalories, should result in gaining extra weight that comprises very little body fat. For success in a weight gain program, athletes should do the following:

- Set realistic weight gain goals.
- Allow adequate time to reach the goals.
- Assess energy and nutrient levels required for weight maintenance.
- Assess daily energy expenditure.
- Increase total energy intake, emphasizing high-quality proteins and carbohydrates.
- Incorporate strength training into the exercise regimen.
- Use a recovery mixture (fluid, electrolytes, carbohydrate, and protein) after strength training to promote rehydration, repletion of muscle glycogen, and most importantly, muscle protein synthesis.

Just as it is unrealistic to expect to lose significant amounts of body fat in a short period, gaining weight cannot be accomplished overnight.

Realistic weight gains of 0.5 to 2.0 lb/week (0.2-0.9 kg/week) can be expected based on reasonable increases in energy intake. It is important to document the energy intake, expenditure, and composition of the diet being consumed at the level of weight maintenance. Once these levels have been established, appropriate recommendations for increases in energy intake can be made.

Carbohydrate intake should be maintained at a level appropriate for the sport (~45% to 65% of energy), with fat at 25% to 35% of energy. Protein intake of 12% to 15% (or 1-2 g/kg body weight) should be adequate to assist with lean tissue accretion. "Gaining Muscle Mass: How Much Energy Is Required?" discusses some of the issues associated with making energy recommendations for weight gain. Timing of nutrient intake after exercise is also important. An athlete should aim to consume high-quality protein soon after exercise is over.

For athletes who are already consuming 4000 to 5000 kcal/day, weight gain can be quite challenging. These athletes must consume excess energy even if they feel no hunger. Consuming excess solid food can lead to gastrointestinal distress, and many athletes find that they do not have enough time during the day to eat extra food. For these people, sport supplement drinks or bars between meals and immediately after exercise may increase energy intake to levels sufficient to cause weight gain.

Numerous over-the-counter supplements purport to increase body weight and lean tissue. Chapter 16 describes in detail the use of ergogenic

Highlight

Gaining Muscle Mass: How Much Energy Is Required?

The exact number of kilocalories needed to gain 1 lb of muscle tissue is not known. One pound of muscle is equal to 454 g (~0.45 kg), but muscle tissue contains mostly water (70-75%), with protein, fat, carbohydrate, and minerals constituting the remaining components. Thus, in 1 lb (454 g) of muscle tissue, only approximately 113.5 to 136.2 g (assuming that 25-30% is protein-containing tissue) is actually protein tissue. To gain 1 lb of muscle tissue, which is high in protein, one could suggest an excess intake of 454 to 545 kcal (assuming 4 kcal/g of protein). However, Bouchard and colleagues (1990) have shown that consuming excess energy results in a highly variable thermic effect of food. Thus, it is important to keep in mind that the amount of excess weight one can gain will be influenced by the thermic response to overfeeding. It has been suggested that 8 kcal/g is required to support weight gain in adults (Forbes et al. 1986). Considering all this information, a reasonable recommendation for excess energy intake, necessary to result in gaining 1 lb (or 454 g) of muscle mass, ranges from 1000 to 3500 kcal.

The following is a brief illustration of recommendations for weight gain. The individual who wishes to gain weight is a 25-year-old man. His body weight is 135 lb (61.4 kg) and his height is 67 in. (170.2 cm). He wants to weigh 150 lb (68.2 kg), which means a gain of 15 lb or 6.8 kg. Analysis of this individual's diet and activity records indicates that he requires approximately 3000 kcal/day to maintain his current weight.

According to the recommendations previously mentioned, this person would need to consume an excess of 1000 to 3500 kcal to gain 1 lb of lean tissue. Assuming a gain of 1 lb (454 g) per week, this would translate into consuming an excess of 143 to 500 kcal/day over a 15-week period. He could easily accomplish this level of additional energy intake by consuming 16 fl oz (0.5 L) of 1% or 2% milk (200-240 kcal); one can of a sport supplement drink (360 kcal); or a large bagel, a banana, and 1 tbsp of low-fat peanut butter (420 kcal).

In addition to consuming excess energy, this person could manipulate his energy expenditure to achieve increased FFM. He could perform more strength training and limit endurance exercise to three times a week for 30 min per session (enough to maintain cardiovascular health without burning excessive energy).

aids in sport and includes a review of creatine, a popular weight gain supplement. Other reported weight gain supplements on the market include β-hydroxy-β methylbutyrate (HMB) (Slater and Jenkins 2000; Palisin and Stacy 2005), anabolic steroids and growth hormone (Smurawa and Congeni 2007), and chromium picolinate (Vincent 2003; Pittler et al. 2003). As you recall, earlier in the chapter we discussed dietary supplements marketed for weight loss. One category of weight loss supplements includes those that are purported to change nutrient partitioning by changing the way the body uses either carbohydrate or fat. These products are said to reduce fat storage, increase fat oxidation, or both, thus altering body composition and increasing the proportion of lean tissue to fat mass. For a more complete review of ergogenic aids and methods for weight gain, see the reviews by Juhn (2003) and Rankin (2002).

WEIGHT CONCERNS OF ATHLETES

The casual observer of athletic events sees young, healthy individuals with lean and muscular bodies. Many people not involved in competition give little thought to the rigorous training it takes for an athlete to achieve and maintain the body needed for optimal performance. While it may appear easy for athletes to maintain their lean physiques due to their high levels of training, there are a number of sports in which body weight and percentage of body fat are major concerns. The pressures to achieve and maintain a low body weight and low body fat can lead to unhealthy— and often dangerous—behaviors on the part of athletes.

Lean-Build Sports

Several sports could be classified as "lean-build sports," meaning that a lean build is associated with successful performance (e.g., diving, track and field, dance, swimming, gymnastics, cross-country skiing, and bodybuilding). In addition to increasing the athlete's individual performance, a lean body may facilitate scoring in sports such as diving, gymnastics, and bodybuilding. In diving and gymnastics, judgments about the "look" of an individual are incorporated into performance evaluations; and in bodybuilding, the "look" is the sole criterion within the competition. The weight concerns of athletes in these sports can lead to unhealthy behaviors that threaten not only athletic performance but also the athlete's health.

Consequences of competing in lean-build sports can include the following:

- **Poor eating habits:** Result from concerns about keeping body weight and fat low and from inattention to healthy eating due to heavy training schedules and a busy lifestyle.
- **Increased risk for eating disorders:** Results from a combination of poor eating habits; pressure from self, peers, and coaches to maintain low body weight; and psychosocial stressors within family and social environments.
- **Increased risk for injury:** Results from poor eating habits, disordered eating, failure to take adequate rest periods to allow for recovery, or poor nutritional status.

Muscular injuries and stress fractures in these types of sports have been linked to poor diet, eating disorders, and failure to rest. Stress fractures and increased risk for premature osteoporosis are major concerns for female athletes in these sports (Nattiv et al. 2007; Manore et al. 2007). Chapters 13 and 15 provide more detailed discussions of nutrition, bone health, and eating disorders.

It is widely believed that people for whom physical appearance is a major concern are at higher risk than others for eating disorders. The incidence of disordered eating is higher for female than for male athletes, although the incidence is growing in males (Beals 2004). Depending on the sport, between 15% and 60% of female athletes may employ pathogenic techniques for weight loss (including fasting, self-induced vomiting, laxatives, and diuretics) (Sundgot-Borgen 1993). Among female athletes considered at high risk for eating disorders, the incidence of use of **pathogenic weight loss techniques** can be very high (80%). Athletes who are more likely to use these techniques are those in aesthetic, weight-dependent, and endurance sports (Sundgot-Borgen 1993; Beals and Manore 2002). It is well known that using diuretics and laxatives can lead to cardiac disorders and gastrointestinal damage. Athletes should avoid these products except under medical supervision.

Research with elite gymnasts demonstrates how poor nutrition relates to menstrual dysfunction and increased incidence of eating disorders and injuries. Sundgot-Borgen (1996) compared 12 females (age range 13-20 years) on the Norwegian national rhythmic gymnastics team with an age-matched control group for incidence of eating disorders and menstrual dysfunction. Only one third of the gymnasts had reached menarche, compared with 100% of the controls. Of the athletes who had reached menarche, all reported either irregular menstrual cycles or amenorrhea. Eight of the 12 athletes reported overuse injuries; all were dieting, the primary motivation being improved performance. While both athletes and controls self-defined their ideal weight at a value lower than their present weight, the athletes had much higher scores on the eating disorder inventory. Four of the 12 athletes had either overt or subclinical eating disorders. When the athletes were interviewed regarding their dietary practices, it became apparent that both the athletes and the coaches could benefit from nutritional education. The athletes reported adhering to nutritional myths such as these:

- Never eat after 5 p.m.
- Rhythmic gymnasts need only 800 kcal/day.
- Eat only cold food.
- Do not eat meat, bread, or potatoes.
- Drinking during training will destroy your practice.

Some of the preoccupation with weight and body image may change for female athletes after they discontinue competing. For example, O'Connor and colleagues (1996) found that former college gymnasts (mean age 36.6 ± 3.8 years) were more preoccupied with thinness during their collegiate gymnastics career but were more satisfied with their bodies years later than a nonathletic matched control group. Interestingly, the former gymnasts were leaner and closer to their self-reported ideal body weight after college than the control group.

Bodybuilding has also been associated with many behaviors that could be viewed as unhealthy:

- Consuming low-kilocalorie diets to decrease body weight and fat
- Use of diuretics and practice of extreme fluid restriction to achieve a more "cut" look
- Use of multiple drugs (including anabolic steroids) and heavy consumption of protein and amino acid supplements in an attempt to achieve large, rapid gains of muscle mass

The incidence of amenorrhea in female bodybuilders has been reported to range from 25% to 81%. Unhealthy practices, however, are not necessary for success in bodybuilding. Results of a case study of a drug-free bodybuilder illustrate how one athlete was able to achieve desirable changes in body composition by employing healthy recommendations (see "Weight Loss in a Bodybuilder," p. 196) (Manore et al. 1993).

Sports That Require "Making Weight"

A number of sports require "making weight," or achieving a weight goal within a strictly defined weight class. These sports include horse racing (jockeys), wrestling, boxing, and crew (rowers). Athletes in these sports commonly seek to compete in a weight class lower than their typical body weight to give them an advantage over people who are naturally smaller, to minimize weight that must be carried during an event, or both.

There are two primary concerns about athletes who must make weight:

1. They frequently "weight cycle," that is, engage in repeated cycles of weight loss and weight gain. Some researchers suspect that weight cycling results in a permanent decrease in RMR, which in turn could increase an athlete's risk of becoming overweight and make future attempts at weight loss more difficult. Weight cycling may also increase a person's risk of early mortality.

2. Weight cycling may increase the risk of eating disorders. Sports involving weight cycling are associated with an increased incidence of bingeing and purging behaviors in addition to the abuse of diuretics.

Does the scientific literature support the theories associated with weight cycling?

The well-controlled studies of weight cycling in humans do not show any evidence that weight cycling results in a permanent decrease in RMR (McCargar and Crawford 1992; McCargar et al. 1993, 1996; Wadden et al. 1996). While the RMR of weight-cycling athletes has been shown to decrease during the competitive season, it increases back to preseason levels once the athletes resume normal eating behaviors (Melby et al. 1990). Whether weight cycling can lead to early death is still controversial. Epidemiological studies suggest that people who experience large fluctuations in weight have increased mortality risk (Hamm et al. 1989). Data from the Framingham Study (Ashley and Kannel 1974) suggest that blood pressure declines with weight loss, while weight gain is associated with a disproportionate increase

Highlight

Weight Loss in a Bodybuilder

A unique case of a drug-free world-class bodybuilder illustrates how healthy dietary practices and a rigorous training regimen can achieve favorable changes in body composition. This athlete was following a program designed to maintain FFM and decrease body fat. He performed weight training to maintain FFM and increased his amount of endurance exercise to reduce body fat. He made no attempt to decrease energy intake. He performed 2 h of endurance exercise daily, consisting of 1 h of stationary cycling and 1 h of stair stepping (at ~60% $\dot{V}O_2$max). He performed 3 h of strength training, which included a morning and an evening workout using light, medium, and heavy weight and working all the muscle groups. He followed the dietary regimen shown here over an 8-week precompetition training period. He used medium-chain triglycerides (MCTs) as a supplement. The table below provides the energy and nutrient information for his diet with and without MCTs.

Mean Energy and Nutrient Intakes of a Male Bodybuilder: With and Without Medium-Chain Triglyceride (MCT)

Nutrient intake	Diet without MCT*	Diet + MCT**
Energy (kcal/day)	3674 ± 279	4952 ± 279
Protein (g/day)*	175 ± 17	175 ± 17
% of kcal/day	19	14
g/kg body weight per day	1.9	1.9
Carbohydrate (g/day)	696 ± 63	696 ± 63
% of kcal/day	76	56
g/kg body weight per day	7.5	7.5
Fat (g/day)	22 ± 4	176 ± 4
% of kcal/day	5	30
Cholesterol (mg/day)	182 ± 61	182 ± 61

Data are presented as means and standard deviations (±). *Diet included carbohydrate (CHO)-containing sport beverage (Exceed, Ross Lab., Columbus, OH): 24 to 36 oz/day; 1 oz = 7.1 g CHO and 28.4 kcal. An additional 12.8 g/day of protein was consumed each day in amino acid supplements; thus, protein intake from diet alone was 162 g/day or 1.75 g/kg body weight. **MCT = medium-chain triglyceride: MCT provides 8.3 kcal/g; 1 tbsp (15 mL) weighs 14 g. Mean MCT consumed per day was 154 g, which represented 26% of the energy consumed.

Reprinted, by permission, from M.M. Manore, J.L. Thompson, and M. Russo, 1993, "Diet and exercise strategies of a drug-free world class bodybuilder," *International Journal of Sport and Nutrition* 3: 76-86.

This dietary regimen was self-imposed, not recommended by a nutritionist. Note the minimal use of protein supplements and the use of **medium-chain triglyceride (MCT) supplements** (fatty acids with 6 to 12 carbons) (see chapter 3 for more information on MCTs). This athlete's dietary fat intake was extremely low (5% of total energy), and the MCTs provided energy during training. Medium-chain triglycerides are absorbed directly into the circulation and transported to the liver and are rapidly used for energy, with minimal potential for storage in adipose tissue (Bach and Babayan 1982; Johnson et al. 1990; Swift et al. 1990). This diet and exercise regimen is unique since many bodybuilders report consuming low-energy-dense diets that are high in protein and low in carbohydrate. For more details on this case see the study by Manore and colleagues (1993).

in blood pressure. Thus, weight cycling could lead to hypertension. Renal ischemia has also been reported in weight-cycling wrestlers (Tcheng and Tipton 1973; Zambraski et al. 1976), which could lead to future problems with hypertension. Others argue that these findings are misleading, as only one longitudinal study of obese individuals partici- pating in weight-cycling behaviors has been done, and no adverse effects on RMR, body composition, or body fat distribution were observed (Wadden et al. 1996). In addition, there have been no stud- ies of weight cycling and mortality in athletes. As with individuals participating in lean-build sports, athletes attempting to make weight are at an

---

Detrimental Consequences of Unhealthy Weight Loss Practices in Athletes and Recommendations for Avoiding These Consequences

Detrimental Consequences	Recommendations
• Decreased aerobic and anaerobic performance	• Initiate weight control program well in advance of competitive season.
• Glycogen depletion	• Determine body fat levels so that realistic weight goals can be set.
• Dehydration	• Establish a range of acceptable body fat and weight values, and monitor health and performance within this range.
• Impaired thermoregulation	
• Impaired oxygen and nutrient exchange	
• Impaired buffering capacity	• Determine specific target level for body weight associated with optimal performance.
• Increased loss of fat-free mass	

---

increased risk of eating disorders or of exhibiting disordered eating behaviors. Many of these athletes have very low energy intakes, use diuretics, exercise in extremely warm environments to dehydrate themselves, and even purge themselves to avoid gaining weight after an episode of bingeing. These practices are dangerous to bone health and to fluid and electrolyte balance, and they prove detrimental to athletic performance.

Regardless of the sport in which one participates, rapid and extreme weight loss is associated with many detrimental consequences. A list of negative consequences associated with weight loss in athletes is shown on this page, as is a list of healthy recommendations for athletes concerned with body weight. It is critical for athletes and coaches to understand that there is no single ideal body weight or percentage body fat for an athlete. While many people believe that having a woman decrease her body fat from 14% to 11% will dramatically increase her speed, her performance may actually suffer because of the extreme practices she employs to reach this very low level of body fat. Appendix D provides a table of body fat percentages reported in the literature for a variety of athletes. We have included this table to give coaches, athletes, and sport nutrition professionals an idea of the range of body fat values reported within many sports. Also included in the list are the ranges of body fat percentages reported for amenorrheic female athletes.

CHAPTER IN REVIEW

The incidence of obesity is rising in developed countries, including the United States. Many people in the United States are attempting to lose weight, including both obese and nonobese individuals who view their body weight as unacceptable. How do we determine the optimal, or healthy, body weight for each individual? Optimal body weight should be a weight that can be maintained without constant dieting, one that allows physical activity and promotes healthy eating habits, and one that takes into account genetic history of body weight and shape.

The market is flooded with weight loss programs, and sorting fact from fiction can be difficult. Very low-calorie diets and starvation diets result in rapid weight loss but also can cause dangerous dehydration and loss of body protein. In addition, few people maintain the weight lost on these diets. Safer and less rapid weight loss can be achieved with LCDs and moderately low-kilocalorie diets, especially those of low nutrient density. The key to weight loss and maintenance of optimal body weight is participation in regular physical activity. Athletes can achieve healthy and successful weight loss by avoiding use of pathogenic weight loss techniques, setting appropriate body composition goals, and avoiding weight loss during the competitive season. When the desire is to gain weight, it is important to maximize lean tissue by

1. increasing total energy intake above daily energy expenditure,
2. eating a diet high in energy and adequate in protein and nutrient-dense carbohydrates, and
3. incorporating strength training into the exercise program.

Supplements used for weight gain should be reviewed carefully with a sport dietitian and are no substitute for a healthy diet and exercise program.

Key Concepts

1. Discuss the role of diet and exercise in achieving healthy body weight.

Both diet and exercise play critical roles in achieving healthy body weight. Energy expenditure must be greater than energy intake for weight loss to occur. Sound weight loss programs include consumption of a diet that is adequate in carbohydrate for the sport and level of physical activity. A diet high in nutrient-dense carbohydrates (e.g., whole grains, legumes, beans, and whole fruits and vegetables), adequate protein, and healthy fats should be selected. Regular physical activity, especially strength training, can also help prevent some of the decrease in RMR that occurs with a decrease in energy intake. Maintaining a healthy body weight can decrease the risk of morbidity and mortality from some chronic diseases, such as cardiovascular disease, diabetes, stroke, and certain forms of cancer.

2. Describe the recommendations for maintaining a healthy body weight.

The recommendations for achieving and maintaining a healthy body weight are similar. Keys to success in maintaining a healthy body weight are consuming a moderate- to low-fat, high nutrient-dense carbohydrate diet; performing regular exercise; and making appropriate behavioral modifications related to dietary intake and exercise.

3. Discuss the weight concerns of athletes.

Athletes who compete in lean-build sports such as diving, track and field, dance, swimming, gymnastics, and bodybuilding, as well those needing to make weight (e.g., wrestlers and jockeys), are generally quite concerned about their weight. Unfortunately, this intense concern can lead to increased risk for eating disorders and injuries and can threaten athletes' physical, mental, and emotional health. There is no evidence that weight cycling permanently decreases RMR; however, rapid and extreme weight loss can lead to dehydration, reduced performance, and even death.

4. Define the recommendations for weight gain.

People can achieve weight gain safely by setting realistic goals, increasing energy intake (and emphasizing a high nutrient-dense carbohydrate diet that supplies adequate protein), and incorporating strength training into their exercise regimen. Using sport supplement drinks and bars between meals can help athletes increase energy intake.

Key Terms

3-hydroxyacyl coenzyme A dehydrogenase (HADH) 185

body mass index (BMI) 169

computed tomography (CT) 169

fad diet 180

high-carbohydrate diet 180

ketogenic diet 177

ketosis 177

low-calorie diet (LCD) 177

low-energy-dense diet 179

magnetic resonance imaging (MRI) 169

medium-chain triglyceride (MCT) supplement 196

meta-analysis 182

moderate energy restriction diet 179

obesity 169

overweight 169

pathogenic weight loss technique 194

protein-sparing modified fast (PSMF) 176

starvation diet 176

very low-calorie diet (VLCD) 176

waist circumference 169

Additional Information

Astrup A, Buemann B, Flint A, Raben A. Low-fat diets and energy balance: how does the evidence stand in 2002? Proc Nutr Soc 2002;61:299-309.

This article deals with the question of whether a high-fat diet causes weight gain. The authors performed four meta-analyses to address the question.

Bravata DM, Sanders L, Huang J, Krumholz HM, Olkin I, Gardner CD, Bravata DM. Efficacy and safety of low-carbohydrate diets. A systemic review. JAMA 2003;289(14):1837-1850.

The authors systematically reviewed the literature addressing the efficacy and safety of low-carbohydrate diets used in an outpatient setting. They specifically evaluated the research for changes in weight, serum lipids, fasting serum glucose and fasting serum insulin, and blood pressure.

Eckel RH, Grundy SM, Zimmet PA. The metabolic syndrome. Lancet 2005;365:1415-1428.

An overview of the current research related to metabolic syndrome, including the definition, relationship to diabetes and cardiovascular disease, mechanisms, and management.

Freedman MR, King J, Kennedy E. Popular diets: a scientific review. Obesity Res 2001;9(suppl):1S-40S.

The authors performed an in-depth review of currently popular diets by classifying them into one of three categories: high fat, moderate fat, and low fat. They then compared the diets using specific outcomes (weight loss, body composition, nutritional adequacy, metabolic parameters, hunger, and compliance) using an evidence-based approach.

Romijn JA, Coyle EF, Sidossis LS, Gastaldelli A, Horowitz JF, Endert E, Wolfe RR. Regulation of endogenous fat and carbohydrate metabolism in relation to exercise intensity and duration. Am J Physiol 1993;265(3) Pt 1: E380-391.

Classic study demonstrating the change in energy substrate with different intensities and durations of physical activity.

References

Abourashed EA, El-Alfy AT, Khan IA, Walker L. Ephedra in perspective—a current review. Phytother Res 2003;17(7):703-712.

Ainsworth BE, Haskell WL, Leon AS, Jacobs Jr. DS, Montoye HJ, Sallis JF, Paffenbarger Jr. RS. Compendium of physical activities: classification by energy costs of human physical activities. Med Sci Sports Exerc 1993;25(1):71-80.

Andersen RE, Wadden TA, Bartlett SJ, Zemel B, Verde TJ, Franckowiak SC. Effects of lifestyle activity vs structured aerobic exercise in obese women: a randomized trial. JAMA Jan 27 1999;281(4):335-340.

Ashley FW Jr, Kannel WB. Relation of weight change to changes in atherogenic traits: the Framingham Study. J Chron Dis 1974;27(3):103-114.

Astrup A. The role of dietary fat in the prevention and treatment of obesity. Efficacy and safety of low-fat diets. Int J Obesity Relat Metab Disord 2001;25 suppl 1:S46-50.

Astrup A, Astrup A, Buemann B, Flint A, Raben A. Low-fat diets and energy balance: how does the evidence stand in 2002? Proc Nutr Soc 2002;61(2):299-309.

Atkins RC. Atkins for life. New York: St. Martin's Press, 2003.

Bach AC, Babayan VK. Medium-chain triglycerides: an update. Am J Clin Nutr 1982;36(5):950-962.

Ball K, Brown W, Crawford D. Who does not gain weight? Prevalence and predictors of weight maintenance in young women. Int J Obes Relat Metab Disorders. 2002;26(12):1570-1578.

Ballor DL, Katch VL, Becque MD, Marks CR. Resistance weight training during caloric restriction enhances lean body weight maintenance. Am J Clin Nutr 1988;47:19-25.

Barr SI. Increased dairy product or calcium intake: is body weight or composition affected in humans? J Nutr 2003;133:245S-248S.

Beals KA. Disordered eating among athletes. A comprehensive guide for health professionals. Champaign, IL: Human Kinetics, 2004.

Beals KA, Manore MM. Disorders of the female athlete triad among college athletes. Int J Sport Nutr Exerc Metab 2002;12:281-293.

Bell EA, Rolls BJ. Energy density of foods affects energy intake across multiple levels of fat content in lean and obese women. Am J Clin Nutr 2001;73:1010-1018.

Berkel LA, Poston WS, Reeves RS, Foreyt JP. Behavioral interventions for obesity. J Am Diet Assoc 2005;105(5) suppl 1:S35-43.

Blackburn GL, Lynch ME, Wong SL. The very low-calorie diet: a weight-reduction technique. In: Brownell KD, Foreyt JP eds. Handbook of eating disorders: physiology, psychology, and treatment of obesity, anorexia, and bulimia. New York: Basic Books, 1986;198-212.

Bogardus C, LaGrange BM, Horton ES, Sims EA. Comparison of carbohydrate-containing and carbohydrate-restricted hypocaloric diets in the treatment of obesity. Endurance and metabolic fuel homeostasis during strenuous exercise. J Clin Invest 1981;68(2):399-404.

Bouchard C, Tremblay A, Després JP et al. The response to long-term overfeeding in identical twins. N Engl J Med May 24 1990;322(21):1477-1482.

Bravata DM, Sanders L, Huang J et al. Efficacy and safety of low-carbohydrate diets: a systematic review. JAMA Apr 9 2003;289(14):1837-1850.

Bray GA. Pathophysiology of obesity. Am J Clin Nutr 1992;55:488S-494S.

Bray GA, Gray DS. Obesity. Part II—treatment. West J Med 1988;149(5):555-571.

Broeder CE, Burrhus KA, Svanevik LS, Wilmore JH. The effects of either high-intensity resistance or endurance training on resting metabolic rate. Am J Clin Nutr 1992;55(4):802-810.

Brown WJ, Burton NW, Rowan PJ. Updating the evidence on physical activity and health in women. Am J Prev Med 2007;33(5):404-411.

Cabrera C, Artacho R, Gimenez R. Beneficial effects of green tea—a review. J Am Coll Nutr 2006;25(2):79-99.

Calle EE, Thun MJ, Petrelli JM, Rodriguez C, Heath CW Jr. Body-mass index and mortality in a prospective cohort of U.S. adults. N Engl J Med Oct 7 1999;341(15):1097-1105.

Calorie Control Council. Trends and statistics, 2007. www.caloriecontorl.org/trndstat.html. Accessed Jan 2008.

Centers for Disease Control and Prevention (CDC), National Center for Health Statistics. Prevalence of overweight and obesity among adults: United States, 2003-2004; 2007. http://www.cdc.gov/nchs/data/databriefs/db01.pdf. Accessed Dec 2008.

Crowe TC. Safety of low-carbohydrate diets. Obesity Rev 2005;6:235-245.

Curioni CC, Lourenco PM. Long-term weight loss after diet and exercise: a systematic review. Int J Obesity (Lond) 2005;29(10):1168-1174.

de la Hunty A, Ashwell M. Are people who regularly eat breakfast cereals slimmer than those who don't? A systemic review of the evidence. Nutr Bull 2007;32:118-128.

Donnelly JE, Blair S, Jakicic J, Manore M, Rankin J. ACSM position stand: appropriate intervention strategies for weight loss and prevention of weight regain in adults. Med Sci Sports Exerc 2009;41: 459-471.

Donnelly JE, Jacobsen DJ, Jakicic JM, Whatley JE. Very low calorie diet with concurrent versus delayed and sequential exercise. Int J Obesity 1994;18(7):469-475.

Donnelly JE, Pronk NP, Jacobsen DJ, Pronk SJ, Jakicic JM. Effects of a very-low-calorie diet and physical-training regimens on body composition and resting metabolic rate in obese females. Am J Clin Nutr 1991;54:56-61.

Donnelly JE, Smith B, Jacobsen DJ et al. The role of exercise for weight loss and maintenance. Best Pract Res Clin Gastroenterol Dec 2004;18(6):1009-1029.

Duncan KH, Bacon JA, Weinsier RL. The effects of high and low energy density diets on satiety, energy intake, and eating time of obese and nonobese subjects. Am J Clin Nutr 1983;37(5):763-767.

Dunn AL, Marcus BH, Kampert JB, Garcia ME, Kohl HW 3rd, Blair SN. Comparison of lifestyle and structured interventions to increase physical activity and cardiorespiratory fitness: a randomized trial. JAMA Jan 27 1999;281(4):327-334.

Dwyer JT, Allison DB, Coates PM. Dietary supplements in weight reduction. J Am Diet Assoc 2005;105:S80-S86.

Eckel RH, Grundy SM, Zimmet PZ. The metabolic syndrome. Lancet Apr 16-22 2005;365(9468):1415-1428.

Ello-Martin JA, Ledikwe JH, Rolls BJ. The influence of food portion size and energy density on energy intake: implications for weight maintenance. Am J Clin Nutr 2005;82(suppl):236S-241S.

Ello-Martin JA, Roe LS, Ledikwe JH, Beach AM, Rolls BJ. Dietary energy density in the treatment of obesity: A year-long trial comparing 2 weight-loss diets. Am J Clin Nutr 2007;85:1465-1477.

Epstein LH, Wing RR. Aerobic exercise and weight. Addict Behav 1980;5(4):371-388.

Field AE, Austin SB, Taylor CB, Malspeis S, Rosner B, Rockett HR, Gillman MW, Colditz GA. Relation between dieting and weight change among preadolescents and adolescents. Pediatrics 2003;112:900-906.

Flatt JP. The biochemistry of energy expenditure. In: Bjorntorp P, Brodoff BN eds. Obesity. Philadelphia: Lippincott, 1992;100-116.

Forbes GB, Brown MR, Welle SL, Lipinski BA. Deliberate overfeeding in women and men: energy cost and composition of the weight gain. Br J Nutr 1986;56(1):1-9.

Ford ES, Mokdad AH, Giles WH. Trends in waist circumference among U.S. adults. Obesity Res 2003;11(10);1223-1231.

Foster GD, Wyatt HR, Hill JO et al. A randomized trial of a low-carbohydrate diet for obesity. N Engl J Med May 22 2003;348(21):2082-2090.

Freedman MR, King J, Kennedy E. Popular diets: a scientific review. Obesity Res 2001;9(suppl):1S-40S.

Fugh-Berman A, Myer A. *Citrus aurantium,* an ingredient of dietary supplements marketed for weight loss: current status of clinical and basic research. Exp Biol Med 2004;229:698-704.

Gades MD, Stern JS. Chitosan supplementation and fat absorption in men and women. J Am Diet Assoc 2005;105:72-77.

Gaesser GA. Thinness and weight loss: beneficial or detrimental to longevity? Med Sci Sports Exerc 1999;31(8):1118-1128.

Garrow JS, Summerbell CD. Meta-analysis: effect of exercise, with or without dieting, on the body composition of overweight subjects. Eur J Clin Nutr 1995;49(1):1-10.

Gorin AA, Phelan S, Wing RR, Hill JO. Promoting long-term weight control: does dieting consistency matter? Int J Obesity Relat Metab Disord 2004;28(2):278-281.

Grundy SM. Drug therapy of the metabolic syndrome: minimizing the emerging crisis in polypharmacy. Nature Rev 2006;5:295-309.

Haller CA, Jacob P 3rd, Benowitz NL. Enhanced stimulant and metabolic effects of combined ephedrine and caffeine. Clin Pharmacol Ther 2004;75(4):259-273.

Hamm P, Shekelle RB, Stamler J. Large fluctuations in body weight during young adulthood and twenty-five-year risk of coronary death in men. Am J Epidemiol 1989;129(2):312-318.

Heaney RP. Normalizing calcium intake: projected population effects for body weight. J Nutr 2003;133(1):268S-270S.

Heymsfield SB, Allison DB, Vasselli JR, Pietrobelli A, Greenfield D, Nunez C. Garcinia cambogia (hydroxycitric acid) as a potential antiobesity agent. JAMA 1998;280(18):1596-1600.

Heymsfield SB, Casper K, Hearn J, Guy D. Rate of weight loss during underfeeding: relation to level of physical activity. Metabolism 1989;38(3):215-223.

Hill JO, Thompson H, Wyatt H. Weight maintenance: what's missing? J Am Diet Assoc 2005;105(5) suppl 1:S63-66.

Hill JO, Wing R. The National Weight Control Registry. Permanente J 2003;7(3):34-37.

Hollenbeck CB, Coulston AM, Quan R, Becker TR, Vreman HJ, Stevenson D, Reaven GM. Effects of a commercial starch blocker preparation on carbohydrate digestion and absorption: in vivo and vitro studies. Am J Clin Nutr 1983;38(4):498-503.

Institute of Medicine, Food and Nutrition Board. Dietary reference intakes for energy, carbohydrate, fiber, fat, fatty acids, cholesterol, protein, and amino acids. Washington, DC: National Academy Press, 2005.

Jakicic JM, Clark K, Coleman E, Donnelly JE, Foreyt J, Melanson E, Volek J, Volpe SL. Position stand. Appropriate intervention strategies for weight loss and prevention of weight regain for adults. Med Sci Sports Med 2001;22(12):2145-2156.

Johnson RC, Young SK, Cotter R, Lin L, Rowe WB. Medium-chain-triglyceride lipid emulsion: metabolism and tissue distribution. Am J Clin Nutr 1990;52(3):502-508.

Juhn M. Popular sports supplements and ergogenic aids. Sports Med 2003;33(12):921-939.

Karlic H, Lohninger A. Supplementation of L-carnitine in athletes: Does it make sense? Nutrition 2004;20:709-715.

Keim NL, Barbieri TF, Van Loan MD, Anderson BL. Energy expenditure and physical performance in overweight women: response to training with and without caloric restriction. Metabolism Jun 1990;39(6):651-658.

Klein S, Allison DB, Heymsfield SB, Kelley DE, Leibel RL, Nonas C, Kahn R. Waist circumference and cardiometabolic risk: a consensus statement from Shaping America's Health: Association for Weight Management and Obesity Prevention; NAASO, the Obesity Society; the American Society of Nutrition; and the American Diabetes Association. Am J Clin Nutr 2007;85:1197-1202.

Klem ML, Wing RR, Lang W, McGuire MT, Hill JO. Does weight loss maintenance become easier over time? Obesity Res 2000;8(6):438-444.

Klem ML, Wing RR, McGuire MT, Seagle HM, Hill JO. A descriptive study of individuals successful at long-term maintenance of substantial weight loss. Am J Clin Nutr 1997;66(2):239-246.

Kovacs EMR, Westerterp-Plantenga MS, Saris WHM. The effects of 2-week ingestion of (-)-hydroxycitrate and (-)-hydroxycitrate combined with medium-chain triglycerides on satiety, fat oxidation, energy expenditure and body weight. Int J Obesity 2001;25:1087-1094.

LaMonte MJ, Blair SN. Physical activity, cardiorespiratory fitness, and adiposity: contributions to disease risk. Curr Opin Clin Nutr Metab Care 2006;9(5):540-546.

Larsen TM, Toubro S, Astrup A. Efficacy and safety of dietary supplements containing CLA for the treatment of obesity: evidence from animal and human studies. J Lipid Res 2003;44:2234-2241.

Ledikwe JH, Blanck HM, Khan LK, Serdula MK, Seymour JD, Tohill BC, Rolls BJ. Dietary energy density is associated with energy intake and weight status in US adults. Am J Clin Nutr 2006;83:1362-1368.

Lee CD, Blair SN, Jackson AS. Cardiorespiratory fitness, body composition, and all-cause and cardiovascular disease mortality in men. Am J Clin Nutr 1999;69(3):373-380.

Lissner L, Levitsky DA, Strupp BJ, Kalkwarf HJ, Roe DA. Dietary fat and the regulation of energy intake in human subjects. Am J Clin Nutr 1987;46:886-892.

Manore MM. Keeping the weight off: how can you maintain your weight loss after the diet is over? ACSM's Health Fit J 2004;8(3):23-24.

Manore MM, Kam LC, Loucks AB. The female athlete triad: components, nutrition issues and health consequences. J Sports Sci 2007;25(S2):S61-S71.

Manore MM, Thompson JL. Body weight regulation and energy needs. In: Wolinsky I, Driskell JA, eds. Sports Nutrition: Energy Metabolism and Exercise. Boca Raton, FL: CRC Press 2008; 241-260.

Manore MM, Thompson JL, Russo M. Diet and exercise strategies of a drug-free world class bodybuilder. Int J Sport Nutr 1993;3:76-86.

Manson JE, Willett WC, Stampfer MJ et al. Body weight and mortality among women. N Engl J Med Sep 14 1995;333(11):677-685.

Mattes R. Fluid calories and energy balance: the good, the bad, and the uncertain. Physiol Behav 2006;89:66-70.

Mattes RD, Bormann L. Effects of (-)-hydroxycitric acid on appetitive variables. Physiol Behav 2000;71(1-2):87-94.

McCargar LJ, Crawford SM. Metabolic and anthropometric changes with weight cycling in wrestlers. Med Sci Sports Exerc 1992;24(11):1270-1275.

McCargar LJ, Sale J, Crawford SM. Chronic dieting does not result in a sustained reduction in resting metabolic rate in overweight owmen. J Am Diet Assoc. 1996;96(11):1175-1177.

McCargar L, Taunton J, Birmingham CL, Pare S, Simmons D. Metabolic and anthropometric changes in female weight cyclers and controls over a 1-year period. J Am Diet Assoc 1993;93(9):1025-1030.

McCracken M, Jiles R, Blanck HM. Health behaviors in the young adult US population: behavioral risk factor surveillance system, 2003. Preventing chronic disease. Web journal from the Centers for Disease Control and Prevention, Apr 2007. www.cdc.gov/pcd/issues/2007/apr/06_0090.htm.

McGuire MT, Wing RR, Klem ML, Seagle HM, Hill JO. Long-term maintenance of weight loss: do people who lose weight through various weight loss methods use different behaviors to maintain their weight? Int J Obesity Relat Metab Disord 1998;22(6):572-577.

Melby CL, Schmidt WD, Corrigan D. Resting metabolic rate in weight-cycling collegiate wrestlers compared with physically active, noncycling control subjects. Am J Clin Nutr 1990;52(3):409-414.

Mhurchu CN, Dunshea-Mooij C, Bennet D, Rodgers A. Effect of chitosan on weight loss in overweight and obese individuals: a systemic review of randomized control trials. Obesity Rev 2005;6:35-42.

National Adolescent Student Health Survey. The national adolescent student health survey: a report on the health of America's youth. Oakland, CA: Third Party, 1989. Reported by CDC: www.cdc.gov/mmwr/preview/mmwrhtml/00001362.htm. Accessed Aug 2008.

National Heart, Lung and Blood Institute (NHLBI). Clinical guidelines on the identification, evaluation, and treatment of overweight and obesity in adults. The evidence report. National Institutes of Health, U.S. Department of Health and Human Services, Jun 1998. www.nhlbi.nih.gov/guidelines/obesity/index.htm. Accessed Aug 2008.

National Heart, Lung and Blood Institute (NHLBI). The practical guide. Identification, evaluation, and treatment of overweight and obesity in adults. National Institutes of Health, U.S. Department of Health and Human Services, NIH pub. no. 02-4084, Jan 2002. www.nhlbi.nih.gov/guidelines/obesity/practgde.htm. Accessed Aug 2008.

Nattiv A, Loucks AB, Manore MM, Sanborn CF, Sundgot-Borgen J, Warren M. American College of Sports Medicine position stand. The female athlete triad. Med Sci Sports Exerc 2007;39(10):1867-1882.

Niakaris K, Magkos F, Geladas N, Sidossis LS. Insulin sensitivity derived from oral glucose tolerance testing in athletes: disagreement between available indices. J Sports Sci 2005;23(10):1065-1073.

Nutrition Business Journal. Sports nutrition and weight-loss. VI, Sep 2006;1-12.

O'Connor PJ, Lewis RD, Kirchner EM, Cook DB. Eating disorder symptoms in former female college gymnasts: relations with body composition. Am J Clin Nutr 1996;64(6):840-843.

Ogden CL, Carroll MD, Curtin LR, McDowell MA, Tabak CJ, Flegal KM. Prevalence of overweight and obesity in the United States, 1999-2004. JAMA 2006;295(13):1549-1555.

Palisin T, Stacy JJ. Beta-hydroxy-beta-methylbutyrate and its use in athletes. Curr Sports Med Rep 2005;4(4):220-223.

Pasman WJ, Saris WHM, Westerterp-Plantenga MS. Predictors of weight maintenance. Obesity Res 1999;7(1):43-50.

Phelan S, Roberts M, Lang W, Wing RR. Empirical evaluation of physical activity recommendations for weight control in women. Med Sci Sports Exerc 2007;39(10):1832-1836.

Phelan S, Wyatt HR, Hill JO, Wing RR. Are the eating and exercise habits of successful weight losers changing? Obesity 2006;14(4):710-716.

Phinney SD. Ketogenic diets and physical performance. Nutr Metab 2004;1:2. doi:10.1186/1743-7075-1-2. www.nutrition-andmetabolism.com/content/1/1/2.

Pittler MH, Ernst E. Guar gum for body weight reduction: meta-analysis of randomized trials. Am J Med 2001;110:724-730.

Pittler MH, Ernst E. Dietary supplements for body-weight reduction: a systemic review. Am J Clin Nutr 2004;79:529-536.

Pittler MH, Schmidt K, Ernst E. Adverse events of herbal food supplements for body weight reduction: systemic review. Obesity Rev 2005;6:93-111.

Pittler MH, Stevinson C, Ernst E. Chromium picolinate for reducing body weight: meta-analysis of randomized trials. Int J Obesity 2003;27:522-529.

Rader DJ. Effect of insulin resistance, dyslipidemia, and intra-abdominal adiposity on the development of cardiovascular disease and diabetes mellitus. Am J Med 2007;120(3A):S12-S18.

Rajpathak SN, Rimm EB, Rosner B, Willett WC, Hu FB. Calcium and dairy intakes in relation to long-term weight gain in US men. Am J Clin Nutr 2006;83(3):559-566.

Rankin JW. Weight loss and gain in athletes. Curr Sports Med Rep Aug 2002;1(4):208-213.

Raynor DA, Phelan S, Hill JO, Wing RR. Television viewing and long-term weight maintenance: results from the National Weight Control Registry. Obesity (Silver Spring) Oct 2006;14(10):1816-1824.

Reaven GM. Syndrome X: 6 years later. J Intern Med Suppl 1994;736:13-22.

Reaven GM. The individual components of the metabolic syndrome: is there a raison d'etre? J Am Coll Nutr 2007;26(3):191-195.

Rolls BJ, Barnett RA. The volumetrics weight-control plan: feel full on fewer calories. New York: HarperCollins, 2000.

Rolls BJ, Roe LS, Meengs JS. Salad and satiety: energy density and protion size of a first-course salad affect energy intake at lunch. J Am Diet Assoc 2004;104: 1570-1576.

Rolls BJ, Drewnowski A, Ledikwe JH. Changing the energy density of the diet as a strategy for weight management. J Am Diet Assoc 2005;105:S98-S103.

Rolls BJ, Roe LS, Meengs JS. Reduction in portion size and energy density of foods are additive and lead to sustained decreases in energy intake. Am J Clin Nutr 2006;83:11-17.

Romijn JA, Coyle EF, Sidossis LS, Gastaldelli A, Horowitz JF, Endert E, Wolfe RR. Regulation of endogenous fat and carbohydrate metabolism in relation to exercise intensity and duration. Am J Physiol 1993;265(3) Pt 1:E380-391.

Ross R, Dagnone D, Jones PJ et al. Reduction in obesity and related comorbid conditions after diet-induced weight loss or exercise-induced weight loss in men. A randomized, controlled trial. Ann Intern Med Jul 18 2000;133(2):92-103.

Saltzman E. Obesity as a health issue. In: Bowman BA, Russell RM eds. Present knowledge in nutrition, 9th ed., vol. II. Washington, DC: ILSI Press, 2006;637-648.

Saper RB, Eisenberg DM, Phillips RS. Common dietary supplements for weight loss. Am Fam Physician 2004;70:1731-1738.

Schutz Y, Flatt JP, Jequier E. Failure of dietary fat intake to promote fat oxidation: a factor favoring the development of obesity. Am J Clin Nutr 1989;50:307-314.

Shaw K, Gennat H, O'Rourke P, Del Mar C. Exercise for overweight or obesity. Cochrane Database Syst Rev 2006;(4):CD003817.

Shekelle FG, Hardy ML, Morton SC et al. Efficacy and safety of ephedra and ephedrine for weight loss and athletic performance. A meta-analysis. JAMA 2003;289(12):1537-1545.

Shick SM, Wing RR, Klem ML, McGuire MT, Hill JO, Seagle H. Persons successful at long-term weight loss and maintenance continue to consume a low-energy, low-fat diet. J Am Diet Assoc 1998;98(4):408-413.

Slater GJ, Jenkins D. Beta-hydroxy-beta-methylbutyrate (HMB) supplementation and the promotion of muscle growth and strength. Sports Med 2000;30(2):105-116.

Smurawa TM, Congeni JA. Testosterone precursors: use and abuse in pediatric athletes. Pediatr Clin North Am 2007;54(4):787-796, xii.

Soni MG, Carabin IG, Griffiths JC, Burdock GA. Safety of ephedra: lessons learned. Toxicol Lett Apr 15 2004;150(1):97-110.

Stiegler P, Cunliffe A. The role of diet and exercise for the maintenance of fat-free mass and resting metabolic rate during weight loss. Sports Med 2006;36(3):239-262.

Strauss RS, Mir HM. Smoking and weight loss attempts in overweight and normal-weight adolescents. Int J Obesity 2001;25:1381-1385.

Sundgot-Borgen J. Prevalence of eating disorders in elite female athletes. Int J Sport Nutr 1993;3:29-40.

Sundgot-Borgen J. Eating disorders, energy intake, training volume, and menstrual function in high-level modern rhythmic gymnasts. Int J Sport Nutr 1996;6(2):100-109.

Svendsen OL, Hassager C, Christiansen C. Effect of an energy-restrictive diet, with or without exercise, on lean tissue mass, resting metabolic rate, and cardiovascular risk factors, and bone in overweight postmenopausal women. Am J Med 1993;95:131-140.

Swift LL, Hill JO, Peters JC, Greene HL. Medium-chain fatty acids: evidence of incorporation into chylomicron triglycerides in humans. Am J Clin Nutr 1990;52:834-836.

Tangney CC, Gustashaw KA, Stefan TM, Sullivan C, Ventrelle J, Filipowski CA, Heffernan AD, Hankins J. A review: which dietary plan is best for your patients seeking weight loss and sustained weight management? Dis Mon 2005;51:284-326.

Tcheng TK, Tipton CM. Iowa wrestling study: anthropometric measurements and the prediction of a "minimal" body weight for high school wrestlers. Med Sci Sports 1973 Spring;5(1):1-10.

Teegarden D. Calcium intake and reduction of weight or fat mass. J Nutr 2003;122:249S-251S.

Thomas PR. Dietary supplements for weight loss? Nutr Today 2004;40(1):6-16.

Thompson JL, Gylfadottir UK, Moynihan S, Jensen CD, Butterfield GE. Effects of diet and exercise on energy expenditure in postmenopausal women. Am J Clin Nutr 1997;66:867-873.

Thompson JL, Manore MM, Thomas JR. Effects of diet and diet-plus-exercise programs on resting metabolic rate: a meta-analysis. Int J Sport Nutr 1996;6:41-61.

Tremblay A, Fontaine E, Poehlman ET, Mitchell D, Perron L, Bouchard C. The effect of exercise-training on resting metabolic rate in lean and moderately obese individuals. Int J Obesity 1986;10:511-517.

Tremblay A, Plourde G, Després J-P, Bouchard C. Impact of dietary fat content and fat oxidation on energy intake in humans. Am J Clin Nutr 1989;49:799-805.

Tremblay A, Simoneau JA, Bouchard C. Impact of exercise intensity on body fatness and skeletal muscle metabolism. Metabolism 1994;43(7):814-818.

Tsai AG, Wadden TA. The evolution of very-low-calorie diets: An update and meta-analysis. Obesity 2006;24(8):1283-1293.

U.S. Food and Drug Administration (FDA). Sales of supplements containing ephedrine alkaloids (ephedra) prohibited, 2004. www.fda.gov/oc/initiatives/ephedra/february2004/. Accessed Jan 2008.

U.S. Food and Drug Administration (FDA). FDA statement on tenth circuit's ruling to uphold FDA decision banning dietary supplements containing ephedrine alkaloids, 2006. www.fda.gov/bbs/topics/NEWS/2006/NEW01434.html. Accessed Jan 2008.

van Dale D, Beckers E, Schoffelen PFM, ten Hoor F, Saris WHM. Changes in sleeping metabolic rate and glucose induced thermogenesis during a diet or a diet/exercise treatment. Nutr Res 1990;10:615-626.

Van Itallie TB. Health implications of overweight and obesity in the United States. Ann Intern Med 1985;103:983-988.

Van Itallie TB. Body weight, morbidity, and longevity. In: Bjorntorp B, Brodoff BN eds. Obesity. Philadelphia: Lippincott, 1992.

Van Itallie TB, Yang M-U. Cardiac dysfunction in obese dieters: a potentially lethal complication of rapid, massive weight loss. Am J Clin Nutr 1984;39:695-702.

Villani RG, Gannon J, Self M, Rich PA. L-Carnitine supplementation combined with aerobic training does not promote weight loss in moderately obese women. Int J Sport Nutr Exerc Metab 2000;10:199-207.

Vincent JB. The potential value and toxicity of chromium picolinate as a nutritional supplement, weight loss agent and muscle development agent. Sports Med 2003;33(3):213-230.

Volek JS, VanHeest JL, Forsythe CE. Diet and exercise for weight loss. A review of current issues. Sports Med 2005;35(1):1-9.

Wadden TA, Foster GD, Stunkard AJ, Conill AM. Effects of weight cycling on the resting energy expenditure and body composition of obese women. Int J Eating Dis 1996;19:5-12.

Wei M, Macera CA, Hornung CA, Blair SN. Changes in lipids associated with changes in regular exercise in free-living men. J Clin Epidemiol 1997;50:1137-1142.

Westman EC, Feinman RD, Mavropoulos JC, Vernon MC, Volek JS, Wortman JA, Yancy WS, Phinney SD. Low-carbohydrate nutrition and metabolism. Am J Clin Nutr 2007;86:276-284.

Whigham LD, Watras AC, Schoeller DA. Efficacy of conjugated linoleic acid for reducing fat mass: a meta-analysis in humans. Am J Clin Nutr 2007;85:1203-1211.

Willett WC, Dietz WH, Colditz GA. Guidelines for healthy weight. New Engl J Med 1999;341:427-434.

Williams PT, Thompson PD. Dose-dependent effects of training and detraining on weight in 6406 runners during 7.4 years. Obesity 2006;24(11):1975-1984.

Woo R, Garrow JS, Pi-Sunyer FX. Voluntary food intake during prolonged exercise in obese women. Am J Clin Nutr 1982;36:478-484.

Wyatt HR, Grunwald GK, Mosca CL, Klem ML, Wing RR, Hill JO. Long-term weight loss and breakfast in subjects in the National Weight Control Registry. Obesity Res 2002;10(2):78-82.

Zambraski EJ, Foster DT, Gross PM, Tipton CM. Iowa wrestling study: weight loss and urinary profile of collegiate wrestlers. Med Sci Sports 1976;8:105-108.

Zemel MG. Role of calcium and dairy products in energy partitioning and weight management. Am J Clin Nutr 2004;79(suppl):907S-912S.

CHAPTER 7

Body Composition

Chapter Objectives

After reading this chapter you should be able to

- understand the relationship between body composition and health,
- describe the relationship between body composition and sport performance,
- compare body composition assessment models and methods,
- understand the accuracy of body composition assessment measurements,
- identify selection criteria for field methods for estimating body composition,
- discuss body composition status of athletes, and
- explain the relationship between body composition standards and health.

What is the ideal level of body fat? How do my weight and body fat levels affect my athletic performance or health? What is the best way to measure body composition? These are questions frequently asked by athletes and fitness enthusiasts. Understanding how body composition relates to health and athletic performance and how to accurately and reliably measure body composition can help you answer these questions.

Although a scale can accurately measure body weight, weight alone provides no information about the body's composition. For example, a male bodybuilder or football player may weigh more for his height than standard weight tables recommend simply because he is very muscular and not because he has excess body fat. Measuring body composition provides information on the absolute and relative amounts of the components that make up the human body. Direct measurement of body composition in living humans is not feasible, since it requires the dissection and chemical analysis of the body. Scientists have therefore developed various models and methods for indirect estimation of body components.

This chapter briefly summarizes the relationships among body composition, health, and sport performance; reviews the strengths and limitations of body composition assessment models and methods; and presents guidelines for making and interpreting body composition measurements.

BODY COMPOSITION AND HEALTH

The human body contains more than 30 major components at the elemental (atomic), molecular, cellular, and tissue-system levels (Wang et al. 1992). Chemical components of body composition that can be estimated include relative **fat mass (FM), fat-free mass (FFM)**, and the major components of FFM—water, mineral, and protein. Although FM is the component of body composition most often assessed, FFM and its components have an equal, if not more important, relationship to health and athletic performance. Fat-free mass includes the organs, soft tissues, and skeletal tissues. Low levels of FFM and loss of FFM are related to impaired functional capacity and decreased energy expenditure for physical activity and thus lead to increased risk for gain of FM. Muscle wasting that occurs with certain diseases and with aging not only decreases muscle strength and the capacity to perform even routine activities, but also is strongly related to mortality (Going and Davis 1998). Low bone mineral mass and density are key predictors of osteoporotic fracture risk (Heaney 1999).

BODY COMPOSITION AND SPORT PERFORMANCE

Although various researchers have reported ranges of relative body fat (%BF) for successful athletes within specific sports, body composition by itself cannot accurately predict athletic performance. All the components of physique—body size, structure, and composition—are significant determinants of athletic success. Each is related to performance in a logical and predictable way. More massive individuals, for example, have an advantage over their lighter counterparts when an activity demands that the inertia of another

body or an external object be overcome (e.g., tackling a runner in football). People with less body mass have the advantage when the goal is to move the body, especially over moderate to long distances (e.g., marathon run). Taller people, with longer levers (limbs) and a higher center of gravity, have the advantage in jumping and throwing events (e.g., javelin throw or long jump), whereas shorter persons have the advantage when the body must be rotated around an axis (e.g., diving and tumbling).

Fat Mass and Performance

There generally appears to be an inverse relationship between FM and performance of physical activities requiring movement of the body either vertically (as in jumping) or horizontally (as in running) (Boileau and Lohman 1977; Malina 1992; Pate et al. 1989). Excess fatness is detrimental to these types of activities because it adds non-force–producing mass to the body. Since acceleration is proportional to force but inversely proportional to mass, excess fat at a given level of force can result in slower changes in velocity and direction (Boileau and Lohman 1977; Harman and Frykman 1992). Excess fat also increases the metabolic cost of physical activities requiring movement of the total body mass (Buskirk and Taylor 1957). In most activities involving movement of the body mass, therefore, a relatively low %BF should be advantageous both mechanically and metabolically (Boileau and Lohman 1977).

Cross-sectional data indicate that %BF is inversely related both to aerobic capacity ($\dot{V}O_2$max) expressed relative to body weight and to distance running performance (Cureton 1992). Only a few experimental studies have addressed the effects of altered body composition on physical performance. Running performance of fit, normal-weight people in these studies decreased with increasing weight added by a weight belt and shoulder harness (Cureton and Sparling 1980; Cureton et al. 1978; Sparling and Cureton 1983). Their performances were similar to those of obese individuals with similar FFM but greater body weight.

In contrast, in some sports for which absorbing force or momentum is important (such as contact sports), adequate amounts of appropriately distributed FM are advantageous. Long-distance swimmers also benefit from a relatively high FM compared to other athletic groups because of the role fat plays in thermal insulation and its contribution to buoyancy (Sinning 1985).

Highlight: Body Fat and Health

There is a strong association between excess body fat—especially excess intra-abdominal (visceral) fat—and increased risk of coronary artery disease, non-insulin-dependent diabetes, hypertension, and certain types of cancers (Going and Davis 1998). This means that obese people with android, or central body, fat distribution (apple shape), who store excess fat in their trunk region, are at greater risk for certain diseases than those with a gynoid fat distribution in which excess fat is stored in the hips and thighs (pear shape) (see figure 7.1).

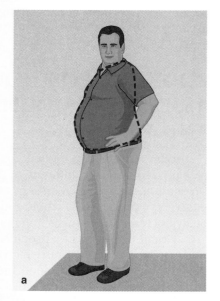
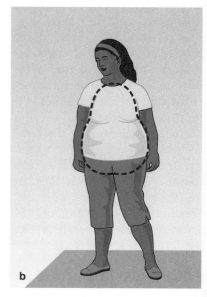

Figure 7.1 *(a)* Upper body (android) and *(b)* lower body (gynoid) obesity.

Reprinted, by permission, from J.H. Wilmore, D.L. Costill, and W.L. Kenney, 2008, *Physiology of sport and exercise*, 4th ed. (Champaign, IL: Human Kinetics), 504.

The ratio between waist circumference and hip circumference has often been used as an index of the distribution of adipose tissue. An elevated waist:hip ratio (WHR) is usually considered an indication of proportionally more abdominal adipose tissue and is associated with an increased risk for some cardiovascular diseases and diabetes. The usefulness of WHR as an indicator of relative adipose tissue distribution has been established in adults but not in children and youth (Malina 2005). More recent research has established that waist circumference (WC) measurements alone can help predict abdominal and nonabdominal fat as well as overall obesity-related health risk (Janssen et al. 2004, 2002). Among adults, it has been suggested that higher WC measurements are related to health risk in a graded fashion (Janssen et al. 2004). The ease of measuring WC makes it a practical tool for assessing health risk; and its predictive value, especially for heart disease, may be improved when coupled with a person's body mass index measurement (i.e., the ratio of a person's weight to his or her height) (Zhu et al. 2002). Additional research is needed to separate effects of fat distribution from those of total body fat and to assess fat distribution as an independent factor for health risks. See chapter 6 for more information related to body fat and health.

Fat-Free Mass and Performance

Performance of activities that require application of force, particularly against external objects (e.g., throwing, pushing, and weightlifting), is positively related to the absolute amount of FFM and therefore to body size (Boileau and Lohman 1977; Harman and Frykman 1992). On the other hand, a large absolute amount of FFM and large body size can negatively affect performance that requires translocation of body weight—such as running, jumping, or rotation of the body about an axis (as in gymnastics or diving). It is obvious that an elite gymnast would not perform well as an offensive lineman in football and vice versa.

The best positive correlations of physical performance in military-related physical tasks are with FFM rather than %BF. In investigations of the relationship of body composition to performance of military tasks, FFM was the best predictor of performance as assessed by maximal aerobic capacity; treadmill run time; 12 min run distance; and the ability to push, carry, and exert torque (Harman and Frykman 1992). For most sports, high FFM:FM ratios at a given body weight are associated with better performance, although too little body fat results in deterioration of both health and performance (Houtkooper 1998; Sinning 1985; Wilmore 1992).

Problems of Extreme Leanness

Athletes in sports such as gymnastics, dancing, diving, bodybuilding, distance running, and track are typically very lean. They follow rigorous training programs and often restrict their dietary intake in order to control their weight. Male athletes who have the lowest levels of FM are in sports for which participants must make weight (e.g., wrestling, boxing, horse racing, lightweight rowing, or football). The potential advantage of a low %BF for successful performance in these types of sports is evident. However, there are negative health and performance implications related to extreme weight loss (Sinning 1996). Minimal levels of %BF considered compatible with good health are 5% for males and 12% for females (Lohman 1992a).

Athletes whose weight drops below a certain desirable level are likely to experience decreases in performance and increases in both minor and major illnesses and injuries (Sinning 1996; Wilmore 1992). Severe weight cutting, secondary to severe short-term starvation and dehydration, can reduce isometric and dynamic strength; over the long term, it can contribute to abnormal kidney function (Sinning 1985).

Athletes who constantly strive to reach or maintain an inappropriate weight or %BF are at risk for developing eating disorders. At the elite or world-class level of several sports, the prevalence of eating disorders in females is estimated to be between 1% and 62% (Beals 2004). Female athletes prone to eating disorders are also at high risk of developing a triad of interrelated disorders that includes anorexia nervosa or bulimia nervosa, menstrual dysfunction, and bone demineralization (Houtkooper 1998; Wilmore 1992; Beals 2004). This triad of disorders is termed the Female Athlete Triad and is discussed in more detail in chapter 15. Eating disorders occur among male athletes as well, with a prevalence estimated between 0% and 57% (Beals 2004).

BODY COMPOSITION ASSESSMENT MODELS AND METHODS

Methods of assessing body composition can be categorized as direct, indirect, or double indirect. **Direct methods** such as dissection and chemical analysis of tissues or of whole cadavers are obviously not feasible for living humans. However, they are critical because they provide the basic data that are the foundation from which indirect assessment techniques are developed. **Indirect methods** can be based on either properties or components (Heymsfield et al. 2005). **Property-based methods** measure specific properties such as body volume, decay properties of specific atomic isotopes, or bioelectrical resistance. For example, neutron activation analysis of living humans (Ellis 2005) has made possible nondestructive chemical analysis of the human body via measurement of radiation given off during decay of excited atoms. A more common property-based method is estimation of **total body water (TBW)** from deuterium dilution, which involves measuring the dilution in the body of a known dose of deuterium isotope using a sample of body fluid.

Component-based methods depend on well-established models that usually represent ratios of measurable quantities of body components that are assumed constant both within and between individuals. With component-based methods, the measured quantity of one component is first estimated by a property-based method, and then another body component is estimated using a body composition model. For example, FFM can be estimated using deuterium dilution to measure the TBW component—the observed TBW value is

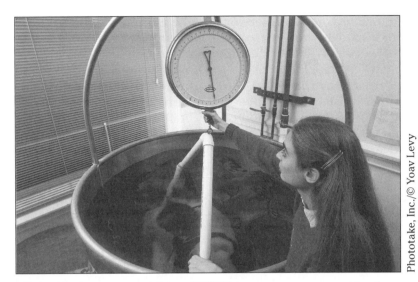

Phototake, Inc./© Yoav Levy

Figure 7.2 Underwater weighing (UWW) is a two-component body composition model (FFM and FM) that uses the principle of densitometry. It is considered one of the criterion methods for body composition assessment.

converted to FFM based on the assumed constant relationship between TBW and FFM. Since this ratio in healthy adults is about 0.74 (74% of FFM is TBW), FFM = TBW × 1.35 (Brozek et al 1963). While it is known that the ratio is higher in children and youths, studies to determine values in aging adults are equivocal, with some showing that it increases slightly with age and others showing no significant increase (Baumgartner 2005).

Two types of mathematical functions are used to estimate body composition with property- and component-based methods (Going and Davis 1998). The **model approach,** which depends on a known ratio between a specific constituent and the component of interest, was illustrated in the preceding paragraph. In the other approach, **regression analysis** of experimental data provides a prediction equation that relates a measured property or component to an "unknown" (estimated) component. Usually, the prediction equation is developed via measurement of the unknown component using a reference method in a defined group of subjects. For example, you can use **densitometry (underwater weighing)** as a reference method to measure body volume (see figure 7.2) and a weight scale to measure body mass on land; then you calculate body density using the simple equation body density = mass / volume. The property of a known component related to body composition is also measured in these same subjects. For example, the known component can be skinfold thicknesses. Regression analysis then provides equations relating the known component (in this case skinfold thicknesses) to the unknown component (body density). This approach has yielded equations for estimating body fat from skinfolds, circumferences, or bioelectrical resistance. Because they generally depend on a combination of property-based and component-based methods and are then used to estimate an unknown component, these assessment methods are considered "doubly indirect."

Two-Component Models and Methods

The two-component chemical model has been the primary model used to study the relationship between body composition and physical performance. This model divides the body into FM and FFM. Fat is a molecular-level chemical component, not to be confused with fat cells or adipose tissue, which are cellular and tissue-system components of body composition. The terms fat and lipid are often confused and inappropriately interchanged (Heymsfield and Wang 1993). Fat refers to the family of chemical compounds called triacylglycerols (triglycerides), whereas lipid is the more general term that includes triacylglycerols and many other compounds (Gurr and Harwood 1991). In the two-component chemical model, the fat component historically has included all lipids; all other body constituents are included in the FFM. The FM is the weight of all the lipids in the body that can be chemically extracted using ether as the solvent. Fat-free mass is the weight of all tissues in the body minus the FM. In more complex three- or four-component chemical models, the FFM is subdivided into its major constituents—water, mineral, and protein (Boileau and Lohman 1977).

This two-component model is based on the assumptions that FFM and FM each have a constant density and a constant composition of constituents for all individuals in a given population (Siri 1961). The density of adult human fat is relatively constant within and among individuals at 0.900 g/cm³ (Lohman 1986). Considerable data demonstrate that the density and composition of FFM are not constant in growing children, and studies are in progress to assess changes in FFM in adults during aging. Chemical maturity of FFM in humans (i.e., chemical stability in the constituents of FFM) does not occur until after puberty (Lohman 1986, 1989). A person is considered to be **chemically mature** when FFM composition reaches the reference values for a chemically mature adult male: 73.8% water, 6.8% mineral, and 19.4% protein, with a density of 1.100 g/cm³ (Brozek et al. 1963). This usually happens between 16 and 18 years of age, with girls maturing earlier than boys (Lohman et al. 1984). Prepubescent and pubescent children deviate considerably from adults in FFM composition and density—generally having relatively higher water content and lower mineral and protein contents, which together result in an FFM density lower than the 1.100 g/cm³ of chemically mature adults (Boileau et al. 1984; Hewitt et al. 1993; Lohman 1986).

Multiple-Component Body Composition Criterion Models and Methods

In theory, the more constituents of the FFM (water, mineral, protein) that can be accurately measured,

the more accurate the FFM and FM estimates. This theory has been the basis for development of multiple-component "criterion" methods for estimating body composition in youths. Such methods, which are considered the "gold standard" of methods, are referred to as **criterion methods** because they provide more accurate estimates of body composition—especially of chemically immature youths—than those based on two-component models (Lohman 1992a; Siri 1961). (See "Criterion Methods of Assessing Body Composition".)

Multiple-component models minimize potential errors in estimates of %BF associated with variability in FFM composition. Historically, the ideal laboratory procedure combined measures of **whole-body density (D_b)** with measures of body water and bone mineral to estimate body composition using an equation based on a four-component model. This approach eliminates the need for assumptions about the proportions of FFM constituents and provides the best estimate of body composition against which to validate field methods of body composition assessment.

Alternatively, D_b can be combined with measures of body water or bone mineral, and equations based on three-component models can be derived. Although more accurate than the two-component equations, these equations assume a constant protein:mineral ratio or protein:water ratio—and individual deviations from the assumed ratios introduce error, although less than in the two-component model.

A concern about multicomponent models has been the increased potential for measurement error when individual components of the FFM are measured. Several investigators have assessed the extent to which measurement errors for individual techniques in the multicomponent model

Highlight

Criterion Methods of Assessing Body Composition

There are many different ways to assess body composition. Those methods that to date are considered the most accurate are called "criterion methods" or "gold standard" methods. Since the measurement of body composition can involve different models (two-, three-, and four-component models), each model has its own criterion method(s). For example, densitometry (underwater weighing) is considered a criterion method for the two-component model of assessing body composition. Thus, it has been used as the criterion method to develop another two-component model of assessing body composition, the skinfold method.

are passed on (propagated) in the assessment of body composition (Friedl et al. 1992; Fuller et al. 1992; Lohman 1992a). The data suggest that the improved accuracy of three-component and four-component models is not compromised by errors arising from individual techniques if measurements are carefully made.

Validation of Body Composition Assessment Methods

A new or existing method is considered valid if it provides an estimate of body composition that is close to the value obtained using a criterion method (described previously) and if the estimate is reproducible (Lohman 1992a). The relative *accuracy* of the method being tested is determined by the size of the prediction error (standard error of the estimate, or root-mean-square error). *Reliability* (also referred to as *precision*) is assessed by the magnitude of the standard deviation for repeated measurements, or magnitude of the coefficient of variation for the measurements.

Cross-validation is the final aspect of validating a new or existing assessment method. In the cross-validation process, the assessment method being evaluated is used to estimate body composition in an independent group to determine how closely the method predicts body composition compared to the criterion method. An indepen-

dent group ideally comprises a new, representative sample of individuals. In the most rigorous cross-validation studies, the tests are done in a laboratory run by investigators other than the ones who conducted the original validation study but using the same techniques as employed in the original study. Alternative cross-validation studies are conducted in the same laboratory that developed the new method or equation, using either a separate sample of subjects or the subjects in the original study but with statistical adjustments. The body composition assessment method being tested is considered accurate and reliable or precise if the results of the cross-validation study indicate that the prediction errors and reliability estimates for the body composition variables are within acceptable ranges. A later section of this chapter presents the criteria for acceptable ranges of prediction errors.

Criterion Methods of Body Composition Assessment

The most widely applied criterion methods or gold standard methods of measuring body composition are densitometry, dual-energy X-ray absorptiometry (see figure 7.3), computed tomography, and magnetic resonance imaging. In the past, hydrometry and ^{40}K spectroscopy were used more extensively as criterion methods for measuring

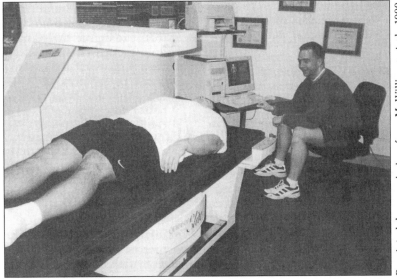

Reprinted, by permission, from M. Williams et al., 1999, *Creatine: The power supplement* (Champaign, IL: Human Kinetics).

Figure 7.3 Dual-energy X-ray absorptiometry (DXA) is a three-component body composition model (FFM, FM, and bone mineral). It is considered one of the criterion methods for body composition assessment.

body composition, but these have been replaced by new methodologies. Each of these methods has been described in detail by others and will be briefly reviewed in this chapter (Brozek et al. 1963; Ellis 2005; Going 1996; Lohman 1986, Lohman and Chen 2005; Lukaski 1987; Ross and Janssen 2005; Siri 1961).

Densitometry The densitometry approach to body composition assessment is based on the relationship between whole-body density (D_b) and the respective densities of the body compartments, regardless of how they are defined. The general principle is that D_b varies inversely with FM:

$$F = f\,(1/D_b) \qquad (7.1)$$

where F is the ether-extractable lipid fraction of body mass (FM), and f is the function describing the relationship between FM and D_b.

To derive simple, useful solutions of equation 7.1, one must assume that the densities of the two compartments (FM and FFM) are constant. Siri's well-known equation for predicting %BF (Siri 1961) represents the simplest solution of equation 7.1. In these equations, %BF is calculated from D_b, and fat and fat-free constituents, respectively, are assumed to have densities of 0.900 g/cm³ and 1.100 g/cm³:

$$1/D_b = F/d_F + FFM/d_{FFM} \qquad (7.2)$$

where $1/D_b$ is body mass; D_b is whole-body density; and F/d_F and FFM/d_{FFM} are the fractions of body mass that are fat and fat-free divided by their respective densities (Brozek et al. 1963; Fidanza et al. 1953).

In the simplest chemical model, FFM comprises primarily water (W), protein (P), and mineral (M) components, and d_{FFM} is derived from the proportions of W, P, and M divided by constant values for their densities (Lohman 1992a; Siri 1956, 1961):

$$d_{FFM} = W/d_W + P/d_P + M/d_M. \qquad (7.3)$$

Thus, for d_{FFM} to be constant, the proportions of W, P, and M must be constant—or they must vary in such a way that d_{FFM} does not change.

In the adult two-component densitometric approach, any deviation of D_b from the d_{FFM} of 1.100 g/cm³ is assumed to be due to the addition of body fat. Thus, %BF may be overestimated in people with lower than average bone mineral mass and underestimated in people with more than average bone mass. These errors in the densitometric criterion method for fat estimation are then passed on to other body composition assessment methods when they are validated against this two-component criterion method.

When densitometry is used for assessment of body composition, underwater weighing is typically used to measure body volume, and D_b is then estimated using the following equation:

$$D_b = BM\,/\,V \qquad (7.4)$$

where D_b is whole-body density, BM is body mass (weight) measured on a scale, and V is body volume.

The usefulness of densitometry as a criterion method for children is limited because of the changes in relative water and bone mineral content of FFM that occur during growth and development. These differences between children and adults result in overestimation of body fatness in children when %BF estimates are made using adult two-component models (e.g., the Siri [1961] and Brozek [1963] equations). These equations can be problematic for estimating %BF in adults—they can be even more invalid for younger youth and those who mature very late. The Siri equation is

$$\%BF = \left[\frac{4.95}{D_b} - 4.50\right]100 \qquad (7.5)$$

where D_b is whole-body density. This equation was derived from the following equation, using the density constants of 1.100 g/cm³ for d_{FFM} and 0.900 g/cm³ for d_{FM}.

Siri (1961) has published the complete derivation of equation 7.6.

$$\%BF = \left[\frac{1}{D_b}\left(\frac{d_{FFM}d_{FM}}{d_{FFM} - d_{FM}}\right) - \frac{d_{FM}}{d_{FFM} - d_{FM}}\right]100 \qquad (7.6)$$

In youths, %BF can be estimated more accurately from measured D_b using modified versions of the Siri equation, which are derived from estimates of FFM composition in youths at different ages. In the same way that the Siri equation was derived based on the adult reference male constants for fractions and densities of components of FFM and FM, Lohman (1989) derived equations for youths for predicting %BF from D_b, using constants based on average measured values for fractions of the water and mineral components of FFM. The result was a set of average FFM density values for boys and girls in nine age groups. For example, the equation for 9- to 11-year-old boys is

$$\%BF = \left[\frac{5.30}{D_b} - 4.89\right]100. \qquad (7.7)$$

The terms in this equation came from solving equation 7.6, substituting 1.084 for d_{FFM} (the average FFM density for 9- to 11-year-old boys), and using 0.900 g/cm³ for d_{FM} (the same density of the

FM for adults). Using Lohman's (1989) gender- and age-specific constants instead of the constants in the Siri equation (equation 7.5) permits one to use D_b (measured via underwater weighing or skinfolds) to estimate %BF values for youths more accurately than is possible with the Siri equation.

There are limitations to this approach because values for youths of the same gender differ to some extent from the average measured water and mineral fraction of the FFM. These deviations lead to increased errors in %BF estimation when these gender- and age group–specific average values for constants are used in prediction equations (Lohman 1989, 1992b). Unfortunately, there has been no systematic attempt to define these constants in different ethnic groups of physically active youths or older adults, and estimation of %BF from density can be confounded by variability in FFM composition and density in youths and adults. A better description of these parameters in different groups of youths, adults, and older adults, including athletes, is an important focus for future research.

Hydrodensitometry and Air Displacement Plethysmography Hydrodensitometry (HD) and **air displacement plethysmography (ADP)** are methods of measuring body size. They are based on the same principle, displacement—of air for ADP and of water (Archimedes' principle) for HD—to measure body volume. Comprehensive reviews of the basic principles behind measuring body composition with ADP and HD have been previously published (Fields et al. 2002; Going 2005). Hydrodensitometry was long considered the gold standard in body composition assessment, but with newer and more advanced multicomponent techniques, this status has changed. When performed correctly, HD can estimate %BF within approximately 2% error (Going 2005). It is limited for use in all populations because the procedure requires submersion of the body under water and measurement of the residual lung volume. Each error of 100 mL for measured residual lung volume can translate into a %BF estimation error of 0.7%. Errors of 100 to 200 mL and 300 to 400 mL are not uncommon when residual lung volume is measured on land or is estimated, respectively (Going 2005).

Air displacement plethysmography is a newer technique that is used to measure body composition by means of a specially designed closed vessel commercially known as the Bod Pod (figure 7.4). The Bod Pod has two chambers; the subject sits in one, and the other is a reference chamber.

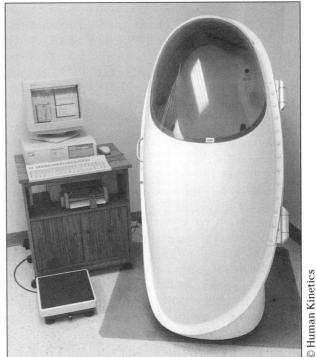

Figure 7.4 The Bod Pod.

© Human Kinetics

Once a person is seated in the vessel, chamber air pressure changes can be measured. These changes in air pressure allow for calculations of body volume that can be translated into measurements of body composition (Ballard et al. 2004).

The authors of a review paper concluded that ADP measures percent body fat for children and youth within 1% to 2% of the %BF measurements made by reference methods such as HD or **dual-energy X-ray absorptiometry (DXA)** (Fields et al. 2002). Further research has shown that the accuracy of ADP may not be as high as previously reported and that ADP may overestimate percent body fat in lean females and in males as weight increases (Ball 2004; Vescovi et al. 2002).

The accuracy of ADP for measuring body composition in athletes varies among athletic groups. Among female collegiate athletes, ADP was found to overestimate percent body fat by 8% when compared with underwater weighing (Vescovi et al. 2002). This overestimation increased in very lean female athletes (Vescovi et al. 2002). Conversely, in a separate sample of collegiate female athletes and nonathletes, no difference was found between %BF estimates from ADP and DXA (Ballard et al. 2004). Differences in reference measures could explain these conflicting results. Among male Division I football players, ADP was found to underestimate %BF when compared with HD (Collins et al. 1999). In contrast, among male collegiate wrestlers, no significant difference was found between %BF measurements from ADP and HD in both euhydrated and dehydrated athletes (Utter et al. 2003). Since ADP is a fairly new body composition assessment methodology, determining its accuracy in various types of athletes, particularly by sport and gender, will require more research.

Anthropometry—Skinfolds Many prediction equations have been developed for estimating whole-body density (D_b) from relatively simple anthropometric measurements such as skinfolds. Although these skinfold-based prediction equations may give accurate estimates of D_b, substantial errors in the estimation of body composition values can occur when D_b is converted to %BF using prediction equations based on adult two-component models such as the Siri or Brozek equations. An alternative approach is to directly predict %BF using skinfold equations developed specifically for the group or individual you are measuring, employing a multicomponent approach (Lohman 1989; Heyward and Wagner 2004. Accuracy of skinfolds for estimating body composition has improved because newer, more accurate techniques for measuring body composition (i.e., computed tomography) can now be used as standards for creating and validating skinfold equations (Wang et al. 2000). Heyward and Wagner (2004) have provided "decision trees" (tables that summarize published research regarding appropriate methods and equations for body composition assessment based on a person's age, ethnicity, gender, level of body fatness, and sport) to help one quickly locate the most appropriate skinfold equations for estimating body composition in different populations.

Computed Tomography and Magnetic Resonance Imaging Computed tomography (CT) and magnetic resonance imaging (MRI) are considered the most accurate assessment methodologies to date for directly measuring body composition (Ross and Janssen 2005). Both procedures also have high reproducibility. The principles behind measuring body composition with CT and MRI image analyses have been described in detail elsewhere (Ross and Janssen 2005). In general, CT produces cross-sectional scans of the body. The CT scan has an X-ray tube and receiver that rotate around a person's body. The tube sends X rays that attenuate through body tissues, producing data that can then be applied to algorithms to create images that help determine body composition (Ross and Janssen 2005; New Fitness 2005).

Magnetic resonance imaging measures body composition by utilizing a magnetic field. The magnetic field "excites" water and fat molecules in the body, producing a measurable signal that is used to create cross-sectional images; these can then be analyzed for body composition assessment. A whole-body analysis using MRI takes as little as 30 min to complete (Ross and Janssen 2005; New Fitness 2005). Both MRI and CT are noninvasive, but they require high levels of technical skill and have high equipment costs; and CT also requires exposure to radiation. Computed tomography and MRI have been used to measure adipose tissue (particularly abdominal adipose tissue for assessment of its relationship with obesity and other health risks) and skeletal muscle in infants through the elderly and in people with diabetes, multiple sclerosis, HIV, and AIDS (Ross and Janssen 2005). To date, neither method has been assessed in relation to estimation of body composition in athletic populations. Interestingly, CT scans have been shown to provide valuable quantitative data on skeletal muscle composition, particularly adipose tissue distribution, which in an athletic population may prove useful for evaluating how intramuscular levels of fat hinder or benefit athletic performance, especially endurance performance (Goodpaster et al. 2000; Bruns and van der Vusse 1998). Magnetic resonance imaging is quickly emerging as an accurate, noninvasive method for measuring skeletal muscle composition and therefore has potential for assessing body composition in relation to strength and performance in athletic populations (Ross et al. 2000).

Dual-Energy X-Ray Absorptiometry Measurement of body composition using dual-energy X-ray absorptiometry (DXA) is based on differential attenuation by body tissues of two low-dose X rays of differing energy levels transmitted through the body, which allows for assessment of regional and total bone mineral content as well as regional and total fat and fat-free content of soft body tissues (Lohman and Chen 2005). Dual X-ray absorptiometry is safe to use in all populations and age groups, with the exception of pregnant women because of the involvement of radiation. A pregnancy test is required for all women of childbearing age before a DXA scan is conducted. The radiation exposure from a total body DXA scan is less than the radiation dose a person would be exposed to during a transcontinental airline flight. Special software to account for hydration of lean tissue has been created for use in measurement of infants, and other software for measurement in children has also been created (Lohman and Chen 2005). Precision of whole-body fat assessment using DXA, in general, is between 1% and 3% (Lohman and Chen 2005), and recently this technique has been shown to have good reproducibility (Kiebzak 2000). The accuracy of DXA to measure changes in body composition during weight loss may be limited. Recent research demonstrated that compared with CT, DXA underestimated changes in lean soft tissue mass while overestimating changes in FM in overweight adults who were actively losing weight (Tylavsky et al. 2003). While CT may be more accurate in estimating body composition, DXA is more practical because it is less expensive and involves a much lower exposure to radiation; therefore more research comparing these two methods and creating adjustment factors to improve accuracy of estimation is warranted.

A few researchers have compared DXA as measure of body composition in athletes with other methodologies. In one study of 43 well-trained adult male athletes, DXA provided significantly higher estimates of %BF compared with skinfolds and bioelectrical impedance analysis (De Lorenzo et al. 2000). In another study, DXA estimates of %BF in professional male soccer players were slightly higher (12.2 ± 3.1 vs. 9.5 ± 4.9) than estimates from skinfolds in other elite male soccer players (Wittch et al. 2001). Since the assumptions underlying skinfold and bioelectrical impedance analysis methods (assuming constant density of FM and FFM) may not be valid in athletic populations due to changes in water and bone mineral content of FFM in athletes, the three-component model provided by DXA may be a more accurate assessment technique (De Lorenzo et al. 2000).

Hydrometry and Spectroscopy In some research and clinical situations, hydrometry and ^{40}K spectroscopy have been the criterion methods used to measure body composition. The validity of both methods depends largely on the appropriateness of the identified conversion constants for the individual to which they are applied. One can estimate FFM via hydrometry by first estimating TBW using isotopically labeled water dilution techniques. Fat-free mass is then calculated from TBW on the basis of the average hydration of FFM, which is assumed to be about 73.8% in the chemically mature reference adult male (Brozek et al. 1963). Once TBW is known, one can calculate FFM using the equation FFM = TBW / (Constant for water fraction of FFM). For example, in adults the equation is FFM = TBW / 0.738.

Since the average relative hydration of FFM in children is higher than in adults, use of the adult constant for the fraction of water in the FFM (73.8%) leads to underestimates of FFM and overestimates of %BF in children. Clearly, the predicted %BF values for youths using hydrometry are more accurate if prediction equations are based on data from youths rather than adults (Lohman 1989). For example, the average values for the water fraction of FFM range from 77% at 7 to 10 years of age to 74% for youths 15 to 17 years old.

Fat-free mass can also be calculated from total body potassium (TBK), which is measured using ^{40}K spectroscopy (Forbes 1987). Once TBK is determined, FFM is calculated from the average concentration of potassium (K) in FFM. In adult males, with TBK expressed in grams, FFM = TBK / 2.66 g K/kg FFM; and in adult females, FFM = TBK / 2.55 g K/kg FFM (Forbes 1987). Total body potassium concentration constants for girls and boys, respectively, ranged from 2.32 to 2.40 g K/kg FFM at 7 to 9 years of age to 2.40 to 2.61 g K/kg FFM at 15 to 17 years (Forbes 1987).

Field Methods of Body Composition Assessment

Field methods are relatively simple techniques for estimating body composition. The techniques are validated and cross-validated using one or more criterion methods. Field methods include anthropometry, bioelectrical impedance, and near-infrared reactance. The anthropometric measures of height, weight, and body mass index have been the most common means of evaluating relative body weight (Deurenberg et al. 1991; Guo et al. 1994; Lohman 1992a; Bellisari and Roche 2005). Skinfolds and circumferences, along with bioelectrical impedance, have been used to assess body composition and fat distribution (Guo et al. 1989; Kaplowitz et al. 1989; Houtkooper et al. 1996; Lohman 1992a; Malina 2005; Mueller and Kaplowitz 1994; Thorland et al. 1983). More recently, handheld or segmental bioelectrical impedance has been used as a method of assessing body composition (Chumlea and Sun 2005).

Anthropometry Body mass index (BMI) is less accurate than skinfolds for assessing %BF (Lohman 1992a) because body weight (the numerator) is influenced by the weight of muscle, organs, and bones as well as FM in the body. A person with a large musculoskeletal system in relation to height can have a high-percentile BMI without having a high %BF level. Conversely, people with a small musculoskeletal mass relative to height can have a low-percentile BMI even if their %BF is not extremely low.

Interpreting BMI across age ranges in children is particularly difficult because growth of the musculoskeletal system is adding weight relative to height as well as fat weight. For example, the 50th percentile for BMI in boys changes from 15.4 at 6 years of age to 21.5 in 17-year-olds—but the sum of two skinfolds (triceps plus subscapular) increases on average only from 12 mm to 15 mm (Lohman 1992a).

Anthropometric measurements, including skinfold thicknesses, bone dimensions, and limb circumferences, can be used in equations to directly predict %BF or to predict D_b, which in turn can be used to estimate %BF (Lohman 1992a; Bellisari and Roche 2005). The skinfold method is the most commonly used anthropometric method for estimating %BF (figure 7.5). It is based on the assumptions (1) that the thickness of the subcutaneous adipose tissue reflects a constant proportion of the total FM and (2) that the sites selected for measurement represent the average thickness of the subcutaneous adipose tissue (Lukaski 1987).

Accurate estimation of %BF from skinfolds depends on several factors. A key factor is the selection of a prediction equation appropriate for the individual being assessed. The skinfold sites used in the prediction equation should reflect the expected location of most subcutaneous fat deposits for the individual. It is also important to use the same type of skinfold caliper that was used to develop the prediction equation because different calipers yield systematic differences in skinfold thickness measurements (Heyward and Wagner 2004). Additionally, variations between people in thickness of skin can affect the validity of a skinfold measurement (Bellisari and Roche 2005). Finally, it is critical to measure accurately the same skinfold sites that were used in developing the prediction equation (Lohman 1992a). It is also important to acknowledge that the significant increases in overweight and obesity in America and other countries over the past few decades may limit the applicability of prediction equations developed many decades ago (Bellisari and Roche 2005).

The preferred skinfold prediction equations are those used to estimate %BF directly from anthropometric measurements and those that have been validated using three- or four-component criterion models. Unfortunately, few such equations have been published and cross-validated for youths (Janz et al. 1993; Slaughter et al. 1988). Heyward and Wagner (2004) provide "decision trees" for selecting the most appropriate skinfold equation for different populations.

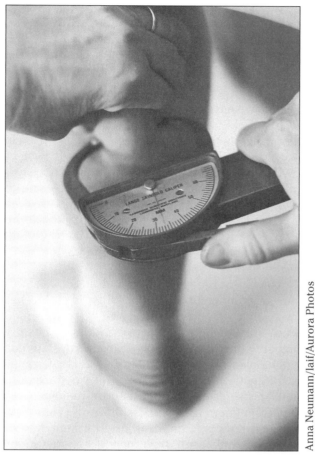

Figure 7.5 Skinfold measurements are an example of a field method of body composition assessment.

One can also track changes in body fat by measuring skinfold thicknesses without conversion to %BF. Careful measurement of skinfolds at specific body sites at regular intervals can indicate if the thicknesses of subcutaneous body fat are changing. A limitation of this technique in children and youths is that skinfold thicknesses increase with normal growth, independent of changes in relative body fatness.

Bioelectrical Impedance Bioelectrical impedance analysis (BIA) is based on the relationship between the volume of a conductor (in this case the body), the conductor's length (an individual's height in this case), and its impedance (i.e., the resistance to the flow of an electric current) (Chumlea and Sun 2005). Whole-body impedance measurements can be made with an individual lying flat on a nonconducting surface (figure 7.6). With electrodes attached to specific sites on the wrist and ankle of the right side of the body, a technician measures resistance while passing a low-dose, single-frequency current through the person's body. Fat-free mass is estimated using a prediction equation that includes measurements of both impedance and height squared as well as other variables including body weight and age. Validity of BIA values is significantly compromised if measurements are not made using standard technique and if appropriate prediction equations are not used (Houtkooper et al. 1996). Standard technique includes having the subject recline on a nonconducting surface, restricting the subject's food intake 3 to 4 h prior to measurements, ensuring the subject's normal hydration status, and placing electrodes at standard locations.

One can improve the accuracy of FFM prediction equations derived from BIA by using population-specific equations that have been validated and cross-validated with multicomponent criterion methods (Houtkooper et al. 1996; Lohman 1992a). Heyward and Wagner (2004) provide "decision trees" for selecting the most appropriate BIA equations for different populations. Overall, the validity of BIA can be affected by hydration status as well as the body itself (i.e., limb shape, body size) (Chumlea and Sun 2005). Both of these are key considerations in the assessment of body composition in athletes. Research has indicated that BIA and equations derived from anthropometric measurements do not accurately estimate %BF in bodybuilders and other power athletes (Huygens et al. 2002).

Bioelectrical impedance analysis devices that measure regional impedance in either the upper or lower body only, and then translate these measurements into estimation of whole-body composition, are gaining popularity in body composition assessment due to their simplicity and the portability of their design (see figure 7.7). Unfortunately, current models have been shown to both under- and overestimate %BF when compared with the traditional full-body BIA or other reference methodology (i.e., DXA, ADP) (Lukaski and Siders 2003; Gartner et al. 2004). Additionally, upper and lower body BIA measurement devices have been shown to give significantly different body composition values within the same person. Possible reasons for these discrepancies could be that direct contact from the foot (lower body device) is more consistent than contact from the handgrip (upper body device) since the handgrip depends upon consistent squeezing throughout measurement (Lukaski and Siders 2003). Three separate segmental BIA analyzers that varied by frequency (single vs. multi-) and number of tactile electrodes (four vs. eight) were evaluated in a recent study. Two of the analyzers measured both leg-to-hand electrical frequencies to estimate whole-body composition (the devices are similar to scales with handles). Results showed that the segmental BIA analyzer with eight tactile electrodes estimated %BF in highest agreement with

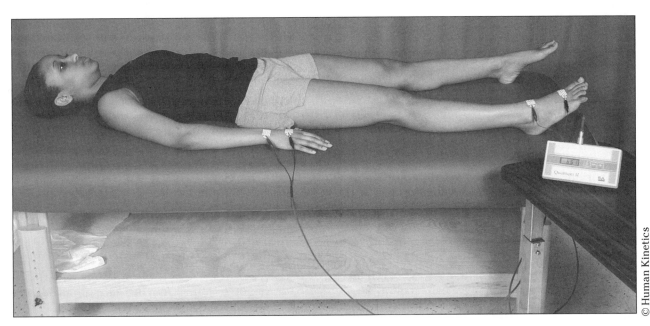

© Human Kinetics

Figure 7.6 Bioelectrical impedance (BIA) is a field method for assessing body composition. Impedance measurements are made while a person lies flat on a nonconducting surface; electrodes are attached to specific sites on the wrist and ankle.

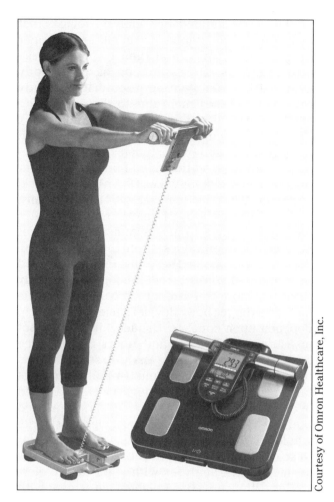

Courtesy of Omron Healthcare, Inc.

Figure 7.7 Bioelectrical impedance analysis.

the reference method, DXA (Demura et al. 2004). The future of segmental BIA analyzers is bright; and as the accuracy of segmental BIA analyzers improves, their role in estimating body composition, especially in nonclinical settings, will likely increase.

Near-Infrared Reactance Near-infrared reactance (NIR) is based on the principles of light absorption and reflection. A fiber optic probe positioned at midbiceps emits an infrared light beam; the beam penetrates subcutaneous fat and muscle, is reflected off the bone, and is finally conducted to the probe's optical detector. Limited validation research with youths and adults has been conducted using this method. Research has shown that NIR overestimates %BF in male athletic and nonathletic children and adolescents and should not be used until new, population-specific equations are developed and validated (Housh et al. 2004). More well-designed studies are needed to validate and cross-validate this technique in

order to determine whether it can accurately and reliably estimate body composition in youths and adults (Cassady et al. 1993; Heyward and Wagner 2004).

ACCURACY OF BODY COMPOSITION ASSESSMENT METHODS

The size of errors from prediction equations represents a compounding of errors from variations in FFM composition and from the measurement errors within criterion and field methods. For example, when D_b is estimated from skinfolds, the total prediction error includes (1) deviations of the individual's body water and minerals from the standards assumed in the criterion model and (2) the technical errors in measuring skinfolds. Additional errors are possible if the measured skinfold sites are not representative of the subject's fat distribution and if the ratio of external to internal fat is different from that of the group in which the equation was developed. One can minimize the magnitude of errors by selecting a prediction equation developed and cross-validated using an appropriate multicomponent criterion model for the group whose body composition is being estimated, and by carefully following standardized techniques when making all measurements.

It is possible to determine %BF or FFM with sufficient accuracy to monitor exercise-induced changes in body composition that are larger than prediction errors for the assessment method. Using D_b as the criterion variable for determining FFM, Lohman (1992a) published guidelines for evaluating the magnitude of the standard errors of estimates in young adult men and women. Prediction errors (standard errors of estimate [SEE]) for FFM of 4.4 to 7.7 lb (2.0-3.5 kg) for men and 4.0 to 6.2 lb (1.8-2.8 kg) for women are rated from ideal to good. Standard errors of estimate between 2.0% and 3.5% are rated as ideal to good for %BF.

With carefully applied skinfold or bioelectrical impedance measurements, one can estimate %BF with an error of approximately 3% and estimate FFM with an error of 5.5 lb (2.5 kg) (Lohman 1992a; Lukaski 1987). This means that if %BF is actually 15%, predicted values may be as high as 18% or as low as 12%; and if the actual FFM value is 66 lb (30 kg), predicted values could range from 60.5 to 71.5 lb (27.5-32.5 kg). With inappropriate prediction equations and poor measurement technique, prediction errors will be much larger.

If you are recommending body composition goals to a client, always consider the potential errors in the data you are using. Recommend a range of goals for %BF or FFM rather than a single value. If a client's body composition falls at the low or high end of the recommended %BF range, perform additional assessments in order to confirm the %BF values by more than one method.

SELECTION CRITERIA FOR FIELD METHODS

Skinfolds and BIA provide similar estimates of %BF that can be within 3% to 4% of criterion values, *if* the measurements are made using established techniques and the appropriate prediction equations are used. Obtaining accurate and reliable skinfold measurements requires more skill than measuring bioelectrical impedance—but the cost of equipment for BIA is much greater than for skinfold measurements. The choice of whether to use skinfolds or BIA depends in part on available funds and available expertise, including the potential cost of training to develop adequate technical skills for measuring skinfolds.

Several authors have recommended equations for estimating body composition using anthropometry and BIA (Heyward and Wagner 2004; Houtkooper and Going 1994; Lohman 1992a) and have also summarized the reasons for selecting these equations (Going and Davis 1998; Heyward and Wagner 2004). Heyward and Wagner's (2004) "decision trees" simplify the selection of equations for different field methods as well as for people of different gender, age, ethnicity, and activity level.

BODY COMPOSITION OF ATHLETES

Athletes often want to know their "ideal" body weight or "ideal" body composition for peak performance—implying the existence of some "universal," optimal combination of body FM and FFM. There is no such thing. It is difficult even to define ideal *relative* FM or FFM for a particular athlete in a specific sport since all aspects of physique, plus many other factors, contribute to successful performance. Recommendations for athletes' body weight and body composition are usually based on average %BF and FFM values obtained from representative athletes in a given sport (Sinning 1985; Wilmore 1992). In other words, they are best guesses within a reasonable range.

Table 7.1 summarizes reported %BF values of elite female and male athletes in various sports (Going and Mullins 2001; Modlesky and Lewis 2000).

Few data have been published on the body composition of athletes less than 18 years of age. Malina and Bouchard (1991) and Fleck (1983) reported %BF values for young athletes and nonathletes based on two-component densitometric estimates. The data indicated that young athletes have lower %BF levels than nonathletes of the same age and gender. These studies included swimmers, runners, gymnasts, football players, and wrestlers. The range of %BF was 13% to 23% for girls and 4% to 15% for boys. Remember always to consider errors inherent in the measurement methods when you interpret such values. Overall, the key determinant of an individual athlete's most desirable body composition is the body composition at which she or he performs best.

BODY COMPOSITION STANDARDS AND HEALTH

There are no accepted %BF standards for all ages (Going and Davis 1998). Most body composition studies use small groups of volunteers who are usually healthy young adults. These studies have shown that body fat levels typically range between 10% and 20% for men and between 20% and 30% for women. Based on these studies, past recommendations for desirable levels of body fat have been 15% for men and 25% for women (Lohman et al. 1997). These standards represent no more than the average percent fat values for relatively small samples of young, healthy adults; their usefulness in other age groups has not been established.

Adult Standards

In the National Health and Nutrition Examination Survey (NHANES III), BIA measurements were performed on a large representative sample of 15,903 U.S. men and women 12 to 80 years of age (Chumlea et al. 2002). The previous methodology for developing body fatness standards had used skinfolds (NHANES II). Standard whole-body BIA prediction equations for males and females were used to estimate FM and FFM for participants (Chumlea et al. 2002). Mean %BF values for American males and females in different age groups and varying ethnicities are presented in table 7.2. The values do not serve as standards or ideal values, but instead reflect average body composition measurements for American adults

Table 7.1 Reported Ranges of Body Mass and % Body Fat (%BF) of Female and Male Athletes From Various Sports

Sport	Body mass(kg)	%BF
Females		
Ballet	48-60	12-22
Basketball	60-74	15-24
Cross-country skiing	56	16
Cycling	61	15
Distance running	47-57	14–21
Field events (throwing)	60-102	19 35
Gymnastics	53-55	17-18
Soccer	60-62	20-22
Softball	54-65	14-24
Sprinting and hurdling	46-62	7-15
Swimming	53-64	16-19
Tennis	55-64	20-24
Triathlon	55-56	13-17
Volleyball	65-76	14-22
Males		
Basketball	80-95	7-14
Canoeing	76-80	10–12
Cross-country skiing	73	8
Cycling	67-71	8–9
Distance running	60-64	1–8
Football (defensive back)	80-90	5-14
Football (defensive line)	107-127	13-24
Football (offensive back)	82-99	5-13
Football (offensive line)	106-119	12-19
Football (quarterback)	79-101	8-21
Gymnastics	62-70	4-9
Rowing	71-82	9-15
Soccer	73-77	9-12
Sprinting and hurdling	66-68	3-14
Swimming	72-79	9-12
Tennis	67-81	6-17
Triathlon	65-82	7-18
Volleyball	66-90	7-13

Adapted from S.B. Going and V. Mullins, 2001, Body composition of the endurance performer. In *Endurance in sport* (IOC Encyclopedia, Vol. II), edited by R. J. Shephard (Oxford, UK: Blackwell Science), 2:346-365; C.M. Modlesky and R.D. Lewis, 2000, Assessment of body size and composition. In *Sports nutrition: A guide for professionals working with active people,* 3rd ed., edited by C.A. Rosenbloom (Chicago, IL: The American Dietetics Association), 185-222.

and also highlight how weight has shifted upward over the past few decades.

Proposed body composition standards include some increase in %BF with age rather than imposing the current young adult standard on all age groups (Lohman et al. 1997). For example, a young adult male at 24% fat would be encouraged to lower his %BF, while a middle-aged man at 24% would be in the healthy range (table 7.3). Future testing of these proposed standards will lead to their further refinement. The recommended adjustments of these fat standards with age are based on studies

showing that in middle age, a lower level of body fat or decreasing body fat is associated with lower bone mineral content—which puts a person at greater risk for osteoporosis and bone fractures (Lohman et al. 1997). Thus, the emphasis on lower levels of %BF to prevent heart disease, especially in women, must be balanced against the increased risk of bone fractures, particularly if bone mineral content is already low.

Standards have also been proposed for %BF in physically active men and women (table 7.4). Although the lower values may not improve

Table 7.2 Mean Percent Body Fat by Age, Gender, and Ethnicity

Age (years)	Non-Hispanic white	Non-Hispanic black	Mexican American
Males			
12-13.9	18.4	19.5	22.0
14-15.9	18.4	17.8	18.8
16-17.9	17.7	18.6	21.3
18-19.9	19.6	19.9	22.7
20-29.9	21.8	23.7	24.1
30-39.9	23.6	23.6	25.4
40-49.9	24.2	24.9	26.6
50-59.9	25.1	25.1	26.7
60-69.9	26.2	24.9	26.7
70-79.9	25.1	24.3	26.1
Females			
12-13.9	24.8	26.9	28.6
14-15.9	29.1	30.9	31.8
16-17.9	30.7	32.6	33.3
18-19.9	30.8	33.3	33.5
20-29.9	31.0	35.5	35.8
30-39.9	33.0	38.0	38.0
40-49.9	35.4	39.4	39.9
50-59.9	37.3	40.0	39.4
60-69.9	36.9	39.8	39.4
70-79.9	35.9	38.5	37.8

Adapted from Chumlea et al., 2002, *National health and nutrition examination survey* (NHANES) III.

Table 7.3 Health Standards for Percent Body Fat

	Recommended percent body fat levels				
	Not recommended	Low	Mid	Upper	Obesity
Men					
Young adult	<8	8	13	22	→
Middle adult	<10	10	18	25	→
Elderly	<10	10	16	23	→
Women					
Young adult	<20	20	28	35	→
Middle adult	<25	25	32	38	→
Elderly	<25	25	30	35	→

Reprinted from T.G. Lohman, L. Houtkooper, and S.B. Going, 1997, "Body fat measurement goes high-tech: Not all are created equal," *ACSM's Health Fitness Journal* 7: 30-35.

Table 7.4 Fitness Standards for Percent Body Fat in Active Men and Women

	Recommended body fat levels		
	Low	Mid	Upper
Men			
Young adult	5	10	15
Middle adult	7	11	18
Elderly	9	12	18
Women			
Young adult	16	23	28
Middle adult	20	27	33
Elderly	20	27	33

Reprinted from T.G. Lohman, L. Houtkooper, and S.B. Going, 1997, "Body fat measurement goes high-tech: Not all are created equal," *ACSM's Health Fitness Journal* 7: 30-35.

health, they may be associated with improved physical performance.

Reference %BF levels corresponding to BMI thresholds of underweight (BMI <18.5 kg/m²), overweight (BMI ≥25 kg/m²), and obese (BMI ≥30 kg/m²) from African Americans, Asians, and whites indicated that %BF levels in 20- to 39-year-old women with BMI values ≥25 kg/m² ranged from 32% to 35% and from 20% to 23% in men of the same age (Gallagher et al. 2000). These values were based on healthy subjects and may not accurately reflect population means. Further research with larger, more diverse populations is needed to evaluate population mean %BF values.

Standards for Children and Youth

Because it is difficult to estimate body composition in young people, definitions of obesity and extreme leanness in this population typically depend on ratios of weight to height or on percentiles of skinfold measurements. For example, when triceps skinfolds are used to assess body composition, children have typically been considered obese if they are in the 85th to 95th percentiles (Dietz and Gortmaker 1984; Gortmaker et al. 1987). Dietz and Gortmaker (1984), who used the 85th percentile to define obesity, observed that more children 6 to 11 years old and 12 to 17 years old were above the 85th percentile in 1971-1974 and 1976-1980 as compared

to 1963-1965. The authors concluded that the prevalence of obesity had increased for boys and girls 6 to 11 years old by 61% and 46%, respectively. For youths 12 to 17 years old, the reported increase in the prevalence of obesity was 18% for boys and 58% for girls. When the 95th percentile was used as the definition of obesity, an even greater increase in the prevalence of obesity for children was reported. According to data from NHANES (1999-2002), obesity prevalence in children 6 to 19 years old had increased from 11% (NHANES 1988-1994) to 16% (Hedley et al. 2004).

Clear interpretation of these data requires determination of %BF values, for a given age group, that correspond to the 85th and 95th percentiles (Dietz and Gortmaker 1984; Gortmaker et al. 1987). Lohman (1992a) developed such tables, calculating %BF from the sum of two skinfolds using equations of Slaughter and colleagues (1988) that were developed specifically for youths using a multicomponent criterion model (table 7.5).

The data in these tables show that boys at the 85th percentile for the triceps plus subscapular skinfolds have equivalent %BF values that range from a low of only 15.6% at 6 years of age to a high of 23.6% at 12 years. For girls, the equivalent %BF values for the 85th percentile in skinfolds range from a low of only 18.1% at 6 years to 32.6% at 16 years (Lohman 1992a). Note that the same skinfold percentile at a given age varies considerably in equivalent %BF value. If the 85th percentile defines

Table 7.5 Percent Fat Corresponding to the 50th, 85th, and 95th Percentiles for Triceps Plus Subscapular Skinfolds (SK)

	Male percentiles						Female percentiles					
	50th		85th		95th		50th		85th		95th	
Age (years)	Σ2SK	% fat	Σ2SK	% fat	Σ2SK	% fat	Σ2SK	% fat	Σ2SK	% fat	Σ2SK	% fat
6	12	11.7	16	15.6	20	19.6	14	13.5	19	18.1	27	23.9
8	13	12.7	19	18.4	28	25.9	16	15.5	25	22.6	36	29.4
10	14	12.7	24	21.9	33	28.8	18	17.2	31.6	26.5	43	33.2
12	14.5	12.5	27	23.6	44	35.0	19.5	18.5	34	27.7	47.3	35.5
14	14	11.0	26.5	22.0	39	30.5	23.5	21.6	37.5	30.2	52.6	38.4
16	14	9.0	24	18.9	39	29.3	25.5	23.0	42	32.6	58	41.4

Males: For 6- and 8-year-olds, the intercept was –1.7; for 10-year-olds, –2.5; for 12-year-olds, –3.4; for 14-year-olds, –4.4; for 16-year-olds, –5.5; the equation is % fat = 1.21 (Σ2SK) – 0.008 (Σ2SK) 2 + 1. For males with skinfolds greater than 35 mm, % fat = 0.783 (Σ2SK) + 2.2 (6- to 8-year-olds), 0.6 (10- to 12-year-olds), and –1.2 (14- to 16-year-olds). Females: % fat = 1.33 (Σ2SK) – 0.013 (Σ2SK) 2 – 2.5 (one intercept for all ages). For females with skinfolds greater than 35 mm, % fat = 0.546 (Σ2SK) + 9.7; all ages.

Note: Calculations were derived using National Healthy Examination Survey (NHES) norms (1963-1965), computed from data obtained from the NHES (1973).

Centers for Disease Control (CDC). Growth Charts, 2005.

obesity in children, a 6-year-old boy would be classified as obese if his %BF was only 15.6%, and a 16-year-old girl would not be classified as obese until she had a %BF value of 32.6%. This large variation in the equivalent %BF values for a given skinfold percentile demonstrates the limitation of using such data to assess body composition or as criteria for defining obesity in children (Going and Williams 1989).

The BMI for age-specific and gender-specific growth charts are another tool for assessing body weight status in children and adolescents. A BMI ≤5% would classify a child or adolescent as underweight; a BMI between 85% and <95% would indicate risk of overweight, and a BMI of ≥95% would indicate overweight (Centers for Disease Control and Prevention 2005).

Lohman (1992a) has published guidelines for evaluating the estimated %BF values for youths. Table 7.6 summarizes these guidelines for girls and boys. These guidelines offer an approach to interpreting estimated %BF values in youths.

In this approach, obesity for boys is defined as a %BF >25%; for girls it is >32%. The concept supporting this approach is sound, but the classifications for the actual %BF levels require further research to determine what levels of body fatness are related to increased risks for diseases. Some researchers have proposed using a single %BF standard for defining obesity in boys and girls of all ages (Hoerr et al. 1992; Lohman 1992a). The current availability of equations for predicting %BF for children using skinfolds makes it possible to use a %BF value as a guideline to define obesity for boys and girls of all ages (Janz et al. 1993; Slaughter et al. 1988).

Table 7.6 Guidelines for Interpreting Percent Body Fat Values for Children

Ratings	Percent body fat	
	Boys	Girls
Very low	<5	<12
Low	5-10	12-15
Optimal	11-20	16-25
Moderately high	21-25	26-30
High	26-31	31-36
Very high	>31	>36

Reprinted, by permission, from L.B. Houtkooper 1996, "Assessment of body composition in youth and relationship to sport," *International Journal of Sports Nutrition* 6(2): 146-164; Adapted, by permission, from T.G. Lohman, 1987, *Moving body fat using skinfolds* (videotape) (Champaign, IL: Human Kinetics).

Instead of using percentile-referenced standards to derive %BF standards for children and youths, Williams and colleagues (1992) used criterion-referenced standards. They assessed the risks for high levels of blood pressure, total cholesterol, and low-density lipoprotein (LDL)-cholesterol and for low levels of high-density lipoprotein (HDL)-cholesterol in males and females aged 6 to 18 years at different levels of body fatness. They found no excess risk until %BF values exceeded 25% in males and 30% in females. Age and ethnicity were not significant predictors of risk in this age group. Thus, these researchers have proposed >25% BF in males and >30% BF in females as useful health standards for black and white girls and boys aged 6 to 18 years. A similar criterion-referenced approach would be useful in adults to determine whether "risk" varies with age and %BF, or whether one %BF standard is valid for all ages and ethnic groups.

Future research that helps more clearly define the relation between body fatness and health status or sport performance will improve the interpretation of body composition status.

CHAPTER IN REVIEW

Over the last 35 years, much research has focused on the development of body composition methods for more accurate and reliable measurement of %BF and FFM. Yet there is little research on the relationship between body composition and athletic performance. We know that excess body fat negatively influences performance in some sports, and that a high ratio of FFM to FM at a given body weight is generally positively related to sport performance. However, very low levels or high levels of body fat can negatively affect health and exercise performance. Perhaps the most useful functional measure of FFM in athletes is assessments of strength and performance.

Practitioners working with athletes need to be aware of the inherent errors associated with body composition assessment and should not attempt to define an exact level of optimal %BF or FFM for an individual athlete. It is reasonable, however, to define a %BF or FFM *range* associated with athletes who are top performers in their sports. These ranges can then be used to establish reasonable training goals for weight, %BF, and FFM, as long as the goals are realistic and are compatible with good health for an individual athlete. More emphasis needs to be placed on defining optimal ratios of FFM and FM for various sports to replace the body weight goals that many currently use.

Key Concepts

1. Understand the relationship between body composition and health.

There is a strong association between excess body fat—especially excess intra-abdominal fat—and increased risk of coronary artery disease, non-insulin-dependent diabetes, hypertension, and certain types of cancers. Low levels of FFM and loss of FFM are related to impaired functional capacity and decreased physical activity and energy expenditure, and increase the risk of gaining FM.

2. Describe the relationship between body composition and sport performance.

High ratios of FFM to FM at a given body weight are generally positively related to physical performance, but too little body fat results in deterioration in health and performance. The ideal relative FM or FFM for an athlete in a specific sport is difficult to define—body size and structure as well as many other factors also contribute to successful athletic performance.

3. Compare body composition assessment models and methods.

Body composition refers to the amounts of constituents in the body at atomic, molecular, cellular, tissue-system, and whole-body levels. The simplest and most common model of body composition partitions the body into two major components (compartments)—FM and FFM.

4. Understand the accuracy of body composition assessment measurements.

Accuracy of field methods for estimation of athletes' body composition depends upon selection of appropriate models and measurement methods, the skill of individuals taking the measurements, and use of appropriate gender- and age-specific prediction equations.

5. Identify selection criteria for field methods for estimating body composition.

Appropriate field methods and careful measurements make it possible to estimate relative body fat with an error of approximately 3% fat and to estimate FFM with an error of about 5.5 lb (2.5 kg).

6. Discuss body composition status of athletes.

The relative body fat ranges of top athletes vary by sport and by gender within a sport. Excess body fat negatively influences physical performance.

7. Explain the relationship between body composition standards and health.

There are no universally acceptable percent body fat standards for adults or children, nor is there a universally accepted upper or lower limit of percent body fat at which health problems will occur. In general, a high %BF is associated with diabetes, hypertension, and heart disease, while a low %BF is associated with osteoporosis, bone fractures, menstrual dysfunction, eating disorders, and muscle wasting. Future research will help to more clearly define the relationship between body fatness and health.

Key Terms

air displacement plethysmography (ADP) 213

bioelectrical impedance analysis (BIA) 216

body mass index (BMI) 215

chemically mature 210

computed tomography (CT) 214

criterion method 210

densitometry (underwater weighing) 209

direct method 208

dual-energy X-ray absorptiometry (DXA) 213
fat mass (FM) 206
fat-free mass (FFM) 206
hydrodensitometry (HD) 213
indirect method 208

magnetic resonance imaging (MRI) 214
model approach 209
property-based method 208
regression analysis 209
total body water (TBW) 208
whole-body density (D_b) 210

Additional Information

Heymsfield SB, Lohman TG, Wang Z, Going SB eds. Human body composition. Champaign, IL: Human Kinetics, 2005.

This is the most complete text in the burgeoning field of body composition research. The book covers the full range of methods to assess body composition, including dual-energy X-ray absorptiometry, electrical impedance, and imaging techniques. This book is an excellent research guide for body composition and incorporates the newest information on methods and topics of biological importance.

Heyward VH, Wagner DR eds. Applied body composition assessment. Champaign, IL: Human Kinetics, 2004.

This book addresses the principles underlying the skinfold, bioelectrical impedance, near-infrared interactance, and anthropometric methods of body composition assessment. It also discusses how to control for potential errors in measurement, different equations for different populations, and much more. The topics covered include the most recently validated equations, the latest developments in body composition methods, and information on measuring the body composition of clinical populations.

References

Ball SD. Inter-device variability in percent fat estimates using the BOD POD. Med Sci Sports Exerc 2004;36(5) suppl:S72.

Ballard TP, Fafara L, Vukovich MD. Comparison of Bod Pod® and DXA in female collegiate athletes. Med Sci Sports Exerc 2004;36:731-735.

Baumgartner RN. Aging In: Heymsfield SB, Lohman TG, Wang Z, Going SB eds. Human body composition. Champaign, IL: Human Kinetics, 2005;259-269.

Beals KA. Prevalence of disordered eating among athletes. In: Beals KA ed. Disordered eating among athletes—a comprehensive guide for health professionals. Champaign, IL: Human Kinetics, 2004;21-40.

Bellisari A, Roche AF. Anthropometry and ultrasound. In: Heymsfield SB, Lohman TG, Wang Z, Going SB eds. Human body composition. Champaign, IL: Human Kinetics, 2005;109-128.

Boileau RA, Lohman TG. The measurement of human physique and its effect on physical performance. Orthop Clin North Am 1977;8:563-581.

Boileau RA, Lohman TG, Slaughter MH, Ball TE, Going SB, Hendrix MK. Hydration of the fat-free body in children during maturation. Hum Biol 1984;56:651-666.

Brozek JF, Grande F, Anderson JT, Keys A. Densitometric analysis of body composition: revision of some quantitative assumptions. Ann NY Acad Sci 1963;110:113-40.

Bruns F, van der Vusse GJ. Utilization of lipids during exercise in human subjects: metabolic and dietary constraints. Br J Nutr 1998;79(2):117-128.

Buskirk E, Taylor HL. Maximal oxygen intake and its relation to body composition with special reference to chronic physical activity and obesity. J Appl Physiol 1957;11:727-728.

Cassady SL, Nielsen DH, Janz KF, Wu WT, Cook JS, Hansen JR. Validity of near infrared body composition analysis in children and adolescents. Med Sci Sports Exerc 1993;25:1185-1191.

Centers for Disease Control and Prevention. Growth charts, 2005. www.cdc.gov. Accessed May 21, 2005.

Chumlea WC, Guo SS, Kuczmarski RJ, Flegal KM, Johnson CL, Heymsfield SB, Lukaski HC, Friedl K, Hubbard VS. Body composition estimates from NHANES III bioelectrical impedance data. Int J Obesity 2002;26:1596-1611.

Chumlea WC, Sun SS. Biolelectrical impedance analysis. In: Heymsfield SB, Lohman TG, Wang Z, Going SB eds. Human body composition. Champaign, IL: Human Kinetics, 2005;79-88.

Collins MA, Millard-Stafford ML, Sparling PB, Snow TK, Rosskopf LB, Webb SA et al. Evaluation of the BOD POD for assessing body fat in collegiate football players. Med Sci Sports Exerc 1999;31:1350-1356.

Cureton KJ. Effects of experimental alterations in excess weight on physiological responses to exercise and physical performance. In: Marriott BM, Grumstrup-Scott J eds. Body composition and physical performance: applications for the military services. Washington, DC: National Academy Press, 1992;71-88.

Cureton KJ, Sparling PB. Distance running performance and metabolic responses to running in men and women with excess weight experimentally equated. Med Sci Sports Exerc 1980;12:288-294.

Cureton KJ, Sparling PB, Evans PW, Johnson SM, Kong UD, Purvis JW. Effect of experimental alterations in excess weight on aerobic capacity and distance running performance. Med Sci Sports Exerc 1978;15:218-223.

De Lorenzo A, Bertini I, Iacopino L, Pagliato E, Testolin C, Testolin G. Body composition measurement in highly trained male athletes. A comparison of three methods. J Sports Med Phys Fit 2000;40:178-183.

Demura S, Sato S, Kitabayashi T. Percentage of total body fat as estimated by three automatic bioelectrical impedance analyzers. J Physiol Anthropol Appl Human Sci 2004;23:93-99.

Deurenberg P, Westrate JA, Seidell JC. Body mass index as a measure of body fitness: age- and sex-specific prediction formulas. Br J Nutr 1991;65:105-114.

Dietz WH, Gortmaker SL. Factors within the physical environment associated with childhood obesity. Am J Clin Nutr 1984;39:619-624.

Ellis KJ. Whole-body counting and neutron activation analysis. In: Heymsfield SB, Lohman TG, Wang Z, Going SB eds. Human body composition. Champaign, IL: Human Kinetics, 2005;51-62.

Fidanza FA, Keys A, Anderson JT. Density of body fat in man and other animals. J Appl Physiol 1953;6:252-256.

Fields DA, Goran MI, McCrory MA. Body-composition assessment via air-displacement plethysmography in adults and children: a review. Am J Clin Nutr 2002;75:453-467.

Fleck SJ. Body composition of elite American athletes. Am J Sports Med 1983;11:398-403.

Forbes GB. Human body composition: growth, aging, nutrition and activity. New York: Springer-Verlag, 1987.

Friedl KE, DeLuca JP, Marchitelli LS, Vogel JA. Reliability of body-fat estimations from a four-component model by using density, body water, and bone mineral measurements. Am J Clin Nutr 1992;55:764-770.

Fuller NJ, Jebb SA, Laskey MA, Coward WA, Elia M. Four-component model for the assessment of body composition in humans: comparison with alternative methods, and evaluation of the density and hydration of fat-free mass. Clin Sci 1992;82:687-693.

Gallagher D, Heymsfield SB, Heo M, Jebb SA, Murgatroyd PR, Sakamoto Y. Healthy percentage body fat ranges: an approach for developing guidelines based on body mass index. Am J Clin Nutr 2000;72(3):694-701.

Gartner A, Dioum A, Delpeuch F, Maire B, Schutz Y. Use of hand-to-hand impedancemetry to predict body composition of African women as measured by air displacement plethysmography. Eur J Clin Nutr 2004;58:523-531.

Going SB. Densitometry. In: Roche AF, Heymsfield SB, Lohman TG eds. Human body composition. Champaign, IL: Human Kinetics, 1996;3-23.

Going SB. Hydrodensitometry and air displacement plethysmography. In: Heymsfield SB, Lohman TG, Wang Z, Going SB eds. Human body composition. Champaign, IL: Human Kinetics, 2005;17-33.

Going SB, Davis R. Body composition. In: Roitman JL ed. ACSM's resource manual for guidelines for exercise testing and prescription. American College of Sports Medicine. Baltimore: Williams & Wilkins, 1998.

Going SB, Mullins V. Body composition of the endurance performer. In: Shephard RJ ed. Endurance in sport (IOC encyclopedia, vol. II, chap. 24). Oxford, UK: Blackwell Science, 2001;2:346-365.

Going SB, Williams D. Understanding fitness standards. JOPHERD 1989;60:34-38.

Goodpaster BH, Thaete FL, Kelley DE. Composition of skeletal muscle evaluated with computed tomography. Ann NY Acad Sci 2000;904:18-24.

Gortmaker SL, Dietz WH, Sobal AM, Wehler CA. Increasing pediatric obesity in the United States. Am J Dis Child 1987;141:535-540.

Guo SS, Roche AF, Chumlea WC, Gardner JD, Siervogel RM. The predictive value of childhood body mass index values for overweight at age 35 y. Am J Clin Nutr 1994;59:810-819.

Guo SS, Roche WC, Houtkooper L. Fat-free mass in children and young adults predicted from bioelectric impedance and anthropometric variables. Am J Clin Nutr 1989;50:435-443.

Gurr MI, Harwood JL. Lipid biochemistry. London: Chapman and Hall, 1991.

Harman EA, Frykman PN. The relationship of body size and composition to the performance of physically demanding military tasks. In: Marriott BM, Grumstrup-Scott J eds. Body composition and physical performance: applications for the military services. Washington, DC: National Academy Press, 1992;105-118.

Heaney R. Bone biology in health and disease: a tutorial. In: Shils M, Olson J, Shike M, Ross A eds. Modern nutrition in health and disease. Baltimore: Williams & Wilkins, 1999.

Hedley AA, Ogden CL, Johnson CL, Carroll MD, Curtin LR, Flegal KM. Overweight and obesity among US children, adolescents, and adults, 1999-2002. JAMA 2004;291:2847-2850.

Hewitt MJ, Going SB, Williams DP, Lohman TG. Hydration of the fat-free body mass in children and adults: implications for body composition assessment. Am J Physiol 1993;265:E88-E95.

Heymsfield SB, Lohman TG, Wang Z, Going SB eds. Human body composition. Champaign, IL: Human Kinetics, 2005.

Heymsfield SB, Wang Z. Measurement of total-body fat by underwater weighing: new insights and uses for old method. Nutrition 1993;9:472-473.

Heymsfield SB, Wang ZM, Withers RT. Multicomponent molecular level models of body composition. In: Heymsfield SB, Lohman TG, Wang Z, Going SB eds. Human body composition. Champaign, IL: Human Kinetics, 2005;163-176.

Heyward VH, Wagner D. Applied body composition assessment, 2nd ed. Champaign, IL: Human Kinetics, 2004.

Hoerr SL, Nelson RA, Lohman TG. Discrepancies among predictors of desirable weight for black and white obese adolescent girls. J Am Diet Assoc 1992;92:450-453.

Housh TJ, Johnson GO, Housh DJ, Cramer JT, Eckerson JM, Stout JR, Bull AJ, Rana SR. Accuracy of near-infrared interactance instruments and population-specific equations for estimating body composition in young wrestlers. J Strength Cond Res 2004;18:556-560.

Houtkooper LB. Assessment of body composition in youth and relationship to sport. Int J Sport Nutr 1996;146-164.

Houtkooper LB. Exercise and eating disorders. In: Lamb D, Murray R eds. Perspectives in exercise science and sports medicine. Exercise, nutrition, and control of body weight. Carmel, IN: Cooper, 1998.

Houtkooper LB, Going SB. Body composition: how should it be measured? Does it affect sport performance? Sports Sci Exch 1994;7:1-8.

Houtkooper LB, Lohman TG, Going SB, Howell WH. Why bioelectrical impedance analysis should be used for estimating adiposity. Am J Clin Nutr 1996;64:436S-448S.

Huygens W, Claessens AL, Thomis M, Loos R, Van Langendonck L, Peeters M, Philippaerts R, Meynaerts E, Vlietinck R, Beunen G. Body composition estimations by BIA versus anthropometric equations in body builders and other power athletes. J Sports Med Phys Fit 2002;42:45-55.

Janssen I, Katzmarzyk PT, Ross R. Body mass index, waist circumference, and health risk. Arch Intern Med 2002;162:2074-2079.

Janssen I, Katzmarzyk PT, Ross R. Waist circumference and not body mass index explains obesity-related health risk. Am J Clin Nutr 2004;79:379-384.

Janz KF, Nielsen DH, Cassady SL, Cook JR, Wu YT, Hansen JR. Cross-validation of the Slaughter skinfold equations for children and adolescents. Med Sci Sports Exerc 1993;25:1070-1076.

Kaplowitz H, Martorell R, Mendoza FS. Fatness and fat distribution in Mexican-American children and youths from the Hispanic health and nutrition examination survey. Am J Hum Biol 1989;1:631-648.

Kiebzak G, Leamy L, Pierson L, Nord R, Zhang Z. Measurement precision of body composition variables using the Lunar DPX-L densitometer. J Clin Densitom 2000;3:35-41.

Lohman TG. Applicability of body composition techniques and constants for children and youth. In: Pandolf KB ed. Exercise and sports science reviews. New York: Macmillan, 1986;325-357.

Lohman TG. Assessment of body composition in children. Pediatr Exerc Sci 1989;1:19-30.

Lohman TG. Basic concepts in body composition assessment (1-5); Body density, body water, and bone mineral: controversies and limitations of the two-component system (7-24); Estimating body composition in children and the elderly (65-78); The prevalence of obesity in children in the United States (79-90). In: Roche AF, Heymsfield SB,

Lohman TG eds. Advances in body composition assessment. Champaign, IL: Human Kinetics, 1992a.

Lohman TG. Exercise training and body composition in childhood. Can J Sports Sci 1992b;17:284-287.

Lohman TG, Chen Z. Dual-energy x-ray absorptiometry. In: Heymsfield SB, Lohman TG, Wang Z, Going SB eds. Human body composition. Champaign, IL: Human Kinetics, 2005;63-78.

Lohman TG, Houtkooper L, Going SB. Body fat measurement goes high-tech: not all are created equal. ACSM's Health Fit J 1997;7:30-35.

Lohman TG, Slaughter MH, Boileau RA, Bunt J, Lussier L. Bone mineral measurements and their relation to body density in children, youth, and adults. Hum Biol 1984;56:667-669.

Lukaski HC. Methods for the assessment of human body composition: traditional and new. Am J Clin Nutr 1987;46:537-556.

Lukaski HC, Siders WA. Validity and accuracy of regional bioelectrical impedance devices to determine whole-body fatness. Nutrition 2003;19:851-857.

Malina RM. Physique and body composition: effects on performance and effects on training, semistarvation, and overtraining. In: Brownell KD, Rodin J, Wilmore JH eds. Eating, body weight, and performance in athletes. Philadelphia: Lea & Febiger, 1992;94-114.

Malina RM. Variation in body composition associated with sex and ethnicity. In: Heymsfield SB, Lohman TG, Wang Z, Going SB eds. Human body composition. Champaign, IL: Human Kinetics, 2005;271-298.

Malina RM, Bouchard C. Characteristics of young athletes. In: Malina RM, Bouchard C eds. Growth, maturation and physical activity. Champaign, IL: Human Kinetics, 1991;443-463.

Modlesky CM, Lewis RD. Assessment of body size and composition. In: Rosenbloom CA ed. Sports nutrition: a guide for professionals working with active people, 3rd ed. Chicago: American Dietetic Association, 2000;185-222.

Mueller WH, Kaplowitz HJ. The precision of anthropometric assessment of body fat distribution in children. Ann Hum Biol 1994;21:267-274.

National Health Examination Survey (NHES). Sample design and estimation procedures for a national health examination survey of children. National Center for Health Statistics Publication No. HRA 74-1005. Rockville, MD: Health Resource Administration, 1973.

New Fitness. Comparing methods for measuring body fat, 2005. www.new-fitness.com/body_fat_analyzing.html. Accessed March 2009.

Pate RR, Slentz CA, Katz DP. Relationships between skinfold thickness and performance of health related fitness test items. Res Q Exerc Sport 1989;60(2):183-189.

Ross R, Goodpaster B, Kelley D, Boada F. Magnetic resonance imaging in human body composition research: from quantitative to qualitative tissue measurement. Ann NY Acad Sci 2000;904:12-17.

Ross R, Janssen I. Computed tomography and magnetic resonance imaging. In: Heymsfield SB, Lohman TG, Wang Z, Going SB eds. Human body composition. Champaign, IL: Human Kinetics, 2005;89-108.

Sinning WE. Body composition and athletic performance. In: Clark DH, Eckert HM eds. Limits of human performance. American Academy of Physical Education Papers, no. 18, 1985;45-56.

Sinning WE. Body composition in athletes. In: Roche AF, Heymsfield SB, Lohman TG eds. Human body composition. Champaign, IL: Human Kinetics, 1996;257-274.

Siri WE. The gross composition of the body. Adv Biol Med Physiol 1956;4:239-280.

Siri WE. Body composition from fluid spaces and density: analysis of methods. In: Brozek J, Henschel A eds. Techniques for measuring body composition. Washington, DC: National Academy of Science, 1961;223-244.

Slaughter MH, Lohman TG, Boileau RA et al. Skinfold equations for estimation of body fatness in children and youth. Hum Biol 1988;60:709-723.

Sparling PB, Cureton KJ. Biological determinants of sex difference in 12 min run performance. Med Sci Sports Exerc 1983;15:218-222.

Thorland WG, Johnston GO, Housh TJ, Refsell MJ. Anthropometric characteristics of elite adolescent competitive swimmers. Hum Biol 1983;55:735-48.

Tylavsky FA, Lohman TG, Dockrell M, Lang T, Schoeller DA, Wan JY, Fuerst T, Cauley JA, Nevitt M, Harris TB. Comparison of the effectiveness of 2 dual-energy X-ray absorptiometers with that of total body water and computed tomography in assessing changes in body composition during weight change. Am J Clin Nutr 2003;77:356-363.

Utter AC, Goss FL, Swan PD, Harris GS, Robertson RJ, Trone GA. Evaluation of air displacement for assessing body composition of collegiate wrestlers. Med Sci Sports Exerc 2003;35(3):500-505.

Vescovi JD, Zimmerman SL, Miller WC, Fernhall B. Effects of clothing on accuracy and reliability of air displacement plethysmography. Med Sci Sports Exerc 2002;34(2):282-285.

Wang J, Thornton JC, Kolesnik S, Pierson RN. Anthropometry in body composition. An overview. Ann NY Acad Sci 2000;904:317-326.

Wang Z, Pierson Jr RN, Heymsfield SB. The five-level model: a new approach to organizing body-composition research. Am J Clin Nutr 1992;56:19-28.

Williams DP, Going SB, Lohman TG, Hewitt MJ, Haber AE. Estimation of body fat from skinfold thicknesses in middle-aged and older men: a multiple component approach. Am J Human Biol 1992;4:595-605.

Wilmore JH. Body weight standards and athletic performance. In: Brownell KD, Rodin J, Wilmore JH eds. Eating, body weight, and performance in athletes. Philadelphia: Lea & Febiger, 1992;315-329.

Wittch A, Oliveri MB, Rotemberg E, Mautalen C. Body composition of professional football (soccer) players determined by dual X-ray absorptiometry. J Clin Densitom 2001;4:51-55.

Zhu SK, Wang ZM, Heshka S, Heo M, Faith MS, Heymsfield SB. Waist circumference and obesity-associated risk factors among whites in the third National Health and Nutrition Examination Survey: clinical action thresholds. Am J Clin Nutr 2002;76:743-749.

CHAPTER 8

Fluid and Electrolyte Balance

Chapter Objectives

After reading this chapter you should be able to

- understand the function and regulation of water and electrolyte balance within the body and the adverse performance and health effects of dehydration, hypohydration, hyperhydration, and hyponatremia,

- identify the fluid and electrolyte recommendations for exercise,

- assess fluid balance using changes in weight from pre- to postexercise,

- understand the role of sport drinks in preventing and maintaining fluid balance before, during, and after exercise,

- understand the effects of heat and cold on fluid needs in athletes and active individuals, and

- identify fluid balance issues and replacement strategies in children.

Although we often do not think of water as an essential nutrient, it is! It is the most abundant constituent of the body. Abnormal decreases in body water (dehydration) can cause death more quickly than the removal of any other essential nutrient from the diet. One can go weeks without eating food, while death from dehydration can occur within three to four days. Water provides more than just fluid to bathe our cells. Most of the water we drink, depending on its source, also contains numerous electrolytes and minerals, including sodium, chloride, magnesium, potassium, fluoride, and calcium. Thus, the water we drink can contribute to our intake of these important nutrients. Because exercise increases the loss of body water and electrolytes, and because these losses can impair exercise performance and the ability and desire to perform work, it is important to understand how to maintain water and electrolyte balance during exercise. This is especially true for exercise in a hot environment. In sports in which dehydration is used to reduce body weight before competition or "weigh-in," the effect on health and performance can be extremely detrimental or even deadly. This was tragically demonstrated late in 1997 when three collegiate wrestlers died trying to make weight through dehydration (Remick et al. 1998). In this chapter, we provide background information on water and electrolyte balance, outline body water and electrolyte losses, and discuss the factors influencing fluid uptake at rest and during exercise. Then we review the importance of consuming adequate fluids before, during, and after exercise, along with recommendations for assessment of fluid balance, for fluid consumption in different types of exercises and sports and environmental conditions, and for fluid consumption in children and adolescents. Finally, we discuss the composition and role of various commercial fluid replacement beverages and sport drinks.

WATER AND ELECTROLYTE BALANCE

Total body weight comprises about 60% (range 45-70%) water (Sawka and Pandolf 1990). People with more muscle mass have a higher percentage of body water than those with more body fat since water composes ~74% of muscle and organ weight but only ~20% to 30% of adipose tissue. Because men generally have a higher percentage of lean body mass than women, they typically have a higher percentage of water in their total body weight. For example, men less than 40 years of age average ~60% to 65% water, while women of the same age average ~50% to 55% (Lorenz and Kleinman 2003). Thus, as a percentage of total body weight, a very lean male may have a body water content of 70%, while an obese man may have only 50%. As people age, muscle mass usually declines, decreasing total body water content.

Function of Water

Water serves a number of functions within the body:

- Water acts as a lubricant that bathes every tissue and cell of the body. It is a transport medium in which many compounds (e.g., nutrients, drugs, hormones, and peptides) can be transported to the cells. It is the medium in which waste materials are removed from the body via the kidneys and the medium in which many body solutes, both organic and inorganic, are dissolved.
- Water is necessary for numerous chemical reactions within the body, especially metabolic reactions involved in energy production.
- Water is a structural part of body tissues such as proteins and glycogen.
- Water is extremely important in the regulation of body temperature. If the body is not cooled properly through sweating, severe metabolic consequences can occur, including death.

Body Water Compartments and Composition

Total body water can generally be divided into intracellular and extracellular components (Lorenz and Kleinman 2003). Intracellular water includes all the water enclosed within cell membranes, while extracellular water is all the water outside cells. Some of the extracellular water compartments include the water in the plasma (intravascular water); water around the cells (interstitial fluid); and water normally present in the gastrointestinal and urinary tracts, the humor of the eye, and the cerebrospinal fluid (transcellular water) (Lorenz and Kleinman 2003). Extracellular water constitutes the medium through which all metabolic exchanges occur, while intracellular water constitutes the medium in which all chemical reactions of cellular metabolism occur. Table 8.1 indicates the compartment volumes in liters for each of the major body water pools. As you can see from this table, a 154 lb (70 kg) man must maintain ~42 L of body water in order to achieve optimal fluid balance. But to maintain fluid balance, the body needs more than just water.

Electrolytes such as sodium, chloride, potassium, calcium, and magnesium ions, as well as many small molecules, play an important role in fluid balance. We must consume electrolytes in food and beverages in order to maintain fluid balance. Since water can easily diffuse across cell membranes, it is the chemical activity and concentrations of the ions and small molecules (e.g., glucose, albumin) that determine body water distribution within the various compartments. The more concentrated the solutes are within a particular compartment, the greater their osmotic pressure (and thus the greater their ability to attract water). For example, if two adjacent compartments

Table 8.1 Distribution of Body Water Volume Into Various Compartments

	Percentage (%) of body weight	Percentage (%) of total body water	Volume in 70 kg man
Total body water	60	–	42 L
Extracellular water	20	33	14 L
Plasma	5	8	3.5 L
Interstitial fluid	15	25	10.5 L
Intracellular water	40	67	28 L

From *Clinical chemistry: Theory, analysis and correlation*, L.A. Kaplan, A.I. Pesce, and S.C. Kazmierczak, editors, Physiology and pathophysiology of body water and electrolytes, I.M. Lorenz and L.I. Kleinman, pgs. 444, Copyright 2003, with permission from Elsevier.

contain differing amounts of sodium, water will be attracted into the compartment with more sodium. **Osmotic pressure** is defined as the force necessary to exactly oppose osmosis (movement) of water into a solution across a semipermeable membrane (Lorenz and Kleinman 2003). Another way to view osmotic pressure is to think of it as the force that tends to move water from dilute solutions to concentrated solutions. If a membrane is permeable to a solute, then the solute exerts no osmotic pressure across the membrane. The effective osmotic pressure of a solution depends on (1) the total number of solute particles in the solution and (2) the permeability characteristics of the membrane through which the solute must pass (Lorenz and Kleinman 2003).

The **osmolarity** of a fluid or solution is a measure of the total number of solute particles (moles) per unit volume. The more solutes found in a fluid, the greater its osmolarity or concentration. Thus, electrolytes help maintain fluid balance within the body by keeping water within a particular body water compartment. If excess loss of electrolytes occurs, the body loses its ability to maintain fluid balance. For example, sodium attracts water; therefore, sodium intake can increase fluid retention within the body. The effect of sodium on water retention may be beneficial for some people and detrimental for others. For someone who wants to rehydrate after strenuous exercise, moderate amounts of sodium in postexercise sport drinks or foods are beneficial. But for a person who retains body fluid due to salt sensitivity, additional dietary

sodium may not be beneficial. Therefore, in addition to adequate water intake, a proper electrolyte balance is necessary to ensure proper fluid balance within the body. **Osmolality** refers to the number of moles or particles per kilogram of water (1 L of water weighs 1 kg). This term is used when the osmotic characteristics of a beverage such as a sport drink are measured (Horswill 1998).

Body Water and Electrolyte Losses

Under normal conditions, daily body water losses come from urine, feces, sweat, and respiration, with the greatest losses coming from urine (~1-2 L/day depending on fluid intake and environmental conditions). Blood losses also decrease total body water since blood is 80% water by weight. For example, donating 1 pint of blood (473 mL) depletes the body of 378 mL of fluid. Table 8.2 outlines normal fluid losses under various conditions. Note that under exercise conditions, especially in the heat, the amount of water lost in sweat can dramatically increase to 1 to 2 L/h, compared to the 100 to 200 mL/day typically lost on nonexercise days in a cool or temperate environment. Exercise increases total body metabolism by 5 to 20 times above resting conditions, depending on the exercise intensity and a person's level of physical conditioning. Much of this increase in metabolic rate, anywhere from 70% to 100%, results in heat that must be dissipated from the body in order to maintain normal body temperature. The amount of sweat produced depends on (1) environmental conditions—air temperature, humidity, wind speed, and radiant load (heat given off by the sun and by surrounding objects); (2) clothing (insulation and moisture permeability); (3) exercise intensity; (4) level of physical conditioning; and (5) acclimation to the environment (Sawka and Pandolf 1990). In addition, women, children, and older adults differ in their sweat response to exercise (Sawka et al. 2007). Figure 8.1 shows hourly sweat rates in liters per hour when a person runs at various speeds in different types of environmental conditions. Sweat rate increases as metabolism increases (i.e., a person is running faster) and as the environment becomes hotter and more humid. If this fluid is not replaced, the body becomes dehydrated. Since the body cannot adapt to dehydration, even though some individuals may tolerate dehydration better than others, the loss of body water can severely affect physiological function, the ability to do work, and overall health.

Table 8.2 Water Balance in Average Adults Under Various Conditions

	Normal	Hot environment	Strenuous work
Fluid intake (mL/day)			
Drinking water	1200	2200	3400
Water from food	1000	1000	1150
Water of oxidation	300	300	450
Total	2500	3500	5000
Fluid output (mL/day)			
Urine	1400	1200	500
Insensible water			
Skin	400	400	400
Lungs	400	300	600
Sweat	100	1400	3300
Stool (feces)	200	200	200
Total	2500	3500	5000

From *Clinical chemistry: Theory, analysis and correlation*, L.A. Kaplan, A.I. Pesce, and S.C. Kazmierczak, editors, Physiology and pathophysiology of body water and electrolytes, I.M. Lorenz and L.I. Kleinman, pgs. 452, Copyright 2003, with permission from Elsevier.

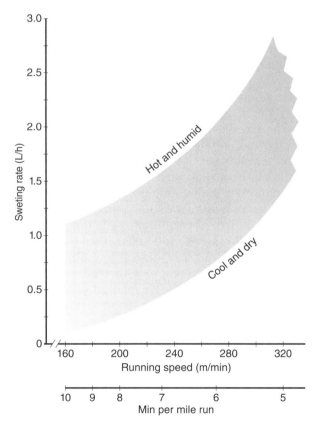

Figure 8.1 Approximation of hourly sweating rates (L/h) for runners at various exercise intensities.

Reprinted, by permission, from M.N. Sawka and K.B. Pandolf, 1990, Effects of body water loss in physiological function and exercise performance. In *Perspectives in exercise and science and sport medicine: Fluid homeostasis during exercise*, edited by D.R. Lamb and C.V.Gisolfi (Traverse City, MI: Cooper Publishing Group), 4.

Electrolyte losses in sweat appear to be highly variable, depending on when the sweat sample is taken and from which part of the body during exercise, the subject's state of acclimatization, and even physiological differences between individuals. Research methods for collecting sweat during exercise and estimating total electrolyte losses are very cumbersome and time-consuming. It is not surprising that values for sweat electrolyte concentrations in the research literature vary dramatically. Although many minerals are lost in sweat, including sodium, chloride, potassium, magnesium, calcium, and iron, the primary electrolytes lost are sodium and potassium. In general, typical values for sweat sodium concentrations range from 10 to 80 mmol/L (to convert mmol or mEq of sodium to mg of sodium, multiply the mmol by 23 [the molecular weight of sodium]; IOM, 2005), with potassium values about 5 to 10 mmol/L (to convert mmol of potassium to mg of potassium, multiply mmol by 39.1 [the molecular weight of potassium]; IOM, 2005) and chloride values about 10 to 60 mmol/L (Maughan and Shirreffs 1997). Sodium is the main electrolyte lost in sweat. Interestingly, sodium is reabsorbed by the sweat glands. The amount reabsorbed is sweating rate dependent; at low sweating rate, more sodium is absorbed than when sweating rate is high. A recent study by Montain and colleagues (2007) characterized the sweat mineral element responses during a 7 h exercise stress protocol. Seven heat-acclimated subjects completed five 60 min treadmill exercise bouts, with 20 min rest between each bout, in two different weather conditions. The purpose was to determine the effect of multiple hours of exercise heat stress on sweat mineral concentrations. The authors collected sweat from sweat collection pouches attached to the upper back during bouts 1, 3, and 5. The results showed that sweat sodium, potassium, and calcium losses during multiple hours of sustained sweating can be predicted from initial sweat composition measured at baseline. This may have substantial practical applicability in sports because an initial sweat sample may be all that is needed to predict losses during exercise. This in turn could assist in determining the electrolyte replacement strategy in the form of a formulated sport drink for exercise.

Regulation of Water and Electrolyte Balance

How does the body know it needs water? What triggers the thirst response? How does the body know when fluid and electrolyte needs have been met? The body has an intricate way of regulating body water—via the stimulation of thirst and via the regulation of fluid loss through the kidneys (e.g., increasing or decreasing output as necessary). The body is constantly assessing fluid balance and adjusting both intake and output to maintain total body water at an optimal level. For example, if blood volume decreases due to increased fluid loss in sweat, the body responds by constricting the blood vessels to increase blood pressure, reducing fluid loss via the kidney, and stimulating the thirst mechanism. All these responses help increase blood pressure and restore fluid balance by decreasing the total vascular space, reducing the probability of continued fluid losses in the urine, and increasing fluid intake. The details of fluid and sodium regulation, including the endocrine and neurological control mechanisms, are reviewed elsewhere (Greenleaf 1992; Heer 2008; Orlov and Mongin 2007; Stachenfeld 2008; Wade 1996; Zambraski 1996).

Gastric Emptying and Intestinal Absorption

Optimal fluid balance, especially during exercise, depends on the effectiveness of oral rehydration to maintain plasma volume and electrolyte balance—which in turn depends on the rates of fluid ingestion, gastric emptying, and intestinal fluid absorption (Puhl and Buskirk 1998; Schedl et al. 1994).

Because little water and few nutrients are absorbed in the stomach, these substances must enter the small intestine for absorption. Water is absorbed readily in the small intestine, while other nutrients (glucose, fructose, and sodium) are absorbed at various rates. Therefore, the rate at which water and nutrients empty into the small intestine from the stomach is an important limiting factor to absorption and determines to a great extent the benefit derived from drinking a particular beverage. A good oral rehydration fluid or sport drink should empty rapidly from the stomach, enhance intestinal absorption, and promote fluid retention (Gisolfi et al. 1995). These issues have prompted a number of research questions related to fluid replacement before, during, and after exercise.

- What type of fluid is absorbed most rapidly?
- What is the optimal composition of this fluid?
- Do warm fluids absorb more quickly than cold fluids?
- Is sodium required for fluid absorption and retention? If so, how much?
- What effect do different types of sugars and carbohydrates have on fluid absorption?
- Are sport drinks absorbed more quickly than water or fruit juices?
- Are there other constituents in sport drinks that can enhance fluid absorption?

A number of factors influence the rate of gastric emptying and the subsequent absorption of fluid from the small intestine. Figure 8.2 shows some of the factors known to affect gastric emptying. The primary factors are fluid volume, osmolality, carbohydrate type and concentration, and exercise intensity (Costill 1990; Gisolfi and Ryan 1996). Individual variability in gastric emptying is also important, as Gisolfi and Duchman (1992) discovered. They found that one subject emptied 80% of a 500 mL solution of water in 15 min, while another emptied only 20% of the solution in 15 min. However, the two subjects had emptied similar amounts of the solution by 30 min. This type of individuality in gastric emptying emphasizes two points:

1. Methods for assessing gastric emptying need to measure gastric emptying rates repeatedly over a designated period.

2. Fluid recommendations for athletes need to be individualized based on gastrointestinal complaints, past experience with fluid intake during exercise, sweat rates, and fluid needs.

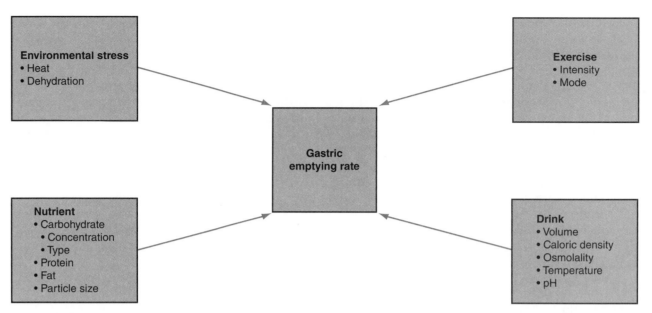

Figure 8.2 Factors influencing gastric emptying rate.

BODY FLUID BALANCE: EXERCISE AND SPORT by C.V. Gisolfi and A.J. Ryan, edited by E.R. Buskirk and S.M. Puhl. Copyright 1996 by Taylor & Francis Group LLC - Books. Reproduced with permission of Taylor & Francis Group LLC - Books in the format Textbook via Copyright Clearance Center.

Gastric Volume

Gastric volume is one of the strongest regulators of gastric emptying. The greater the volume of fluid consumed, the greater the rate of gastric empty-ing. This relationship apparently holds true up to a volume of about 600 mL (Costill 1990; Leiper 2001). Above this point, a further increase in volume may not increase the rate of gastric emptying. Since an average person can empty approximately 40 mL of water per minute from the stomach, or 2.4 L/h, consuming too much fluid during exercise is usu-ally not a limiting factor for most athletes (Gisolfi and Ryan 1996). In fact, most athletes have trouble drinking enough fluids during exercise. Note that consuming a large volume of fluid helps speed gas-tric emptying compared to sipping small amounts of fluids over the same time period.

Osmolality

Osmolality is negatively correlated with gas-tric emptying—adding carbohydrates or other nutrients to a solution generally slows emptying from the stomach compared to **isotonic solu-tions** (those containing electrolytes equivalent in osmolarity to that of body fluid). Since most oral rehydration solutions and sport beverages are low in sodium (35-110 mg/8 oz, or 132-416 mg/L) and in osmolality (<400 mOsm/L), they do not inhibit water absorption (Gisolfi et al. 1995). For example, when Brouns and colleagues (1995)

compared six solutions with equal carbohydrate content but different osmolalities, ranging from 240 to 390 mOsm/L, they found that all drinks emptied from the stomach at a similar rate. The effects of different carbohydrates on osmolality have also been studied, since glucose polymers (frequently used in sport drinks) have a lower osmolality than glucose. The formulation of a rehydration beverage must balance a number of factors: The beverage must be low in osmolality to maintain gastric emptying and absorption, yet must provide carbohydrates for energy and salts to enhance palatability and fluid retention.

Carbohydrate Concentration and Type

The effects of carbohydrate on gastric empty-ing and fluid absorption in the small intestine have been extensively studied, since sport and rehydration beverages include various types of carbohydrates. Because little fluid is absorbed in the stomach, it must leave the stomach and move to the small intestine where fluid absorption can occur. Any factor that decreases gastric emptying may also decrease absorption, since a fluid cannot be absorbed until it leaves the stomach. In gen-eral, as the carbohydrate concentration of a fluid increases, gastric emptying decreases. Depend-ing on the research examined, the effect of low concentrations of carbohydrate solutions (2-8%) on gastric emptying is variable. These differences in gastric emptying rates can be explained by the differing research methods used in various studies—for example, the type of test drink, the volume consumed, types of carbohydrates and electrolytes used, time of administration, varying osmolalities, and sample timing. For example, Vist and Maughan (1994) found that even low concentrations of glucose (2% solution) slowed gastric emptying compared to water (but the difference was not statistically significant); higher glucose concentrations (>2%) significantly decreased gastric emptying. In a follow-up study, Vist and Maughan (1995) reported that both osmolality and carbohydrate content influenced gastric emptying, but that carbohydrate content had a greater influence than osmolality.

It appears that the type of carbohydrate may have less effect than the amount of carbohydrate added to a solution. Although carbohydrate may slow gastric emptying, it appears to enhance fluid and sodium absorption in the small intestine (Gisolfi and Duchman 1992; Gisolfi et al. 1991, 1995). Glucose is actively transported in the gut by a sodium energy-dependent transport system. As carbohydrate and sodium are absorbed, water follows. Thus, transported carbohydrate, cotransported with sodium, is the primary method for promoting water absorption from a sport drink or oral rehydration solution (Schedl et al. 1994). Although the composition of a beverage can affect gastric emptying, solutions containing 2% to 6% simple carbohydrate of various types (glucose, sucrose, fructose, maltodextrins, or various combinations of these sugars) are generally emptied quickly from the stomach and absorbed as well as or better than water (Gisolfi and Ryan 1996; Gisolfi et al. 1992). Therefore, carbohydrate-electrolyte beverages of low concentration (~6% carbohydrate) should not compromise fluid replenishment during exercise (Ryan et al. 1998). Research also shows that a variety of sugars in a sport drink (i.e., glucose and fructose), compared to one type of sugar in a similar dose (i.e., glucose only), is more readily absorbed from the intestinal tract. This appears to be mostly due to different transport mechanisms of sugars such as fructose and glucose across the intestinal wall (Jentjens et al. 2004a, 2004b). Moreover, numerous research studies indicate that these substances improve exercise performance by providing additional energy substrate (see chapter 2, which also discusses intestinal absorption of different types of carbohydrates). Finally, Ploutz-Snyder and colleagues (1999) studied the gastric emptying rates of various carbohydrate-electrolyte replacement beverages with and without carbonation. They found that noncarbonated carbohydrate-electrolyte beverages and water leave the gut sooner than lightly carbonated carbohydrate-electrolyte beverages or carbonated cola.

Exercise Intensity and Type

Although low- to moderate-intensity exercise (~30-70% $\dot{V}O_2$max) for 60 to 90 min appears to have little effect on gastric emptying and intestinal absorption (Gisolfi et al. 1991; Schedl et al. 1994), high-intensity exercise (>70% $\dot{V}O_2$max) delays gastric emptying (Gisolfi and Ryan 1996). Different types of physical activity may also alter the ability to consume fluids, the ease of consuming them, and the way in which they are emptied from the stomach. For example, runners typically have lower fluid intakes than cyclists because it is more difficult to drink while running and because fluid movement in the stomach can be uncomfortable. This lower consumption of fluid in runners can in turn affect gastric emptying. On the other hand, running may aid gastric emptying by increasing mechanical movement of fluids in the stomach and thereby increasing intragastric pressure (Puhl and Buskirk 1998). Running intensity may also influence intestinal permeability (Pals et al. 1997) and reduce blood flow to the gut—both of which may explain some of the gastrointestinal distress associated with intense running. Thus, the amounts of fluid consumed, as well as the effect of a particular sport on gastric emptying and gastrointestinal distress, depend on the nature and intensity of the sport, the type of movement involved, and the amount of fluid consumed.

Euhydration, Hypohydration, Dehydration, and Hyponatremia

Hypohydration refers to a reduction of body water as the body progresses from a normally hydrated (euhydrated) to a dehydrated state. For example, during exercise, **dehydration** can occur because most active people tend to drink too little to offset the water losses that take place due to sweating. In fact, many athletes consume only ~16 oz (0.5 L) of fluid per hour. The amount of fluid they consume is not enough to maintain a state of **euhydration** (normal hydration). Most exercisers end a workout in a state of dehydration that will eventually be corrected by eating and drinking during the postexercise period.

Whether dehydration has performance consequences is a matter of current debate (Sawka and Noakes 2007). According to the American College of Sports Medicine (ACSM), dehydration that exceeds a 2% body weight loss deters aerobic exercise performance in a temperate, warm or hot environment (Sawka et al. 2007). The International Olympic Committee concluded in a consensus statement that dehydration impairs performance in most events, and athletes should consume adequate fluid to limit dehydration to < 2% body weight (Shireffs et al. 2004). Greater levels of dehydration will have a greater effect, although the performance effects are likely dependent on the environmental factors (heat and humidity), the exercise task, and the individual's tolerance to dehydration. Some people are more tolerant of dehydration than others. Dehydration has a marginal effect on aerobic exercise in the cold, (IOM, 2005; Sawka et al. 2007) and according to some research, dehydration (3-5% body weight loss) probably does not impair strength (Eve-tovich et al. 2002; Greiwe et al. 1998) or anaerobic performance (Cheuvront et al. 2006). Dehydration also has various effects on cognitive function (Maughan et al. 2007b; Sawka et al. 2007). The effects of dehydration are summarized in "Physiological Responses to Dehydration."

Dehydration increases hemoconcentration, blood viscosity and osmolality, core body temperature, and heart rate while decreasing stroke volume (Montain and Coyle 1992). Dehydration also hastens the onset of fatigue and makes any given exercise intensity appear harder than if the individual was well hydrated (Sawka et al. 2007). According to Maughan (1992), dehydration is one of the most common nutritional problems that athletes face. Drinking adequate fluids is imperative for good exercise performance (Maughan 1992). In addition, glycogen is used more rapidly when a person exercises while dehydrated. The most serious effect of progressive dehydration, however,

Physiological Responses to Dehydration

Increases In:
- Gastrointestinal distress
- Plasma osmolality
- Blood viscosity
- Heart rate
- Core temperature at which sweating begins
- Core temperature at which blood flow increases in skin
- Muscle glycogen use

Decreases In:
- Plasma volume
- Splanchnic and renal blood flow
- Central blood volume
- Central venous pressure
- Stroke volume
- Cardiac output
- Sweat rate at a given core temperature
- Maximal sweat rate
- Skin blood flow at a given core temperature
- Performance
- Endurance capacity (exercise to exhaustion)

Reprinted, by permission, from R. Murray, 1995, "Fluid needs in hot and cold environments," *International Journal of Sport Nutrition* 5: S62-S73.

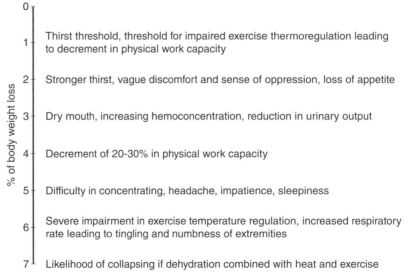

Figure 8.3 Adverse effects of dehydration on work capacity.
Reprinted, by permission, from J.E. Greenleaf, 1992, "Problem: thirst, drinking behavior and involuntary dehydration," *Medicine and Science in Sports and Exercise* 24: 645-656.

is that reduced blood flow to the skin limits the body's ability to sweat. This in turn reduces the body's ability to cool itself, which increases core body temperature and the risk of heat illness and collapse—and, in rare situations, life-threatening exertional heatstroke (Sutton 1990). "Heat-Related Disorders" outlines various types of heat-related disorders, as well as factors that increase the risk for heat illness.

Dehydration can cause significant reductions in cardiac output since the reduction in stroke volume can be greater than the increase in heart rate (Convertino et al. 1996; Sawka et al. 2007). Figure 8.3 provides an overview of the effects of

Highlight

Heat-Related Disorders

Several severe heat disorders can deteriorate exercise performance and may lead to adverse health effects and even death.

Exercise-Associated Muscle Cramps (Exertional Heat Cramps)

Skeletal muscle spasms occur after prolonged, strenuous exercise in the heat when sweat losses are high, urine volume is low, and sodium intake is inadequate to replace the losses. Muscle cramps occur most often in American football and tennis (Bergeron 2003a), probably because these activities are played over a prolonged period of time and are accompanied by large fluid and electrolyte losses. However, these types of cramps are also common in athletes participating in long-distance races, in which duration and intensity often exceed what has been experienced in training. Cramps usually occur in the legs, arms, or abdominal wall (Bergeron 1996, 2003a, 2003b). Factors predisposing individuals to these cramps include exercise-associated muscle fatigue, body water loss, and a large sweat sodium loss (Bergeron 1996, 2003a). It is hypothesized that the primary mechanism behind these muscle cramps is the extreme loss of sweat sodium (Sutton 1990; Bergeron 2003a). Stofan and colleagues (2005) studied National Collegiate Athletic Association (NCAA) Division I football players in action on the field during summer training. In a matched-pair design ("crampers" matched to "noncrampers"), sweat loss was not different between crampers and noncrampers, but crampers lost 10.4 g of sodium over the course of the day (two practices, 2.5 h each)—more than twice as much as the noncrampers. This amount of sodium equals about 5 tsp of salt lost in one day of college football practice. Significant quantities of calcium, magnesium, and potassium are not lost during exercise, and thus cramps are most likely related to the extreme sodium losses, which are then insufficiently replaced (Bergeron 2003a). In a case study of a tennis player who suffered from recurring episodes of muscle cramps, treatment with a higher amount of sodium in his diet in the form of table salt resolved the disorder (Bergeron 1996).

When a cramp occurs, the best treatment is to stretch the muscle group at full length and add sodium to fluid (add 1/8 to 1/4 tsp table salt to 300-500 mL water or sport drink). Alternative solutions might include consuming one or two salt tablets with 300 to 500 mL of fluid; eating salty snacks such as pretzels, pickles, or jerky combined with water; or sipping broth (Armstrong et al. 2007b). As with many things, prevention is better than treatment. Muscle cramps can be prevented through the maintenance of fluid and salt balance. Athletes who have a history of **exercise-associated muscle cramps** may need extra sodium when exercising in the heat. They can obtain the extra sodium by increasing the consumption of dietary salt to 5 to 10 g/day when exercising in the heat, especially during the phase of heat acclimatization. This topic is addressed in more detail later in the chapter. Heat cramps per se are thought to be somewhat different from exercise-associated muscle cramps and are characterized by different signs and symptoms. Heat cramps are possible with prolonged exposure to heat or physical activity (or both) in temperatures between 90° and 105° F (~32-41° C) (National Weather Service 2006).

Exertional Heat Exhaustion and Heatstroke

Plasma volume decreases during exercise, reducing blood flow from the muscles to the skin—which in turn compromises the body's ability to dissipate the heat generated during exercise and to adequately

(continued)

cool itself. The result is that the body's heat production exceeds its ability to dissipate heat—and core body temperature rises to >104° F (>40° C). Dehydration exacerbates these physiological changes and contributes to heat-related problems. Think of these two illnesses as on a continuum—**exertional heat exhaustion** can lead to **exertional heatstroke** (exertional heat exhaustion is less severe than heatstroke, which can lead to a loss of consciousness and even death). Early symptoms of heat injury are excessive sweating, headache, nausea, dizziness, a gradual impairment of consciousness, and difficulty concentrating. Almost all individuals suffering from exertional heatstroke exhibit sweat-soaked and pale skin at the time of collapse (Armstrong et al. 2007b). This is markedly different from the classic type of heatstroke, which is nonexertion related and is characterized by dry, hot, and flushed skin (Sutton 1986). Environmental conditions that predispose exercisers to heat exhaustion or exertional heatstroke are hot, humid, windless conditions or unseasonably hot conditions to which they are not acclimatized. People are more susceptible to heatstroke if they are unfit, overweight, dehydrated, sleep deprived, unacclimatized to the heat, or ill (with an infection, diarrhea, vomiting, or fever). Nevertheless, exertional heatstroke can also occur in a well-trained, healthy, and heat-acclimated athlete who is exercising at high intensity if heat loss is insufficient to balance metabolic heat production (Armstrong et al. 1994).

Finally, children and people who are elderly are more susceptible than other groups to heat-related injury because they have less sensitive homeostatic mechanisms for fluid balance (Sutton 1990). The greatest risk for exertional heatstroke exists when the wet bulb globe temperature (WBGT) exceeds 82° F (28° C) during high-intensity exercise. See p. 240 for an explanation of WBGT and table 8.3 for safe exercise guidelines under dangerous environmental conditions.

In American football, exertional heatstroke usually happens during the first four days of preseason practice in the month of August, when the days are hottest and most humid and when the players are the least fit. These athletes' risk for a heatstroke dramatically rises if they experience a multitude of stressors such as a sudden increase in training, long initial heat exposure, wearing a heavy uniform, getting too little sleep, being dehydrated, and eating a poor diet. In addition, repetitive training days with a similar environmental stress and physical demand can raise the risk for a heatstroke (read more on this topic on p. 242). Lately, several cases of collapse in football have also pointed at the use of dietary supplements such as ephedrine, synephrine, and ma huang, as well as the use of other stimulants, drugs (e.g., ecstasy), or medications (e.g., antidepressant), that may increase the body's heat production. In any case, it should be clear that exertional heatstroke is probably a consequence of a variety of compounding factors. Treatment of exertional heatstroke requires immediate whole-body cooling with cold water and ice water immersion therapy. For more information, refer to ACSM's position stand on exertional heat illness during training and competition (Armstrong et al. 2007b) and read "ACSM's Position Stand on Exercise and Fluid Replacement" on p. 246.

Rhabdomyolysis

Rhabdomyolysis is a syndrome that occurs with novel, strenuous exercise and is characterized by the release of skeletal muscle contents. Rhabdomyolysis is defined as the breakdown of muscle fibers (Armstrong et al. 2007b). It occurs most commonly in unaccustomed exercisers who experience eccentric and concentric muscle overuse. But it can also occur in exertional heat illness in trained athletes when muscle tissue exceeds the critical temperature threshold of cell membranes (Armstrong et al. 2007b). Indeed, hyperthermia increases the permeability of muscle membranes, and heat can decompose cell membranes so that myoglobin leaks out, increasing the risk of toxicity and obstruction of the kidney. Research indicates that dehydration can exacerbate the symptoms of rhabdomyolysis, mainly due to the acute kidney failure seen with rhabdomyolysis (Armstrong et al. 2007b). Reports come predominantly from the military, relating to soldiers who were hospitalized for serious heat illness. Twenty-five percent had rhabdomyolysis, and 13% had acute kidney failure (Carter et al. 2005). It appears that heat stress, dehydration, and unaccustomed training can lead to severe health problems such as rhabdomyolysis, which can be fatal. However, rhabdomyolysis can also occur in marathon runners (Clarkson 2007); and a recent case study described dehydration, muscle cramping, and rhabdomyolysis in a high school football player (Cleary et al. 2007).

continued dehydration on thirst, on the ability to perform work, and on physiological functions. This figure presents the possible progression of dehydration and thirst in relation to performance and health. It is unclear whether it is thirst or the loss of total body water that initially deters exercise performance (Sawka and Noakes 2007). Dr. Timothy Noakes, a physician and scientist at Capetown University in South Africa, hypothesizes that what impairs exercise performance is thirst rather than the progressive loss of total body water. He suggests that athletes who drink sufficiently to prevent thirst during exercise will optimize performance regardless of the extent to which they become dehydrated (Sawka and Noakes 2007). Regardless of what actually impairs performance, thirst or loss of body water, fluid replacement recommendations during exercise need to be made on an individual basis. Athletes should estimate sweat loss from weight loss (% of body weight). This topic is addressed in greater detail later in the chapter (see p. 245).

As one becomes progressively dehydrated, which body water pools does the water come from? According to an early study by Costill and colleagues (1976), who dehydrated subjects using a combination of cycling exercise and heat exposure, low levels of dehydration remove water primarily from the extracellular space. As body water losses increase, a proportionally greater percentage of water comes from the intracellular spaces. When Costill's subjects lost 9% of their body weight due to dehydration, ~50% of the lost water was intracellular water. This means that body cells, especially muscle cells that are 70% water, were being depleted of the water necessary to maintain metabolic functions—perhaps this is one of the reasons dehydration hinders exercise performance. Researchers have also examined the effect of exercise, without prior dehydration, on change in body water compartments (Maw et al. 1998). When subjects cycled for 50 min at moderate intensity (50% $\dot{V}O_2$max) in a cool environment (60° F or 14.4° C), fluid losses came primarily from the extracellular fluid. When they repeated the protocol in a hot environment (97° F or 36.2° C), 23% of the fluid losses came from the intracellular environment. Thus, progressive dehydration in well-hydrated people doing moderate exercise primarily depletes extracellular fluid; when the stress of heat is added, some fluid is drawn from the intracellular space.

Environmental conditions have a dramatic effect on fluid loss. As temperature and humidity rise, exercising becomes harder and the risks of heat-related problems increase. Table 8.3 outlines

Table 8.3 Wet Globe Temperature Levels for Modification or Cancellation of Workouts or Athletic Competition for Healthy Adults[a]

WBGT[b], °F	WBGT, °C	Risk to exercise	Comments
≤50 and 50.1-65.0	≤10 and 10.1-18.3	Generally safe	Exertional heat illness can occur associated with individual factors during continuous activity and competition.
65.1-72.0	18.4-22.2	Increased risk of heat illness for high-risk individuals	High-risk individuals should be monitored or should not compete, and coaches should increase rest/work ratio and adjust exercise duration and intensity and monitor fluid intake.
72.1-82.0	22.3-27.8	Increased risk of heat illness for all competitors	High-risk individuals should be monitored or should not compete, and coaches should increase rest/work ratio and adjust exercise duration and intensity and monitor fluid intake in all athletes.
82.1-86.0	27.9-30.0	High risk	Coaches should increase rest/work ratio to 1:1 and adjust exercise duration and intensity of high-risk individuals and also watch and plan activity for acclimated[c] individuals carefully. All athletes' fluid balance should be monitored, and athletes should be watched carefully.
86.1-90.0	30.1-32.2	Very high risk	Cancel or stop practice or competition in high-risk individuals and limit intense exercise and heat exposure in acclimated[c] individuals; watch for signs and symptoms of heat stress.
≥90.1	>32.3	Very high risk	Cancel exercise for all athletes.[d]

[a] Revised from Casa and Eichner 2005; [b] wet bulb globe temperature; [c] acclimated to training in the heat for at least three weeks; [d] internal heat production exceeds heat loss.

Adapted, by permission, from L.E. Armstrong et. al., 2007, "American College of Sports Medicine position stand: Exertional heat illness during training and competition, *Medicine and Science in Sports and Exercise* 39: 556-572.

the effects of air temperature, relative humidity, and solar radiation on potential environmental heat hazards. As the **wet bulb globe temperature (WBGT)** rises, the risks of exercising in the heat also rise. **Wet bulb** is an index of relative humidity (the method for calculating WBGT follows). **Dry bulb** is an index of ambient temperature (the actual air temperature measured on a thermometer). If the dry bulb and wet bulb temperatures are the same, the air has a humidity of 100% and evaporation is impossible. The **black bulb** is an index of heat radiation from the environment (e.g., from the sun). The combination of these three temperatures into a single factor is known as the wet bulb globe temperature.

WBGT = 0.7 (Wet bulb temperature) + 0.2 (Black bulb temperature) + 0.1 (Dry bulb temperature).

The greatest contributor to the WBGT is humidity (wet bulb), whereas the ambient temperature (dry bulb) contributes the least. Thus, it is easier and safer to exercise in a hot environment with a low humidity than in a hot environment with a high humidity. For example, it is easier to exercise in the Southwest of the United States or the Mediterranean countries when the temperature is 90° F (32° C) with 10% humidity (heat index <90° F) than it is to exercise in the South of the United States or China when the temperature is 90° F with 90% humidity (heat index = 122° F). The greatest risk for exertional heatstroke exists when the WBGT exceeds 82° F (28° C) during high-intensity exercise or strenuous exercise exceeding 1 h (Armstrong et al. 2007b). As the humidity rises, it is harder for the body to cool itself through evaporation of sweat from the skin. If you do not have access to wet and black bulb temperatures, you can use the heat index chart in figure 8.4 to calculate a rough index of the WBGT by using just the air temperature and relative humidity. The one part of the WBGT that this chart does not include is the effect of radiated heat. For this reason, it is important to remember that exercising in direct sunlight increases the temperature. The U.S. National Weather Service

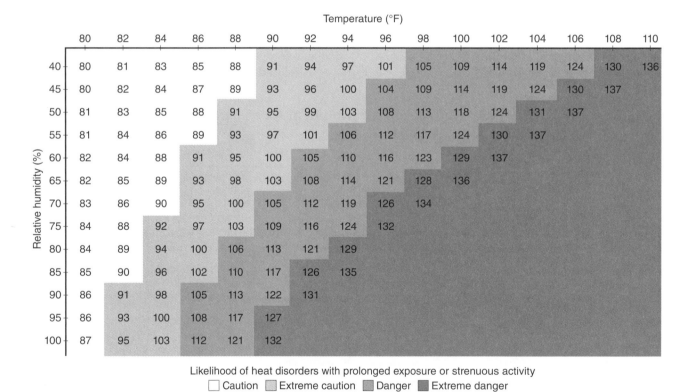

Likelihood of heat disorders with prolonged exposure or strenuous activity
☐ Caution ☐ Extreme caution ▨ Danger ■ Extreme danger

Figure 8.4 This heat index chart provides general guidelines for assessing the potential severity of heat stress. Individual reactions to heat will vary. It should be remembered that heat illness can occur at lower temperatures than indicated on the chart. In addition, studies suggest that the susceptibility to heat illness tends to increase with age.

Reprinted from National Weather Service, National Oceanic and Atmospheric Administration, Dept. of Commerce, Heat Index Chart. June, 2006. Available: www.nws.noaa.gov.

(2006) developed this chart to alert Americans to the dangers of developing heat-related illnesses when temperatures rise. As the air temperature and the humidity rise, the heat index values increase. For example, when the air temperature is 86° F (~30° C) and the relative humidity is 40%, it feels like 85° F (~29° C). If the air temperature is 86° F (~30° C) and the relative humidity is 95%, it feels like 108° F (~42° C). As indicated by the heat index chart, exercising outside on such a day can pose real health risks. The heat index values were devised for shady, light-wind conditions; and exposure to full sunshine can increase heat index values by up to 15° F (~6° C). Strong winds, especially combined with very hot dry air, can also increase heat index values.

How to Use the Heat Index Chart

1. Across the top, locate the air temperature (°F).
2. Down the left side of the chart, locate the relative humidity (%).
3. Follow down and across to find the apparent temperature. Apparent temperature is the combined index of heat and humidity. It is an index of the body's sensation of heat caused by the temperature and humidity. In other words, it is what the temperature "feels like" to the body.
4. Note that the exposure to full sunshine can increase heat index values by up to 15° F.

Reprinted from National Weather Service, National Oceanic and Atmospheric Administration, Dept. of Commerce, Heat Index Chart. June, 2006. www.nws.noaa.gov.

The term hypohydration is also frequently used to refer to **voluntary dehydration** that many athletes self-impose before a competitive exercise event. Athletes usually do this in order to make weight for a particular sport (e.g., wrestling, rowing, boxing, or horse racing) or to improve muscle definition and physical appearance (e.g., bodybuilders before competition). Hypohydration can negatively affect exercise performance and health because, in this case, the individual *begins* the competition depleted of body water and then experiences further dehydration during the competition. The result can be muscle fatigue, loss of concentration, and poor exercise performance. For example, a wrestler may lose 6 to 11 lb (3-5 kg) of his body weight three days prior to weigh-in and another 2.2 lb (1 kg) or more during the match. While most wrestlers try to rehydrate after weigh-in but before their match begins, total rehydration is not always possible. Their ability to

rehydrate depends on the level of hypohydration earlier imposed and the amount of time between weigh-in and competition. Some wrestlers experience severe dehydration by the end of the match, especially if they are competing indoors under conditions that increase sweat rate and water loss. Using dehydration to lose weight can have serious consequences. "Dehydration-Related Deaths in Three Collegiate Wrestlers in 1997" (see highlight on p. 242) demonstrates the potential lethality of severe dehydration. One of the outcomes of the dehydration-related deaths in college and high school wrestling was a rule change that requires all athletes to undergo hydration status assessment prior to establishing the minimum weight for competition (Wrestling Rules Committee, NCAA 2003; Wrestling Rules Committee, NFSHSA, 2003). The purpose of these new rules is to prevent extreme methods of weight loss and their potential health risks, as well as to promote competitive sportsmanship among the athletes.

Exercise-associated hyponatremia (EAH) refers to abnormally low plasma sodium concentrations (< 135 mmol/L) before, during, or after exercise. This condition usually occurs when excess water accumulates, relative to sodium, in the extracellular water compartments of the body. The primary factor responsible for EAH appears to be the consumption of fluids (water or sport drink) in excess of total body fluid loss (i.e., transcutaneous, respiratory, gastrointestinal, sweat, and renal fluid loss) (Hew-Butler et al. 2008). Early symptoms of hyponatremia include bloating, "puffiness," nausea, vomiting, and headaches. With plasma sodium levels <125 mmol/L and falling, symptoms of hyponatremia become increasingly more severe and include headache, vomiting, swollen hands and feet, restlessness, undue fatigue, confusion and disorientation (due to the progressive encephalopathy), and wheezy breathing (due to pulmonary edema) (Sawka et al. 2007). Victims of hyponatremia may have seizures, fall into a coma, or even die (Hew-Butler et al. 2008). While there are many clinical causes of hyponatremia, during exercise it usually seems to result from excessive consumption of hypotonic (low sodium) fluid that exceeds a person's sweating rate (Sawka et al. 2007). Besides excessive fluid consumption (>1.5 L/h of exercise), weight gain during exercise, low body weight, exercise duration >4 h or slow running pace, female gender, availability of fluids, and extreme cold or hot temperatures represent additional risk factors for hyponatremia (Rosner and Kirven 2007; Hew-Butler et al. 2008).

Dehydration-Related Deaths
in Three Collegiate Wrestlers in 1997

During late autumn of 1997, three previously healthy collegiate wrestlers living in different states died while engaging in programs of rapid weight loss to qualify for competition. In the hours before the official weigh-in, all three wrestlers engaged in weight loss regimens that promoted dehydration. They also restricted fluid and food intake and tried to maximize sweat losses by wearing vapor-impermeable suits under cotton warm-ups and by exercising vigorously in hot environments. Remick and colleagues (1998) compiled the complete details of these three cases for the Centers for Disease Control and Prevention.

Case 1

In North Carolina, a 19-year-old wrestler attempted to lose 15 lb (6.8 kg) in a 12 h period so he could compete in the 195 lb (88.6 kg) weight class of a wrestling tournament. His preseason weight was 233 lb (106 kg), and over the next 10 weeks he lost 23 lb (10.5 kg). Using the weight loss regimen described, this wrestler lost 9 lb (4 kg) in 8 h. After a 2 h rest, he exercised for another hour, at which time he felt poorly and stopped exercising. Within an hour he went into cardiac arrest and died.

Case 2

In Wisconsin, a 22-year-old wrestler attempted to lose 4 lb (1.8 kg) in a 4 h period so he could compete in the 153 lb (69.5 kg) weight class of a tournament. His preseason weight was 178 lb (81 kg); over the next 10 weeks he lost 21 lb (9.5 kg), of which 8 lb (3.6 kg) were lost over the three days prior to his death. On the day of his death, he initiated the weight loss regimen described and lost 3.6 lb (1.6 kg) in 3 h. During this time he complained of shortness of breath but continued to exercise. After resting for 30 min, he resumed exercising again but stopped 30 min later because he was not feeling well. He then became unresponsive, went into cardiac arrest, and could not be resuscitated.

Case 3

In Michigan, a 21-year-old wrestler attempted to lose 6 lb (2.7 kg) in a 3 h period in order to compete in the 153 lb (69.5 kg) weight class of a wrestling tournament. His preseason weight was 180 lb (82 kg); over the next 13 weeks he lost 21 lb (9.5 kg), of which 11 lb (5 kg) were lost over the two days prior to his death. On the day of his death, he initiated the weight loss regimen described, lost 2.3 lb (1 kg) in 1.5 h, and weighed 156.7 lb (71.2 kg). He then participated in wrestling practice; after practice, he continued the same weight loss regimen. Within the next 75 min, he lost another 2 lb (0.9 kg). He then took a 15 min rest and continued to exercise for another hour, at which time he stopped to weigh himself. A few minutes later, his legs became unsteady. He became incommunicative, went into cardiac arrest, and died.

Dehydration-Related Deaths in Football Players
During Preseason Conditioning

From 1960 to 2007 in the United States, 114 football players died from heatstroke. Particularly during preseason conditioning, heat- and dehydration-related problems seem to persist despite heightened awareness and prevention strategies. Striking were the reports in 2006, when five young athletes, from 11 to 17 years old, died of heatstroke. Several other deaths were reported in the same year, but they were not clearly attributable to heatstroke. In 2007, two cases of heatstroke deaths at the high school level were reported (National Center for Catastrophic Sport Injury Research 2008; Bergeron et al. 2005), and this reduction is probably due to increased caution and better training and hydration strategies in the preseason. When core temperature rises to 103° or 104° F (~40° C), the brain's hypothalamus loses its ability to regulate the heat. The heart begins to beat faster to increase the blood flow to the skin and aid in heat dissipation. This leads to a decrease in blood flow to the heart and muscle. Brain death begins around a body core temperature of 106° F (41° C). But death from heatstroke is not always sudden. In fact, it is possible for an athlete to gradually deteriorate over the course of several training days when organs begin to fail (National Center for Catastrophic Sport Injury Research 2008). This was the case with U.S. pro football player Corey Stringer, who died in a training camp. He was the first professional football player to die from heatstroke in the 82-year history of the National Football League (NFL). Stringer apparently was unable to complete practice on the day before he died. He also showed other signs of heat exhaustion, such as vomiting, but continued to train the following day. Unfortunately, Stringer died of heatstroke at a heat index of 109° F (~43° C). Stringer's body temperature was 108° F (~42° C) on the field, and he died 15 h later in the hospital (Randall 2001).

The National Center for Catastrophic Sport Injury Research (NCCSI) is a center that conducts the Annual Survey of Football Injury Research. The primary purpose of the survey is to make football a safer and more enjoyable game. Many rule changes and prevention strategies have gradually reduced the number of injuries, including those related to heat stress. Both exertional heatstroke and heat exhaustion can be prevented by the control of various factors during preseason conditioning. In hot weather, the NCCSI recommends the following precautions:

1. Athletes need to be evaluated by a physician before starting to play.

2. Athletes need to be acclimatized to the heat gradually over the course of 7 to 10 days.

3. The heat index determines the heat stress on the athlete. One should carefully evaluate the heat index when planning preseason training, and practice should be altered at a wet bulb temperature exceeding 78° F (25.5° C).

4. Rest periods should be frequent and should be offered in the shade, and athletes should be able to temporarily remove clothing and pads.

5. Cool fluids should be available at all times, and coaches should provide fluids regularly.

6. Salt should be replaced daily through dietary and not pharmaceutical means.

7. Athletes should weigh in each day before and after practice; losing more than 3% body weight through fluid loss is approaching the danger zone for dehydration in the sport of football during preseason training.

8. Clothing should be breathable, and athletes should not wear long-sleeved shirts, long stockings, or any excess clothing.

9. Athletes at risk for heat injury, those who are overweight, are undertrained, or have a history of heat-related problems and dehydration, should be watched closely.

10. Signs of heat illness include nausea, incoherence, fatigue, weakness, vomiting, cramps, a rapid pulse, flushed appearance, visual disturbances, and unsteadiness. Heatstroke victims may sweat quite strongly. A physician should be contacted immediately if any of these signs are apparent.

11. Treatment for heat illness may include cool water immersion, fanning, or the use of ice baths, all of which reduce the athlete's core temperature.

National Center for Catastrophic Sport Injury Research, *Annual survey of football injury research 1931-2007.* January, 2008. Available: http://unc.edu/depts./nccsi/SurveyofFootballInjuries.htm.

Exercise-associated hyponatremia can occur in a variety of settings. For example, in 1996 a woman developed hyponatremia during an all-day hike in the heat of the Grand Canyon in Arizona, consuming only bottled water and low-sodium foods (Richards 1996). Noakes and colleagues (1990) reported that in the 1986 and 1987 Comrades Marathon in South Africa, 9% of collapsed runners had hyponatremia. Almond and colleagues (2005) found that in the 2002 Boston Marathon, 13% of the 488 runners examined had hyponatremia. Exercise-associated hyponatremia also occurs in football and tennis as too much fluid may be ingested to treat or prevent exercise-associated heat cramps (Herfel et al. 1998; Dimeff 2006). There are also several reports of hospitalizations due to hyponatremia that appeared to have been mistreated with intravenous fluids (Sawka et al. 2007) or recommendations to drink large volumes of fluid (O'Brien et al. 2001). To prevent hyponatremia, athletes should avoid overconsumption of fluid before, during, and after exercise. It is important that fluid assessment include the measurement of body weight before and after exercise to estimate sweating rate and to individualize fluid replacement. While losing weight during exercise is normal due to a mismatch of fluid intake and sweat loss, gaining weight from too much drinking is not normal and can have severe consequences. Thirst can also be used as an indicator to drink during exercise, especially in mature athletes. It is important to note that sport drinks by themselves cannot prevent hyponatremia because their sodium content is lower than 135 mmol/L; if excess fluid is consumed and retained in the body during exercise, it will still cause a dilution of plasma sodium levels (Hew-Butler et al. 2008). Athletes should participate in educational workshops in which fluid replacement strategies are discussed and in which they have the opportunity to estimate their sweating rate and calculate fluid needs (see table 8.4 for estimating your sweating rate).

FLUID AND ELECTROLYTE RECOMMENDATIONS FOR EXERCISE

Exercise increases the loss of water and electrolytes from the body. Dehydration can increase cardiovascular stress and limit the body's ability to cool itself (Sawka et al. 2007). These physiological changes increase the probability that exercise performance may be compromised. This section outlines fluid recommendations for before, during, and after exercise. The recommendations assume that the active person, regardless of skill level, is beginning the exercise event well fed and hydrated. Anyone who has dehydrated prior to exercise in order to make weight, or who has been ill or dieting prior to the event, should change the recommendations given here to account for his or her current state of hydration and nutrition. Since people typically are weak and dehydrated following illness and dieting, they should do all they can to nourish and hydrate themselves before exercise.

Fluid Needs Before Exercise

Because most athletes do not match fluid intake to their sweat loss during exercise, it is essential that athletes and active individuals begin exercise in a well-hydrated state. Athletes in weight-class sports (with weigh-ins) and people training or racing in environments to which they have not yet acclimatized are at greatest risk to begin exercise in a dehydrated state; thus, athletes in these situations need to pay extra attention to hydration before beginning their event or training session. The ACSM has recently published an update of its position stand on exercise and fluid replacement from 1996 (Sawka et al. 2007) (see p. 246). The recommendation is that athletes and active individuals consume 5-7 mL/kg body weight 4 h before exercise.

One way to check the level of hydration before exercise is to monitor urine volume and color. If urine volume is very small and the color of the urine is dark, the recommendation is to drink another 3-5 mL/kg body weight about 2 h before exercise (Sawka et al. 2007). These recommendations are given in metric units, and it is not realistic to convert them to fluid ounces because the amounts per pound of body weight are so small that they are difficult to measure (1 fl oz of water = 28.4 mL of water). It is best that athletes get into the habit of using water bottles that are labeled in cups, ounces, liters, and milliliters. Even the calculations of "estimated" sweating rate are much simpler and quicker with the use of kilograms and liters versus pounds and ounces. The level of fluid intake before exercise suggested in the preceding paragraph should ensure adequate hydration and allow time for the excretion of excess fluid as urine before the session begins. It should also help to correct any fluid imbalance that may have been present before exercise and help delay or avoid the negative effects of large fluid shifts during

Table 8.4 Estimating the Sweating Rate for an Athlete From Pre- and Postexercise Weight Changes

Date	Temp	Relative humidity	Weight pre	Weight post	Weight change	Fluid intake	Urine output	Total sweat loss[a]	Exercise duration	Hourly sweating rate	Weight change (%)	Thirst (1-10)	Heart rate	RPE (1-10)
7/08	75° F	50%	130 lb (59 kg)	128 lb (58.2 kg)	2 lb (0.8 kg)	12 oz (~350 ml)	0	0.8 + 0.350 = 1.15	1.5 h	1.15 / 1.5 = 0.75 L (24 oz)	1.6	4	150	6
Comments for session: 7/08 Workout was running on flat terrain, it was windy, did not feel extremely thirsty, a bit dry at the end, felt I could pull it through well. Felt that my fluid intake was good. RPE was what coach wanted me to do. Felt comfortable.														
Comments for session:														
Comments for session:														

[a] Total sweat loss: weight change + fluid intake; RPE: Rating of Perceived Exertion.

Steps to estimate hourly sweating rate:

1. Make sure you are hydrated before the exercise session.

2. Warm up for 5 to 10 min or until you begin to sweat. Urinate if necessary.

3. Take a nude body weight on a stable scale with an accuracy of 0.1 kg before exercise, and repeat the process after exercise.

4. Use a heart rate monitor and measure your heart rate.

5. Subtract weight post from weight pre to calculate weight change; if you are converting from pounds to kilograms, divide pounds by 2.2.

6. Measure and add fluid consumed (Fluid intake) to weight change; if you are converting from ounces to milliliters and liters, divide ounces by 28.4 to convert to milliliters (ml) and then by 1000 to convert to liters (L).

7. If no urine was passed, leave this blank or it is equal to 0. If you collected urine, subtract it in liters from weight change (number 6 above: use same conversion as in number 5 above: converting fluid ounces to ml and then to L).

8. Divide total sweat loss (weight change + fluid intake − urine output) by exercise duration in hours to get an hourly sweating rate.

9. Convert your weight change from pounds or kilograms to % weight change. Did you exceed 2%?

10. Rate the thirst you perceived during exercise: 1 = not thirsty; 10 = highly thirsty with a dry mouth

11. Record your heart rate.

12. Rate the effort you perceived during exercise (RPE); 1 = no effort; 10 = the highest effort)

13. Consider your fluid intake. Was it enough to maintain your effort?

14. Whereas thirst, heart rate, and RPE are not used to calculate your sweating rate, these factors are important for evaluating your fluid replacement strategy for this particular exercise session and environment. It may be that you exceeded a 2% body weight loss by replacing fluid in an amount lower than the amount you lost through sweat, but that you were able to complete your session with the RPE set by you or your coach. In addition, you did not feel thirsty and your heart rate responded normally to the intensity of the workout. As you can see, this spreadsheet could include more information such as total work accomplished, type of fluid, other energy sources from food or fluids, and possible sources of error to consider for this calculation. It's best to make your own spreadsheet that you can tweak in accordance with your needs. The goal of this spreadsheet is to monitor your fluid balance and to identify the range of fluid intake that best fits your sport in various environments. Ultimately, this should help you to optimize your race strategies!

Highlight

ACSM's Position Stand on Exercise and Fluid Replacement

This position statement replaces the 1996 position stand on exercise and fluid replacement (Sawka et al. 2007). Position stands by professional organizations are evidence based (see Highlight "What Does Evidence Based Mean?") and serve as a valued resource for health professionals, professional organizations, and governmental agencies. The new position stand on exercise and fluid replacement includes a *strength of recommendation taxonomy* to document the strength of evidence for recommendations and conclusions related to exercise and fluid replacement. The following statements are based on category A evidence and may serve as solid facts based on current research. If you are interested in reading statements from category B or category C, go to www.acsm.org.

- Exercise can elicit high sweating rates and substantial water and electrolyte losses during exercise, particularly in warm-hot weather.
- There is considerable variability for water and electrolyte losses between individuals and between different activities.
- If sweat water and electrolyte losses are not replaced, the person will dehydrate.
- Body weight changes can reflect sweat losses during exercise and can be used to calculate individual fluid replacement needs for specific exercise and environmental conditions.
- Dehydration increases physiologic strain and perceived effort to perform a given exercise task and is accentuated in warm-hot weather.
- Dehydration (>2% body weight) can degrade aerobic exercise performance, especially in warm-hot weather.
- Dehydration (3-5% body weight) does not degrade either anaerobic performance or muscular strength (A and B evidence category).
- Dehydration is a risk factor for both heat exhaustion and exertional heatstroke (A and B evidence category).
- Symptomatic exercise-associated hyponatremia can occur in endurance events.
- Fluid consumption that exceeds sweating rate is the primary factor leading to exercise-associated hyponatremia.
- Women generally have lower sweating rates than men.
- Older adults have age-related decreased thirst sensitivity when dehydrated, making them slower to voluntarily establish euhydration.
- Meal consumption promotes euhydration.
- Sweat electrolyte (sodium and potassium) losses should be fully replaced to reestablish euhydration.

Adapted, by permission, from M.N. Sawka et al., 2007, "American College of Sports Medicine position stand: Exercise and fluid replacement," *Medicine and Science in Sports Exercise* 39: 377-390.

exercise. In hot weather, however, it may be wise to add ~8 to 16 oz (250-500 mL) prior to exercise (Murray 1998). Consuming fluids containing sodium (20-50 mmol/L) before exercise or having a small salted snack such as pretzels (or both) will also help stimulate thirst and retain consumed fluids (Sawka et al. 2007).

Athletes and active individuals do well when training their bodies to absorb larger fluid volumes. One of the factors influencing gastric emptying is the volume of fluid and related stomach distension. To achieve optimal fluid delivery, it may be best to begin exercise with a comfortably large amount of fluid in the stomach. During exer-

Highlight

What Does "Evidence Based" Mean?

An abundance of information regarding nutrition and exercise is communicated over the Internet and through magazines, newspapers, scientific publications, books, and TV specials. When do you know whether a source of information is reliable and trustworthy? When do you know that your approach when working with a client is **evidence based?** The term "evidence based" refers to the systematic review of scientific evidence. This includes the evaluation and synthesis of the best available evidence from research, national guidelines, policies, consensus statements, expert opinion, and quality improvement data (American Dietetic Association 2006). Both the American Dietetic Association and ACSM have used an evidence based approach to summarize important research questions pertaining to nutrition and exercise. These publications are presented as position statements and typically provide a hierarchy of evidence (see the following list) from strongest (A) to weakest (D), depending on the extent to which a research question has been investigated and the methodology used (i.e., types of research designs).

- A: Randomized controlled trials: rich body of data or evidence. Definition: A consistent pattern of findings is provided from substantial studies.

- B: Randomized controlled trials: limited body of data or evidence available. Definition: Few randomized trials exist, or they are small in size and the results are inconsistent.

- C: Nonrandomized trials or observational studies. Definition: Outcomes are from uncontrolled, nonrandomized, or observational studies.

- D: Panel consensus judgment. Definition: Panel's expert opinion is that the evidence is insufficient to place the research in categories A through C.

For more information go to http://www.nhlbi.nih.gov/guidelines/obesity/

An excerpt of a recent position statement on exercise and fluid replacement published by ACSM in 2007 (Sawka et al. 2007) was presented earlier in the chapter. To the practitioner, these statements provide a highly reliable source of information to use for recommending sport nutrition strategies to athletes and active individuals.

---

cise, it is important to maintain a good strategy of fluid replacement (Noakes et al. 1991), of course not neglecting one's sweating rate and individual thirst response to exercise (Sawka and Noakes 2007). Most athletes will tolerate a fluid bolus of 10.5 to 14 fl oz (300-400 mL) about 15 to 20 min before exercise begins (Noakes et al. 1991).

Little work has focused on hydration in the week prior to competition in a hot environment. However, researchers in one study doubled fluid intake in heat-acclimated subjects for one week and found a significant increase in fluid retention and balance prior to the event (Kristal-Boneh et al. 1995). Despite the benefits of **hyperhydration** (e.g., increased sweating rate and reduced cardiovascular and thermal stress; Moroff and Bass 1965; Greenleaf 1992; Nadel et al. 1980), hyperhydration often leads to a quick elimination of water through the kidney, which minimizes the time period during which the body can maintain an

increased level of water (Freund 1996). Because of this effect, researchers have studied the potential for hyperhydrating agents such as glycerol and creatine to help the body retain the extra fluid ingested during hyperhydration. In the following paragraphs, we discuss these two agents and their efficacy to improve fluid balance and thermoregulation before and during exercise.

Glycerol, a hyperhydrating agent, is typically consumed in small amounts (1-1.5 g/kg body weight) in combination with a large volume of fluid (25-35 mL/kg body weight) 2.5 to 4 h before exercise (Burke 2006). From the chapter on fat, you may remember that glycerol is a by-product of fat metabolism. In fact, glycerol builds the backbone of triglyceride and is made up of a three-carbon alcohol. Glycerol acts as a hyperhydrating agent because it is quickly absorbed and distributed among tissues, exerting an osmotic pressure that results in greater fluid retention (Robergs and

Griffin 1998). Research has shown that glycerol supplementation has produced a fluid retention of 400 to 700 mL (Riedesel et al. 1987; Magal et al. 2003), but whether hyperhydration with glycerol improves performance in sport is presently unclear. There are a few promising studies in cyclists (Hitchins et al. 1999; Anderson et al. 2001), showing improved time trial performance with glycerol versus water alone. A recent meta-analysis examined whether glycerol was more effective as a hyperhydrating strategy than water (Goulet et al. 2007). (Read "What Is a Meta-Analysis?" in chapter 6 to understand how this type of research is done.) This meta-analysis pooled 28 studies, 14 of which met the inclusion criteria set up by the authors. The researchers found that compared with fluid alone, added glycerol significantly improved fluid retention by 7.7 mL/kg body weight and resulted in a 2.6% performance improvement. Unfortunately, glycerol has side effects that include nausea, vomiting, and other gastrointestinal symptoms and can be detrimental to performance if not trialed before competition.

Creatine has also been examined as a hyperhydrating agent (Kern et al 2001; Kilduff et al. 2004; see Ganio et al. 2007 for a review). Unlike glycerol, creatine retains fluid predominantly intracellularly. Supplementation with creatine has produced fluid retention of 400 to 800 mL (Kern et al. 2001; Volek et al. 2001). Creatine ingestion of ~20 g/day dissolved with 0.5 L of water for one week can effectively attenuate the rise in heart rate and core temperature during endurance exercise in the heat (Kilduff et al. 2004). These effects are most likely due to an increase in intracellular water, improving the body's capacity to deal with heat (Kern et al. 2001; Kilduff et al. 2004).

Researchers have also examined the combined effect of creatine and glycerol on fluid retention and in preparation for exercise in the heat. Easton and colleagues (2007) matched 24 subjects for body mass and randomly assigned them to a creatine or a placebo group (glucose). Subjects in both groups also received 1 g of glycerol per kilogram of body weight twice daily in either the first or the second supplementation regimen. The design was double blinded and counterbalanced, which means that all subjects received all treatments but did not know, nor did the researchers, which treatment they received. This design allowed four possible combinations to be studied: (1) placebo/placebo, (2) placebo/glycerol, (3) placebo/creatine, and (4) creatine/glycerol. Both placebo/creatine and creatine/glycerol resulted in significant reductions in heart rate, rectal temperature, and rating of perceived exertion during exercise at 86° F (30° C) and 70% relative humidity. The addition of glycerol to creatine significantly increased total body water retention over creatine alone but had no further effect on thermal and cardiovascular responses. However, hyperhydrating before exercise through creatine, glycerol, or a combination of the two did not result in any significant improvement of the 16.1 km time trial compared with euhydration. It may be that the time trial was too short to reflect any benefits of this supplemental strategy or that the effects of hyperhydration are minimal. In addition, as with the ingestion of large volumes of fluid, the risk for hyponatremia and additional weight gain needs to be considered, especially in sports with a large power-to-weight component such as cycling (see highlight on p. 252). Athletes experimenting with hyperhydration and the use of agents such as creatine and glycerol to increase preexercise fluid retention should consult with a professional.

Optimizing hydration status before exercise should include the following considerations:

1. The last meal before exercise should be eaten 1 to 4 h before the start of exercise. The recommendation is to drink 5-7 mL/kg body weight 4 h before exercise, and this may be best paired with the preexercise meal. If urine volume is low or color is dark, additional fluid; 3-5 mL/kg body weight should be ingested.

2. Sport drinks containing electrolytes are more palatable and help retain ingested fluids better than water. However, whether a sport drink over water is preferred prior to exercise depends on the nutritional status of the athlete, individual preference, the goal of the exercise session, and whether carbohydrates are available during the activity (see chapter 2 on carbohydrates for more information).

3. For exercise in the heat, an additional bolus of 10.5 to 14 fl oz (300-400 mL) prior to exercise may be advantageous.

4. Athletes should attempt hyperhydration in training first, especially if they experiment with agents such as glycerol or creatine. It is also likely that athletes respond differently to these strategies before and after acclimatization to a hot environment.

Useful Hydration Assessment Methods for Athletes

When it comes to hydration recommendations, "one size fits all" no longer applies. New hydration guidelines underline the importance of individual hydration status assessment. This section reviews the current methods for hydration assessment and indicates which measures are feasible for athletes and active individuals.

Urine Color

According to recent research, which involved monitoring athletes and active individuals over a 24 h period, urine color is a good field indicator of hydration and was as effective as or better than urine volume in predicting fluid balance in athletes (Armstrong et al. 1998). People should continue to drink until their urine is either "very pale yellow" or "pale yellow." The body mass of an athlete with this urine color should be within 1% of the well-hydrated baseline body mass (Armstrong et al. 1998). However, Kovacs and colleagues (1999) found that urine color was not a good indicator of hydration up to 6 h postexercise. The length of time required for urine color to indicate good hydration status after exercise varies depending on the level of dehydration that occurs during exercise, the amount of fluid consumed postexercise, and environmental conditions. Illness and various food and sport supplements—especially vitamin supplements—can produce dark or neon-like urine color with a strong odor; in these cases, urine color cannot be used as a guide to hydration level.

Daily Body Weight Changes

Total body water (first morning body weight after urination and measured in the nude) is normally regulated to fluctuate between ±0.2% and 0.5% of daily body mass, although females experience much larger deviations due to their menstrual cycle, as body mass can increase by >4.4 lb (>2 kg) during the luteal phase (Bunt et al. 1989). In athletes, glycogen loading may also produce small increments in total body water, although this is not always seen (Zderic et al. 2004). There is also extra water storage from the normal storage of muscle glycogen on a daily basis; however, this amount of water is rather small (~200 mL) (Sherman et al. 1982). Daily body weight measurements, therefore, provide a simple and useful tool to assess and monitor daily fluid balance.

Urine Specific Gravity and Osmolality

Urine specific gravity (USG) and osmolality are good indicators of hydration status if used in the morning along with the first morning body weight after voiding. Urine specific gravity should be <1.020, whereas urine osmolality should be <700 m_{osm}/kg; both values indicate euhydration. During the rehydration period after exercise, USG, osmolality, and urine color are *not* good indicators of hydration status because athletes typically ingest large volumes of fluid that temporarily dilute the plasma and increase urinary volume (Shirreffs et al. 1996), and both of these measures may lag behind plasma and serum measures.

Plasma and Serum Osmolality

Plasma and serum osmolality are also good for the assessment of hydration status; however, they require a more invasive method, blood sampling. Urinary measures, on the other hand, lag behind the plasma and serum values. A plasma osmolality of <290 m_{osm}/kg indicates euhydration (Sawka et al. 2007).

Acute Changes in Body Weight

Acute changes in body weight before and after exercise can be used to estimate sweat rate. This approach assumes that 1 mL of sweat equals 1 g of body weight loss because the specific gravity of sweat is 1 g/mL (Sawka et al. 2007). Weight (preferably nude) is measured before and after exercise; one accounts for urine volume and fluid intake by subtracting and adding them to the calculation, respectively (see table 8.4). Sources of errors when one is estimating sweating rate from acute body weight changes include respiratory loss and metabolic water gain. We will discuss this topic more in the next section. For exercise durations exceeding 3 h, corrections should be made in order to increase the accuracy of the estimate (Sawka et al. 2007). Table 8.4 on p. 245 shows an example of how to estimate an athlete's sweating rate from changes in body weight from pre- to postexercise.

Fluid Needs During Exercise

The goal of drinking fluids during exercise is to maintain plasma volume and electrolytes, prevent abnormal elevations in heart rate and core body temperature, and provide fuel to the working muscles. This in turn may delay fatigue and prevent severe fluid imbalances that may occur during exercise when no fluid is consumed. As mentioned earlier, the most serious effect of exercise-induced dehydration is the abnormal rise in core body temperature (i.e., >104° F or 40° C) due to the inability to dissipate heat. The effectiveness of a fluid in replacing sweat loss depends on factors such as exercise duration and intensity, the volume and composition of the fluid, environmental conditions, drinking frequency, and the nutritional status of the individual before exercise. No single beverage and no single volume can meet the needs of all active individuals in all exercise situations.

Sweating rates vary among sports and individuals and between genders, and also differ depending on environmental factors, intensity of exercise, fitness status, age, and level of acclimatization. On average, sweating rates in athletes range from as little as 0.2 L/h to up to 2 L/h. Figure 8.5 shows a compilation of sweating rates among different sports and in males and females exercising in different environmental and competitive conditions.

Sweating rates vary most dramatically according to gender, environmental temperature, and exercise intensity (Sawka et al. 2007). Females have lower sweating rates than males, primarily because of the smaller body size and lower metabolic rates during engagement in a given exercise task (Sawka et al. 1983). Whether the athlete is male or female, the environmental temperature and exercise intensity can change sweating response dramatically. A runner weighing 110 lb (50 kg) may sweat as little as 0.4 L/h running at 8.5 km/h (5.3 mph) in a cool-temperate environment (64° F; 18° C) and up to 1 L/h—almost twice as much—running at 15 km/h (9.5 mph) in a warm (82° F; 28° C) environment. As can be expected, body mass has a very strong effect on sweating rate, with the heavier athlete sweating more in both of these scenarios (Sawka et al. 2007).

Sweating rates also vary by age. Young athletes (prepubescent) have a lower sweating rate than adults; values typically do not exceed 0.4 L/h (Bar-Or 1989; Meyer et al 1992). Factors such as smaller body mass and lower metabolic rate probably account for this difference (more on children and fluid replacement at the end of the chapter).

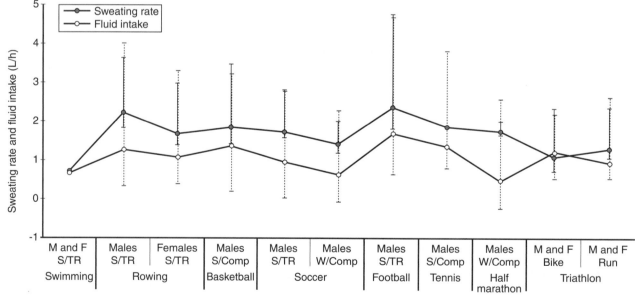

Figure 8.5 Sweating rate and fluid intake. It is obvious that sweating rate varies according to sport, gender, and environmental condition (summer vs. winter). Data represent mean sweating rates estimated from changes in body weight (pre- to postexercise weight). Bars represent ranges (from minimum to maximum) and show the large variability within and among sports. Training environments: S/TR = summer training; S/Comp = summer competition; W/comp = winter competition. Gender: m (males); f (females).

Data from M.N. Sawka et al., 2007, "American College of Sports Medicine position stand: Exercise and fluid replacement," *Medicine and Science of Sports and Exercise* 39: 377-390.

Conversely, older individuals have a blunted thirst response, a lower glomerular filtration rate, and a more sluggish response to the need to restore fluid balance. Older individuals are also at risk for retaining sodium because of the slower process by which water and sodium are excreted. This is important to consider when one is recommending sodium-containing fluids as a hydration strategy in older individuals with hypertension (Luft et al. 1987).

It is no longer possible to recommend the amount an athlete should drink during exercise without a thorough assessment of fluid loss during a variety of exercise tasks in different environments. Fluid replacement strategies during exercise need to be adapted to the individual's sweating rate for a given exercise session, and should also take into account the accessibility of fluid and the feasibility of strategic, regular fluid replacement during the session. Because sweating rates vary between and within individuals on a daily basis according to factors just discussed, athletes need to begin to measure their body weight before and after exercise to estimate sweating rate. Fluid replacement strategies should be based on the goal of preventing excessive dehydration and hyponatremia as well as large daily body weight fluctuations. Fluid replacement strategies should be predominantly guided by the experience of the athlete in the sport, and by signs and symptoms of dehydration such as the degree of body weight loss (% body weight loss from body weight measures), level of thirst, and performance indices or a measure of perceived exertion. Although thirst lags behind changes in hydration, thirst should still be integrated into a daily or weekly log for identification of the optimal fluid replacement strategy along with other information. It is probably not reasonable to suggest to athletes that they always drink enough to prevent a body weight loss of 2%; however, in the heat, this strategy is most likely key to preventing dangerous levels of dehydration, especially if athletes are not yet acclimatized. It is also worthwhile to compile other signals, such as thirst and particularly the subjective perception of performance or perceived effort of the session, in a spreadsheet or daily fluid log to take a more integrated approach to establishing an athlete's fluid replacement scheme. Table 8.4 provides the steps involved in estimating sweating rate from pre- to postexercise weight changes and ideas for a spreadsheet design.

Body weight changes can reflect sweat losses during exercise and may be used to calculate individual fluid replacement needs for specific exercise and environmental conditions (Sawka et al. 2007). However, there are multiple issues and major sources of error when one is calculating sweating rate from pre- and postexercise body weight measures. These errors were summarized by Maughan and colleagues (2007a):

1. Water loss due to respiration: Respiratory water loss can be high, particularly in a dry climate because expired air has to be humidified. It is estimated that under physically hard work at high altitude in dry air, approximately 1500 mL of body water may be lost due to respiration (Ladell 1965). According to Maughan and colleagues (2007a), respiratory water loss may approximate 2.7 and 3 mL/min during high-intensity work in hot (95° F, 35° C) and cold (32° F, 0° C;) but dry conditions, respectively. In humid conditions in the heat, respiratory water loss will be relatively small. Considering that this error can be significant, it should be taken into account during high-intensity work in dry climates. This volume of fluid would need to be subtracted from the pre- and postexercise body weight calculation.

2. Water produced due to substrate oxidation: When carbohydrate, protein, and fat are oxidized, water is formed. This water is not lost as in the case of sweat; it is added to the total body water pool.

3. Water produced due to substrate mass loss: When substrates are oxidized, body mass will slightly change because substrates that were stored have been oxidized as fuel. The weight associated with the water formed, due to substrate oxidation and the loss of substrate, depends on a number of factors such as exercise intensity, substrate storage, fitness level, and carbohydrate intake during exercise. Any factor that determines fuel selection during exercise can affect this variable. It would be a daunting task to quantify this for each exercise condition when estimating fluid needs from weight changes! It is important, however, to note that both of these sources of error contribute to changes in body weight from pre- to postexercise but have nothing to do with actual sweat loss—and may be cancelled out with the loss of fluid from respiration illustrated in point 1.

4. Water stored with substrate such as glycogen: Whether 3 g of water is actually stored with each gram of glycogen is still a matter of debate (Maughan et al. 2007a); however, body mass

changes do occur according to acute manipulations of the diet (Sherman et al. 1982; Olsson and Saltin 1970). Considering the potential to overestimate sweating rate from changes in weight due to glycogen, it may be wise to choose training scenarios rather than the preparation for an event to estimate fluid replacement strategies.

5. Water balance changes due to fluid intake: Although we would expect fluid intake to improve the total body water pool regardless of when it is consumed during exercise, this may not necessarily be the case. If the fluid is consumed late during exercise or if a hypertonic fluid is ingested, both of which can slow absorption, then fluid ingestion may not immediately improve the total body water pool. In general, only part of the fluid intake may become part of the available total body water pool, since some fluid may be held in the gastrointestinal tract. Although this is an important point, it is almost impossible to quantify.

6. Water loss due to feces, urine, or both: The rate of urine production is reduced by about 20% to 60% during exercise (Zambraski 1996); however, many athletes still have to urinate and sometimes even defecate during exercise. Fecal water loss is variable and relatively small, whereas daily urine output may be between 1 and 2 L or 40 and 80 mL/h (Shirreffs and Maughan 2001), which would amount to about 50 to 100 mL in a 2 to 3 h exercise period.

Fluid replacement during exercise lasting longer than 60 min should be common practice for most athletes, and fluid volumes should be adjusted to individual requirements as previously highlighted. Water is a better strategy than drinking no fluids. Hargreaves and colleagues (1996) studied five trained men during 2 h of cycling at 67% $\dot{V}O_2$max on two different cycling tests—one with water provided, one with no fluids. Compared to what happened in the trial with no fluid intake, exercise with water intake significantly decreased heart rate, rectal temperature, muscle temperature, and muscle glycogen utilization. Net muscle glycogen utilization also decreased by 16% when water was ingested, which may help explain why fluid intake during exercise can improve exercise performance. Beyond just using water, ingesting a carbohydrate-containing sport drink may do an even better job in enhancing performance, particularly under exercising conditions longer than 60 min, when muscle and liver glycogen stores become limited; the additional, exogenous source of carbohydrate from the sport drink assists in maintaining blood glucose during

---

Highlight

Is the Weight Loss Associated With Hypohydration Beneficial in Increasing Hill-Climbing Performance in Cyclists?

Researchers at the Australian Institute of Sport examined this question in well-trained cyclists (Ebert et al. 2007). Using a randomized crossover design, they had eight well-trained cyclists ($\dot{V}O_2$peak: 66.2 ± 5.8 mL · kg^{-1} · min^{-1}) perform a 2 h ride at 53% $\dot{V}O_2$peak immediately followed by a cycling hill climb to fatigue at 88% $\dot{V}O_2$peak at 86° F or 30° C. During the 2 h ride, the cyclists received either 2.4 L (HIGH) of a carbohydrate drink (7%) or 0.4 L (LOW) of water with carbohydrate gels to match the carbohydrate content of the carbohydrate drink trial. The LOW volume trial resulted in a significant loss of body weight (–2.5%) versus the HIGH trial (+0.3%) before the hill climb. In addition, rectal temperature was significantly higher in the LOW versus the HIGH trial before and after the hill climb. Despite being almost 2 kg (4.4 lb) lighter, athletes in the LOW trial fatigued about 5 min earlier (LOW: 13.9 ± 5.5 min vs. 19.5 ± 6.0 min), a 30% difference between HIGH and LOW trials. These findings suggest that dehydration in a warm climate is detrimental to cycling hill-climbing performance. If a cyclist's goal is to influence his or her power-to-weight ratio, the best way to do it is via a dietary strategy during the off-season and the preparatory phase, targeting fat loss during high-volume, low-intensity training. Using dehydration strategies to manipulate weight acutely is not effective. It is likely that endurance performance will suffer, particularly in the heat.

exercise (Costill et al. 1973; Erickson et al. 1987; Pirnay et al. 1982).

The idea that carbohydrate supplementation in the form of sport drinks enhances performance is nothing new. An abundance of studies show this positive performance effect in endurance (Coggan and Coyle 1991; Tsintzas et al. 1993, 1995; Coyle, 2004) and intermittent and team sport (Davis et al. 1997; Nicholas et al. 1995; Vergauwen et al. 1998; Welsh et al. 2002; for a review see Shirreffs et al. 2006) exercise protocols. Sports involving intermittent exercise are usually team or individual sports in which high-intensity exercise is interspersed with rest or with lower-intensity exercise. Typical team sports include volleyball, soccer, basketball, American football, and ice hockey; individual, intermittent sports include sports such as ice skating, gymnastics, alpine skiing, swimming, and tennis. The duration and intensity of these sports vary dramatically; the activity can last anywhere from a few minutes to 2 h. These sports can produce sweat rates as high as or higher than those seen in endurance sports and usually involve high-intensity exercise that relies heavily on muscle glycogen. Many of the individual, intermittent sports are characterized by one short performance bout; however, warm-up and cool-down may make the actual time spent in activity relatively long or on the order of 2 to 3 h. It is also important to consider that many of these sports have training schemes that are markedly different from the actual competition—and these could probably be characterized as intermittent-type activities and at least hypothetically may result in various degrees of fluid imbalances and glycogen utilization. Moreover, many of these sports are played indoors, where higher temperatures can contribute to increased sweat losses.

Unlike endurance sports, in which the athlete usually dictates fluid intake, intermittent sports usually restrict fluid consumption to breaks in play or between events. Research on the effect of fluid intake during intermittent or high-intensity exercise (>80% $\dot{V}O_2$max) has shown that beverages containing electrolytes and carbohydrate can improve exercise performance and prevent dehydration. Laboratory researchers have attempted to mimic the team sport environment by interspersing high-intensity work with lower-intensity exercise over an extended period. Davis and colleagues (1997) had subjects repeatedly cycle for 1 min at 120% to 130% $\dot{V}O_2$max, with the cycling bouts separated by 3 min of rest, until fatigued. They repeated this protocol on two different occa-sions, in one using a carbohydrate-electrolyte replacement beverage and in the other using a water placebo. In the carbohydrate trial, subjects received an 18% carbohydrate solution before exercise began and a 6% carbohydrate solution during exercise. In the carbohydrate trial, time to fatigue was 27 min longer than with the water placebo. In addition, during the carbohydrate trial, subjects were able to complete 21 high-intensity exercise bouts, 1 min each, compared to only 14 bouts with the water placebo. Nicholas and colleagues (1995) conducted a similar study using shuttle running. Participants completed 75 min of exercise, which included five 15 min periods of intermittent running (sprinting interspersed with periods of jogging and walking). This was then followed by a run to fatigue. Consumption of a beverage containing electrolytes and 6.9% carbohydrate during the shuttle running increased time to fatigue by 33% compared to a noncarbohydrate placebo.

Researchers have also examined the effect of fluid intake on exercise performance, as well as the physiological factors associated with dehydration, in high-intensity exercise protocols (usually ~80% $\dot{V}O_2$max) lasting ~1 h. Ball and colleagues (1995) found that in a 50 min simulated cycle time trial, a 7% carbohydrate solution increased subjects' peak power and mean power output compared with a water placebo. These data were supported by a study by Jeukendrup and colleagues (1997), who fed a 7.6% carbohydrate-electrolyte beverage or a water placebo to athletes during cycling time trials lasting approximately 1 h. Participants cycled faster and achieved more work when drinking a carbohydrate solution versus a water placebo. These studies tested athletes after an overnight fast; the results in well-fed athletes might be different.

In summary, it appears that consuming fluids—especially carbohydrate-electrolyte beverages—increases endurance performance. Improvement in performance is also seen in high-intensity exercise and in team sports in which intermittent play occurs over an extended period. The effect on performance may be especially profound if high-intensity exercise is done in a hot environment that increases sweat loss (Morris et al. 1998), because in these environments, smaller degrees of body weight loss due to fluid loss may have a more profound effect on performance (Walsh et al. 1994). Consumption of a sport drink may be especially beneficial for the athlete who is dehydrated, who has fasted, or who has poor glycogen stores before a high-intensity event. A number of excellent review articles have addressed the role of fluids in intermittent exercise, team sports, and high-intensity protocols (Burke and Hawley 1997; Coyle 2004; Shi and Gisolfi 1998; Shirreffs, Casa, and Carter 2007).

Fluid Needs After Exercise

What level of fluid is required to return an athlete to a euhydrated state after exercise is over? The goal of postexercise rehydration is to replace the water and electrolytes lost during exercise. This is particularly critical if a second training session is planned for the day or if the next event is only 4 to 8 h away. Full restoration of fluid may take between 4 and 24 h (Greenleaf 1992) depending on the degree of dehydration that occurred before (in the case of weigh-ins) or during exercise. As we now know, how much an athlete loses during exercise depends on many factors; and even within a given person, sweating rates and fluid intake vary according to exercise intensity, environmental conditions, and accessibility of fluid. How much sodium an athlete loses is even more difficult to assess, and athletes lose sweat electrolytes at highly different rates. It is believed that typical sweat sodium losses range from 20 to 80 mmol/L in exercising humans (Armstrong et al. 1987). It is generally thought that athletes should be able to replace water and electrolytes by consuming adequate water and food during the recovery period. If no food is available, either by choice or by circumstance, then any fluid consumed should contain electrolytes, especially sodium (~50 mmol/L), and some carbohydrate (Maughan and Shirreffs 1997). The sodium improves fluid retention in the body, while the carbohydrate enhances intestinal uptake of sodium and water and helps replace muscle and liver glycogen. Most sport drinks contain only a moderate amount of sodium (10-20 mmol/L), which is probably not enough to optimize fluid retention during the recovery period. In fact, there seems to be a direct relationship between the fluid retained and the amount of sodium ingested, at least up to a concentration of 100 mmol/L (Maughan and Leiper 1995). Thus, amounts in the range of 50 to 60 mmol/L are more likely to restore fluid and electrolyte balance after exercise. However, such high sodium levels often compromise the palatability of a fluid, which affects the voluntary fluid intake; people generally drink less of a fluid with a high sodium concentration.

Nevertheless, higher sodium levels should be targeted when limited time is available to restore fluid balance to a euhydrated state before the next exercise session. An easy strategy for athletes is to combine a commercial sport drink with salted pretzels or another salty snack. Failure to replace sodium losses will make it difficult to return to a euhydrated state because the fluid ingested will result in greater urine production (Maughan and Leiper 1995; Shirreffs and Maughan 1998). If enough time is available to restore fluid balance, athletes may begin their immediate recovery with a sport drink, followed by a meal containing electrolytes and more fluid in the form of water ingested within 1 h postexercise. In fact, studies have shown that the ingestion of additional sodium through food, along with plenty of water, enhances fluid retention to a greater extent than a sodium-containing sport drink alone (Maughan et al. 1996).

The volume of fluid consumed should be greater than the volume of sweat lost because losses of fluid in the urine and in respiration also need to be recovered (Shirreffs et al. 1996). Shirreffs and colleagues (1996) found that athletes needed to consume at least 150% of the body mass loss that occurred during exercise, in the form of a high-sodium fluid, to reach euhydration 6 h after exercise ended. These athletes were dehydrated by 2% of body mass by exercise in a hot, humid environment at approximately 60% $\dot{V}O_2$max for 35 to 40 min (figure 8.6). Besides the volume of fluid, how an athlete consumes the fluid after exercise may make a difference in restoration of fluid balance. Spacing fluid intake over several hours of recovery appears to be more effective than consuming a large amount of fluid immediately after exercise (Archer and Shirreffs 2001). However, this may depend on the time available for fluid restoration, with the longer recovery period probably providing plenty of opportunity to achieve euhydration (Kovacs et al. 2002).

A number of studies have examined the effect of various electrolyte replacement beverages, water, and other fluids on restoration of fluid balance after exercise. Gonzalez-Alonso and colleagues (1992) found that a dilute carbohydrate-electrolyte solution (6% carbohydrate, 20 mmol/L sodium, 3 mmol/L potassium) was more effective in promoting postexercise rehydration than plain water or Diet Coke. The carbohydrate-electrolyte beverage produced the smallest urine volume, indicating that it promoted the greatest retention of fluid. Brouns and colleagues (1998) confirmed these

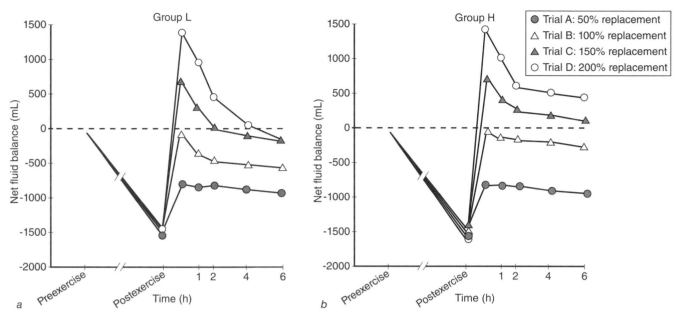

Figure 8.6 Net fluid balance calculated from the volumes of sweat loss, fluid ingestion, and urine output in 12 male volunteers, dehydrated by 2.06% of body mass by intermittent cycle exercise, who consumed four different drink volumes equivalent to 50% (trial A), 100% (trial B), 150% (trial C), and 200% (trial D) of body mass lost. Subjects consumed these four different drink volumes in four separate weeks; in each trial, six subjects received drink L (low sodium: 23 mmol/L sodium) and six received drink H (61 mmol/L of sodium). The left panel shows the results for group L (a) and the right panel shows the results for group H (b).

Reprinted, by permission, from S.M. Shirreffs et al., 1996, "Post-exercise rehydration in man: effects of volume consumed and drink sodium content," *Medicine and Science in Sports and Exercise* 28: 1260-1271.

results. They examined the effect of three different fluid replacement beverages—a European carbohydrate-electrolyte drink (Isostar; 7% carbohydrate per liter), a low-sodium mineral water, or a caffeinated soft drink (Coca-Cola)—on fluid replacement in the first 2 h following cycling in the heat. The cola and the water trials produced the greatest urinary losses of sodium, potassium, chloride, magnesium, and calcium during the 2 h recovery period; the carbohydrate-electrolyte drink resulted in better sodium, magnesium, and calcium retention with no difference in potassium and chloride retention. The researchers concluded that ingesting either water or caffeinated cola after exercise resulted in a negative electrolyte balance and that a carbohydrate-electrolyte drink containing moderate amounts of sodium, magnesium, and calcium helped maintain electrolyte balance. Although this study looked at a variety of electrolytes and minerals, it is the consensus of the International Olympic Committee (2003) that there is no convincing justification for the addition of electrolytes other than sodium to recovery fluids (Shirreffs et al. 2004). Most of these nutrients, along with others, are best ingested in the postexercise meal. Athletes who have time to eat and drink after exercise can effectively restore fluid balance without even consuming a carbohydrate-electrolyte sport drink (Maughan et al. 1996).

From the above studies, it should be clear that caffeinated sport drinks or energy drinks are probably not suitable for the recovery period when the main goal is to restore fluid balance. The diuretic effect of caffeine has probably been overstated, considering the limited amount of research, and hydration status does not seem to be affected with caffeine intake (Armstrong 2002; Armstrong et al. 2005, 2007a; Ganio et al. 2007). Nevertheless, after exercise, because fluids such as water and soda increase urine production to a larger extent than a sodium-containing sport drink, it may be best to recommend fluids that primarily contain carbohydrate, adequate sodium, and potassium and to defer caffeinated products to a different time (i.e., before and during exercise) in order to achieve their ergogenic effects (see p. 260 for more information on caffeine).

A recent study focused on milk as an effective recovery drink due to its relatively high sodium content apart from its ability to deliver carbohydrate and protein—two important ingredients in an athlete's contemporary postexercise recovery mixture (Shirreffs, Watson, and Maughan 2007). The researchers used four experimental drinks: (1) water only, (2) a commercial sport drink, (3) milk, and (4) milk + extra sodium. Table 8.5 shows the composition and energy content of the four experimental drinks.

Eleven healthy participants received the four experimental drinks four times in a crossover fashion, in random order, in amounts equal to 150% of their fluid loss after an intermittent exercise session in a warm environment (temperature: 95° F or 35° C; relative humidity 56%), which produced an average of 1.8% body mass loss. Drinks were consumed in bolus feedings every 15 min postexercise, providing a total drinking time of 60 min. Urine samples were collected over a 5 h period postexercise. To ensure equal metabolic conditions for each of the testing sessions, participants were asked to keep a two-day dietary and physical activity record before the first trial and to repeat the same protocol for each trial. Trials were separated by at least seven days, and participants reported to the testing lab in a fasted state; however, they were allowed to drink 500 mL of water 90 min prior to each trial. Results showed significantly better fluid retention for the milk trials compared with the water and sport drink trials. Moreover, both milk trials resulted in net positive fluid balance already after the first hour of fluid replacement, whereas the water and sport drink trials led to a net negative fluid balance after

the first hour postexercise. The researchers concluded that milk can be an effective postexercise rehydration drink and can be used by anyone except those with lactose intolerance.

A few concerns, however, have been discussed regarding the methodology of this study that put the results into perspective. Milk has a much higher energy density (kilocalories per gram) than water or a sport drink, and it could be expected that the milk did not leave the stomach or intestinal tract as rapidly as the other drinks, especially during the measurement period. This would lead to the lower urine output in the milk trials, misinterpreted as having led to better fluid retention. The researchers should have provided some objective measure of gastric emptying or intestinal absorption to rule out this possibility. Further, it may be surprising that the sport drink was not superior to water in retaining fluid, since it contained a level of sodium previously shown to be advantageous (Shirreffs, Watson, and Maughan 2007; Gonzales-Alonso et al. 1992). Finally, if drinking milk is a good rehydration strategy for athletes, its effect on subsequent exercise performance should also have been tested. Nevertheless, and despite the critique of this study, it seems feasible to combine a sport drink and a snack containing milk to optimize multiple aspects of the recovery process, including rehydration, glycogen resynthesis, and repair of muscle tissue.

Whereas milk seems to be a good option to include in the recovery from exercise, alcohol is not! In fact, alcohol has a strong diuretic effect and can interfere with recovery. Alcohol increases urinary volume because of the diuretic effect, especially at an alcohol concentration of 4% or higher (Shirreffs and Maughan 1995, 1997). Further, alcohol delays the recovery process, in particular glycogen resynthesis, which is particularly important when timely recovery between training sessions is of key importance.

In summary, these are the rehydration recommendations postexercise:

- Sodium should be consumed either in food or in a carbohydrate-electrolyte beverage after exercise is over. Fluids should be palatable and at the temperature appropriate for the occasion. Cool (50-60° F; 10-15° C), flavored fluids tend to increase fluid intake.

- Water or caffeinated beverages with a low sodium content are not recommended unless these fluids are ingested along with food and coincide with the culture and habits of the athlete.

Table 8.5 Composition and Energy Content of Four Experimental Drinks

	Water	Sport drink	Milk	Milk + sodium
Carbohydrate (g/L)	0	60	50	50
Protein (g/L)	0	0	36	36
Fat (g/L)	0	0	3	3
Energy (kcal/L)	0	244	354	354
Sodium (mmol/L)	0.3	23.0	38.6*	58.0
Potassium (mmol/L)	0	2.0	45.2	47.0

*Sodium content in milk from the United Kingdom; sodium content in U.S. milk is lower.

Adapted from S.M. Shirreffs, P. Watson, and R.J. Maughan, 2007, "Milk as an effective post-exercise rehydration drink," *British Journal of Nutrition* 98: 173-180. Adapted with permission of Cambridge University Press.

- The amount of fluid consumed should equal 150% of the fluid lost in sweat—that is, for every pound (0.45 kg) of body weight lost due to sweating, ~24 oz (~750 mL) of fluid needs to be consumed. The athlete should monitor changes in body weight before and after exercise to set up a good strategy for fluid replacement after exercise. Reliance on thirst for rehydration is not a good approach.

- Fluid replacement after exercise may be spaced over several hours, with the initial intake occurring immediately after exercise, most preferentially in the form of a sport drink followed by a meal with additional fluids within 1 or 2 h postexercise.

- Alcoholic beverages (4% or more of volume) interfere with rehydration and recovery and are not recommended.

Throughout the last few years, many organizations have published guidelines for fluid replacement in sport. These organizations, their published materials, and the corresponding Web site are listed on this page. Many materials are free to download, and several of these organizations keep abreast of the research and keep their materials up-to-date.

SPORT DRINKS AND FLUID REPLACEMENT BEVERAGES

There is no general agreement among researchers on the optimal formulation of a sport drink; neither is there an "ideal" beverage that will satisfy all conditions (Gisolfi and Duchman 1992). Ideally, the optimal sport drink for any one person would depend on the duration and intensity of the

Current Hydration Guidelines Available Through National and International Organizations

Organization	Sports	Web site
International Olympic Committee (IOC)	Olympic summer and winter sport nutrition booklets released in 2003 with update in 2007 Full consensus report published in *Journal of Sports Sciences* in 2004	www.olympic.org/uk (search for nutrition documents)
International Federation of Football Associations (FIFA)	Nutrition booklet for football released in 2006 Full consensus report published in *Journal of Sports Sciences* in 2006	www.fifa.com
International Association of Athletics Federations (IAAF)	Nutrition booklet for athletics released in 2008; Consensus statement released in 2007; full report to be published in *Journal of Sports Sciences*	www.iaaf.org
American Academy of Pediatrics (AAP)	Consensus statement on climatic heat stress and the exercising child and adolescent (Anderson et al. 2000)	www.aap.org
National Athletic Trainers' Association (NATA)	Position statement on fluid replacement for athletes (Casa et al. 2000)	www.nata.org
American Medical Athletic Association (AMAA)	Updates on fluid and hydration strategies for running	www.amaasportsmed.org
American College of Sports Medicine (ACSM)	Position stands: "Exercise and Fluid Replacement" (Convertino et al. 1996 and Sawka et al. 2007) "Exertional Heat Illness during Training and Competition" (Armstrong et al. 2007b) "Prevention of Cold Injuries during Exercise" (Castellani et al. 2006) "ACSM Roundtable on Hydration and Physical Activity: Consensus Statements" (Casa et al. 2005)	www.acsm.org

exercise, the environmental conditions, and the characteristics of the individual (Maughan 1992). Table 8.6 lists the energy and nutrient contents of selected sport drinks. Although we do not have an "optimal" sport drink or oral rehydration solution, any drink listed in table 8.6 that contains both electrolytes and carbohydrate can enhance fluid balance. The sport drink or fluid replacement solution should contain 4% to 8% carbohydrate from multiple sugars such as glucose, sucrose, fructose,

and maltodextrin and 500 to 700 mg (20-50 mmol) of sodium per liter.

Depending on the fluid replacement strategy, more or fewer carbohydrates will be consumed from the sport drink. In many cases, athletes add extra carbohydrates from gels, blocs, jelly beans, bars, or food, targeting a total carbohydrate intake from various sugars of approximately 60 to 70 g/h, which results in carbohydrate oxidation rates of 1 to 1. 3 g/min (Jentjens et al. 2004a, 2004b). The

Table 8.6 Sport Drink Comparison Table

Sport drink Ingredients per 8 oz	Carbohydrate content (%)	Carbohydrate (g)	Carbohydrate type	Calories (kcal)	Sodium (mg)	Potassium (mg)	Protein (g)	Caffeine
Gatorade	6	14	Sucrose syrup, high-fructose corn syrup	50	110	30	0	No
Gatorade EF	5	14	Sucrose syrup, high-fructose corn syrup	50	200	90	0	No
Propel	1	3	Sucrose, sucralose	10	35	0	0	No
Powerade	7	17	High-fructose corn syrup, maltodextrin	60	55	30	0	No
Accelerade	6	15	Sugar, trehalose	80	120	15	4	No
Amino Vital	3	8	Fructose	35	10	35	<750 mg amino acids	No
ClifShot electrolyte drink	8	19	Organic brown rice syrup, organic evaporated cane juice	80	200	50	0	Yes, in some
Cytomax	5	13	Fructose, dextrose, maltodextrin	50	55	30	0	Yes, in some
GU20	5	13	Maltodextrin, fructose	50	120	20	0	No
HEED (1 scoop)	10	25	Maltodextrin	100	62	16	0	No
Ultima Replenisher (1 scoop)	2	6	Maltodextrin	50	75	150	0	No

carbohydrate provides energy and maintains blood glucose levels during exercise, whereas the sodium improves palatability and replaces lost electrolytes. These fluids should also be cool and flavor enhanced to increase consumption. Ideally, fluid intake should begin early during exercise and occur frequently. The beneficial effect of carbohydrate-containing sport drinks on exercise performance has been well established and is discussed in detail in chapter 2. Athletes should become familiar with their own sweating rate during exercise under various environmental conditions by measuring weight before and again after exercise. They should then strive to consume enough fluid from water or sport drink during exercise to avoid significant dehydration.

Whether or not to use a sport drink depends on many factors. The primary reasons for using a beverage containing electrolyte and carbohydrate are to maximize fluid intake, replace electrolyte losses, and provide carbohydrate for energy and to maintain blood glucose during exercise (Marriott 1994). These beverages can be helpful in a number of situations, depending on the individual, his or her nutritional status in general and before exercise, and the intensity and duration of exercise, as well as the environment. Here we list eight situations in which athletes are better off using a sport drink over water:

- During prolonged exercise lasting >60 to 90 min
- During high-intensity or intermittent exercise
- During exercise in the heat
- During preseason training or two-a-days
- In competition, during games, and during events
- During phases of poor nutrition
- During phases of compromised immune status
- During exercise at altitude and in the cold

In a number of exercise situations you may want to recommend *not* using a sport drink but water instead:

- If exercise intensity is low and the session lasts <60 to 90 min
- If the goal of the fitness program (active individual) is weight loss and the person engages in moderate exercise lasting <60 to 90 min
- If the goal of the training program (endurance athlete) is optimization of fat metabolism

- If the athlete is well fed and is training at low to moderate intensity in a temperate or cool environment
- During the off-season and on recovery days

Lately, sport drinks have become highly sophisticated beverages packing more than just electrolytes and carbohydrates. The addition of protein, single amino acids, caffeine, and various levels of sodium has been trialed and tested. Here we briefly review the potential benefits of protein and caffeine and their postulated mechanisms when they are added to a sport drink.

Protein

Several studies have examined additional protein (2%) in the sport drink using a variety of methodologies, with equivocal outcomes. In a recent study by Van Essen and colleagues (2006), cyclists received a carbohydrate drink (6%), a carbohydrate drink (6%) plus protein (2%), or a placebo during a cycling task that lasted 2 to 2.5 h and included a performance trial (in which cyclists were to cover a fixed distance as fast as possible, as in a race). Even though the two sport drink mixtures showed improved performance over placebo, there were no significant differences between the carbohydrate-only and carbohydrate plus protein drinks. The addition of protein had no effect on the performance trial but also did not hurt it.

Other studies have used slightly different protocols. In an investigation by Ivy and colleagues (2003), the carbohydrate plus protein drink contained more calories than the carbohydrate drink alone. Problematic was that the carbohydrate drink delivered only 47 g of carbohydrate per hour, whereas Van Essen and colleagues (2006) maximized carbohydrate delivery in both conditions to elicit higher carbohydrate oxidation rates. In addition, Ivy and colleagues (2003) measured time to exhaustion, which is very different from a performance trial. This type of outcome measure is also an index of endurance capacity or how long an individual can keep going until fatigued. This type of outcome is typically more sensitive to different treatments; however, it does not necessarily apply to the performance edge an athlete is looking for in a race. Nevertheless, the cyclists using the carbohydrate plus protein drink in the study by Ivy and colleagues (2003) improved their endurance capacity by 30%, probably due to the added calories of the drink. Subsequent studies showed that if carbohydrate content is higher

(Luden et al. 2007; Saunders et al. 2007; Valentine et al. 2008) and the two drinks contain the same number of calories (Romano-Ely et al. 2006; Valentine et al. 2008), endurance performance differences no longer exist.

Consumption of a protein-containing sport drink versus a traditional carbohydrate-containing sport drink has also been associated with decreased markers of muscle damage or disruption, indicated by reduced plasma creatine kinase (Luden et al. 2007; Romano-Ely 2006; Saunders et al. 2004, 2007; Valentine et al. 2008), serum myoglobin (Valentine et al. 2008), lactate dehydrogenase (Romano-Ely 2006), and subjective ratings of muscle soreness (Luden et al. 2007; Romano-Ely et al. 2006). And recently, Valentine and colleagues (2008) showed that these lower levels of muscle damage or disruptions may also be associated with greater muscle strength 24 h postexercise. Thus, the addition of protein may not necessarily boost endurance performance, but it may be that protein protects the exercising muscle from excess damage or disruption or helps in the recovery process. More data are definitely needed to identify the mechanisms behind the potential benefit from a protein-containing carbohydrate-electrolyte sport drink. It may also be that protein in a sport drink results in better fluid retention due to the osmotic effect of protein in the plasma (Seifert et al. 2006), although some critical views suggest that the sport drink containing protein may have a delayed rate of absorption.

Caffeine

It is well known that caffeine increases performance, particularly endurance performance (for a comprehensive review, see Rogers 2005). Recently, caffeine has been added to sport drinks, and it has been shown that performance effects tend to be enhanced when sport drinks contain caffeine compared with carbohydrate and electrolytes alone. It appears that the most likely mechanism behind this effect is increased glucose absorption (Van Nieuwenhoven et al. 2000), leading to increased glucose oxidation in the muscle (Yeo et al. 2005).

Caffeine is still regarded as a diuretic despite the evidence that this is not so (Armstrong 2002; Armstrong et al. 2005; Ganio et al. 2007). If caffeine did act as a diuretic, it could interfere with normal fluid homeostasis and thus heat tolerance during exercise in a hot environment. However, this does not seem to be the case (Millard-Stafford et al. 2007; Armstrong et al. 2007a). Nevertheless, a word of caution is needed regarding athletes who like the boost of multiple, caffeine-laden energy drinks prior to or during high-intensity exercise. Using these drinks in heat to which they are not acclimatized may raise their risk for heat-related illness (Armstrong et al. 2007b).

When or if a sport drink with protein, caffeine, or other constituents should be used during exercise is an individual decision. The most important factors to consider in the selection of a sport drink are individual preferences and whether the drink is well tolerated by the athlete, particularly during racing. Carbohydrate and electrolytes should form the foundation of a sport drink before the athlete experiments with protein, caffeine, or other ingredients. Keep in mind that athletes often consume sport drinks, gels, bars, and food during prolonged activity. The compounding of macro- and micronutrients plus caffeine could be counterproductive. When one is selecting the fuel for exercise, simplicity can go a long way.

FLUID NEEDS IN HOT ENVIRONMENTS

Exercise stresses the body's ability to regulate body heat and fluid balance. Exercise in the heat increases the risk of dehydration as core body temperature and sweat rates rise. Core body temperature exceeding 102° to 104° F or 39° to 40° C is known as **hyperthermia,** a condition in which exercise performance is severely impaired. Trained subjects become exhausted at relatively similar levels of internal temperature (around 104° to 105.8° F or 40° to 41° C) and cardiovascular strain (heart rate 196 to 198 bpm, cardiac output 20 L/min, rating of perceived exertion 19 [Borg Scale units]) (Gonzalez-Alonso et al. 1999). As hyperthermia progresses, cardiac output declines; perfusion pressure and leg blood flow are reduced, which leads to a rapid suppression of oxygen delivery and uptake by muscle. Brain blood flow and oxygen extraction also decline, eventually impairing mental performance. Exercising in the heat also increases the use of glycogen as a fuel source (Murray 1995). Particularly the hot and humid environment can challenge the thermoregulatory system due to the difficulty with which heat is exchanged between the body and the environment when the air is saturated with water vapor. Dehydration challenges the system even further. Interestingly, hyperthermia and dehydration have independent mechanisms in relation to the cardiovascular system, but their effects are additive. Of course, all these physiologic changes can result in decreased physical performance—or, in some cases, exertional heat exhaustion or heatstroke (see "Heat-Related Disorders," p. 237).

Heat acclimatization (the process of adapting to environmental stress) and nutritional strategies (especially through proper hydration) as interventions are the most effective in dealing with exercise in hot environments (Wendt et al. 2007). Heat acclimatization results in several physiological adaptations that permit more effective cooling and less physiological strain during exercise in the heat. These adaptations include a lower body core temperature at rest, decreased heart rate during exercise, increased sweat rate and sweat sensitivity, decreased sodium loss (increased sodium reabsorption) in sweat and urine, and plasma volume expansion (Armstrong and Maresh,1991). **Heat acclimation** (condition once the person has acclimated to the environmental stress), and to some extent endurance training, can increase sweating rates by 10% to 20% (Gisolfi 1993) or to 200 to 300 mL/h more than the 1 to 2 L/h of sweat typically lost during high-intensity exercise. Table 8.7 shows the approximate time required for some of these systems to adapt to heat exposure.

During heat acclimatization, it appears that the elevated core temperature and the stimulation of sweating are most critical, which implies that training sessions must be prolonged (90-120 min) and somewhat intense (including some intervals) to stimulate adaptation (Wendt et al. 2007). Accomplishing heat acclimatization requires a smart nutritional intervention. Optimal strategies relating to fluid replacement for heat acclimatization include the following:

1. Measuring daily morning weights to ensure body weight stability. If body weight is reduced by 2% to 3%, extra fluids are needed. If body weight is reduced by 4% to 6%, a reduction in exercise training and additional fluid intake may be required (Armstrong and Maresh 1991).

2. Checking urine color before exercise. Recommendations include drinking 5 to 7 mL/kg body weight 4 h before exercise, and if urine is dark, an additional 3 to 5 mL/kg body weight 2 h before exercise (Sawka et al. 2007).

3. Estimating sweating rate and replacing lost fluids to avoid losing more than 1.5% to 2% of body weight. Overdrinking should be avoided; athletes should not gain weight from drinking too much.

4. Beginning to drink early during exercise because of the time lag until fluid is absorbed and distributed.

5. Using a sport drink with a variety of sugars, sodium, and potassium. If an athlete is a salty sweater, extra sodium may be needed (e.g., higher sodium content in sport drink, sodium chloride tablets, sodium-containing gels).

6. Rehydrating immediately after exercise by ingesting 150% of lost fluid over the course of 1 h in the form of a sport drink and eating some salty snacks; eating a meal and drinking plenty of water a bit later after exercise. Sodium intake should be increased if total daily sodium from food and beverages is less than 3 g/day (Armstrong and Maresh 1991). One way to increase sodium and fluid intakes is to use a carbohydrate-electrolyte sport drink before, during, and after exercise in the heat. Other ways to increase sodium intake are to eat adequate amounts of food, including foods high in sodium (pickles, salty snacks, processed foods such as canned soups, stews, chili), and adding table salt to food.

7. Knowing the signs and symptoms of heat stress and illness—prevention is the best treatment.

Table 8.7 Range of Days Required for Different Adaptations to Occur During Heat Acclimatization

Adaptation	Days of heat acclimatization
Decrease in heart rate during exercise	3-6
Plasma volume expansion	3-6
Decrease in sweat Na+ and Cl- concentrations	5-10
Increase in sweat rate and sweat sensitivity	7-14
Increase in cutaneous vasodilation	7-14

Reprinted, by permission, from D. Wendt, L.J. van Loon, W.D. Lichtenbelt, 2007, "Thermoregulation during exercise in the heat: strategies for maintaining health and performance," *Sports Medicine* 37:669-682.

FLUID NEEDS IN COLD ENVIRONMENTS

Less has been written on the body's response to cold weather exercise compared to activity in warmer weather; however, exercising in cold environments stresses the body's thermoregulation mechanisms. If exercise in the cold is combined with high altitude, the metabolic stresses on the body are extremely high, escalating the demand for adequate fuel and fluid intake. Fluid requirements are higher in cold compared to temperate environments, as cold air contains less water than warmer air even if relative humidity is the same. Thus, cold exposure leads to a small but significant increase in respiratory water loss, which is on the order of ~0.2 to 1.5 L/day (Freund and Sawka 1996). In addition, cold temperatures can result in an impaired thirst response (Askew 1995) and increased **cold-induced diuresis,** possibly leading to hypohydration and subsequent dehydration (Freund and Sawka 1996). In soldiers marching for 4.5 h at 5100 ft (1700 m) in cold temperatures (32° F, 0° C), marked voluntary dehydration was noticed, along with evidence of decreased glomerular filtration rate and urinary volume (Dann et al. 1990). Other military research demonstrated that water consumption of less than 2 L/day led to dehydration, while forced drinking reestablished fluid balance. Interestingly, fluid consumption correlated positively with energy intake in this population (Edwards and Roberts 1991).

In cross-country skiers, the ingestion of a sport drink resulted in greater fluid retention, better maintenance of fluid balance, and a 70% reduction in urine output compared with the ingestion of plain water (Seifert et al. 1998). In alpine skiers, 2 h of slalom skiing in the cold resulted in nearly 1% body mass loss. Athletes ingesting water were better able to maintain fluid balance than athletes who did not ingest fluids (Seifert et al. 2000). Nevertheless, many alpine skiers, particularly females, continue to drink very little fluid during on-snow training (Meyer et al. 1999; Meyer and Parker-Simmons 2007). One of the issues relates to the accessibility of bathroom facilities in glacier areas above 9000 ft (3000 m). Further, athletes are geared up and often unwilling to remove clothing and interrupt training for a bathroom break (Meyer 2003). While alpine skiing is a sport that does not necessarily lead to sweating in the cold, other outdoor sports may lead to heavy sweating due to physical exertion, cumbersome movement patterns in heavy snow, and insulated clothing (e.g., snow shoeing, backcountry skiing, freestyle snowboarding with hiking). Sweating rates are expected to be higher in these winter sports.

Few data are available on dehydration and its effects on performance in the cold. Dehydration in the cold was shown to result in a greater level of peripheral vasoconstriction compared to that with euhydration (Young et al. 1987). Physical work capacity was reduced, probably through compromised blood flow to working muscles. In addition, cold-induced dehydration has been shown to impair cognitive function (Banderet 1986). Similar to what occurs during exercise in a thermoneutral environment, a loss of 1% to 2% body weight can lead to decreased mechanical efficiency and shortened time to exhaustion in the cold (5° C) (Rintamäki et al. 1995).

Optimal fluid replacement strategies for exercise in the cold include the following:

1. When exercise starts, the athlete should be well hydrated and should have a clear urine color and a stable morning body weight. If urine volume is small, more fluid should be ingested prior to exercise (Castellani et al. 2006).

2. Warm sport drinks or tea with honey and a pinch of salt may be beneficial for people exercising in the cold. The temperature of the drink can help keep up core temperature, especially in sports in which maintaining thermoregulation is difficult (e.g., alpine skiing). The sodium will help to retain fluid and minimize the cold-induced diuresis typically experienced in these environments (Castellani et al. 2006).

3. Fluid replacement strategies during winter sport activities are similar to those for summer sports; however, a higher degree of dehydration may be possible without compromise to physical performance (Castellani et al. 2006). This depends, though, on the sport and its physical demand, as well as the change in core temperature and sweating rate experienced. One should be aware of the data of Rintamäki and colleagues (1995) showing impaired performance at 1% to 2% body weight loss, similar to that in temperate

environments. Meyer and Parker-Simmons (2007) suggest drinking 8 to 16 oz or 250 to 500 mL/h for activities such as alpine skiing; however, these recommendations may be higher for snowboarders who also hike along the half-pipe.

4. Fluid replacement strategies after exercise in the cold are similar to those for exercise in temperate environments.

5. Be aware of the signs and symptoms of dehydration and hyponatremia. They too may occur in winter sport athletes and others who exercise in the cold.

FLUID AND ELECTROLYTE NEEDS FOR CHILDREN AND ADOLESCENTS

Probably over 50% of children and adolescents participate in some type of competitive athletics, either at school or in the community (Squire 1990). Health professionals are constantly encouraging schools and communities to keep children active to prevent obesity and promote good health. However, children and adults respond differently to exercise and have different fluid requirements. Dr. Oded Bar-Or and colleagues at McMaster University in Ontario have extensively studied the responses of children to exercise, especially in the heat (Bar-Or and Unnithan 1994; Wilk and Bar-Or 1996; Wilk et al. 1998). They found that children are less efficient thermoregulators than adults, especially when exercising in warm environments. Compared to adults, children acclimatize more slowly. In fact, a child may need as many as 8 to 10 exposures (30-45 min each) to a new climate in order to acclimatize adequately. Exposures can occur every day, or every other day for a more conservative approach (Anderson et al. 2000). Children also have a higher **set point** (i.e., change in rectal temperature at which sweating starts) and a lower sweating rate, produce more metabolic heat per kilogram of body weight during exercise, and have greater physiological impairment from dehydration. Playing in the heat stresses a child's thermoregulatory mechanisms much more than is the case for an adult who is playing with the child. And if the child is dehydrated, this heat stress affects the child much more, potentially leading to heat-related illness. If you as an adult feel hot, your child is probably *very* hot! And like adults, when children and adolescents exercise they often do not drink adequate amounts of fluid to maintain fluid balance—leading to involuntary dehydration. For these reasons, active children need to learn the importance of adequate fluid intake before, during, and after exercise. "Keeping Children and Adolescents Well Hydrated During Exercise" provides some important guidelines for anyone who works with children and adolescents.

Children overheat and become dehydrated more quickly than adults. They should be encouraged to drink adequate fluids before, during, and after exercise. In conditions of prevailing high temperature, humidity, and radiation, sweating rates are expected to be high; and if an athlete is dehydrated for whatever reason or is not heat acclimatized, extra precautions should be taken to ensure a safe training environment. A few tips may help prevent the collapse on the field of a young athlete in training:

- Athletes should start exercise well-hydrated and well-fed. The last meal should be consumed between 1 and 4 h prior to practice. The closer to practice the athlete eats, the smaller the meal should be. Examples of pretraining snacks are a bowl of cereal with nonfat milk and water, a sandwich with turkey and water, an energy bar and a sport drink. These meals and snacks should be accompanied by plenty of fluid, flavor enhanced if needed.

- During exercise, athletes should have frequent fluid breaks in the shade and have access to cool sport drinks.

- After exercise, rehydration should occur immediately. Athletes should drink a sport drink and grab a snack rich in carbohydrates, electrolytes, and some protein. Examples include pretzels, orange wedges, bananas, low-fat milk, or a smoothie.

- An athlete who is participating in sport after having had an illness, vomiting, or diarrhea should ingest a sport drink before, during, and after practice. This will ensure the replacement of electrolytes and the retention of fluid, both of which may have been lost in high quantities through means other than sweating.

Highlight

Keeping Children and Adolescents Well Hydrated During Exercise

Children can maintain euhydration during prolonged and intermittent exercise if they drink 4 oz of fluid (120 mL) every 15 to 20 min (Bar-Or and Unnithan 1994). Children should be encouraged to drink fluids (~4-8 oz or roughly 120-240 mL) before exercise in order to be well hydrated; and after exercise they should drink ~16 oz of fluid (roughly 0.5 L) for every pound (0.5 kg) lost. Adolescents are also encouraged to measure their weight before and after exercise and to drink according to their sweat loss, or at least to replace fluid loss, to prevent a significant level of dehydration. After exercise, replacing about 150% of lost fluid also applies to youth. The American Academy of Pediatrics (2000) recommends that adolescent athletes weighing about 60 kg (132 lb) drink 9 oz (250 mL) every 20 min and be careful not to rely on thirst to drink (Anderson et al. 2000). Although adolescents have a better-adapted thermoregulatory system than children, it still lags behind that of adults. Both children and adolescents should be reminded that thirst may not be a good indicator of fluid needs. Like adults, children can learn to monitor their urine color as an indicator of fluid balance. Daily weight measurements, especially during two-a-day preseason practice in high school athletes, can have the advantage that athletes are monitored before they go out on the field for exercise.

Two-a-day practice in the summer heat as currently practiced in sports such as football can be hazardous for young people, especially if they are not acclimatized to the heat, are unfit, and are dehydrated. Clothing and equipment such as pads should be worn in progression, starting with light clothing, before the full uniform is worn in the heat. In addition, providing shaded areas for breaks, incorporating frequent fluid breaks, and selecting practice times during the cooler part of the day are all important precautions coaches should enforce during this type of training. The American Academy of Pediatrics (2000) also recommends reducing all activities that last 15 min or more whenever relative humidity, solar radiation, and air temperature are above critical levels (WBGT > 79° F; >26° C). Further they recommend canceling all athletic activities above a WBGT of 85° F (>29° C) (Anderson et al. 2000). Remember that WBGT is not air temperature; it is an index of climatic heat stress and takes into account radiation, humidity, and temperature.

Fluids offered to children and adolescents should be flavored, palatable, and cool. Research shows that particularly children aged 9 to 13 years prefer flavored beverages (especially grape) over water (Meyer et al. 1994). Compared to unflavored or flavored water, flavored beverages containing sodium and carbohydrate better promote fluid intake and help maintain fluid balance during exercise in the heat (Rivera-Brown et al. 1999; Wilk and Bar-Or 1996; Wilk et al. 1998). However, water is a good beverage, especially if other fluids are not available or if the exercise intensity is low and of short duration. It is also important to be aware of the early signs of dehydration in active children: dry lips and tongue, dark yellow urine, fatigue and apathy, muscle cramps, infrequent urination, and sunken eyes.

CHAPTER IN REVIEW

There is no question that maintaining fluid balance during exercise is important for exercise performance and good health. The amount, type, and timing of fluid intake both before and during exercise depend on a number of factors related to a person's level of fitness and general health and to the exercise environment. After exercise is over, it is also impor-

tant to make sure that adequate energy, fluids, and electrolytes are available in the food and drink consumed; this will replenish the body and prepare for the next exercise session or event. Inadequate fluid intake before, during, and after exercise is one of the most common nutritional problems facing athletes, especially those who work and train in extreme environments such as in the heat. It should be a priority to teach athletes the importance of fluid balance, how to monitor their own level of hydration, and how to adequately replace fluid. Before recommending an oral rehydration solution or sport drink to an athlete, one should evaluate the formulation and the extent to which the fluid will influence gastric emptying and intestinal absorption. In addition, the fluid should fit the athlete's requirements for fluid, energy, and electrolytes before, during, and after exercise, and should be well tolerated and liked by the athlete. Finally, exercise duration and intensity should be considered so that fluid replacement strategies match the goal of the athlete's training session (for example, when water should be preferred over a sport drink; at what intensity a sport drink should be mixed; if a sport drink should contain components besides carbohydrates and electrolytes; how it should be ingested).

In general, a sport drink should provide low concentrations of carbohydrate for energy and sodium for electrolyte replacement, and it should taste good. However, because today's marketplace is filled with fluid replacement beverages, sport drinks, fruit juices, energy drinks, soda, and bottled fitness water, selecting the right drink for the situation can be confusing. All of these beverages provide fluid, whereas some provide energy, electrolytes, protein, caffeine, and other ergogenic substances. Whether other ingredients are to be included should be based on a systematic decision-making process that should integrate factors such as nutritional and fitness status of the athlete, training and competition phase, exercise duration and intensity, and environmental conditions. After exercise, if athletes cannot or will not consume food, sport drinks are an excellent source of fluid, energy, and important electrolytes that help with effective rehydration.

◆

Key Concepts

1. **Understand the function and regulation of water and electrolyte balance within the body and the adverse health effects of dehydration, hypohydration, and hyponatremia.**

   Body water makes up a significant proportion of body weight (~60%); it functions as a transport medium, as a structural part of body tissues, as a lubricant, and as a component of chemical reactions. Body water is found both inside (intracellular) and outside (extracellular) the cells. Electrolytes help maintain this distribution of water within and outside the cells. Balance of water and electrolytes within the body is maintained by endocrine and neurological control mechanisms. Especially during exercise, optimal fluid balance is required to maintain plasma volume and electrolyte balance; and fluid balance depends on the rate and content of fluid intake and on the rates of gastric emptying and of intestinal absorption. Dehydration, which occurs when there is a decrease in total body water, hastens the onset of fatigue and degrades exercise performance. Hypohydration in weight-class sports can occur when athletes voluntarily dehydrate before a competitive event to make weight or improve aesthetic appearance. Hypohydration can also negatively affect exercise performance and health because it eventually may lead to substantial losses of body water. During exercise, hyponatremia (low plasma sodium concentrations) occurs when excess water is consumed and sodium intake is low or sodium losses are high. General symptoms of mild hyponatremia are fatigue and nausea.

2. **Identify the fluid and electrolyte recommendations for exercise.**

   Four hours before exercise, athletes should consume ~5 to 7 mL of fluid per kilogram body weight along with their last meal; more fluid is needed if the weather is hot or the individual is poorly hydrated. During exercise, athletes should consume fluid based on their sweating rate—enough to prevent a substantial fluid loss. The goal of the postexercise rehydration period is to replace the water and electrolytes lost during exercise. Athletes can achieve this by consuming both food and beverages during the postexercise period. The amount of fluid consumed should be 150% of the fluid lost during exercise. Consuming a sport beverage during the postexercise period helps replace fluid and electrolyte losses and provides carbohydrate for energy and glycogen replacement.

3. Assess fluid balance using changes in weight from pre to postexercise.

No one fluid recommendation fits all athletes. Fluid assessment should occur in all athletes to determine optimal fluid replacement strategies during and after exercise. Assessments of daily morning body weight, urine color, and urine volume, as well as changes in body weight before and after exercise, are currently the most practical measures athletes can take to evaluate their own hydration status. Monitoring body weight changes before and after exercise (and % body weight loss), level of thirst, and perceived exertion in a daily fluid log may assist in identifying the most optimal fluid replacement strategy for different environments and exercise regimens.

4. Understand the role of sport drinks in preventing and maintaining fluid balance before, during, and after exercise.

The primary reasons for using a sport drink before, during, and after exercise are to maximize fluid balance and replace electrolyte losses; to provide carbohydrate for energy and maintenance of blood glucose during exercise; and to rapidly replace muscle and liver glycogen after exercise.

5. Understand the effects of heat and cold on fluid needs in athletes.

Exercise in the heat increases sweat rate, fluid loss, and the risk of dehydration, especially if fluid intake does not match fluid loss. The body's core temperature rises quickly under such circumstances and can lead to hyperthermia. Performance decreases as a result, and the compounding effect of dehydration and hyperthermia can also lead to exertional heat illness. Acclimatization to exercise in the heat is the process of adapting thermoregulatory responses. A heat-acclimated athlete will sweat more heavily and sooner than one who is not acclimatized and thus will more effectively adapt to severe environmental stressors such as heat and humidity.

As one would expect, exercise in the cold results in a lower sweat response than exercise in the heat. However, maintaining fluid balance during exercise in the cold involves several challenges. First, in cold and dry environments, respiratory fluid loss can be substantial, leading to accelerated fluid loss and increasing the risk of dehydration. In addition, cold-induced diuresis, a reduced thirst response, and limited access to fluids as well as rest room facilities can lower voluntary fluid intake, increasing the risk of dehydration.

6. Identify fluid balance issues and replacement strategies in children.

Children have different fluid requirements than adults. Children are less efficient thermoregulators, especially when exercising in the heat, and have a higher sweat threshold. Overall, children have sweat rates that are lower than those of adults. During exercise, children often forget to replace fluids and need to be encouraged by adults to do so. Children should drink approximately 4 oz of fluid (120 mL) every 15 to 20 min of exercise, and they should drink a beverage that is palatable so that fluid consumption is encouraged.

Key Terms

black bulb 240
cold-induced diuresis 262
dehydration 235
dry bulb 240
euhydration 235
evidence based 247
exercise-associated hyponatremia
  (EAH) 241
exercise-associated muscle cramp 237
exertional heat exhaustion 238
exertional heatstroke 238
extracellular water 230
heat acclimation 261
heat acclimatization 261
hyperhydration 247
hyperthermia 260

hypohydration 235
interstitial fluid 230
intracellular water 230
intravascular water 230
isotonic solution 234
osmolality 231
osmolarity 231
osmotic pressure 231
rehydration 254
rhabdomyolysis 238
set point 263
transcellular water 230
Urine specific gravity (USG) 249
voluntary dehydration 241
wet bulb 240
wet bulb globe temperature (WBGT) 240

Additional Information

Burke L. Practical Sports Nutrition. Champaign, IL: Human Kinetics, 2007.

> Provides sport-specific guidelines for rehydration for road cycling and triathlon, middle- and long-distance running, swimming and rowing, sprint and jumping, field-based team sports, court and indoor team sports, racket sports, strength and power sports, weight-making sports, gymnastics, and winter sports.

Australian Institute for Sport (AIS): http://www.ausport.gov.au/ais

> Fact sheets for different sports provide data on sweating rates for a variety of sports, collected in AIS athletes.

Sodium balance and exercise (suppl). Curr Sports Med Rep 2008;7(4):S1-S55.

> A supplemental issue of *Current Sports Medicine Reports* for July/August. This supplement covers the topics of sodium balance and exercise, sodium regulation in the body, acute effects of sodium ingestion, fluid balance, exertional heat illness, strategies to prevent hyponatremia during prolonged exercise, determinants of sweat sodium, muscle cramps, and intravenous versus oral rehydration.

Fluid calculators for estimating sweat rates are available from these commercial Web sites:

> Gatorade: http://www.gatorade.co.uk/
>
> Accelerade: www.accelerade.com/team/Tools/Default.aspx

References

Almond CS, Shin AY, Fortescue EB, Mannix RC, Wypij D, Binstadt BA, Duncan CN, Olson DP, Salerno AE, Newburger JW, Greenes DS. Hyponatremia among runners in the Boston Marathon. N Engl J Med 2005;352:1550-1556.

American Academy of Pediatrics. Climatic heat stress and the exercising child and adolescent. Pediatrics 2000;106:58-59.

American Dietetic Association. Definitions and descriptions of key considerations and evidence-based dietetics practice,

2006. http://www.eatright.org/cps/rde/xchg/ada/hs.xsl/advocacy_11991_ENU_HTML.htm. Accessed December 2008.

Anderson MJ, Cotter JD, Garnham AP, Casley DJ, Febbraio MA. Effect of glycerol-induced hyperhydration on thermoregulation and metabolism during exercise in the heat. Int J Sport Nutr Exerc Metab 2001;11:315-333.

Anderson SJ, Griesemer BA, Johnson MD, Martin TJ, McLain LG, Rowland TW, Small E. American Academy of Pediatrics (AAP) position statement: climatic heat stress and the exercising child and adolescent. Pediatrics 2000;106:158-159.

Archer DT, Shirreffs SM. Effect of fluid ingestion rate on post-exercise rehydration in man. Proc Nutr Soc 2001;60:200A.

Armstrong LE. Caffeine, body fluid-electrolyte balance, and exercise performance. Int J Sport Nutr Exerc Metab 2002;12:189-206.

Armstrong LE, Casa DJ, Maresh CM, Ganio MS. Caffeine, fluid-electrolyte balance, temperature regulation, and exercise-heat tolerance. Exerc Sport Sci Rev 2007a;35:135-140.

Armstrong LE, Casa DJ, Millard-Stafford M, Moran DS, Pyne SW, Roberts WO. American College of Sports Medicine (ACSM) position stand: exertional heat illness during training and competition. Med Sci Sports Exerc 2007b;39:556-572.

Armstrong LE, Costill DL, Fink WJ. Changes in body water and electrolytes during heat acclimation: effects of dietary sodium. Aviat Space Environ Med 1987;58:143-148.

Armstrong LA, Maresh CM. The induction and decay of heat acclimatization in trained athletes. Sports Med 1991;12:302-312.

Armstrong LE, Maresh CM, Crago AE, Adams R, Roberts WO. Interpretation of aural temperatures during exercise, hypothermia, and cooling therapy. Med Exerc Nutr Health 1994;3:9-16.

Armstrong LE, Pumerantz AC, Roti MW, Judelson DA, Watson G, Dias JC, Sokmen B, Casa DJ, Maresh CM, Lieberman H, Kellogg M. Fluid, electrolyte, and renal indices of hydration during 11 days of controlled caffeine consumption. Int J Sport Nutr Exerc Metab 2005;15:252-265.

Armstrong LA, Soto JAH, Hacker FT, Casa DJ, Kavouras SA, Maresh CM. Urinary indices during dehydration, exercise, and rehydration. Int J Sport Nutr 1998;8:345-355.

Askew EW. Environmental and physical stress and nutrient requirements. Am J Clin Nutr 1995;61:631S-637S.

Ball TC, Headley SA, Vanderburgh PM, Smith JC. Periodic carbohydrate replacement during 50 min of high-intensity cycling improves subsequent sprint performance. Int J Sport Nutr 1995;5:151-158.

Banderet LE, MacDougall DM, Roberts DE, Tappan D, Jacey M, Gray P. Effects of hypohydration or cold exposure and restricted fluid intake upon cognitive performance. Natick, MA: U.S. Army Research Institute of Environmental Medicine, 1986;T15-86.

Bar-Or O. Temperature regulation during exercise in children and adolescents. In: Gisolfi C, Lamb D eds. Perspectives in exercise science and sports medicine: youth, exercise and sport. Indianapolis: Benchmark Press, 1989;335-367.

Bar-Or O, Unnithan VB. Nutritional requirements of young soccer players. J Sports Sci 1994;12:S39-S42.

Bergeron MF. Heat cramps during tennis: a case report. Int J Sport Nutr 1996;6:626-628.

Bergeron MF. Exertional heat cramps. In: Armstrong LE ed. Exertional heat illnesses. Champaign, IL: Human Kinetics, 2003a;91-102.

Bergeron MF. Heat cramps: fluid and electrolyte challenges during tennis in the heat. J Sci Med Sport 2003b;6:19-27.

Bergeron MF, McKeag DB, Casa DJ, Clarkson PM, Dick RW, Eichner ER, Horswill CA, Luke AC, Mueller F, Munce TA, Roberts WO, Rowland TW. Youth football: heat stress and injury risk. Med Sci Sports Exerc 2005;37:1421-1430.

Brouns F, Kovacs EMR, Senden JMG. The effect of different rehydration drinks on post-exercise electrolyte excretion in trained athletes. Int J Sports Med 1998;19:56-60.

Brouns F, Senden J, Beckers EJ, Saris WH. Osmolarity does not effect the gastric emptying rate of oral rehydration solutions. J Parenter Enteral Nutr 1995;19:403-406.

Bunt JC, Lohman TG, Boileau RA. Impact of total body water fluctuations of body fat from body density. Med Sci Sports Exerc 1989;21:96-100.

Burke LM. Preparation for competition. In: Burke LM, Deakin V eds. Clinical sports nutrition. Sydney, Australia: McGraw-Hill, 2006;355-384.

Burke LM, Hawley JA. Fluid balance in team sports. Guidelines for optimal practices. Sports Med 1997;24:38-54.

Carter RI, Chevront SN, Wray DW, Kolka MA, Stephenson LA, Sawka MN. Hypohydration and exercise-heat stress alters heart rate variability and parasympathetic control. J Thermal Biol 2005;30:495-502.

Casa DJ, Armstrong LE, Hillman SK, Montain SJ, Reiff RV, Rich BS, Roberts WO, Stone JA. National Athletic Trainers' Association position statement: fluid replacement for athletes. J Athl Train 2000;35:212-224.

Casa DJ, Clarkson PM, Roberts WO. American College of Sports Medicine roundtable on hydration and physical activity: consensus statements. Curr Sports Med Rep 2005;4:115-127.

Casa DJ, Eichner ER. Exertional heat illness and hydration. In: Starkey C, Johnson G eds. Athletic training and sports medicine. Boston: Jones and Bartlett, 2005;597-615.

Castellani JW, Young AJ, Ducharme MB, Giesbrecht GG, Glickman E, Sallis RE. American College of Sports Medicine (ACSM) position stand: prevention of cold injuries during exercise. Med Sci Sports Exerc 2006;38:2012-2029.

Cheuvront SN, Carter R 3rd, Haymes EM, Sawka MN. No effect of moderate hypohydration or hyperthermia on anaerobic exercise performance. Med Sci Sports Exerc 2006;38:1093-1097.

Clarkson PM. Exertional rhabdomyolysis and acute renal failure in marathon runners. Sports Med 2007;37:361-363.

Cleary M, Ruiz D, Eberman L, Mitchell I, Binkley H. Dehydration, cramping, and exertional rhabdomyolysis: a case report with suggestions for recovery. J Sport Rehab 2007;16:244-259.

Coggan AR, Coyle EF. Carbohydrate ingestion during prolonged exercise: effects on metabolism and performance. Exerc Sport Sci Rev 1991;19:1-40.

Convertino VA, Armstrong LE, Coyle EF, Mack GW, Sawka MN, Senay LC, Sherman WM. American College of Sports Medicine (ACSM) position stand: exercise and fluid replacement. Med Sci Sports Exerc 1996;28:i-vii.

Costill DL. Gastric emptying of fluids during exercise. In: Gisolfi CV, Lamb DR eds. Perspectives in exercise and science and sport medicine: fluid homeostasis during exercise. Indianapolis: Benchmark Press, 1990;97-121.

Costill DL, Bennett A, Branam G, Eddy D. Glucose ingestion at rest and during prolonged exercise. J Appl Physiol 1973;34:764-769.

Costill DL, Cote R, Fink W. Muscle water and electrolytes following varied levels of dehydration in man. J Appl Physiol 1976;40:6-11.

Coyle EF. Fluid and fuel intake during exercise. J Sports Sci 2004;22:39-55.

Dann EJ, Gillis S, Burstein R. Effect of fluid intake on renal function during exercise in the cold. Eur J Appl Physiol Occup Physiol 1990;61:133-137.

Davis JM, Jackson DA, Broadwell MS, Query JL, Lambert CL. Carbohydrate drinks delay fatigue during intermittent, high-intensity cycling in active men and women. Int J Sport Nutr 1997;7:261-273.

Dimeff RK. Seizure disorder in a professional American football player. Curr Sports Med Rep 2006;5:173-176.

Easton C, Turner S, Pitsiladis YP. Creatine and glycerol hyperhydration in trained subjects before exercise in the heat. Int J Sport Nutr Exerc Metab 2007;17:70-91.

Ebert TR, Martin DT, Bullock N, Mujika I, Quod MJ, Farthing LA, Burke LM, Withers RT. Influence of hydration status on thermoregulation and cycling hill climbing. Med Sci Sports Exerc 2007;39:323-329.

Edwards JS, Roberts DE. The influence of a calorie supplement on the consumption of the meal, ready-to-eat in a cold environment. Mil Med 1991;156:466-471.

Erickson MA, Schwarzkopf RJ, McKenzie RD. Effects of caffeine, fructose, and glucose ingestion on muscle glycogen utilization during exercise. Med Sci Sports Exerc 1987;19:579-583.

Evetovich TK, Boyd JC, Drake SM, Eschbach LC, Magal M, Soukup JT, Webster MJ, Whitehead MT, Weir JP. Effect of moderate dehydration on torque, electromyography, and mechanomyography. Muscle Nerve 2002;26:225-231.

Freund BJ, Sawka MN. Influence of cold stress on human fluid balance. In: Marriott BM, Carlson SJ eds. Nutritional needs in cold and in high-altitude environments. Washington, DC: National Academy Press, 1996.

Ganio MS, Casa DJ, Armstrong LE, Maresh CM. Evidence-based approach to lingering hydration questions. Clin Sports Med 2007;26:1-16.

Gisolfi CV. Water requirements during exercise in the heat. In: Marriott BM ed. Nutritional needs in hot environments. Washington, DC: National Academy Press, 1993;87-96.

Gisolfi CV, Duchman SM. Guidelines for optimal replacement beverages for different athletic events. Med Sci Sports Exerc 1992;24:679-687.

Gisolfi CV, Ryan AJ. Gastrointestinal physiology during exercise. In: Buskirk ER, Puhl SM eds. Body fluid balance: exercise and sport. Boca Raton, FL: CRC Press, 1996;19-51.

Gisolfi CV, Spranger KJ, Summers RW, Schedl HP, Bleiler TL. Effects of cycling exercise on intestinal absorption in humans. J Appl Physiol 1991;71:2518-2527.

Gisolfi CV, Summers RW, Schedl HP, Bleiler TL. Intestinal water absorption from select carbohydrate solutions in humans. J Appl Physiol 1992;73:2142-2150.

Gisolfi CV, Summers RW, Schedl HP, Bleiler TL. Effect of sodium concentration in a carbohydrate-electrolyte solution in intestinal absorption. Med Sci Sports Exerc 1995;27:1414-1420.

Gonzalez-Alonso J, Heaps CL, Coyle EF. Rehydration after exercise with common beverages and water. Int J Sports Med 1992;13:399-406.

Gonzalez-Alonso J, Teller C, Andersen SL, Jensen FB, Hyldig T, Nielsen B. Influence of body temperature on the development of fatigue during prolonged exercise in the heat. J Appl Physiol 1999;86:1032-1039.

Goulet ED, Aubertin-Leheudre M, Plante GE, Dionne IJ. A meta-analysis of the effects of glycerol-induced hyperhydration on fluid retention and endurance performance. Int J Sport Nutr Exerc Metab 2007;17:391-410.

Greenleaf JE. Problem: thirst, drinking behavior and involuntary dehydration. Med Sci Sports Exerc 1992;24:645-656.

Greiwe JS, Staffey KS, Melrose DR, Narve MD, Knowlton RG. Effects of dehydration on isometric muscular strength and endurance. Med Sci Sports Exerc 1998;30:284-288.

Hargreaves M, Dillo P, Angus D, Febbraio MA. Effect of fluid ingestion on muscle metabolism during prolonged exercise. J Appl Physiol 1996;80:363-366.

Heer M. Sodium regulation in the human body. Curr Sports Med Rep 2008;7(4):S3-S6.

Herfel R, Stone CK, Koury SI, Blake JJ. Iatrogenic acute hyponatraemia in a college athlete. Br J Sports Med 1998;32:257-258.

Hew-Butler T, Ayus JC, Kipps C, Maughan RJ, Mettler S, Meeuwisse WH, Page AJ, Reid SA, Rehrer NJ, Roberts WO, Rogers IR, Rosner MH, Siegel AJ, Speedy DB, Stuempfle KJ, Verbalis JG, Weschler LB, Wharam P. Statement of the Second International Exercise-Associated Hyponatremia Consensus Development Conference, New Zealand, 2007. Clin J Sport Med 2008; 18:111-21.

Hitchins S, Martin DT, Burke L, Yates K, Fallon K, Hahn A, Dobson GP. Glycerol hyperhydration improves cycle time trial performance in hot humid conditions. Eur J Appl Physiol Occup Physiol 1999;80:494-501.

Horswill CA. Effective fluid replacement. Int J Sport Nutr 1998;8:175-195.

Institute of Medicine (IOM), Food and Nutrition Board, National Academy of Science. Water. In: Dietary reference intakes for water, sodium, chloride, potassium, and sulfate. Washington, DC: National Academy Press, 2005;73-185.

Ivy JL, Res PT, Sprague RC, Widzer MO. Effect of a carbohydrate-protein supplement on endurance performance during exercise of varying intensity. Int J Sport Nutr Exerc Metab 2003;13:382-395.

Jentjens RLPG, Achten J, Jeukendrup AE. High oxidation rates from combined carbohydrates ingested during exercise. Med Sci Sports Exerc 2004a;36:1551-1558.

Jentjens, RLPG, Venables MC, Jeukendrup AE. Oxidation of exogenous glucose, sucrose, and maltose during prolonged cycling exercise. J Appl Physiol 2004b;96:1285-1291.

Jeukendrup A, Brouns F, Wagenmakers AJM, Saris WHM. Carbohydrate-electrolyte feedings improve 1-h time trial cycling performance. Int J Sports Med 1997;18:125-129.

Kern M, Podewils LJ, Vukovich M, Buono MJ. Physiological response to exercise in the heat following creatine supplementation. JEPonline 2001;4:18-27.

Kilduff LP, Georgiades E, James N, Minnion RH, Mitchell M, Kingsmore D, Hadjicharlambous M, Pitsiladis YP. The effects of creatine supplementation on cardiovascular, metabolic, and thermoregulatory responses during exercise in the heat in endurance-trained humans. Int J Sport Nutr Exerc Metab 2004;14:443-460.

Kovacs EM, Schmahl RM, Senden JM, Brouns F. Effect of high and low rates of fluid intake on post-exercise rehydration. Int J Sport Nutr Exerc Metab 2002;12:14-23.

Kovacs EMR, Senden JMG, Brouns F. Urine color, osmolality and specific electrical conductance are not accurate measures of hydration status during post-exercise rehydration. J Sports Med Phys Fit 1999;39:47-53.

Kristal-Boneh E, Glusman JG, Shitrit R, Chaemovitz C, Cassuto Y. Physical performance and heat tolerance after chronic water loading and heat acclimation. Aviat Space Environ Med 1995;66:733-738.

Ladell WSS. Water and salt (sodium chloride) intakes. In: Edholm O, Bacharach A eds. The physiology of human survival. New York: Academic Press, 1965;235-299.

Leiper JB. Gastric emptying and intestinal absorption of fluids, carbohydrates, and electrolytes. In: Maughan RJ, Murray R eds. Sports drinks: basic science and practical aspects. Boca Raton, FL: CRC Press, 2001;89-128.

Lorenz JM, Kleinman LI. Physiology and pathophysiology of body water and electrolytes. In: Kaplan LA, Pesce AI, Kazmierczak SC eds. Clinical chemistry: theory, analysis and correlation, 4th ed. St. Louis: Mosby, 2003;441-461.

Luden ND, Saunders MJ, Todd MK. Postexercise carbohydrate-protein-antioxidant ingestion decreases plasma creatine kinase and muscle soreness. Int J Sport Nutr Exerc Metab 2007;17:109-123.

Luft FC, Weinberger MH, Fineberg NS, Miller JZ, Grim CE. Effects of age on renal sodium homeostasis and its relevance to sodium sensitivity. Am J Med 1987;26(82):9-15.

Magal M, Webster MJ, Sistrunk LE, Whitehead MT, Evans RK, Boyce JC. Comparison of glycerol and water hydration regimens on tennis-related performance. Med Sci Sports Exerc 2003;35:150-156.

Marriott BM ed. Fluid replacement and heat stress. Committee on Military Nutrition Research, Food and Nutrition Board, Institute of Medicine. Washington, DC: National Academy Press, 1994.

Maughan RJ. Fluid balance and exercise. Int J Sports Med 1992;13:S132-S135.

Maughan RJ, Leiper JB. Sodium intake and post-exercise rehydration in man. Eur J Appl Physiol 1995;71:311-319.

Maughan RJ, Leiper JB, Shirreffs SM. Restoration of fluid balance after exercise-induced dehydration effects of food and fluid intake. Eur J Appl Physiol 1996;73:317-325.

Maughan RJ, Shirreffs SM. Recovery from prolonged exercise: restoration of water and electrolyte balance. J Sports Sci 1997;15:297-303.

Maughan RJ, Shirreffs SM, Leiper JB. Errors in the estimation of hydration status from changes in body mass. J Sports Sci 2007a;25:797-804.

Maughan RJ, Shirreffs SM, Watson P. Exercise, heat, hydration and the brain. J Am Coll Nutr 2007b;26:604S-612S.

Maw GJ, MacKenzie IL, Taylor NAS. Human body-fluid distribution during exercise in hot, temperate and cool environments. Acta Physiol Scand 1998;163:287-304.

Meyer F, Bar-Or O, McDougall D, Heigenhauser G. Sweat electrolyte loss during exercise in the heat: effects of gender and maturation. Med Sci Sports Exerc 1992;24:776-781.

Meyer F, Bar-Or O, Salsberg A, Passe D. Hypohydration during exercise in children: effect of thirst, drink preference and rehydration. Int J Sport Nutr 1994;4:22-35.

Meyer NL. Female winter sport athletes: Nutrition issues during the preparation for the 2002 Olympic winter games in Salt Lake City. Dissertation. University of Utah, Exercise and Sport Science, Salt Lake City, 2003.

Meyer NL, Johnson SC, Askew EW, Lutkemeier ML, Bainbridge C, Shultz BB, Manore MM. Energy and nutrient intake of elite female alpine ski racers during the preparatory phase. Med Sci Sports Exerc 1999;31:S100.

Meyer NL, Parker-Simmons S. Winter sports. In: Burke L ed. Practical sports nutrition. Champaign, IL: Human Kinetics, 2007;335-358.

Millard-Stafford ML, Cureton KJ, Wingo JE, Trilk J, Warren GL, Buyckx M. Hydration during exercise in warm, humid conditions: effect of a caffeinated sports drink. Int J Sport Nutr Exerc Metab 2007;17:163-177.

Montain SJ, Cheuvront SN, Lukaski HC. Sweat mineral-element responses during 7 h of exercise-heat stress. Int J Sport Nutr Exerc Metab 2007;17:574-582.

Montain SJ, Coyle EF. Influence of graded dehydration on hyperthermia and cardiovascular drift during exercise. J Appl Physiol 1992;73:1340-1350.

Moroff SV, Bass DE. Effects of overhydration on man's physiological responses to work in the heat. J Appl Physiol 1965;20:267-270.

Morris JG, Nevill ME, Lakomy HKA, Nicholas C, Williams C. Effect of a hot environment on performance of prolonged, intermittent, high-intensity shuttle running. J Sports Sci 1998;16:677-686.

Murray R. Fluid needs in hot and cold environments. Int J Sport Nutr 1995;5:S62-S73.

Murray R. Fluid needs of athletes. In: Berning JR, Steen SN eds. Nutrition for sport and exercise. Gaithersburg, MD: Aspen, 1998;143-153.

Nadel ER, Fortney SM, Wenger CB. Effect on hydration state of circulatory and thermal regulations. J Appl Physiol 1980;49:715-721.

National Center for Catastrophic Sport Injury Research. Annual Survey of Football Injury Research 1931-2007, January, 2008. http://www.unc.edu/depts/nccsi/FootballAnnual.pdf

National Weather Service, National Oceanic and Atmospheric Administration, Department of Commerce. Heat index chart, June 2006. www.nws.noaa.gov.

Nicholas CW, Williams C, Phillips G, Nowitz A. Influence of ingesting a carbohydrate-electrolyte solution on endurance capacity during intermittent, high intensity shuttle running. J Sports Sci 1995;13:282-290.

Noakes TD, Norman RJ, Buck RH, Godlonton J, Stevenson K, Pittaway D. The incidence of hyponatremia during prolonged ultraendurance exercise. Med Sci Sports Exerc 1990;22:165-170.

Noakes TD, Rehrer NJ, Maughan RJ. The importance of volume in regulating gastric emptying. Med Sci Sports Exerc 1991;23:307-313.

O'Brien KK, Montain SJ, Corr WP, Sawka MN, Knapik JJ, Craig SC. Hyponatremia associated with over-hydration in US Army trainees. Mil Med 2001;166:405-410.

Olsson KE, Saltin B. Variation in total body water with muscle glycogen changes in man. Acta Physiol 1970;80:11-18.

Orlov SN, Mongin AA. Salt-sensing mechanism in blood pressure regulation and hypertension. Am J Physiol Heart Circ Physiol 2007;293(4):H2039-H2053.

Pals KL, Chang R, Ryan AJ, Gisolfi CV. Effect of running intensity on intestinal permeability. J Appl Physiol 1997;82:571-576.

Pirnay F, Crielaard JM, Pallikarakis N, Lacroix M, Mosora F, Krzentowski G, Luyckx AS, Lefebvre PJ. Fate of exogenous glucose during exercise of different intensities in humans. J Appl Physiol 1982;53:1620-1624.

Ploutz-Snyder L, Foley J, Ploutz-Snyder R, Kanaley J, Sagendorf K, Meyer R. Gastric gas and fluid emptying assessed by magnetic resonance imaging. Eur J Appl Physiol 1999;79:212-220.

Puhl SM, Buskirk ER. Nutrient beverages for physical performance. In: Wolinsky I ed. Nutrition in exercise and sport. Boca Raton, FL: CRC Press, 1998;277-314.

Randall K. The NFL meat grinder: US pro football player dies in training camp. www.wsws.org. World Socialist Web site, http://www.wsws.org/articles/2001/aug2001/nfl-a10.shtml. Accessed, Dec 2008.

Remick D, Chancellor K, Pederson J, Zambraski EJ, Sawka MN, Wenger CD. Hyperthermia and dehydration-related deaths associated with intentional rapid weight loss in three collegiate wrestlers—North Carolina, Wisconsin, and Michigan, November-December 1997. MMWR 1998;47:105-108.

Richards L. Disturbing trend: hiker ill from too much water. Arizona Republic, Apr 7, 1996.

Riedesel ML, Allen DY, Peake GT, Al-Quattan K. Hyperhydration with glycerol solutions. J Appl Physiol 1987;63:2262-2268.

Rintamäki HT, Oksa MJ, Latvala J. Water balance and physical performance in cold. Arctic Med Res 1995;54 suppl:32-36.

Rivera-Brown AM, Gutierrez T, Gutierrez JC, Frontera WR, Bar-Or O. Drink composition, voluntary drinking, and fluid balance in exercising, trained, heat-acclimatized boys. J Appl Physiol 1999;86:78-84.

Robergs RA, Griffin SE. Glycerol: biochemistry, pharmacokinetics and clinical and practical applications. Sports Med 1998;26:145-167.

Rogers NL, Dinges DF. Caffeine: implications for alertness in athletes. Clin Sports Med 2005;24(2):e1-13, x-xi.

Romano-Ely BC, Todd MK, Saunders MJ, Laurent TS. Effect of an isocaloric carbohydrate-protein-antioxidant drink on cycling performance. Med Sci Sports Exerc 2006;38:1608-1616.

Rosner MH, Kirven J. Exercise-associated hyponatremia. Clin J Am Soc Nephrol 2007;2:151-161.

Ryan AJ, Lambert G, Shi X, Chang RT, Summers RW, Gisolfi CV. Effect of hypohydration on gastric emptying and intestinal absorption during exercise. J Appl Physiol 1998;84:1581-1588.

Saunders MJ, Kane MD, Todd MK. Effects of a carbohydrate-protein beverage on cycling endurance and muscle damage. Med Sci Sports Exerc 2004;36:1233-1238.

Saunders MJ, Luden ND, Herrick JE. Consumption of an oral carbohydrate-protein gel improves cycling endurance and prevents postexercise muscle damage. J Strength Cond Res 2007;21:678-684.

Sawka MN, Burke LM, Eichner ER, Maughan RJ, Montain SJ. American College of Sports Medicine (ACSM) position stand: exercise and fluid replacement. Med Sci Sports Exerc 2007;39:377-390.

Sawka MN, Noakes TD. Does dehydration impair exercise performance? Med Sci Sports Exerc 2007;39:1209-1217.

Sawka MN, Pandolf KB. Effects of body water loss in physiological function and exercise performance. In: Lamb DR, Gisolfi CV eds. Perspectives in exercise and science and sport medicine: fluid homeostasis during exercise. Indianapolis: Benchmark Press, 1990;1-38.

Sawka MN, Toner MM, Francesconi RP, Pandolf KB. Hypohydration and exercise: effects of heat acclimation, gender, and environment. J Appl Physiol 1983;55:1147-1153.

Schedl HP, Maughan RJ, Gisolfi CV. Intestinal absorption during rest and exercise: implications for formulating an oral rehydration solution (ORS). Med Sci Sports Exerc 1994;26:267-280.

Seifert JG, Luetkemeier MJ, White AT, Mino LM. The physiological effects of beverage ingestion during cross country ski training in elite collegiate skiers. Can J Appl Physiol 1998;23:66-73.

Seifert JG, Lutkemeier MJ, White AT, Mino LM, Miller D. Fluid balance during slalom training in elite collegiate alpine racers. In: 2nd International Congress on Skiing and Science. St. Christoph, Austria: Verlag Dr. Kovac, 2000;634-640.

Seifert J, Harmon J, DeClercq P. Protein added to a sports drink improves fluid retention. Int J Sport Nutr Exerc Metab 2006;16:420-429.

Sherman WM, Plyley MJ, Sharp RL, Van Handel PJ, McAllister RM, Fink WJ, Costill DL. Muscle glycogen storage and its relationship with water. Int J Sports Med 1982;3:22-24.

Shi X, Gisolfi CV. Fluid and carbohydrate replacement during intermittent exercise. Sports Med 1998;25:157-172.

Shirreffs SM, Armstrong LE, Cheuvront SN. Fluid and electrolyte needs for preparation and recovery from training and competition. J Sports Sci 2004;22:57-63.

Shirreffs SM, Casa DJ, Carter R. Fluid needs for training and competition in athletes. J Sports Sci 2007;25(S1):S83-S91.

Shirreffs SM, Maughan RJ. The effect of alcohol consumption on fluid retention following exercise-induced dehydration in man. J Physiol 1995;489:33P-34P.

Shirreffs SM, Maughan RJ. Restoration of fluid balance after exercise-induced dehydration: effects of alcohol consumption. J Appl Physiol 1997;83:1152-1158.

Shirreffs SM, Maughan RJ. Volume repletion after exercise-induced volume depletion in humans: replacement of water and sodium losses. Am J Physiol 1998;274:F868-875.

Shirreffs SM, Maughan RJ. Water turnover and regulation of fluid balance. In: Maughan RJ, Murray R eds. Sports drinks: basic science and practical aspects. Boca Raton, FL:CRC Press, 2001;29-44.

Shirreffs SM, Taylor AJ, Leiper JB, Maughan RJ. Post-exercise rehydration in man: effects of volume consumed and drink sodium content. Med Sci Sports Exerc 1996;28:1260-1271.

Shirreffs SM, Sawka MN, Stone M. Water and electrolyte needs for football training and match-play. J Sports Sci. 2006:24:699-707.

Shirreffs SM, Watson P, Maughan RJ. Milk as an effective post-exercise rehydration drink. Br J Nutr 2007;98:173-180.

Squire DL. Heat illness: fluid and electrolyte issues for pediatric and adolescent athletes. Pediatr Clin North Am 1990;37:1085-1109.

Stachenfeld NS. Acute effects of sodium ingestion on thirst and cardiovascular function. Curr Sports Med Rep 2008;7(4):S7-S13.

Stofan JR, Zachwieja JJ, Horswill CA, Murray R, Anderson SA, Eichner ER. Sweat and sodium losses in NCAA football players: a precursor to heat cramps? Int J Sport Nutr Exerc Metab 2005;15:641-652.

Sutton JR. Thermal problems in the masters athlete. In: Sutton JR, Brock R eds. Sports medicine for the mature athlete. Indianapolis: Benchmark Press, 1986;125-132.

Sutton JR. Clinical implications of fluid imbalance. In: Lamb DR, Gisolfi CV eds. Perspectives in exercise and science and sport medicine: fluid homeostasis during exercise. Indianapolis: Benchmark Press, 1990;425-453.

Tsintzas OK, Liu R, Williams C, Campbell I, Gaitanos G. The effect of carbohydrate ingestion on performance during a 30-km race. Int J Sport Nutr 1993;3:127-139.

Tsintzas OK, Williams C, Singh R, Wilson W, Burrin J. Influence of carbohydrate-electrolyte drinks on marathon running performance. Eur J Appl Physiol Occup Physiol 1995;70:154-160.

Valentine RJ, Saunders MJ, Todd MK, St Laurent TG. Influence of carbohydrate-protein beverage on cycling endurance and indices of muscle disruption. Int J Sport Nutr Exerc Metab 2008;18:363-378.

Van Essen M, Gibala MJ. Failure of protein to improve time trial performance when added to a sports drink. Med Sci Sports Exerc 2006;38:1476-1483.

Van Nieuwenhoven MA, Brummer RM, Brouns F. Gastrointestinal function during exercise: comparison of water, sports drink, and sports drink with caffeine. J Appl Physiol 2000;89:1079-1085.

Vergauwen L, Brouns F, Hespel P. Carbohydrate supplementation improves stroke performance in tennis. Med Sci Sports Exerc 1998;30:1289-1295.

Vist GE, Maughan RJ. Gastric emptying of ingested solutions in man: effect of beverage glucose concentration. Med Sci Sports Exerc 1994;26:1269-1273.

Vist GE, Maughan RJ. The effect of osmolality and carbohydrate content on the rate of gastric emptying of liquids in man. J Physiol 1995;486:523-531.

Volek JS, Mazzetti SA, Farquhar WB, Barnes BR, Gómez AL, Kraemer WJ. Physiological responses to short-term exercise in the heat after creatine loading. Med Sci Sports Exerc 2001;33:1101-1108.

Wade CE. Hormonal control of body fluid volume. In: Buskirk ER, Puhl EM eds. Body fluid balance: exercise and sport. Boca Raton, FL: CRC Press, 1996;53-73.

Walsh RM, Noakes TD, Hawley JA, Dennis SC. Impaired high-intensity cycling performance time at low levels of dehydration. Int J Sports Med 1994;15:392-398.

Welsh RS, Davis JM, Burke JR, Williams HG. Carbohydrates and physical/mental performance during intermittent exercise to fatigue. Med Sci Sports Exerc 2002;34:723-731.

Wendt D, van Loon LJ, Lichtenbelt WD. Thermoregulation during exercise in the heat: strategies for maintaining health and performance. Sports Med 2007;37:669-682.

Wilk B, Bar-Or O. Effect of drink flavor and NaCl on voluntary drinking and hydration in boys exercising in heat. J Appl Physiol 1996;80:1112-1117.

Wilk B, Kriemler S, Heidemaire K, Bar-Or O. Consistency in preventing voluntary dehydration in boys who drink a flavored carbohydrate-NaCl beverage during exercise in the heat. Int J Sport Nutr 1998;8:1-9.

Wrestling Rules Committee. National Collegiate Athletic Association wrestling rules. Indianapolis: NCAA, 2003.

Wrestling Rules Committee. National Federation of State High School Associations wrestling rules. Indianapolis: NFSHSA, 2003.

Yeo SE, Jentjens RL, Wallis GA, Jeukendrup AE. Caffeine increases exogenous carbohydrate oxidation during exercise. J Appl Physiol 2005;99:844-850.

Young AJ, Muza SR, Sawka MN, Pandolf KB. Human vascular fluid responses to cold stress are not altered by cold acclimation. Undersea Biomed Res 1987;14:215-228.

Zambraski EJ. The kidney and body fluid balance during exercise. In: Buskirk ER, Puhl EM eds. Body fluid balance: exercise and sport. Boca Raton, FL: CRC Press, 1996;75-96.

Zderic TW, Davidson CJ, Schenk S, Byerley LO, Coyle EF. High-fat diet elevates resting intramuscular triglyceride concentration and whole body lipolysis during exercise. Am J Physiol Endocrinol Metab 2004;286:E217-E225.

CHAPTER 9

B Vitamins Important in Energy Metabolism

Chapter Objectives

After reading this chapter you should be able to

- understand the exercise-related functions and dietary requirements of the B vitamins,
- discuss the rationale for increased need for B vitamins in active individuals,
- identify the dietary and biochemical assessment methods for the B vitamins,
- discuss how exercise may alter B vitamin requirements in active people, and
- explain the relationship between B vitamins and exercise performance.

Do you take vitamin or mineral supplements? If you answer yes, *why* are you supplementing? How did you know which supplement to buy? People give many different reasons for supplementing with vitamins and minerals. If you were to ask friends or clients why they supplement, here are some of the responses you might hear:

- They supplement as an insurance policy because they do not eat right.
- They think the food supply lacks sufficient vitamins and minerals.
- They think supplements will give them extra energy.
- They supplement to prevent disease or to treat a particular health problem.
- They think active people need more vitamins than sedentary individuals.
- They think people under high stress need more vitamins and minerals.

At least 25% of Americans appear to use dietary supplements daily, and as many as 35% to 40% use them occasionally. For people engaged in physical activity, the estimates are as high as 50% (Sobal and Marquart 1994). In some sports, like bodybuilding, 60% to 100% of the participants use supplements. This high use of supplements has created a $4 billion industry that constantly bombards the public with advertisements. In addition, newspapers and TV news programs frequently report studies about nutrients that can prevent cancer, improve health, or prevent fatigue. It is not surprising that American consumers are confused about whether they should use vitamin or mineral supplements. As a health professional, you will be constantly asked about supplements, especially if you are working with active individuals. How do you sort through this information overload? How can you make the best recommendations to people who ask you about supplements? How do you respond to the athlete who wants to know whether exercise increases the need for vitamins, or whether supplementation will improve exercise performance? (See "Guidelines for Recommending Vitamin Supplements")

This chapter addresses these questions, specifically examining whether exercise increases the need for the **B vitamins** (thiamin, riboflavin, vitamin B$_6$, niacin, pantothenic acid, and biotin) required in energy metabolism. Because these vitamins are especially important in the production of energy, they are grouped together in one chapter (vitamin B$_{12}$ and folate are also B vitamins but because of their critical role in blood formation are covered in chapter 12).

First, we review the exercise-related functions and dietary requirements of each vitamin. Then we briefly cover whether active people have increased needs. Next, we review the methods for assessing vitamin status, including the dietary sources of each nutrient, the typical intakes reported in active individuals, and the biochemical assessment parameters typically measured. We then address the impact of vitamin deficiency or marginal vitamin status on exercise performance and work. Finally, we examine whether vitamin supplementation in healthy individuals enhances exercise performance.

Because most B vitamins are cofactors for metabolic reactions that produce energy, it is natural to hypothesize that exercise increases the need for these nutrients. In fact, the 1989 Recommended Dietary Allowances (RDAs) for most of these nutrients were based on intakes of energy (thiamin, riboflavin, and niacin catalyze steps in energy metabolism) and protein (vitamin B$_6$ is involved in protein synthesis and glycogen metabolism) (Food and Nutrition Board 1989). As people become more physically active, it is reasonable to think that they will consume more

Highlight

Guidelines for Recommending Vitamin Supplements

The following questions will help you determine whether you should recommend vitamin supplements for an active person:

- Is current dietary intake of the vitamin adequate?
- Is there any indication for increased need?
- Is the amount recommended below the toxic level?
- Are any nutrient–nutrient or drug–nutrient interactions indicated?
- Why does the athlete want to supplement?
- Is the athlete willing to make dietary changes that would improve vitamin intakes?
- What is the cost of the supplement? What is the cost of getting the nutrient from food?
- Can the nutrient be easily obtained in food by means of simple dietary changes that are acceptable to the athlete?

energy and protein and, in the process, consume more of these vitamins. Yet this is not always true. If people make poor dietary choices, they may not increase their consumption of these micronutrients as much as they increase their energy and protein intakes. Moreover, if they increase physical activity but restrict energy intake (as happens often with people who are dieting), the need for the vitamins may increase while their dietary intake actually declines.

EXERCISE-RELATED FUNCTIONS AND DIETARY REQUIREMENTS

To discuss why exercise might increase the need for these vitamins, we must first understand their role in energy metabolism. Figure 9.1 shows how thiamin, riboflavin, vitamin B_6, niacin, pantothenic acid, and biotin are each cofactors in one or more of the metabolic pathways that produce energy during exercise. Table 9.1 lists each vitamin, its active form in the body, the various metabolic pathways for which it is required, and some of the specific enzymes that require the vitamin as a cofactor. The following section briefly discusses the specific exercise-related function of each of the B vitamins involved in energy metabolism.

Thiamin

Thiamin is an essential cofactor for important enzymes involved in the metabolism of both carbohydrate and amino acids, especially the **branched-chain amino acids (BCAA)**. The active form of thiamin in the body is **thiamin diphosphate (TDP)** (formerly called thiamin pyrophosphate or TPP). Thiamin is a coenzyme for the pyruvate dehydrogenase complex that catalyzes the conversion of pyruvate to acetyl-CoA (see figure 9.1), which can then enter the **tricarboxylic acid (TCA)** cycle for metabolism. Thiamin is also a cofactor for α-ketoglutarate decarboxylase, an enzyme responsible for the formation of succinyl-CoA in the TCA cycle. Thus, thiamin helps in the oxidation of both carbohydrate and fat through this cycle. Thiamin is also required for transketolase, an important enzyme in the pentose pathway. Finally, thiamin is required for the branched-chain α-keto decarboxylases, enzymes responsible for the catabolism of the BCAAs (Butterworth 2006).

Physical activity stresses these energy-producing metabolic pathways. Because thiamin requirements are linked to energy metabolism

(especially carbohydrate metabolism), the 1989 RDA for thiamin was expressed in terms of energy intake (mg/1000 kcal), with 0.5 mg of thiamin required per 1000 kcal consumed per day (Food and Nutrition Board 1989). This value was then extrapolated to the estimated minimum energy requirements for men and women. Thus, the 1989 RDA was 1.5 mg/day for adult men and 1.1 mg/day for adult women, with a minimum of 1.0 mg/day required for all adults. An additional 0.4 and 0.5 mg/day are recommended during pregnancy and lactation, respectively (Food and Nutrition Board 1989). In 1998, the RDA for thiamin was decreased for men but not for women (IOM 1998). The new thiamin RDA for men (19-50 years) is 1.2 mg/day. One reason for the decrease for men was that the new RDA for thiamin was no longer based on energy intake (see "How Does the Dietary Reference Intake Differ From the Recommended Dietary Allowance?" p. 280). However, this does not diminish the importance of thiamin for carbohydrate metabolism. It merely means that active people, especially those consuming high levels of energy or carbohydrate, may need more thiamin than the current RDA.

Riboflavin

Riboflavin is necessary for the synthesis of two important coenzymes in the body—**flavin mononucleotide (FMN)** and **flavin adenine dinucleotide (FAD)**. These coenzymes are especially important in the metabolism of glucose, fatty acids, glycerol, and amino acids for energy. Because exercise stresses the biochemical pathways that metabolize these substrates, it has been hypothesized that riboflavin requirements are higher in people who exercise. Riboflavin is also involved in the conversion of pyridoxine (vitamin B_6) and folate to their coenzyme forms (Leklem 1988). As with thiamin, the 1989 RDA for riboflavin was expressed in terms of energy intake, with 0.6 mg of riboflavin recommended for every 1000 kcal consumed—or 1.7 mg/day for adult men and 1.3 mg/day for adult women, with a minimum recommended intake of 1.2 mg/day. Because pregnancy and lactation increase energy demands, an additional 0.3 mg/day was recommended during pregnancy and an additional 0.4 to 0.5 mg/day during lactation (Food and Nutrition Board 1989).

In 1998, the RDA for riboflavin was revised downward for both adult men and women (19-70 years), to 1.3 mg/day for men and 1.1 mg/day for women (IOM 1998). One of the reasons for the lower RDA was that the new RDA for riboflavin

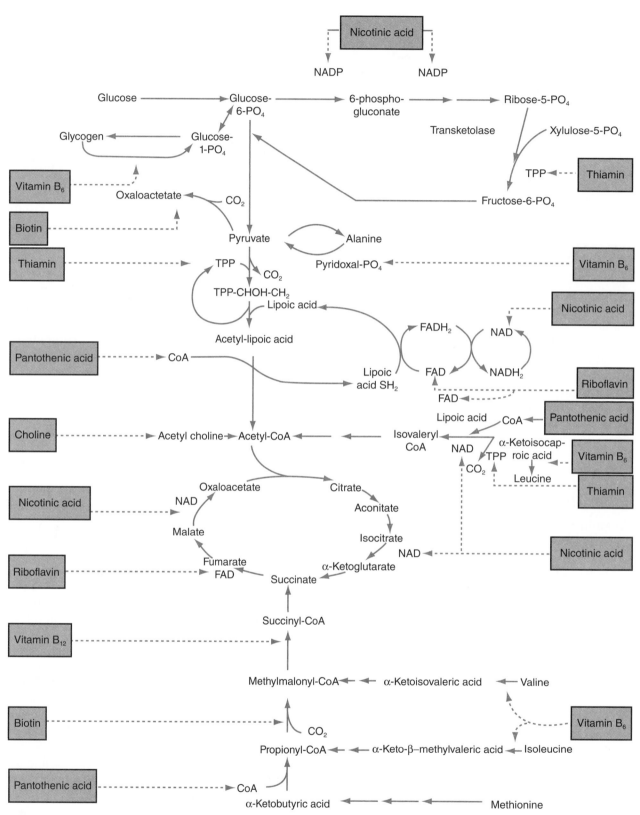

Figure 9.1 Metabolic pathways that require B vitamins.
Thiamin = thiamin diphosphate (TDP); formerly called thiamin pyrophosphate or TPP
Riboflavin = flavin adenine dinucleotide (FAD)
Nicotinic acid = nicotinamide adenine dinucleotide (NAD) and NAD phosphate (NADP)
Pantothenic Acid = coenzyme A (CoA)

Table 9.1 Exercise-Related Metabolic Functions and Examples of Enzymes in These Functions That Require B-Complex Vitamins as Cofactors

Vitamin	Active form of the vitamin	Functions of the vitamin related to exercise	Metabolic pathways that require the vitamin	Major enzymes that require the vitamin as a cofactor
Thiamin (B$_1$)	Thiamin pyrophosphate (TPP)	Energy production from protein, fat, and carbohydrate	Carbohydrate, branched-chain amino acid, and fat metabolism	Pyruvate dehydrogenase, α-keotglutarate decarboxylase, branched-chain keto acid decarboxylase
Riboflavin (B$_2$)	Flavin mononucleotide (FMN); flavin adenine dinucleotide (FAD)	Energy production from protein, fat, and carbohydrate; conversion of vitamin B$_6$ and folate to their active forms	Carbohydrate, protein, and fat metabolism (tricarboxylic acid [TCA] cycle, electron transport)	acyl-CoA dehydrogenase, succinate dehydrogenase, glycerol dehydrogenase, pyruvate dehydrogenase
Vitamin B$_6$	Pyridoxine, pyridoxal, pyridoxamine; pyridoxal-5'-phosphate (PLP) is active cofactor	Transamination of amino acids, release of glucose from glycogen, glucose-alanine cycle, gluconeogenesis	Protein and carbohydrate metabolism	Glycogen phosphorylase, transaminases
Niacin (B$_3$), nicotinic acid	Nicotinamide adenine dinucleotide (NAD), nicotinamide adenine dinucleotide phosphate (NADP)	Energy production from protein, fat, and carbohydrate	TCA cycle, glycolysis, pentose phosphate pathway	Lactate dehydrogenase, glucose-6-phosphate dehydrogenase, 3-phosphoglyceraldehyde dehydrogenase, glutamine dehydrogenase
Pantothenic acid	Coenzyme A (CoA); acyl carrier protein (ACP)	Energy metabolism from fat and carbohydrate	β-Oxidation of fats, TCA cycle, glycolysis	CoA and ACP function as carriers of acyl groups
Biotin		Energy production from protein, carbohydrate metabolism, and fat synthesis	Gluconeogenesis, fatty acid synthesis and amino acid degradation	Pyruvate carboxylase, acetyl-CoA carboxylase, propionyl-CoA carbocylase, 3-methylcrotonyl-CoA carboxylase

was no longer based on energy intake (see "How Does the Dietary Reference Intake Differ From the Recommended Dietary Allowance?" on p. 280). This change was due to limited research on how riboflavin requirements change over a large range of energy intakes and body sizes. It is well known that riboflavin plays an important role in energy metabolism; the new RDAs for riboflavin were adjusted to reflect differences in average energy requirements and in body size and to reflect the energy requirements of pregnancy and lactation. The change does not diminish the importance of riboflavin for energy metabolism in active individuals who may need more riboflavin than the current RDA.

Vitamin B$_6$

Vitamin B$_6$ plays a major role in metabolic pathways required during exercise. It is required in the metabolism of proteins and amino acids and in the release of glucose from stored glycogen. **Pyridoxal-5'-phosphate (PLP),** the most metabolically active form of vitamin B$_6$, can be measured in the blood. Pyridoxal-5'-phosphate is a cofactor for transferases, transaminases, decarboxylases, and other enzymes used in the metabolic transformations of amino acids. During exercise, the gluconeogenic process involves the breakdown of amino acids for energy in the muscle and the conversion of lactic acid to

How Does the Dietary Reference Intake Differ From the Recommended Dietary Allowance?

In 1989, the Food and Nutrition Board of the National Research Council published the last complete set of RDAs for all nutrients, defining RDAs as "the levels of intake of essential nutrients that, on the basis of scientific knowledge, are judged by the Food and Nutrition Board to be adequate to meet the known nutrient needs of practically all healthy persons" (Institute of Medicine [IOM], Food and Nutrition Board 1989). In the past, the RDAs were regularly updated to reflect new scientific knowledge. We have gone through a transition period in which the RDAs are being replaced with a set of **Dietary Reference Intakes (DRIs)**, which include the RDAs but also other measures of nutrient needs. This change was made to reflect the growing body of scientific evidence that nutrient requirements may change in chronic disease. The DRI committee for each group of nutrients establishes reference intakes, periodically updating the recommendations according to newer scientific data (see chapter 1, figure 1.1, for an outline of this process). Currently, we have new guidelines for all the nutrients (vitamins, minerals, macronutrients, energy, and fiber). Since the DRIs were established in 1998 for the B vitamins, we give both the more recent DRIs and the 1989 RDAs for the B vitamins throughout this chapter so that you can see how these values have changed with increased scientific information. The next few paragraphs explain the new guidelines.

Recommended Dietary Allowance

The **Recommended Dietary Allowance (RDA)** is the intake that meets the nutrient need of almost all of the healthy individuals in a specific age and gender group. It should be used in guiding people to achieve adequate nutrient intake aimed at decreasing the risk of chronic disease. It is based on estimates of average requirements, plus an increase to account for the variation within a particular group. Available scientific evidence allowed the DRI committee to calculate RDAs for adults for vitamin A, vitamin E, vitamin C, phosphorus, magnesium, iron, zinc, selenium, iodine, copper, molybdenum, thiamin, riboflavin, niacin, vitamin B_6, folate, and vitamin B_{12}.

Adequate Intake

When sufficient scientific evidence is not available to estimate an average requirement, **Adequate Intakes (AIs)** have been set. Individuals should use the AI as a goal for intake where no RDAs exist. The AI is derived though experimental or observational data showing a mean intake that appears to sustain a desired indicator of health (e.g., calcium retention in bone) for most members of a population group. For example, AIs have been set for infants through 1 year of age using the average observed nutrient intake of populations of breast-fed infants as the standard. The committee set AIs for vitamin D, vitamin K, calcium, manganese, chromium, fluoride, pantothenic acid, biotin, and choline.

Estimated Average Requirement

The **Estimated Average Requirement (EAR)** is the intake that meets the estimated nutrient need of half the individuals in a specific group. This figure is used as the basis for developing the RDA and is used by nutrition policy makers in evaluating the adequacy of nutrient intakes of a group and in planning how much the group should consume.

Tolerable Upper Intake Level

The **Tolerable Upper Intake Level (UL)** is the maximum intake by an individual that is unlikely to pose risks of adverse health effects in almost all healthy individuals in a specified group. It is not a recommended level of intake; there is no established benefit for individuals to consume nutrients at levels above the RDA or AI. For most nutrients, this figure refers to total intakes from food, fortified food, and nutrient supplements.

glucose in the liver. The breakdown of muscle glycogen for energy during exercise is another function of vitamin B_6 that is directly related to energy production. Vitamin B_6 must be present to release glucose-1-phosphate from muscle glycogen (Mackey et al. 2006; Manore 2000). Once you know the functions of vitamin B_6, it is easy to understand why adequate vitamin B_6 is so important for exercise. Because vitamin B_6 is directly involved in amino acid metabolism, the 1989 RDA for vitamin B_6 was expressed in terms of protein intake. This means that the more protein you consume, the more vitamin B_6 you need (milligrams per day). The 1989 RDA for vitamin B_6 was based on a dietary vitamin B_6 intake of 0.016 mg/g of protein. It was determined that this ratio is adequate to ensure good vitamin B_6 status. To establish the 1989 RDA for vitamin B_6, twice the RDA for protein was used (126 g/day for men and 100 g/day for women). The recommendation for adults 25 years of age or older was calculated to be 2.0 mg/day for men and 1.6 mg/day for women. As with thiamin and riboflavin, vitamin B_6 requirements increase slightly with pregnancy and lactation (Food and Nutrition Board 1989; IOM 1998).

In 1998, the RDA for vitamin B_6 was revised downward, to 1.3 mg/day for both men and women (ages 19-50 years) (IOM 1998). One reason for the decrease was that the new RDA was no longer based on protein intake (see "How Does the Dietary Reference Intake Differ From the Recommended Dietary Allowance?"), and the biochemical cutoff points for status were changed. This change was due to discrepancies in the research data on the relationship between protein and vitamin B_6 intake. However, this does not diminish the importance of vitamin B_6 for protein or carbohydrate metabolism. It just means that active individuals, especially active women, may need to consume significantly more vitamin B_6 than the new RDA calls for. In fact, recent research suggests that the vitamin B_6 requirements for women are greater than 0.016 mg/g of protein (Hansen et al. 1997). In this study, sedentary women consuming 85 g/day of protein (1.16 g/kg body weight) required a minimum of 1.3 mg/day of vitamin B_6 to maintain adequate vitamin B_6 status. A second study, by Huang and colleagues (1998), showed that sedentary young women consuming 96 g/day of protein (1.55 g/kg body weight) required 1.94 mg vitamin B_6 per day—or approximately 0.019 mg/g of protein. A subsequent study showed that 1.7 mg/day of vitamin B_6 or 0.018 mg/g of protein was required to maintain good vitamin B_6 status in sedentary young women (Hansen et al. 2001). It should be noted that these research studies were published after the new 1998 vitamin B_6 RDA was set. Thus, new data suggest that the RDA for vitamin B_6 may be too low and that higher amounts of vitamin B_6 are required to maintain good status.

Niacin

Niacin, also known as nicotinic acid and nicotinamide, serves as the precursor for two coenzymes, **nicotinamide adenine dinucleotide (NAD)** and **NAD phosphate (NADP)**. These two coenzymes are found in all cells and are required for production of energy through glycolysis, the TCA cycle, electron transport, and the pentose pathway (figure 9.1). They are also involved in the β-oxidation of fats and the synthesis of proteins.

The body's requirement for niacin can be met in two ways. It can be consumed in the diet from food or made in the body from the essential amino acid tryptophan (hence the RDA for niacin is reported in **niacin equivalents [NE]** instead of just milligrams of niacin per day); it takes about 60 mg of tryptophan to make 1 mg of niacin or 1 NE (see "Calculating Total Niacin Equivalent Intake," p. 282). To calculate total NE in the diet, you need to know the amounts of both preformed niacin and tryptophan consumed.

Because niacin is so involved in energy production, the 1989 RDA for niacin was expressed as NE/1000 kcal (6.6 NE/1000 kcal). For adults 19 to 50 years of age, the 1989 RDA for niacin was 19 NE/day (i.e., the equivalent of 19 mg niacin per day) for men and 15 NE/day for women (Food and Nutrition Board 1989). In 1998, the RDA for niacin was changed to 16 NE/day for men of all ages and to 14 NE/day for women of all ages (IOM 1998). The 1989 RDAs for niacin were based on the dose required to prevent pellagra (11.3-13.3 mg NE/day) (Bourgeois et al. 2006). Although the 1998 RDA for niacin is not based on energy intake, niacin is still important for the oxidation of fuels for energy.

Pantothenic Acid

All tissues can convert pantothenic acid to its biologically functional forms—**coenzyme A (CoA)** and **acyl carrier protein (ACP)**. Coenzyme A and ACP function as carriers of acyl groups. Acetyl-CoA is formed from attachment of acetate to CoA. Pantothenic acid–containing CoA is involved in

Highlight

Calculating Total Niacin Equivalent Intake

Many computerized nutrient analysis programs now calculate the total NE (niacin equivalents) of the diet being analyzed. If you are using an analysis program that does not do this, you can still figure out the total intake of niacin in your diet by using the following calculation. The simple fact to keep in mind is that 1 NE = either 60 mg tryptophan or 1 mg niacin.

Total NE = Niacin intake + (Tryptophan intake / 60)

where both intakes are measured in milligrams per day.
Here is a sample calculation for total NE in a diet containing 1696 kcal/day:

Niacin intake = 18.9 mg/day.

Tryptophan intake = 630 mg/day.

Therefore total NE = 18.9 + (630 / 60) = 29.4 NE/day.

This person is consuming the equivalent of 29.4 mg niacin per day (17.3 mg/1000 kcal); one third of the niacin intake comes from tryptophan. Foods like milk that are low in preformed niacin but high in tryptophan can still significantly add to total niacin intake.

---

many energy-producing metabolic pathways, such as glycolysis, β-oxidation, and the TCA cycle. Pantothenic acid is also involved in gluconeogenesis and in the synthesis of steroid hormones, acetylcholine, fatty acids, and membrane phospholipids. Finally, pantothenic acid is involved in protein degradation and amino acid synthesis (Trumbo 2006). Since pantothenic acid is widely distributed in foods, human deficiencies are rare. No RDA has been set for pantothenic acid; however, there is an estimated Adequate Intake (AI) recommendation of 5 mg/day (IOM 1998).

Biotin

Biotin serves as an essential cofactor for several key carboxylase enzymes required for metabolism of glucose, fat, and protein. For example, in gluconeogenesis, pyruvate carboxylase requires biotin; in fatty acid synthesis, acetyl-CoA carboxylase is the biotin-dependent enzyme. Biotin is also required for the degradation of some amino acids (isoleucine, valine, methionine, and leucine) and odd-carbon fatty acids. The conversion of biotin to its active coenzyme requires both magnesium and adenosine triphosphate (ATP). Like pantothenic acid, biotin is widely distributed in foods; deficiencies are rare since only small amounts are needed daily. There is no RDA for biotin, but an estimated AI of 30 mg/day is recommended (IOM 1998).

RATIONALE FOR INCREASED NEED FOR ACTIVE INDIVIDUALS

Because exercise stresses metabolic pathways that use these B vitamins, it has been suggested that the requirements increase in athletes and active individuals. Theoretically, exercise could increase the need for these nutrients in the following ways:

- Altered absorption of the nutrient due to decreased transit time
- Increased turnover, metabolism, or loss of the nutrient in urine or sweat
- Increased need due to the biochemical adaptations associated with training
- Increased mitochondrial enzymes that require the nutrients as cofactors
- Increased need for the nutrient for tissue maintenance and repair
- Increased need due to biochemical adaptations associated with changes in the composition of the diet (higher intakes of carbohydrate or protein or both)

There is some biochemical evidence of poor vitamin status for these nutrients in active people

Highlight

B Vitamins:
Pharmacological Effects and Toxic Levels

High intakes of some of the water-soluble B vitamins can have pharmacological effects unrelated to the role they play as essential micronutrients. High intakes of these vitamins can be toxic in some cases.

Thiamin

There is no evidence of thiamin toxicity from oral supplementation. Because there appears to be little risk for thiamin toxicity, the new 1998 DRIs set no UL for thiamin (IOM 1998). However, parenteral doses at 100 times the RDA may cause headache, convulsions, weakness, paralysis, cardiac arrhythmia, and allergic reactions (Combs 2008; IOM 1998).

Riboflavin

There is no evidence of riboflavin toxicity from food or supplements since the human gut can absorb only about 20 to 27 mg in a single dose (IOM 1998; McCormick 2006). Thus, there is no UL for riboflavin.

Vitamin B$_6$

Chronic high doses (>500 mg/day) of vitamin B$_6$ in the treatment of some diseases have resulted in increased risk of neurotoxicity (Mackey et al. 2006). Toxicity symptoms include depression, fatigue, irritability, headaches, numbness, damage to nerves leading to loss of reflexes and sensations, and difficulty walking. Because of this risk of neurotoxicity, the 1998 DRIs include a UL of 100 mg/day for vitamin B$_6$ (IOM 1998).

Niacin

For years, physicians have prescribed niacin in doses of 1.5 to 3.0 g/day to treat high blood lipids. Side effects can include flushing of the skin, hyperuricemia, abnormal liver function, and low blood glucose levels (Bourgeois et al. 2006). The high doses of niacin used to lower blood lipids also negatively affect substrate use during exercise, which lowers exercise performance. Niacin supplementation decreases the ability to burn fat during exercise, thus increasing the amount of carbohydrate required for energy (Heath et al. 1993; Murray et al. 1995). Because of the flushing that occurs with high doses of niacin, the 1998 DRIs include a UL of 35 mg/day (IOM 1998).

Pantothenic Acid and Biotin

Since pantothenic acid and biotin appear to be relatively safe even at high intakes, no UL has been set for these two vitamins. For pantothenic acid there is no evidence of toxicity in humans even with relatively high intakes (e.g., 10 g/day).

(see table 9.2), but the research has been limited and equivocal. Poor nutritional status may occur in some active people because of long-term marginal dietary intakes associated with either poor dietary choices or reduced energy intake. Inconsistencies in these studies may also be related to differences in experimental designs, which can vary according to

- degree of dietary control,
- type and intensity of exercise used,
- type and number of status indices measured,
- level of regular physical activity in which subjects engaged,
- type of subjects included, and
- whether or not a control group was included.

Exercise increases both energy and protein needs, which may in turn increase the total daily

Table 9.2 Incidence of Low or Marginal Vitamin B₆, Riboflavin, Thiamin, and Niacin Status in Studies of Nonsupplemented Active Individuals

Study	Assessment indices[1]	No. of subjects	Type of subjects	Low status (%)	Dietary vitamin (mg/day)[2]
Vitamin B$_6$					
Fogelholm, Ruokonen et al 1993	EASTAC (>2.00) EAST basal	42	Active subjects[3]	43	–
Guilland et al. 1989	EASTAC (>1.99) Plasma PLP	55	Male athletes	35 17	1.5 ± 0.1
Telford et al. 1992	EASTAC	86		59	–
Rokitzki et al. 1994	EASTAC (>1.50) Urine 4-PA (<2.73 μmol/g Cr) Whole-blood B$_6$	57	Athletes[3]	5 18	1.36-5.40[4]
Weight et al. 1988	Plasma PLP	30	Female athletes	0[5]	1.7 ± 0.6
Riboflavin					
Fogelholm, Ruokonen et al 1993	EGRAC (>1.30) EGR basal	42	Active subjects[2]	57	–
Guilland et al. 1989	EGRAC (>1.20)	55	Male athletes	4	2.1 ± 0.2
Keith and Alt 1991	EGRAC (>1.20) Urinary riboflavin	13	Female athletes	0[5]	1.9 ± 0.9
Rokitzki et al. 1994	EGRAC (>1.50) Whole-blood riboflavin Urinary riboflavin	62	Athletes[3]	0[5]	1.4-2.5[4]
Weight et al. 1988	EGRAC (>1.15)	30	Male runners	0[5]	1.8 ± 1.8
Thiamin					
Fogelholm, Ruokonen et al 1993	ETKAC (>1.20)	42	Active subjects[2]	12	–
Guilland et al. 1989	ETKAC (>1.20)	55	Male athletes	17	1.5 ± 0.1
Weight et al. 1988	TPP stim. (>25%) ETK basal	30	Male runners	0[5]	1.5 ± 0.5
Niacin					
Weight et al. 1988	Plasma niacin	30	Male runners	0[5]	20.4 ± 5.6

[1] See table 9.3 for description of assessment parameters and normal values. In addition, cutoff values for poor status vary depending on the biochemical assessment parameter used and the laboratory. Telford and colleagues (1992) do not provide the EASTAC cutoff value used to determine poor status.

[2] Mean ± SD or range of intakes.

[3] Included both male and females.

[4] Researchers used seven-day weighed food records.

[5] Zero means that none of the individuals had poor status. Values reported are a range of intakes for various male and female athletes.

EALTAC = erythrocyte alanine transaminase activity coefficient

EAST and EASTAC = erythrocyte aspartate transaminase activity coefficient

EGR and EGRAC = erythrocyte glutathione reductase activity coefficient

ETK and ETKAC = erythrocyte transketolase activity coefficient

TPP = thiamin pyrophosphate

PLP = phyridoxal phosphate

4-PA = urinary 4-pyridoxic acid

need for thiamin, riboflavin, vitamin B_6, and niacin in active people. Dietary intakes of these vitamins even by athletes should be adequate unless the individuals make poor dietary choices or restrict their energy intake. Unfortunately, as people increase their training regimens, they do not always correspondingly increase their consumption of energy, protein, or vitamins and minerals.

ASSESSMENT OF VITAMIN STATUS

To determine a person's vitamin status, one needs to measure a number of assessment parameters. Ideally, these measurements should include biochemical assessments (both direct and indirect) along with dietary intake data (see table 9.3). In this section we discuss the most common assessment parameters—including biochemical, dietary intake, and food source data—for thiamin, riboflavin, vitamin B_6, and niacin. Because dietary intake data are poor for pantothenic acid and biotin, these two nutrients have not often been measured in active people. There are no research data indicating poor status for these two nutrients in healthy active individuals, probably because of their widespread distribution in food.

For premenopausal females, phase of the menstrual cycle can alter energy and nutrient intakes. Because some blood and urinary assessment parameters for vitamins are influenced by recent nutrient intakes, studies of nutrient status should consider the phase of the menstrual cycle. Martini and colleagues (1994) found significant increases in energy, protein, carbohydrate, fat, vitamin D, riboflavin, potassium, phosphorus, and magnesium intakes in the midluteal phases versus the midfollicular phases in women studied over four to six ovulatory menstrual cycles.

Biochemical Assessment of Vitamin Status

Biochemical tests can reflect the body's stores of a nutrient as well as the amount of the vitamin lost from the body in urine, feces, or sweat. (When possible, researchers and clinicians like to include functional measurements of vitamin status—i.e., measurements of the availability of the vitamin to function as a coenzyme within the body.) Biochemical measurements can be direct (measurement of blood, urine, or fecal concentration of the vitamin or its metabolite) or indirect (measurement of an enzyme that requires the vitamin as a cofactor or

measurement of that enzyme's functional activity). The typical dietary intake of the vitamin should also be determined. One should measure as many assessment parameters as possible, using both indirect and direct measurements, plus dietary data. Table 9.3 specifically outlines all the various assessment parameters that might be used in assessing status for the vitamins discussed in this chapter, along with cutoff points for poor status.

Thiamin

Currently, there are no reliable physiologically functional indices of thiamin status (Gibson 2005). Therefore, the most widely used biochemical assessment parameter for thiamin is the measurement of **erythrocyte transketolase activity coefficient (ETKAC). Erythrocyte transketolase** is a thiamin-dependent enzyme; without adequate thiamin, activity of the enzyme declines. To determine ETKAC, one first measures the basal activity of the enzyme (without the added coenzyme) and then measures the enzyme activity (with added coenzyme). To determine the activity coefficient, or percentage of stimulation, the stimulated enzyme activity is divided by the basal enzyme activity. A high activity coefficient indicates poor or marginal nutritional status. The criteria used for interpreting ETKAC depend on the laboratory and the biochemical method used. An activity coefficient close to 1.0 is generally considered normal, while values >1.25 are considered deficient (Gibson 2005). The transketolase activity can be converted to a "percentage of stimulation" or PS effect (%) using the following formula: Percent of stimulation (PS) = (Activity coefficient × 100) – 100. When this is done, a TDP effect >25% is considered deficient (Gibson 2005; Butterworth 2006). Thiamin can also be measured in urine, whole blood, or plasma. Thiamin in the urine does not adequately reflect body stores but is a better index of dietary intake (Gibson 2005).

Riboflavin

Riboflavin status is determined via measurement of a number of blood and urine parameters. The most common measurements are urinary excretion of riboflavin, erythrocyte riboflavin levels, and the determination of **erythrocyte glutathione reductase activity coefficient (EGRAC).** The EGRAC is increasingly used as an index of subclinical riboflavin deficiency. As with thiamin, to calculate the activity coefficient, the enzyme activity (with added cofactor FAD) is divided by the basal enzyme activity (without added

Table 9.3 Assessment Indices for Evaluating Vitamin B_6, Riboflavin, Thiamin, and Niacin Status

Indices	Suggested value for poor status
Vitamin B_6	
Plasma pyridoxal phosphate (PLP)	<30 nmol/L[1] or <20 nmol/L[3]
Plasma total vitamin B_6	<40 nmol/L[1]
Urinary 4-pyridoxic acid (4-PA)	<3.0 μmol/day[1,3]
Urinary total vitamin B_6	<0.5 μmol/day[1]
Erythrocyte alanine transaminase activity coefficient (EALTAC)	>1.25[1,3]
Erythrocyte aspartic transaminase activity coefficient (EASTAC)	>1.80[1] or >1.60[3]
1989 Recommended Dietary Allowance (RDA)[2]	
Adult men (≥15 years)	2.0 mg/day
Adult women (≥15 years)	1.6 mg/day
1998 RDA[3]	
Adult men (19-50 years)	1.3 mg/day
Adult women (19-50 years)	1.3 mg/day
Riboflavin	
Plasma riboflavin	<0.24 μmol/L or <240 nmol/L
Erythrocyte riboflavin	<270 nmol/L[1,3]
Erythrocyte glutathione reductase activity coefficient (EGRAC)	>1.25[1] or >1.4[3]
Urinary riboflavin per gram creatinine (Cr): low status	<30 μg/g Cr[1] or 19-27 μg/g Cr[3]
Urinary riboflavin per gram Cr: deficient status	<19 μg/gCr[3]
Urinary riboflavin	
Per 24 h	<40 μg/day
Per 6 h	<10 μg/6 h[4]
1989 RDA (based on consumption of 0.6 mg riboflavin/1000 kcal)[2]	
Adult men (15-50 years)	1.7 mg/day
Adult women (11-50 years)	1.3 mg/day
1998 RDA[3]	
Adult men (19-70 years)	1.3 mg/day
Adult women (19-70 years)	1.1 mg/day
Thiamin	
Plasma thiamin	<98 nmol/L or <10 ng/mL[1]
Erythrocyte thiamin: marginal deficiency	70-90 nmol/L[3]
Erythrocyte thiamin: deficiency	<70 nmol/L[3]
Thiamin pyrophosphate (TPP) % stimulation: marginal deficiency	15-24%[3]
Thiamin pyrophosphate (TPP) % stimulation: deficiency	≥25%[3]
Erythrocyte transketolase activity coefficient (ETKAC): marginal deficiency	1.20-1.25[3]
ETKAC: deficiency	>1.25[3]
Urinary thiamin per gram Cr: marginal deficiency	40-100 μg/g Cr[3]
Urinary thiamin per gram Cr: deficiency	<5 μg/g Cr[3]
Urinary thiamin	
Per 24 h: marginal deficiency	27-66 μg/day[3]
Per 24 h: deficiency	<27 μg/day[3]
Per 6 h	<10 μg/6 h[4]
1989 RDA (based on consumption of 0.5 mg/1000 kcal)[2]	
Adult men (15-50 years)	1.5 mg/day
Adult women (11-50 years)	1.1 mg/day
1998 RDA[3]	
Adult men (19-50 years)	1.2 mg/day
Adult women (19-50 years)	1.1 mg/day

Indices	Suggested value for poor status
Niacin	
Urinary N'-methylnicotinamide (NMN): low status	5.8-17.5 μmol/day[3]
Urinary NMN: deficient status	<5.8 μmol/day[3]
NMN/N'-methyl-2-pyridone-5-carboxylamide (2-pyridone) ratio[4]	
Niacin deficiency or low status	<1.0
Acceptable niacin status	1.0-4.0
1989 RDA (based on 6.6 niacin equivalents (NE)/1000 kcal)[2]	
Adult men (15-50 years)	19 mg NE/day
Adult women (15-50 years)	15 mg NE/day
1998 RDA[3]	
Adult men (all ages)	16 mg NE/day
Adult women (all ages)	14 mg NE/day

[1] Values are from Fischbach (2000).

[2] Values are the 1989 RDAs for the vitamins (Food and Nutrition Board 1989). For vitamin B_6, the RDA is based on a vitamin B_6:protein ratio of 0.032 mg/day protein for adult males consuming 126 g of protein per day and females consuming 100 g of protein per day.

[3] Values are the 1998 RDAs for the vitamins and the new cutoff values for low or deficient status for urine and blood parameters (IOM 1998).

[4] Values are from Gibson (2005).

cofactor FAD). Thus, a high EGRAC indicates impaired riboflavin status, which has been confirmed using human depletion studies (Soares et al. 1993). The evaluation criteria for EGRAC vary depending on the laboratory. The cutoff value frequently used for adequate status is <1.2, while low status is 1.2 to 1.4 and deficient status is >1.4 (McCormick 2006). Low levels of riboflavin excretion also indicate deficiency (table 9.3) (McCormick 2006). Although some researchers question whether the standard reference values for sedentary individuals are appropriate for active people (Rokitzki et al. 1994), this suggestion has not yet been tested.

Vitamin B_6

As with riboflavin, vitamin B_6 status is determined via measurement of a number of blood and urine parameters. The most relevant direct measures of vitamin B_6 status are plasma PLP, total plasma vitamin B_6, and **urinary 4-pyridoxic acid (4-PA)**. Indirect measures include evaluation of either erythrocyte alanine transaminase stimulation index or erythrocyte aspartate transaminase stimulation index, with activation by PLP (both enzymes require PLP as a cofactor) (Mackey et al. 2006) (see table 9.3). These are also sometimes referred to as **erythrocyte alanine transaminase activity coefficient (EALTAC)** and **erythrocyte aspartate transaminase activity coefficient (EASTAC)**. As with thiamin and riboflavin, high activity coefficients or stimulation index indicate poor status. If possible, at least two biochemical measures should be taken and dietary intakes of vitamin B_6 and protein should be ascertained for determination of vitamin B_6 status.

Niacin

Currently, there are no functional assessment measurements for niacin status. Blood concentrations of niacin and niacin metabolites are quite low and appear to be better indicators of recent dietary intakes than long-term status (Gibson 2005). The best index available for assessing niacin status measures the two major end products of niacin metabolism found in the urine: **N'-methylnicotinamide (NMN)** and **N'-methyl-2-pyridone-5-carboxylamide (2-pyridine)**. Both compounds are derived from either dietary niacin or the nicotinic acid ribonucleotide made from tryptophan within the body. It is estimated that healthy adults excrete about 20% to 30% of niacin as NMN and 40% to 60% as 2-pyridone (Gibson 2005). Both urinary metabolites decrease with niacin deficiency. Urine 2-pyridone can decrease to nearly zero before clinical signs of deficiency appear, while urinary excretion of NMN decreases after clinical signs appear. A low urinary concentration of NMN (<0.8 mg/day) is the standard criterion used to indicate poor niacin status and is much easier to measure clinically than 2-pyridone (Fischbach 2000; Gibson 2005). Sometimes the urinary ratio of 2-pyridone:NMN is used to assess niacin status. A ratio <1.0 indicates low niacin status, while an acceptable ratio is between 1.3 and 2.0 (Bourgeois et al. 2006).

Dietary Intakes of Active Individuals

Few researchers have investigated thiamin, riboflavin, vitamin B_6, or niacin intakes by athletes. As you read these studies, remember that B vitamin data from older research (before about 1989) are usually incomplete because good nutrient databases were not available. In addition, few researchers have looked at intakes of biotin or pantothenic acid in active people. In general, studies examining dietary intakes of active males indicate adequate intakes of thiamin, riboflavin, vitamin B_6, and niacin (Woolf and Manore 2006, 2007; Manore 2000). These adequate intakes can be attributed to the relatively high energy intakes in active males. Only Guilland and colleagues (1989) reported low mean intakes of vitamin B_6 in young male athletes (20 years); 67% of the subjects consumed less than 100% of the 1989 RDA (2 mg/day) and had a vitamin B_6:protein ratio of 0.013. No studies have shown low mean thiamin, riboflavin, or niacin intakes in active males. Only two studies (DeBolt et al. 1988; Faber and Benade 1991) indicated that 5% to 18% of their subjects were consuming less than the 1989 RDA for thiamin and riboflavin. There are no reports of low intakes of thiamin, riboflavin, or niacin expressed as mg/1000 kcal per day. No studies published since 2000 have indicated low intakes of these nutrients in active males. It appears that the high energy consumption of active men keeps dietary intakes of all these vitamins high, usually 1.5 to 2.0 times the RDA.

As expected, dietary intakes of these vitamins are generally lower in active females compared to males; yet most studies indicate adequate intakes for thiamin, riboflavin, and niacin (Manore 2000; Woolf and Manore 2006, 2007). Kaiserauer and colleagues (1989) reported thiamin, riboflavin, and niacin to be low in their amenorrheic runners, while Beals and Manore (1998) reported low niacin intakes (less than two-thirds of the 1989 RDA) in only 10% of their female athletes ($n = 49$). Clark and colleagues (2003) also reported mean intakes of some B vitamins (thiamin, riboflavin, vitamin B_6, and folate) that were less than the RDA in National Collegiate Athletic Association (NCAA) Division I female soccer players at the end of their season. Lower dietary intakes of the B vitamins usually accompany energy intakes <1900 kcal/day (Kaiserauer et al. 1989; Rucinski 1989; Clark et al. 2003). For example, Clark and colleagues (2003) reported adequate mean intakes for the B vita-

mins before the soccer season started when the athletes were consuming ~2300 kcal/day; but by the end of the season energy intake had decreased to 1865 kcal/day, and so had the intake of many micronutrients, including the B vitamins. Unless a person is restricting energy intake or consuming a diet high in refined foods, nutrient intakes of thiamin, riboflavin, vitamin B_6, and niacin appear to be adequate. Mean dietary folate intake is almost always reported to be low in the diets of active females if they do not supplement. This B vitamin is discussed in detail in chapter 12.

Dietary Sources

The water-soluble B vitamins occur in a variety of animal and plant products and in a number of different biochemical forms. Their bioavailability depends on factors such as the dietary form of the vitamin, other substances in the diet, drugs that a person is taking, age, and the person's general health. Several of the B vitamins are sensitive to environmental conditions, which can alter the amount of the vitamin in foods. For example, light easily destroys riboflavin—which is why milk, a food high in riboflavin, is packaged in opaque containers. Other B vitamins, such as biotin, vitamin B_6, thiamin, and pantothenic acid, can easily be destroyed by heating, cooking, and milling processes; or they can be lost in cooking water. Any cooking process that exposes food to heat (canning, heat curing, cooking) or milling, or in which cooling fluids are discarded, may reduce the amounts of these vitamins. The amount of a vitamin absorbed by the gut and made available to the body may be very different from the amount of the vitamin measured in the raw food.

In general, B vitamins are found in the germ and bran portions of whole grains, in meat products, and in fortified or enriched cereals and grains (see "Enriched and Fortified Foods"). More specifically, thiamin is abundant in lean pork, yeast, legumes, and enriched cereals and breads. Riboflavin is found in eggs, lean meats, milk, milk products, broccoli, and enriched breads and cereals. Vitamin B_6 is plentiful in meats (especially chicken and tuna) and in plant foods such as beans, cereals, and brown rice. In the typical American diet, approximately 40% of dietary vitamin B_6 comes from animal products and 60% from plants. The highest amounts of niacin occur in meats and in the bran portion of grains. In the typical American diet, meats, fish, and poultry contribute about half the NE consumed. Other good sources of niacin are whole grains, legumes and seeds (peanuts), enriched and fortified breads and cereals, peaches, potatoes, and mushrooms. Vegetables are rich sources of niacin (per kilocalorie). Since vegetables can provide substantial amounts of niacin if consumed in abundance, vegetarians can obtain adequate amounts of niacin if they choose their foods carefully.

Pantothenic acid and biotin are widespread in foods. Dietary sources particularly high in pantothenic acid are meats (especially liver and heart), baker's yeast, wheat and rice bran, mushrooms, nuts (cashews and peanuts), soybeans, broccoli, and avocados. Grains are good sources of the vita-min, but it is located in the outer layers, which are frequently removed with milling. Like pantothenic acid, biotin is widely distributed in foods but in low concentrations. Foods that contribute most to our dietary intake of biotin are brewer's yeast, milk, cheese, liver, egg yolks, nuts (peanuts and walnuts), lentils, soybeans, and some vegetables (cauliflower, spinach, peas) and grains (oats, wheat bran, sorghum). Small amounts of biotin are also produced in the intestinal tract of humans. A substance in raw eggs, avidin, interferes with biotin absorption and decreases biotin status. But since avidin is unstable in heat, cooked eggs cause no threat to biotin status.

Highlight

Enriched and Fortified Foods

One way federal governments protect the health of their populations is by mandating the enrichment of some foods and allowing for the fortification of other foods. Here we explain the difference between these two processes. In the United States, policy makers and scientists are currently discussing whether the fortification of flour, breads, and grains with folic acid has improved the folate status of the American population. This fortification process was mandated by the U.S. Department of Agriculture (USDA) in 1998.

Enriched Foods

When grain is milled, the germ and bran are removed. Since many of the vitamins and minerals are in this portion of the grain, the refined product is less nutritious than unmilled grain. White flour and white rice have fewer vitamins and minerals than whole wheat flour or brown rice. In the 1940s, the Food and Drug Administration (FDA) mandated that some of the nutrients lost during the milling and refining of flour be replaced by enrichment. In the milling process, these nutrients (thiamin, riboflavin, niacin, and iron) are added back to the refined product at levels specifically established by the FDA. In Canada, all refined flour is also enriched with these nutrients. If you read package labels, you will notice that enriched flour is added to many products like bread, pasta, doughnuts, muffins, and cookies. Besides flour, many milled grain products, such as rice and corn, are also enriched.

Fortified Foods

Fortification is the addition of a vitamin or mineral to a food product during processing. The FDA of the United States does not mandate this process except for folic acid in flour, breads, and grains. Health Canada oversees the fortification process of foods in Canada. In the United States, manufacturers can add any amount of any vitamin or mineral to their products. They can add micronutrients that may not naturally occur in the original product, or they can add additional levels to what is already present. For example, many cereals are fortified with 100% of the RDA for selected vitamins and minerals. Orange juice is now fortified with calcium and additional vitamin C. Even some candies are now being fortified with vitamin C! The manufacturer determines which foods will be fortified and the amount of fortification.

Sport and diet foods have been especially targeted for fortification with vitamins, minerals, or both. The level of fortification depends on the product, but many manufacturers add 25% to 100% of the RDA or DRI of various nutrients to sport bars and meal replacement products. Most fat-free cookies, breakfast bars, muffins, and granola bars are fortified to some extent.

B vitamins are frequently added to commercially prepared foods at 25% to 100% of the RDA per serving. This means that consuming fortified cereals, breakfast bars, sport bars and drinks, or energy shakes or meal replacement products (e.g., Ensure, Boost, Slim-Fast, Gatorade Nutrition Shake) will dramatically increase total dietary intakes. Frequently individuals who "watch their weight" or engage in physical activity use these types of products. In addition, many multivitamin or vitamin-mineral supplements contain 100% or more of the RDA for these nutrients. Since many Americans use dietary supplements, the total intake of these vitamins in the diet may be increasing regardless of dietary choices.

Vitamin Deficiency in Active Individuals

Because B vitamins are important to energy production during exercise, it is assumed that individuals with poor status (poor dietary intakes and poor biochemical assessment values) will have a reduced ability to perform physical activity (see "Vitamin Deficiencies and Their Symptoms"). A number of studies have supported this hypothesis. Van der Beek and colleagues (1994) depleted

24 healthy men of thiamin, riboflavin, and vitamin B_6 over an 11-week metabolic feeding period, then examined the effects of the multiple deficiencies on physical performance. Depletion of these three vitamins had the following effects on exercise performance:

- 12% decrease in maximal work capacity ($\dot{V}O_2$max)
- 7% decrease in **onset of blood lactate accumulation (OBLA)**
- 12% decrease in oxygen consumption at OBLA
- 9% decrease in peak power
- 7% decrease in mean power

This study supports earlier research that identified individuals with subclinical vitamin deficiencies and assessed their ability to do work before and after vitamin supplementation. After measuring vitamin B_6 and riboflavin status in boys (n = 124, ages 12-14 years), Suboticanec and colleagues (1990) found that 24% had poor vitamin B_6 status (EASTAC >2.00) and 19% had poor riboflavin status (EGRAC >1.20). A subgroup (n = 37) of the original sample pool was then given 2 mg of vitamin B_6 (pyridoxine) six days a week for two months. A

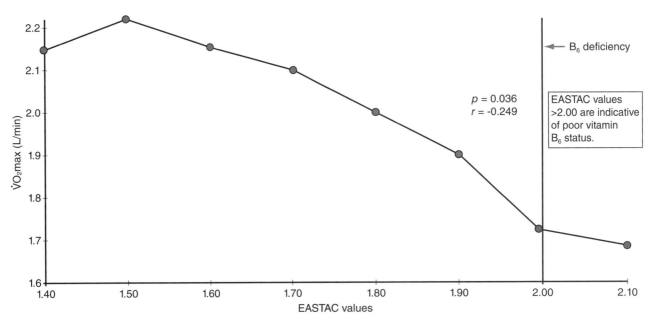

Figure 9.2 Changes in $\dot{V}O_2$max with improved vitamin B_6 status, as determined by EASTAC, in boys 12 to 15 years of age. EASTAC = erythrocyte aspartate transaminase activity coefficient.

Adapted, by permission, from Suboticanec et al., 1990, "Effect of pyridoxine and riboflavin supplementation on physical fitness in young adolescents," *International Journal of Vitamins and Nutrition Research* 60: 81-88.

Highlight

Vitamin Deficiencies and Their Symptoms

The B vitamins discussed in this chapter are essential micronutrients. If inadequate amounts of these nutrients are consumed, deficiency symptoms can result, which can lead to disease and death. Although deficiency diseases are not prevalent in developed countries, subclinical deficiencies of micronutrients are not uncommon and can compromise health and the ability to engage in physical activity.

Thiamin

Beriberi is associated with low dietary intake of thiamin. The disease affects the cardiovascular, gastrointestinal, and nervous systems. Clinical signs and symptoms include mental confusion, altered carbohydrate metabolism, increased levels of tissue and plasma pyruvate, anorexia, muscular weakness, peripheral paralysis, edema, muscle wasting, tachycardia, and enlarged heart (IOM 1998). In the United States, people at greatest risk for thiamin deficiency are alcoholics, renal patients, the chronically ill, and anyone who consumes a diet high in processed foods (which are typically low in thiamin). Enrichment of white flour has eliminated much of the risk for beriberi in the United States.

Riboflavin

No single disease is associated with low dietary intakes of riboflavin. Low intakes are associated with lesions around the mouth, general dermatitis, and normocytic anemia (IOM 1998). Riboflavin is essential for the conversion of vitamin B_6 and niacin to their active forms.

Vitamin B_6

Like riboflavin, vitamin B_6 has no unique clinical deficiency disease associated with low intakes. Deficiency symptoms, which are usually connected with other B vitamin deficiencies, are convulsions, neurological symptoms, dermatitis, and anemia (IOM 1998). If high protein intakes accompany low vitamin B_6 intakes, the deficiency will appear sooner.

Niacin

Pellagra is associated with niacin deficiency. Early symptoms include weakness; lassitude; anorexia; digestive disturbances; and mental symptoms of anxiety, depression, irritability, and forgetfulness (Gibson 2005). Later stages of the disease are characterized by dermatitis, diarrhea, inflammation of the mucous membranes, dementia, and in some cases death (Food and Nutrition Board 1989) (the disease is frequently called the "disease of the four Ds"). The symptoms are due to a lack of energy for muscle control and neural functions. Although prevalent in the southern United States in the early 1900s, pellagra is now rare due to the enrichment of white flour and government programs that provide food to the poor. People still at risk for the disease are malnourished alcoholics, some elderly individuals, and those using isoniazid or 3-mercaptopurine for the treatment of tuberculosis or leukemia, respectively (Gibson 2005). The disease is usually associated with poor intakes of all the B vitamins and poor protein intakes.

Pantothenic Acid and Biotin

There are no deficiency diseases associated with low intakes of pantothenic acid or biotin.

second subgroup (n = 38) was given 2 mg of riboflavin six days a week for two months. At the beginning and end of each treatment period, physical work capacity was measured on a bicycle ergometer. The researchers reported a significant negative correlation (p = 0.036) between $\dot{V}O_2$max and

EASTAC (a measure of vitamin B_6 status) (figure 9.2)—as vitamin B_6 status improved (EASTAC got smaller), work capacity also improved ($\dot{V}O_2$max values increased). Although the results for riboflavin appeared similar to those for vitamin B_6, the negative correlation did not reach statistical significance. These data suggest that subclinical deficiencies of vitamin B_6 (and possibly riboflavin) negatively affect aerobic capacity in young boys. When the vitamin deficiency is corrected through diet or vitamin supplementation, work capacity improves. In summary, these studies suggest that deficiencies of thiamin, riboflavin, or vitamin B_6 may decrease the ability to do work, especially maximal work.

EXERCISE AND VITAMIN REQUIREMENTS

How do you determine if exercise increases the need for vitamins? The most common types of research studies on this question are the following:

- Metabolic diet studies of sedentary and active individuals (for more details, see "What Is a Metabolic Diet Study? How Do These Studies Assess Vitamin Requirements?")
- Cross-sectional studies comparing nutrient intakes and status of active and sedentary individuals
- Intervention studies examining nutrient intakes and status of sedentary people who begin an exercise program, with the aim of determining whether vitamin status decreases as these people become more physically fit
- Intervention studies examining nutrient intakes and status of sedentary people who start a diet (reduced energy intake) and exercise program for weight loss, with the aim of determining if status decreases as the individuals lose weight and become more physically fit

Metabolic Diet Studies

Metabolic studies are the most highly controlled way to answer the question posed earlier. With this approach, a researcher feeds a known amount of the vitamin to both sedentary and active individuals and determines if subsequent nutrient status is different between the two groups. If vitamin status decreases in active people compared to controls, or if more of the vitamin is required to maintain status, it would appear that active individuals need more of the vitamin. In this section,

we evaluate metabolic studies that have examined riboflavin status and vitamin B_6 status of both sedentary and active people under controlled conditions. To date there have been no metabolic studies of thiamin, niacin, pantothenic acid, or biotin status in active and sedentary people.

Based on a series of metabolic studies in active women, it appears that exercise, dieting, and diet plus exercise increase the need for riboflavin above the 1989 RDA (0.6 mg/1000 kcal or 1.3 mg/day). The current RDA is set at 1.1 mg/day (IOM 1998), which is lower than the 1989 RDA. Belko and colleagues (1983) at Cornell University were first to examine riboflavin requirements of active people. Measuring riboflavin status (EGRAC and urinary riboflavin excretion) in young women fed various levels of riboflavin over a 12-week period, they found that weight-stable women who exercised (running) for 20 to 50 min six days per week needed at least 1.1 mg riboflavin/1000 kcal (~2.4 mg/day) to maintain good riboflavin status. Even when the women were not exercising and were receiving the 1989 RDA (0.6 mg/1000 kcal), they demonstrated poor riboflavin status. In the women who exercised, mean EGRAC values remained normal (<1.25) only at the higher intake levels of riboflavin (about 2.3 times the 1989 RDA) (figure 9.3).

This study was followed by two others (Belko et al. 1984, 1985) in which young overweight women were placed on a metabolic diet providing 1200 to 1250 kcal/day and various levels of riboflavin intake (0.8-1.6 mg/1000 kcal) (figure 9.4). Dieting for weight loss increased the amount of riboflavin required to maintain good status in these women; when dieting was combined with exercise, even more riboflavin was required. The researchers concluded that 1.6 mg of riboflavin/1000 kcal is required to maintain good riboflavin status in women who both diet and exercise (3 h/week at 75-85% of maximal heart rate). Finally, Winters and colleagues (1992) examined the effect of moderate exercise (2.5 h/week at 75-85% of maximal heart rate) on riboflavin status of active women 50 to 67 years old. All subjects consumed a metabolic diet that provided adequate energy for weight maintenance (1800-2000 kcal/day) at two levels of riboflavin (0.6 and 0.9 mg/1000 kcal) for five weeks. Exercise increased the amount of riboflavin required to maintain good status (0.9 mg of riboflavin/1000 kcal or ~1.8 mg/day). It appears that both exercise and dieting for weight loss increase riboflavin requirements above the

Highlight

What Is a Metabolic Diet Study? How Do These Studies Assess Vitamin Requirements?

The purpose of a metabolic diet study is to determine how vitamin assessment parameters change under controlled conditions when the dietary intake of a nutrient is closely controlled. In these studies, all foods eaten by study participants are prepared in a metabolic research kitchen. A study may last for weeks or months. All food is weighed to within 0.1 g and carefully recorded. Subjects are usually required to either live at the research facility (all physical activity is monitored) or come to the research facility for all their meals. In addition, body weight is measured daily to prevent any increase or decrease in weight. If weight does change, energy intake is altered so that the subject returns to the baseline weight. This must be done without any change in the intake of the vitamin being studied. Periodically over the course of the study, vitamin biochemical assessment parameters are also measured (such as blood, urine, and fecal material). This may require that the subject collect all 24 h urine and fecal samples throughout the study. The following is an example of a study you might design to determine whether active and sedentary women have different vitamin requirements.

Feed active women (all of equal fitness levels and exercising the same number of hours per week) and sedentary females three different diets that provide three different levels of vitamin B_6: vitamin B_6 below the RDA (1.0 mg/day) for three weeks, vitamin B_6 at the level of the RDA (1.3 mg/day) for three weeks, vitamin B_6 above the RDA (1.6 mg/day) for three weeks. Ideally, you would like to randomly assign these diets, with a six-week "washout" period between diets. (The RDA for vitamin B_6 should provide adequate amounts of the vitamin for normal healthy women.) Feeding a metabolic diet means that subjects are fed all the food they eat during the study period and are monitored to make sure they eat all the food. The amount of vitamin B_6 in the food is determined by biochemical assessment. You would collect blood and 24 h urine samples throughout the study period and make sure that all subjects maintain baseline body weights. You would determine nutritional status for each of the diets to test which of the diets provide adequate vitamin B_6 to keep assessment parameters within normal range. You would also compare vitamin status between groups for each of the diets. If the active women have poor status on 1.3 mg/day of vitamin B_6 while the sedentary subjects have adequate status on this level, you would conclude that the RDA is not adequate for the active individuals.

RDA. Combining exercise (2.5-5 h/week) with dieting (~1250 kcal/day) increases the riboflavin required for good status even more (1.6 mg/1000 kcal, or 2 mg/day). These studies all examined the riboflavin requirements of women engaged in moderate exercise (2.5-5 h/week). No metabolic data are available for people who participate in more strenuous exercise.

A number of metabolic studies have examined vitamin B_6 requirements of active and sedentary people—leading to the conclusion that approximately 1.5 to 2.3 mg/day of vitamin B_6 is required to maintain PLP concentrations above the cutoff value of 30 nmol/L (Leklem 1990). The DRI committee for B vitamins has recommended a cutoff value of 20 nmol/L (IOM 1998); however, more recent research suggests that this value it too low. Shultz and colleagues (2003) found that when plasma

PLP concentrations were 23 nmol/L, participants had more DNA strand breaks, suggesting that adequate vitamin B_6 was not available to protect DNA (Hansen and Manore 2006). The 1989 RDA for vitamin B_6 was 1.6 mg/day for women and 2.0 mg/day for men, while the 1998 RDA is 1.3 mg/day for both men and women (IOM 1998). For example, a metabolic study by Dreon and Butterfield (1986) examined vitamin B_6 status in active and sedentary men consuming 4.2 mg/day of vitamin B_6. The active men were running either 5 or 10 miles/day (8-16 km/day). Although vitamin B_6 status did not change as running mileage increased, the men were consuming three times the current RDA for vitamin B_6. Manore and colleagues (1987) examined vitamin B_6 status in three groups of women (active young, sedentary young, sedentary old) who were fed two levels of vitamin B_6 over

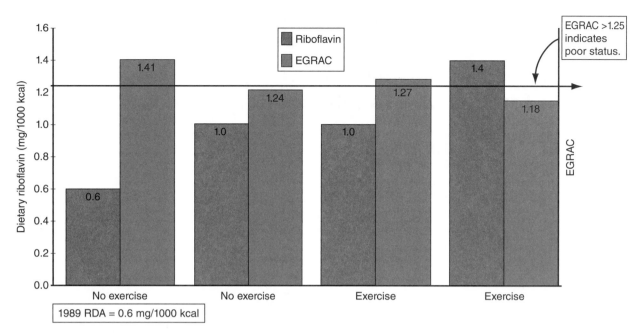

Figure 9.3 Effect of exercise on riboflavin requirements in young women who consumed different levels of riboflavin and either exercised or did not exercise. Each nonexercising period was 2 weeks, and each exercise period was 3 weeks. Blue bars indicate dietary riboflavin intake; gray bars indicate the erythrocyte glutathione reductase activity coefficient (EGRAC). EGRAC values> 1.25 indicate poor riboflavin status.

Adapted from A.Z. Belko et al., 1983, "Effects of exercise on riboflavin requirements of young women," *American Journal of Clinical Nutrition* 37: 509-517.

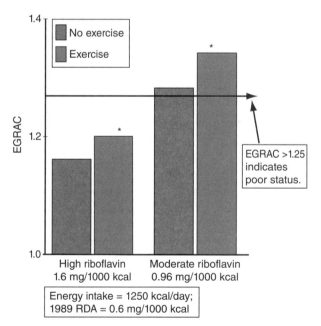

Figure 9.4 Effect of exercise on riboflavin requirements in women consuming a 1250 kcal/day metabolic weight loss diet with either high (1.6 mg/1000 kcal) or moderate (0.96 mg/1000 kcal) riboflavin intake and with and without exercise. Erythrocyte glutathione reductase activity coefficient (EGRAC) was used to determine riboflavin status (EGRAC > 1.25 indicates poor riboflavin status). When this study was done, the 1989 Recommended Dietary Allowance (RDA) for riboflavin was 0.6 mg/1000 kcal/d. Exercise significantly increased EGRAC compared to nonexercise ($p<0.05$). More riboflavin was needed to maintain good riboflavin status during exercise.

*Indicated significantly different from no exercise.

Adapted from A.Z. Belko et al., 1985, "Effects of exercise on riboflavin requirements: biological validation in weight reducing women," *American Journal of Clinical Nutrition* 41: 270-277.

a seven-week period. Throughout the study, the active women continued to exercise (2-4 h/week). At baseline, the young active subjects and the sedentary older subjects had lower plasma PLP concentrations (indicating poor vitamin status) compared to the young sedentary subjects. For all groups, mean plasma PLP concentrations improved when they were fed a metabolic diet providing either 2.3 or 10.0 mg/day of vitamin B_6. The only differences observed between the active and sedentary groups were that the active females lost more vitamin B_6 as 4-PA.

Manore and colleagues (1987) also measured changes in plasma PLP concentrations during a 20 min exercise period at 80% $\dot{V}O_2$max. For all subjects, plasma PLP concentrations increased significantly during exercise (figure 9.5) and then returned to baseline within 60 min. A number of other studies have confirmed this phenomenon (Crozier et al. 1994; Hofmann et al. 1991; Leklem and Schultz 1983) in short-term exercise. However, Leonard and Leklem (2000) found a decrease in plasma PLP concentrations with ultra-endurance running (50 km). This extreme level of exercise may affect plasma PLP concentrations differently than in earlier studies that used exercise bouts of shorter duration (5-120 min). While the

metabolic reason for the increase in plasma PLP concentrations during shorter-duration exercise is not known, animal studies reveal a shift in the vitamin from the liver to the muscle. The increase in plasma PLP concentrations during exercise increases the probability that PLP will be metabolized in the liver to 4-PA and lost in the urine (Crozier et al. 1994). Thus, exercise can increase the turnover and loss of vitamin B_6.

Researchers have documented higher urinary 4-PA losses in active individuals compared to sedentary controls, and after strenuous exercise (Crozier et al. 1994; Manore 1994). Rokitzki and colleagues (1994) calculated, on the basis of urinary 4-PA excretion concentrations, that marathon runners lose approximately 1 mg of vitamin B_6 during a 26.2-mile (42 km) race. Yet no one has documented a decrease in plasma PLP concentrations due to exercise-induced 4-PA losses. In general, any loss of vitamin B_6 due to exercise is small and could easily be replaced via consumption of one or two servings of a high vitamin B_6 food. However, as table 9.4 illustrates, some individuals (especially the elderly) have poor plasma PLP concentrations on their self-selected free-living diets, and numerous studies have documented lower vitamin B_6 status in elderly

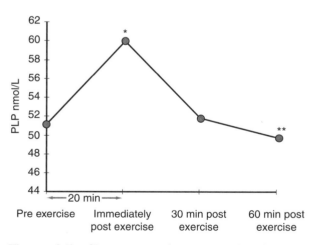

Figure 9.5 Changes in plasma pyridoxal phosphate (PLP) concentration during 20 min of exercise (80% $\dot{V}O_2$max) in active and sedentary females consuming a metabolic diet containing 2.3 mg/day vitamin B_6. Plasma PLP increased with exercise and then decreased to baseline 60 min post-exercise ($p<0.05$).

Adapted from M.M. Manore, J.E. Leklem, and M.C. Walter, 1987, "Vitamin B-6 metabolism as affected by exercise in trained and untrained women fed diets differing in carbohydrate and vitamin B-6 content," *American Journal of Clinical Nutrition* 46: 995-1004.

Table 9.4   Pyridoxal-5'-Phosphate (PLP) in Active and Sedentary Women on Free-Living Diets and Metabolic Diets (~2.3-2.4 or 10 mg/day of Vitamin B_6)

Groups	PLP* (mmol/L)
Active young (n = 5)	
Free-living diet	42 ± 14
2.3-2.4 mg B_6 per day	48 ± 9
10 mg B_6 per day	175 ± 24
Sedentary young (n = 5)	
Free-living diet	35 ± 15
2.3-2.4 mg B_6 per day	61 ± 24
10 mg B_6 per day	203 ± 56
Sedentary young (n = 5)	
Free-living diet	30 ± 12
2.3-2.4 mg B_6 per day	44 ± 18
10 mg B_6 per day	181 ± 41

*All values are mean ± SD fasting plasma concentrations. A plasma PLP concentration <30 mmol/L is considered low.

Adapted from M.M. Manore, J.E. Leklem, and M.C. Walter, 1987, "Vitamin B-6 metabolism as affected by exercise in trained and untrained women fed diets differing in carbohydrate and vitamin B-6 content," *American Journal of Clinical Nutrition* 46: 995-1004.

persons (Lowik et al. 1989; Manore et al. 1989; Ribaya-Mercado et al. 1991) and in individuals with various chronic diseases such as arthritis (Woolf and Manore 2008) and diabetes (Manore et al. 1991; Manore 2000). No one has determined if active individuals with chronic diseases such as diabetes or arthritis have higher requirements for vitamin B_6.

The effect of combining exercise and dieting for weight loss has also been examined to a limited extent for vitamin B_6. Fogelholm, Koskinen, and colleagues (1993) found a significant decrease in vitamin B_6 status in male elite wrestlers after three weeks of dieting (1700 kcal/day) but no changes in thiamin and riboflavin status. However, the authors provided no dietary intake data for vitamin B_6; thus, the poor status may have been due to poor dietary intakes during the dieting period combined with high physical activity. Van Dale and colleagues 1990) examined the effect of a 14-week diet (900 kcal/day) or of diet plus exercise in 12 obese men (mean age = 40 years). Plasma PLP concentrations significantly decreased in the diet plus exercise group (54.5 to 40.0 nmol/L) compared to the diet-only group (49.8 to 48.7 nmol/L). Riboflavin and thiamin status decreased in both groups, but the only statistically significant changes were for riboflavin status in the diet plus exercise group. However, the dietary intakes of vitamin B_6 and thiamin were below the 1989 RDA for the last nine weeks of the study, while riboflavin intake was at the 1989 RDA. Finally, the Committee on Military Nutrition Research (CMNR) recently released a report recommending that soldiers participating in high-intensity combat operations, when the availability of adequate energy may be restricted, increase their daily intake of B vitamins involved in energy metabolism (Erdman et al 2006). The committee recommended that rations have higher levels of thiamin (1.6-3.4 mg), riboflavin (2.8-6.5 mg), niacin (28-35 mg), and vitamin B_6 (2.7-3.9 mg) to accommodate the high level of energy expenditure experienced by these soldiers.

Vitamin Status of Active Individuals

If exercise increases the need for the B vitamins involved in energy metabolism, then active individuals should have poor status while consuming the RDA for these vitamins. This section deals with the research available on the vitamin status (thiamin, riboflavin, vitamin B_6, niacin) of nonsupplementing active individuals consuming free-living diets.

Table 9.2 outlines studies examining the nutritional status of active individuals who consume free-living diets with no supplemental intakes of thiamin, riboflavin, vitamin B_6, or niacin. The number of assessment parameters measured for each study varies, but most studies that indicate poor status used more than one biochemical measurement and dietary intake of the vitamin. For vitamin B_6, the number of active people with poor status ranged from 0% to 60% in five studies. To date, Telford and colleagues (1992) have reported the most athletes with poor vitamin B_6 status. They studied 86 male and female athletes before and after an eight-month training period during which half of the athletes consumed a multivitamin-mineral supplement and a matched group took a placebo. They found that 60% of the athletes had poor vitamin B_6 status before any supplementation occurred. Poor status for the other B vitamins in active people consuming a free-living diet has been reported less often. There are no well-controlled studies of pantothenic acid or biotin status in active people. One report from Finland (Fogelholm, Ruokonen et al. 1993) examined vitamin B_6, riboflavin, and thiamin status in 42 physically active college students (18-32 years) before and after five weeks of vitamin B supplementation. At the beginning of the study, 43% had poor vitamin B_6 status, 57% had poor riboflavin status, and 12% had poor thiamin status. Supplementation significantly improved status measurements for all three vitamins. These data suggest that some active individuals have poor vitamin status while consuming a free-living diet. Frank and colleagues (2000) also reported that 1.7% of their subjects (n = 55 males; n = 5 females; data were pooled) had low thiamin status and 1.8% had low riboflavin status before starting a 100 km (62-mile) walk. However, if you do the calculations, this represents only about one individual out of the 60 with poor status for these two micronutrients. Research also indicates that exercise can decrease vitamin status in people who already have poor or marginal vitamin status (Soares et al. 1993).

VITAMINS AND EXERCISE PERFORMANCE

A number of researchers have examined whether vitamin or mineral supplements, or both, improve exercise performance. These types of studies are difficult to do because so many factors besides diet can affect performance. In addition, there are many ways to measure performance. The major flaw in most studies is that they did not control for nutritional status before adding supplements to athletes' diets; when the study began, some athletes may already have had good nutritional status while others had poor status. If initial nutritional status is not controlled, there is no way to unambiguously determine the effect of the supplement on performance.

The following is an example of an early project that tested whether supplementation improved exercise performance. Barnett and Conlee (1984) examined the effect of a commercial dietary supplement on endurance performance in 20 male runners. For four weeks, subjects were given either a placebo or a supplement containing vitamins, minerals, amino acids, and a fatty acid complex. The study was "double blind"—neither the subjects nor the researchers knew who was on which treatment. Before and after the four-week treatment period, subjects performed a 60 min submaximal treadmill run (65-70% $\dot{V}O_2$max) and a maximal $\dot{V}O_2$ test. There were no differences between groups in blood concentrations of glucose, free fatty acids, and lactate during exercise, or in the amount of glycogen used during exercise. The supplement had no effect on maximum oxygen consumption. The authors concluded that the supplement had no beneficial effect on exercise performance. These were the major problems with the study:

1. The researchers did not determine the subjects' nutritional status before the study began.
2. Neither diet nor exercise training was controlled during the study.
3. The supplement contained 33 different nutrients.

It is not surprising that the supplement had no effect on performance: There were too many uncontrolled variables.

To date there are no data to support improved exercise performance in individuals who supplement with vitamins or minerals as long as nutrient status was good before supplementation began. For example, if you already have good vitamin B_6 status, supplementing with more vitamin B_6 will not improve your exercise performance. However, if your vitamin B_6 status is poor, then improvement in vitamin B_6 status, through either diet or supplements, may increase exercise performance above that seen in the "subclinical" state. Once vitamin status has normalized, additional supplementa-

tion will not continue to improve performance. This does not mean that supplementation may not be beneficial for other health reasons.

CHAPTER IN REVIEW

We started this chapter by asking two questions about vitamin supplementation and exercise. This section summarizes the research available to answer these questions.

Does exercise increase the need for B vitamins in active healthy individuals? Research on the micronutrient needs of active people has been limited, with most of the work done in athletes. It appears that riboflavin requirements increase with exercise, dieting, and dieting plus exercise in both young and older women doing moderate activity. No data are available on men or for individuals exercising more strenuously. Exercise alters vitamin B_6 metabolism by increasing plasma concentrations of PLP during exercise, which in turn may increase the loss of vitamin B_6 through urinary 4-PA excretion. But the amount of vitamin B_6 needed to cover losses or increased need is small (<1 mg/day in individuals running a 26.2-mile [42 km] marathon) and can be easily met through good food choices. In addition, exercise appears to cause a redistribution of vitamin B_6 from the liver to the muscles. The exact reason for this redistribution is not known. The data on changes in thiamin status with exercise are limited, but some cross-sectional studies suggest that a small percentage of active individuals can have poor status. There are few or no data on the effect of exercise on niacin, pantothenic acid, or biotin status.

Little research has been done on the effect of combined diet and exercise for weight loss on micronutrient status of thiamin, riboflavin, vitamin B_6, or niacin. If people are restricting energy intake for weight loss or are making poor dietary choices, dietary intakes of these nutrients will probably be low. Finally, no data are available on the effect of exercise or dieting plus exercise on B vitamin status of people with chronic health problems, such as diabetes or hypertension.

Does supplementation with B vitamins improve exercise performance? In active individuals who already have good nutritional status, there are no data to support improved exercise performance with vitamin or mineral supplementation. However, if a person has marginal nutritional status, supplementation may improve performance by improving nutritional status and the availability of cofactors in the energy metabolism pathways.

Key Concepts

1. Understand the exercise-related functions and dietary requirements of the B vitamins.

The B vitamins (thiamin, riboflavin, vitamin B_6, niacin, pantothenic acid, and biotin) are cofactors for various enzymes in the metabolic pathways that produce energy from protein, carbohydrate, or fat (or some combination of these) during exercise. In 1998, new joint DRIs between the United States and Canada were established for the B vitamins, which included new RDAs for thiamin (1.2 mg/day for men; 1.1 mg/day for women), riboflavin (1.3 mg/day for men; 1.1 mg/day for women), vitamin B_6 (1.3 mg/day for men and women), and niacin (16 NE/day for men; 14 NE/day for women). Pantothenic acid and biotin do not have RDAs, but AIs have been established: 5 mg/day for pantothenic acid and 30 mg/day for biotin.

2. Discuss the rationale for increased need for B vitamins in active individuals.

Theoretically, exercise may increase or alter the need for B vitamins in several ways. Exercise stresses many of the metabolic pathways that require these micronutrients. Exercise training may result in muscle biochemical adaptations that increase micronutrient need. Exercise may also increase the turnover of these micronutrients, increasing their loss from the body. Finally, higher intakes of micronutrients may be required to cover increased needs for the repair and maintenance of lean tissue mass in athletes.

3. Identify the dietary and biochemical assessment methods for the B vitamins.

Determination of vitamin status for an individual requires measurement of a number of parameters, including biochemical markers of status and levels of dietary intake. The biochemical markers should reflect the body's stores of the vitamin and the amount of the vitamin lost from the body in urine, feces, or sweat. If available, functional measurements of vitamin status should be included. The most widely used biochemical assessment parameter for thiamin is ETKAC. The most common biochemical measures of riboflavin status are urinary excretion of riboflavin, erythrocyte riboflavin concentrations, and EGRAC. For vitamin B_6, the most common assessment measures are plasma PLP, total vitamin B_6, and urinary 4-PA. Measurement of EASTAC and EALTAC indirectly assesses vitamin B_6 status. Good biochemical assessment measures for niacin, biotin, and pantothenic acid are not available.

4. Discuss how exercise may alter B vitamin requirements in active people.

Exercise may increase the need for some of the B vitamins (thiamin, riboflavin, vitamin B_6) by one to two times the current RDA, but this increased need can generally be met by the higher energy intakes required of athletes to maintain body weight. Combining dieting for weight loss and exercise may further increase the need for these vitamins. Vitamin supplementation is recommended for active people who consume low-energy diets or diets high in processed foods, or who restrict dietary intake of fruits, vegetables, or whole grains.

5. Explain the relationship between B vitamins and exercise performance.

Vitamin status is one of many factors that can influence an individual's exercise performance. No data are available to support improved exercise performance in people who supplement with B vitamins if vitamin status was good before supplementation. Exercise performance may be improved with supplementation if B vitamin status was poor prior to supplementation.

Key Terms

acyl carrier protein (ACP) 281

Adequate Intake (AI) 280

beriberi 291

branched-chain amino acid (BCAA) 277

B vitamins 276

coenzyme A (CoA) 281

Dietary Reference Intakes (DRI) 280

erythrocyte alanine transaminase activity coefficient (EALTAC) 287

erythrocyte aspartate transaminase activity coefficient (EASTAC) 287

erythrocyte glutathione reductase activity coefficient (EGRAC) 285

erythrocyte transketolase 285

erythrocyte transketolase activity coefficient (ETKAC) 285

Estimated Average Requirement (EAR) 280

flavin adenine dinucleotide (FAD) 277

flavin mononucleotide (FMN) 277

NAD phosphate (NADP) 281

niacin equivalent (NE) 281

nicotinamide adenine dinucleotide 281

N'-methyl-2-pyridone-5-carboxylamide (2-pyridone) 287

N'-methylnicotinamide (NMN) 287

onset of blood lactate accumulation (OBLA) 290

pellagra 291

pyridoxal-5'-phosphate (PLP) 279

Recommended Dietary Allowance (RDA) 280

thiamin diphosphate (TDP) 277

Tolerable Upper Intake Level (UL) 280

tricarboxylic acid (TCA) 277

urinary 4-pyridoxic acid (4-PA) 287

Additional Information

Joubert LM, Manore MM. Exercise, nutrition, and homocysteine. Int J Sport Nutr Exerc Metab Aug 2006;16(4):341-361.

> Physical activity may increase homocysteine, an independent cardiovascular disease (CVD) risk factor. This review examines the influence of nutrition (B vitamins) and exercise on blood homocysteine levels.

Lukaski HC. Vitamin and mineral status: effects on physical performance. Nutrition Jul-Aug 2004;20(7-8):632-644.

> An overview of the current literature examining the impact of vitamin and mineral status on exercise performance and groups at risk for poor status.

Woolf K, Manore MM. B-vitamins and exercise: does exercise alter requirements? Int J Sport Nutr Exerc Metab Oct 2006;16(5):453-484.

> Provides an in-depth review of the current literature on the B vitamins, including folate and vitamin B_{12}, and exercise. Specifically addresses how physical activity may increase the needs for these vitamins.

References

Barnett DW, Conlee RK. The effects of a commercial dietary supplement on human performance. Am J Clin Nutr 1984;40:586-590.

Beals KA, Manore MM. Nutritional status of female athletes with subclinical eating disorders. J Am Diet Assoc 1998;98:419-425.

Belko AZ, Meredith MP, Kalkwarf HJ et al. Effects of exercise on riboflavin requirements: biological validation in weight reducing women. Am J Clin Nutr 1985;41:270-277.

Belko AZ, Obarzanek E, Kalkwarf HJ et al. Effects of exercise on riboflavin requirements of young women. Am J Clin Nutr 1983;37:509-517.

Belko AZ, Obarzanek E, Roach B et al. Effects of aerobic exercise and weight loss on riboflavin requirements of moderately obese, marginally deficient young women. Am J Clin Nutr 1984;40:553-561.

Bourgeois C, Cervantes-Laurean D, Moss J. Niacin. In: Shils ME, Shike M, Ross AC, Caballero B, Cousins RJ eds. Modern nutrition in health and disease, 10th ed. Philadelphia: Lippincott Williams & Wilkins, 2006;442-451.

Butterworth RF. Thiamin. In: Shils ME, Shike M, Ross AC, Caballero B, Cousins RJ eds. Modern nutrition in health and disease, 10th ed. Philadelphia: Lippincott Williams & Wilkins, 2006;426-433.

Clark M, Reed DB, Crouse SF, Armstrong RB. Pre- and post-season dietary intake, body composition, and performance indices of NCAA Division I female soccer players. Int J Sport Nutr Exerc Metab 2003;13:303-319.

Combs GF. The vitamins: fundamental aspects in nutrition and health. New York: Elsevier Academic Press, 2008.

Crozier PG, Cordain L, Sampson DA. Exercise induced changes in plasma vitamin B-6 concentrations do not vary with exercise intensity. Am J Clin Nutr 1994;60:552-558.

DeBolt JE, Singh A, Day BA, Deuster PA. Nutritional survey of the U.S. Navy SEAL trainees. Am J Clin Nutr 1988;48:1316-1323.

Dreon DM, Butterfield GE. Vitamin B-6 utilization in active and inactive young men. Am J Clin Nutr 1986;43:816-824.

Erdman JW, Bistrain BR, Clarkson PM, Dwyer JT, Klein BP, Lane HW, Manore MM, O'Neil PM, Russell RM, Tepper BJ, Tipton KD, Yates AA. Committee on Metabolic Monitoring for Military Field Applications. Nutrient Composition of Rations for Short-term, High-intensity Combat Operations. Standing Committee on Military Nutrition Research (CMNR), Institute of Medicine. National Academies Press, Wash DC, 2006.

Faber M, Benade AJ. Mineral and vitamin intake in field athletes (discus-, hammer-, javelin-throwers and shot-putters). Int J Sports Med 1991;12:324-327.

Fischbach F. A manual of laboratory and diagnostic tests, 6th ed. Philadelphia: Lippincott, 2000.

Fogelholm GM, Koskinen R, Laakso J, Rankinen T, Ruokonen I. Gradual and rapid weight loss: effects on nutrition and performance in male athletes. Med Sci Sports Exerc 1993;25(3):371-377.

Fogelholm M, Ruokonen I, Laakso JT, Vuorimaa T, Himberg JJ. Lack of association between indices of vitamin B-1, B-2 and B-6 status and exercise-induced blood lactate in young adults. Int J Sport Nutr 1993;3:165-176.

Food and Nutrition Board, National Research Council. Recommended dietary allowances, 10th ed. Washington, DC: National Academy Press, 1989.

Frank T, Kühl M, Makowski B, Bitsch R, Jahreis G, Hübscher J. Does a 100-km walking affect indicators of vitamin status? Int J Vitam Nutr Res 2000;70(5):238-250.

Gibson RS. Principles of nutritional assessment, 2nd ed. New York: Oxford University Press, 2005.

Guilland JC, Penaranda T, Gallet C, Boggio V, Fuchs F, Klepping J. Vitamin status of young athletes including the effects of supplementation. Med Sci Sports Exerc 1989;21(4):441-449.

Hansen CM, Leklem JE, Miller LT. Changes in vitamin B-6 status indictors of women fed a constant protein diet with varying levels of vitamin B-6. Am J Clin Nutr 1997;66:1379-1387.

Hansen CM, Manore MM. Vitamin B6. In: Wolinsky I, Driskell JA eds. Sports nutrition. Vitamins and trace minerals. Boca Raton, FL: CRC Press, 2006;81-91.

Hansen CM, Shultz TD, Kwak HK, Memon S, Leklem JE. Assessment of vitamin B-6 status in young women consuming a controlled diet containing four levels of vitamin B-6 provides an estimated average requirement and recommended dietary allowance. J Nutr 2001;131:1777-1786.

Heath EM, Wilcox AR, Quinn CM. Effects of nicotinic acid on respiratory exchange ratio and substrate levels during exercise. Med Sci Sports Exerc 1993;25:1018-1023.

Hofmann A, Reynolds RD, Smoak BL, Villanueva VG, Deuster PA. Plasma pyridoxal and pyridoxal 5'-phosphate concentrations in response to ingestion of water or glucose polymer during a 2-h run. Am J Clin Nutr 1991;53:84-89.

Huang Y, Chen W, Evans MA, Mitchell ME, Shultz TD. Vitamin B-6 requirement and status assessment of young women fed a high-protein diet with various levels of vitamin B-6. Am J Clin Nutr 1998;67:208-220.

Institute of Medicine (IOM), Food and Nutrition Board. Dietary reference intakes: thiamin, riboflavin, niacin, vitamin B-6, folate, vitamin B-12, pantothenic acid, biotin, and choline. Washington, DC: National Academy Press, 1998.

Kaiserauer S, Snyder AC, Sleeper M, Zierath J. Nutritional, physiological, and menstrual status of distance runners. Med Sci Sports Exerc 1989;21:120-125.

Keith RE, Alt LA. Riboflavin status of female athletes consuming normal diets. Nutr Res 1991;11:727-734.

Leklem JE. Physical activity and vitamin B-6 metabolism in men and women: interrelationship with fuel needs. In: Reynolds RD, Leklem JE eds. Vitamin B-6: its role in health and disease. New York: Liss, 1985;221-241.

Leklem JE. Vitamin B-6: of reservoirs, receptors and requirements. Nutr Today 1988;Sept/Oct:4-10.

Leklem JE. Vitamin B-6: a status report. J Nutr 1990;120;1503-7.

Leklem JE, Shultz TD. Increased plasma pyridoxal 5'-phosphate and vitamin B-6 in male adolescents after a 4500-meter run. Am J Clin Nutr 1983;38:541-548.

Leonard SW, Leklem JE. Plasma B-6 vitamin changes following a 50-km ultra-marathon. Int J Sport Nutr Exerc Metab 2000;10(3):302-314.

Lowik MR, van den Berg H, Westenbrink S, Wedel M, Schrijver J, Ockhuizen T. Dose-response relationships regarding vitamin B-6 in elderly people: a nationwide nutritional survey (Dutch Nutritional Surveillance System). Am J Clin Nutr 1989;50(2):391-399.

Mackey AD, Davis SR, Gregory JF. Vitamin B6. In: Shils ME, Shike M, Ross AC, Caballero B, Cousins RJ eds. Modern nutrition in health and disease, 10th ed. Philadelphia: Lippincott Williams & Wilkins, 2006;452-461.

Manore MM. Vitamin B6 and exercise. Int J Sport Nutr 1994;4(2):89-103.

Manore MM. Effect of physical activity on thiamine, riboflavin, and vitamin B-6 requirements. Am J Clin Nutr 2000;72(2) suppl:598S-606S.

Manore MM, Leklem JE, Walter MC. Vitamin B-6 metabolism as affected by exercise in trained and untrained women fed diets differing in carbohydrate and vitamin B-6 content. Am J Clin Nutr 1987;46:995-1004.

Manore MM, Vaughan LA, Carroll SS, Leklem JE. Plasma pyridoxal 5-phosphate concentration and dietary vitamin B-6 intake in free-living, low-income elderly people. Am J Clin Nutr 1989;50:339-345.

Manore MM, Vaughan LA, Leklem JE, Felicetta JV. Changes in plasma pyridoxal phosphate (PLP) in diabetic, hypertensive and hypertensive-diabetic men fed a constant vitamin B-6 diet. FASEB J 1991;5:A586 (abstract).

Martini MC, Lampe JW, Slavin JL, Kurzer MS. Effect of the menstrual cycle on energy and nutrient intake. Am J Clin Nutr 1994;60:895-899.

McCormick DB. Riboflavin. In: Shils ME, Shike M, Ross AC, Caballero B, Cousins RJ eds. Modern nutrition in health and disease, 10th ed. Philadelphia: Lippincott Williams & Wilkins, 2006;434-441.

Murray R, Bartoli WP, Eddy DE, Horn MK. Physiology and performance responses to nicotinic-acid ingestion during exercise. Med Sci Sports Exerc 1995;27:1057-1062.

Ribaya-Mercado JD, Russell RM, Sahyoun N, Morrow FD, Gershoff SN. Vitamin B-6 requirements of elderly men and women. J Nutr 1991;121:1062-1074.

Rokitzki L, Sagredos A, Keck E, Sauer B, Keul J. Assessment of vitamin B2 status in performance athletes of various types of sports. J Nutr Sci Vitaminol 1994a;40:11-22.

Rokitzki L, Sagredos AN, Reub F, Buchner M, Keul J. Acute changes in vitamin B-6 status in endurance athletes before and after a marathon. Int J Sport Nutr 1994b;4:154-165.

Rokitzki L, Sagredos AN, Reub F, Cufi D, Keul J. Assessment of vitamin B-6 status of strength and speedpower athletes. J Am Coll Nutr 1994c;13:87-94.

Rucinski A. Relationship of body image and dietary intake of competitive ice skaters. J Am Diet Assoc 1989;89:98-100.

Schultz TD, Hansen GM, Hunt KC, Hardin K, Leklem JE, Huang A, Ames BN. Lymphocyte DNA strand breaks in smokers and nonsmokers are related to vitamin B-6 intake and metabolite concentrations in plasma and urine. FASEB J 2003;17:A1156.

Soares MJ, Satyanarayana K, Bamji MS, Jacob CM, Ramana YV, Rao SS. The effect of exercise on the riboflavin status of adult men. Br J Nutr 1993;69:541-551.

Sobal J, Marquart LF. Vitamin/mineral supplement use among athletes: a review of the literature. Int J Sport Nutr 1994;4:320-334.

Suboticanec K, Stavljenic A, Schalch W, Buzina R. Effects of pyridoxine and riboflavin supplementation on physical fitness in young adolescents. Int J Vitam Nutr Res 1990;60:81-88.

Telford RD, Catchpole EA, Deakin V, McLeay AC, Plank AW. The effect of 7 to 8 months of vitamin/mineral supplementation on the vitamin and mineral status of athletes. Int J Sport Nutr 1992;2:123-134.

Trumbo PR. Pantothenic acid. In: Shils ME, Shike M, Ross AC, Caballero B, Cousins RJ eds. Modern nutrition in health and disease, 10th ed. Philadelphia: Lippincott Williams & Wilkins, 2006;452-469.

van Dale D, Schrijver J, Saris WHM. Changes in vitamin status in plasma during dieting and exercise. Int J Vitam Nutr Res 1990;60:67-74.

van der Beek EJ, van Dokkum W, Wedel M, Schrijver J, van den Berg H. Thiamin, riboflavin and vitamin B-6: impact of restricted intake on physical performance in man. J Am Coll Nutr 1994;13:629-640.

Weight LM, Noakes TD, Labadarios D, Graves J, Jacobs P, Berman PA. Vitamin and mineral status of trained athletes including the effects of supplementation. Am J Clin Nutr 1988;47:186-191.

Winters LRT, Yoon JS, Kalkwarf HJ et al. Riboflavin requirements and exercise adaptation in older women. Am J Clin Nutr 1992;56:526-532.

Woolf K, Manore MM. B-vitamins and exercise: does exercise alter requirements? Int J Sport Nutr Exerc Metab Oct 2006;16(5):453-484.

Woolf K, Manore MM. Micronutrients important for exercise. In: Spurway N, MacLaren D eds. Advances in sport and exercise science series: nutrition and sport. Philadelphia: Elsevier, 2007;117-134.

Woolf K, Manore MM. Elevated plasma homocysteine and low vitamin B-6 status in nonsupplementing older women with rheumatoid arthritis. J Am Diet Assoc 2008;108(3):443-453.

CHAPTER 10

Antioxidant Nutrients

Chapter Objectives

After reading this chapter you should be able to

- define free radicals,
- list the enzymes involved in antioxidant activities and describe the reactions in which they participate,
- discuss the nutrients involved in antioxidant activities,
- describe the methods used to assess oxidative damage,
- describe the proposed rationale for increased antioxidant need among active people,
- discuss how antioxidants play a role in chronic diseases, and
- discuss the relationship between antioxidants and athletic performance.

The health benefits of antioxidant nutrients are widely published in both scientific and popular literature. Antioxidants have been purported to protect active people from oxidative tissue damage, reduce risks of cancer and heart disease, and even slow or reverse the aging process. Is there scientific evidence to support these claims? Should people, particularly active people, increase their consumption of foods high in antioxidants, take antioxidant supplements, or both? This chapter attempts to answer these questions. We define antioxidants and describe in detail the specific nutrients involved in the antioxidant process. We also examine the claim that consuming antioxidants enhances athletic performance.

ACTIONS OF ANTIOXIDANTS

Antioxidants are nutrients that act to prevent oxidative damage resulting from **free radical** formation (see "Definition of a Free Radical"). Specifically, antioxidants can

- scavenge free radicals;
- remove the catalysts that accelerate oxidative reactions, thus minimizing the formation of free radicals;
- repair the damage resulting from oxidation; and
- bind free metal ions to prevent them from reacting with reactive species.

In order to have a clearer understanding of how antioxidants work, you must understand how free radicals form. Several mechanisms are believed to form free radicals related to exercise. The most commonly cited mechanism of exercise-induced free radical production is increased oxygen flux to the mitochondria during exercise. This is often called the "mitochondrial leak."

Mitochondrial oxidation usually occurs by four single-electron transfer reactions, starting from nicotinamide adenine dinucleotide (NADH) and ending with a final product of water (Alberts et al. 1989) (figure 10.1). The electron transfer occurs within the **electron transport chain (respiratory chain),** which is located in the inner mitochondrial membrane. As figure 10.1 shows, the electron transport chain comprises a series of electron carriers, including **cytochrome-c, ubiquinone** (i.e., **coenzyme** Q_{10}), and the following three enzyme complexes:

- NADH dehydrogenase complex: Accepts electrons from NADH and passes them to ubiquinone, which then transfers its electrons to the b-c_1 enzyme complex.

Highlight

Definition of a Free Radical

A free radical is a molecule with an unpaired electron in its outer orbit, or valence shell. Free radicals are naturally produced during normal respiration and can be generated in response to exposure to toxic substances (e.g., ozone, alcohol, UV rays, etc.). Free radicals are highly reactive and can create a chain reaction that produces even more free radicals! This chain reaction occurs when a free radical reacts with a stable compound in order to pair its unpaired electron with an electron from the stable compound (see "Reactions that Form Free Radicals" on p. 305). If free radicals are produced in excess and not neutralized by the antioxidant systems present in the human body, then cellular damage can occur. A number of free radicals and reactive oxygen species have been identified. Some of these are

- superoxide radical ($O_2 \cdot^-$);
- hydroxyl radical (OH·);
- hydrogen peroxide (H_2O_2)—not a free radical, but can be involved in reactions that cause the production of free radicals;
- singlet oxygen ($^1O_2$);
- hydroperoxyl free radical (ROOH·); and
- nitric oxide free radical (NO·).

"Reactions That Form Free Radicals and Other Reactive Oxygen Species" reviews the processes that form these reactive species, which can damage lipids in membranes **(lipid peroxidation)**, resulting in cell damage and possibly cell death. Free radicals are also purported to cause damage to cell proteins, particularly those associated with genetic material. Free radicals also may destroy endothelial cells that line blood vessels, damage the lungs, and accelerate the aging process (Cutler 1984; Halliwell and Gutteridge 1999; Tate and Repine 1984).

Antioxidant defense systems, including enzymes and nutrients that possess antioxidant properties, help prevent oxidative damage.

Reactions That Form Free Radicals and Other Reactive Oxygen Species

Superoxide radical is formed when an electron is added to an oxygen molecule:

$$O_2 + e^- = O_2 \cdot^-.$$

Hydroxyl radical is formed when hydrogen peroxide reacts with $O_2 \cdot^-$ in the presence of free metal ions (e.g., Fe^{3+} or Cu^{2+}), or when water reacts with $O_2 \cdot^-$:

$$\text{Fe, Cu}$$
$$O_2^- + H_2O_2 = O_2 + OH + OH^-.$$
$$H_2O + 1/2\, O_2^- = 2OH \cdot.$$

Hydrogen peroxide is formed by the joining of two hydroxyl radicals or by superoxide radicals generated in aqueous solutions:

$$OH \cdot + OH \cdot = H_2O_2.$$
$$2O_2 \cdot^- + 2H^+ = H_2O_2 + O_2.$$

Singlet oxygen is formed when one of the six electrons in the outer shell of an oxygen molecule moves into a new extra orbit (Karlsson 1997). This occurs as a result of release of energy from a nearby chemical reaction or because of exposure to radiation.

Hydroperoxyl free radical is formed through a series of reactions occurring at the sites of a lipid, a protein, or a nucleotide (adapted from Karlsson 1997):

- The hydroxyl radical attacks an organic compound (RH), and a carbon-centered radical is formed ($R \cdot$):

$$RH + OH \cdot = R \cdot + H_2O.$$

- A peroxyl radical is formed from $R \cdot$ reacting with oxygen:

$$R \cdot^- + O_2 = ROO \cdot.$$

- A hydroperoxyl radical is formed when the peroxyl radical reacts with a surrounding molecule (either a protein or lipid):

$$ROO \cdot^- + RH = R \cdot + ROOH.$$

Nitric oxide free radical is released from the vascular endothelium (lining of blood vessel) and dilates blood vessels. It can react with other radicals such as the superoxide radical to form peroxynitrate. Peroxynitrate is not a free radical, but an oxidant.

$$NO \cdot + O_2 \cdot^- = ONOO^-.$$

- The b-c$_1$ enzyme complex: Accepts electrons from ubiquinone and passes them to cytochrome-c, which carries its electrons to the cytochrome oxidase complex.
- Cytochrome oxidase complex: Accepts electrons from cytochrome-c and passes them on to oxygen to form water.

Electrons (e^-) can be accepted in the electron transport process in two ways: through tetravalent reduction of oxygen to water and through alternative univalent pathways. No oxygen intermediates are formed during the tetravalent process. During normal cellular respiration, most of the O_2 is reduced to form water via the tetravalent reaction; however, electrons can escape from various locations along the electron transport chain. Oxygen can accept these escaped electrons in an alternate univalent reaction that results in formation of the superoxide radical, which can be further reduced to potentially harmful species—hydrogen peroxide and hydroxyl radical (figure 10.2). It has been estimated that 4% to 5% of the oxygen consumed in mitochondrial oxidation may form oxygen species with unpaired electrons (Jenkins and Goldfarb 1993). These highly reactive oxygen species can produce more free radicals, including other reactive oxygen species.

More recently, oxidative damage has been attributed to a number of other potential sources

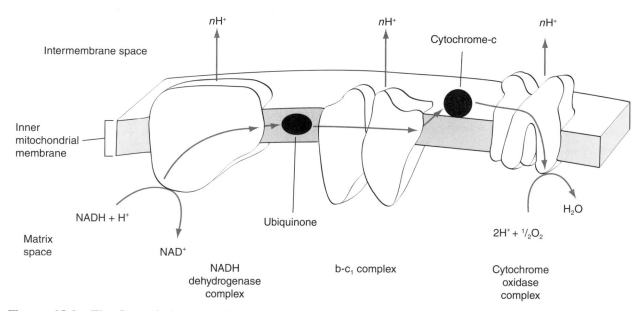

Figure 10.1   The flow of electrons through the three major respiratory enzyme complexes during the transfer of two electrons from nicotinamide adenine dinucleotide (NADH) to oxygen. Ubiquinone and cytochrome-c serve as carriers between the complexes.

Reprinted, with permission of Garland Publishing, from *Molecular Biology of the Cell,* B. Alberts et al., 2nd ed. 1989; permission conveyed through Copyright Clearance Center, Inc.

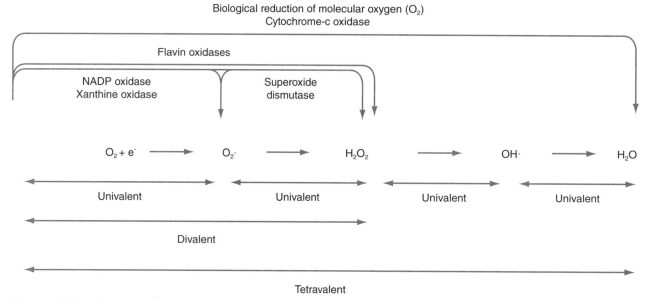

Figure 10.2   Molecular oxygen can participate in univalent, divalent, and tetravalent reactions in mitochondrial metabolism. Respiration and water formation is the normal and tetravalent reaction. Water can also be formed by four consecutive univalent reactions, which produce oxygen-centered radicals as well as hydrogen peroxide (H_2O_2). Hydrogen peroxide provokes hydroxyl radical (OH·) formation from water.

Adapted, by permission, from J. Karlsson, 1997, *Antioxidants and exercise* (Champaign, IL: Human Kinetics).

that may contribute to free radical production even more than mitochondrial oxidation. Most likely many of these mechanisms, listed next, act synergistically, and some may play greater roles depending on the type of exercise involved. For more details on these mechanisms, see the reviews by Powers and colleagues (1999), Vollaard and colleagues (2005), and Finaud and colleagues (2006).

- Ischemia-reperfusion: Temporary hypoxia associated with intense exercise triggers the xanthine oxidase pathway. When the skeletal tissue is reoxygenated, this pathway produces superoxide free radicals.
- Inflammation: Exercise-induced cell damage triggers an inflammatory response. A neutrophil respiratory burst results in superoxide, hydrogen peroxide, and other free radicals.
- Auto-oxidation of heme proteins: The breakdown of hemoglobin and myoglobin produces superoxide and peroxide free radicals.

- Nitric oxide release: Increased nitric oxide, a free radical, is released during exercise, which can combine with the superoxide free radical to form the toxic oxidant peroxynitrite.

ENZYMES INVOLVED IN ANTIOXIDANT ACTIVITIES

Numerous defense systems protect the body against excessive oxidative damage. The defenses include enzymatic systems—such as superoxide dismutase (SOD), catalase (CAT), glutathione peroxidase (GPX), glutathione reductase (GR), and peroxidase—located in the extracellular, membranous, and intracellular components of cells. Figure 10.3 provides a visual representation of the antioxidant defense system in relation to the cell. The defenses are widespread and strategically placed within the cell—for instance, SOD is located in both the cytoplasm and the mitochondrion, where it can convert the superoxide

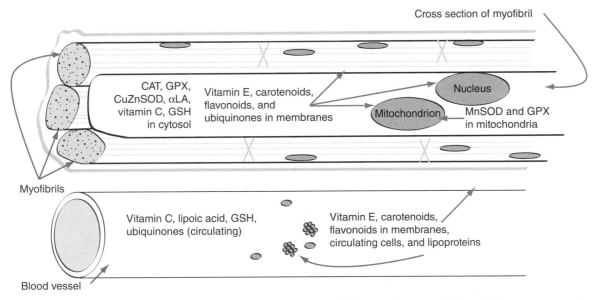

Figure 10.3 The human body contains several intracellular and extracellular defense systems to protect itself from free radical damage. These consist of enzymes and antioxidant nutrients. Within the myofibril, enzymes and antioxidants are located both in the cytosol and in the mitochondria. The enzymes catalase (CAT), glutathione peroxidase (GPX), and superoxide dismutase (SOD) remove free radicals with the help of the micronutrients copper (Cu), zinc (Zn), and manganese (Mn). Fat-soluble antioxidants such as vitamin E (vit E) exist in the cell membranes to prevent lipid peroxidation. Antioxidants such as vitamin C (vit C), α-lipoic acid (αLA), and glutathione (GSH) also circulate in the blood to help protect cells from oxidation.

From S.K. Powers, 2004, "Dietary antioxidants and exercise," *Journal of Sports Science* 22: 81-94. Reprinted by permission of the publisher (Taylor & Francis Ltd, http://www.tandf.co.uk/journals).

radical to hydrogen and oxygen in both lipid and aqueous media.

The antioxidant defense enzymes require minerals as cofactors, including

- copper (Cu), which is part of the structure of cytosolic SOD;
- iron (Fe), which is part of the structure of CAT;
- manganese (Mn), which is part of the structure of mitochondrial SOD; and
- zinc (Zn), which is part of the structure of cytosolic SOD.

Deficiencies of these minerals can result in reduced activities of the corresponding antioxidant enzymes. Note also that unbound forms of certain minerals, such as iron and copper, can enhance oxidative damage.

Enzymes provide an endogenous defense system to protect our cells from free radical damage. As previously mentioned, micronutrients such as copper, manganese, zinc, and iron play key roles in activating these enzymes. The enzyme defense systems are as follows:

- **Superoxide dismutase (SOD):** Accelerates the conversion of superoxide radical to hydrogen peroxide. Superoxide dismutase requires manganese in the mitochondria and zinc and copper in the cytosol.
- **Catalase (CAT):** Removes hydrogen peroxide. Catalase requires iron.
- **Glutathione:** A substrate (not an enzyme) involved in the removal of hydrogen peroxide and the reduction of lipid hydroperoxides. The oxidized form of glutathione is abbreviated GSSG; the reduced form is abbreviated GSH.
- **Glutathione peroxidase (GPX):** Removes hydrogen peroxide and reduces lipid hydroperoxides. Glutathione peroxidase requires selenium.
- **Glutathione reductase (GR):** Converts oxidized glutathione (GSSG) back to reduced glutathione (GSH).
- **Peroxidase:** Rids the body of excess hydrogen peroxide.

Superoxide dismutase provides one line of defense in the mitochondria and cytosol. Found primarily in oxidative muscle, this enzyme acts to accelerate the conversion of the superoxide radical to hydrogen peroxide and oxygen, as illustrated in equation 10.1:

(SOD)

$$2O_2^{\cdot-} + 2H^+ \rightarrow H_2O_2 + O_2. \quad (10.1)$$

Catalase, located in peroxisomes and in smaller amounts in mitochondria, removes hydrogen peroxide by converting it to water and oxygen:

(CAT)

$$2H_2O_2 \rightarrow 2H_2O + O_2. \quad (10.2)$$

Glutathione peroxidase and GR are substrate–enzyme complexes located in the mitochondria and cytosol. Glutathione peroxidase removes hydrogen peroxide by using it to oxidize reduced glutathione (GSH). It also reduces lipid hydroperoxides to hydroxy acids, as in equations 10.3 and 10.4:

(GPX)

$$2GSH + H_2O_2 \rightarrow GSSG + 2H_2O \quad (10.3)$$

(GPX)

$$ROOH + 2GSH \rightarrow ROH + H_2O + GSSG \quad (10.4)$$

where R is any organic backbone of a hydroperoxide.

Equation 10.3 is probably the major reaction that processes the hydrogen peroxide formed in the SOD reaction of equation 10.1 (Gutteridge and Halliwell 1994). Because GPX requires GSH to reduce hydroperoxides, GSH must be regenerated. To do this, GR converts oxidized glutathione (GSSG) back to reduced glutathione (GSH), as illustrated in equation 10.5:

(GR)

$$GSSG + NADPH \rightarrow GSH + NADP \quad (10.5)$$

Although both CAT and GPX remove hydrogen peroxides, GPX has a much higher affinity for these free radicals; therefore, it plays a greater role in hydrogen peroxide removal (Powers et al. 1999).

Peroxidases are enzymes that use hydrogen peroxide to oxidize a given substrate (S), thus ridding the body of excess hydrogen peroxide. This action is illustrated in equation 10.6:

(Peroxidase)

$$SH_2 + H_2O_2 \rightarrow S + 2H_2O \quad (10.6)$$

where S is any reduced substrate.

The reactions in equations 10.1 through 10.6 represent only a few of the functions these enzyme systems perform. Many of these enzyme systems are also involved in the repair of damage caused by free radicals and in regenerating other protective antioxidant nutrients. For instance, GPX metabolizes damaged lipids from membranes, which can then be replaced by healthy fatty acids, and GSH assists in recycling both vitamins E and C (Gutteridge and Halliwell 1994).

NUTRIENTS INVOLVED IN ANTIOXIDANT ACTIVITIES

In addition to enzyme systems, many micronutrients are also involved in the antioxidant process. While vitamins E, C, and β-carotene are well-known antioxidants, other nutrients (including many minerals) also help remove free radicals (table 10.1).

Table 10.1 Nutrients Involved in Antioxidant Activities

Nutrient	Primary antioxidant functions
α-Lipoic acid	Recycles vitamin E
Vitamin E (α-tocopherol)	Halts lipid peroxidation
Vitamin C (ascorbic acid)	Quenches singlet oxygen, regenerates the reduced form of vitamin E
β-Carotene	Quenches singlet oxygen
Ubiquinol (reduced coenzyme Q or Q_{10})	Scavenges peroxyl radicals
Selenium	Is part of the glutathione peroxidase enzyme system
Copper	Is part of the Cu-Zn SOD enzyme complex (in cytosol)
Zinc	Is part of the Cu-Zn SOD enzyme complex (in cytosol)
Iron	Is part of the catalase enzyme system
Manganese	Is part of the Mn-SOD enzyme complex (in mitochondria)
Flavonoids (isoflavones, anthocyananins, catechins)	Inhibit inflammatory enzymes; scavenge superoxide, hydroxyl, and peroxyl radicals

Vitamin E

Vitamin E is an essential fat-soluble vitamin that includes eight compounds classified as tocopherols and tocotrienols, with each compound having a different biological activity (Traber 2006). Of the eight compounds, α-**tocopherol** is found in the greatest amount in tissues and plasma and is considered the most biologically active vitamin E compound. However, in recent years this idea has become controversial. All vitamin E compounds exert biological activity, and some, such as gamma-tocopherol, may exert an even greater antioxidant effect than α-tocopherol (Traber and Blatt 2002). The research has primarily addressed α-tocopherol, which is the focus of this chapter.

Vitamin E performs many antioxidant functions in the body. The following are some of the primary functions of vitamin E (Traber 2006):

- Halts lipid peroxidation
- Quenches singlet oxygen
- Stabilizes the superoxide radical
- Stabilizes the hydroxyl radical
- Spares selenium and protects β-carotene from destruction
- Stabilizes membrane structure

The primary role of vitamin E is to protect the polyunsaturated fatty acids (PUFAs) in biological membranes against oxidative damage. Vitamin E interrupts the chain reaction of lipid peroxidation, helping to maintain membrane stability and fluidity and protecting cellular structures against oxidative damage.

Methods of Assessment

Currently there are no biochemical indices that accurately reflect dietary vitamin E intakes or body stores of vitamin E. Tocopherol values can be measured in serum, erythrocytes, platelets, and tissues such as liver or adipose (Gibson 2005; Traber 2006). Although serum tocopherol concentration is often used as an index of vitamin E status, concentrations can vary significantly and are closely associated with serum lipid levels. Serum tocopherol values vary with age, physiological state, and method of analysis; a wide range of values is reported for apparently healthy individuals.

Measurement of tocopherol in erythrocytes is technically difficult, and there appears to be little justification for using this measure to indicate vitamin E status. Tocopherol concentrations in platelets and tissues appear promising as accurate indicators of vitamin E status, but more research needs to be done to confirm their usefulness; however, assessing tissue tocopherol levels is invasive and not appropriate for use in large populations.

Two indirect assessments of vitamin E status are the **erythrocyte hemolysis test** and **breath pentane measurements** (Gibson 2005). Hemolysis rates are inversely related to serum tocopherol levels; one weakness of this test is that changes in the status of other nutrients, such as folic acid, can also increase erythrocyte hemolysis. The breath pentane test measures exhalation of the aliphatic hydrocarbons ethane and pentane as indirect indicators of linolenic and linoleic acid oxidation—which is positively correlated with vitamin E deficiency. The use of aliphatic hydrocarbons as indicators of oxidative damage is discussed in more detail later in this chapter.

Dietary Sources, Recommended Intakes, and Supplementation Products

Primary food sources for vitamin E include certain vegetable oils, green leafy vegetables, nuts, wheat germ, and whole grains. The results of National Health and Nutrition Examination Survey (NHANES) III showed that fortified breakfast cereals, bakery products, beef, white bread, fats and oils, pasta, nuts, and seeds were the major contributors to vitamin E intake among U.S. adults (Maras et al. 2004). While animal products are generally poor sources of vitamin E, they are consumed more frequently by adults and thus contribute more to vitamin E intakes in the U.S. diet than higher vitamin E content foods such as vegetable oils and nuts.

Although nuts are a good source of vitamin E, their consumption is low in the U.S. diet.

Vitamin E deficiencies are rare in humans and occur primarily in premature infants or people with fat-malabsorption syndromes. The Recommended Dietary Allowance (RDA) for vitamin E is 15 mg α-tocopherol. The RDA is based on the amount of vitamin E needed to prevent hemolysis, the breakdown of PUFA-rich red blood cells. This equates to approximately 22 IU natural or 33 IU synthetic vitamin E (Institute of Medicine [IOM] 2000) (see "Forms of Vitamin E and Units of Expression"). Because vitamin E is needed to protect PUFAs from oxidation, vitamin E requirements rise with higher intakes of PUFAs. Since many athletes and active people consume a diet that is moderately high in fat (25-35% of total kilocalories from fat), and since they utilize more oxygen than sedentary people, vitamin E requirements for active people may be higher than the RDA. While it is possible to consume adequate vitamin E from dietary sources, Maras and colleagues (2004) found that only 8% of men and 2.4% of women were meeting the Estimated Average Requirement (EAR) of 12 mg/day of vitamin E. People can increase vitamin E intake by focusing on increasing monounsaturated fats versus polyunsaturated fats (Traber 2006).

Vitamin E supplements are available to the general public. Unlike supplementation with other fat-soluble vitamins, vitamin E supplementation appears to be safe. However, at high doses vitamin E may act as an anticoagulant, which can increase the risk of hemorrhage. Smokers and those with chronic disease should also use caution if supplementing with vitamin E. Although newer studies suggest that smokers may indeed have higher vitamin E requirements than nonsmokers (Bruno et al. 2005, 2006), the ATBC Cancer Prevention

Highlight

Forms of Vitamin E and Units of Expression

In the body, α-tocopherol is present in the natural form *RRR*-α-tocopherol (*d*-α-tocopherol). The RDA is based on this form. Supplements may contain either natural vitamin E (*RRR*-α-tocopherol or *d*-α-tocopherol) or synthetic vitamin E (*all rac*-α-tocopherol or *dl*-α-tocopherol). Natural vitamin E is more potent than synthetic vitamin E.

Vitamin E is commonly expressed using two primary units of measurement: international units (IU) and milligrams (mg). To convert 1 IU of natural vitamin E to milligrams, multiply by 0.67; to convert 1 IU of synthetic vitamin E to milligrams, multiply by 0.45 (Mastaloudis and Traber 2006). The units used in this chapter are those reported in the cited research papers.

Study showed an increase in hemorrhagic stroke in smokers (Alpha-Tocopherol, Beta-Carotene Cancer Prevention Study Group [ABCPSG] 1994). A well-publicized meta-analysis showed an increase in all-cause mortality with daily vitamin E intakes ≥400 IU (Miller et al. 2005). However, it should be noted that the meta-analysis covered studies in people with chronic disease and included studies that administered vitamin E in doses higher than the Tolerable Upper Limit (UL). Given the potential for bleeding, it is prudent to remain below the UL of 1000 mg/day.

Vitamin C

Vitamin C, also known as ascorbic acid or **ascorbate,** is an essential water-soluble vitamin. While plants and most mammals are capable of synthesizing their own vitamin C, humans (and other primates) lack **gulonolactone oxidase,** the enzyme that catalyzes the final step in vitamin C synthesis (Levine et al. 2006). Scurvy is the primary vitamin C deficiency disease in humans. Vitamin C plays many important roles in the body, including that of an antioxidant.

Vitamin C functions as an antioxidant primarily in the extracellular fluid (Levine et al. 2006). The suggested antioxidant actions of vitamin C include the following:

- Stabilizes the hydroxyl radical
- Quenches singlet oxygen
- Scavenges the superoxide radical
- Reduces the oxidized form of vitamin E
- Reduces nitrosamines to harmless species
- May help protect the lungs from ozone and cigarette smoke (see "Vitamin C and Cigarette Smoking")

Highlight

Vitamin C and Cigarette Smoking

Serum vitamin C concentrations are depressed in smokers and those exposed to secondhand smoke. Cigarette smoke contains numerous oxidants, and vitamin C is depleted in both active smokers and in people exposed to secondhand smoke (Alberg 2002). The RDA for vitamin C is 90 mg/day for men and 75 mg/day for women. Because smokers need more vitamin C, an additional 35 mg/day is recommended for people who smoke. This equals 125 mg/day for men and 110 mg/day for women. Vitamin C helps protect against the harmful effects of cigarette smoking through three mechanisms:

1. Improving endothelium-dependent vasodilation (Heitzer et al. 1996)

2. Reducing adhesiveness of monocytes to endothelium cells (Weber et al. 1996)

3. Decreasing oxidative damage (Dietrich et al. 2003)

All three of these actions can help reduce the risk of cardiovascular disease in smokers. Smokers have a diminished vasodilator response to chemical and mechanical stressors, which affects blood flow and blood pressure. Reducing the adhesiveness of monocytes to endothelial cells may prevent the inflammatory response in the vessel wall resulting from cigarette smoke, which in turn could reduce the initiation and development of atherosclerosis. As oxidation of serum lipids is strongly associated with increased risk of cardiovascular disease, any mechanism by which oxidative damage can be reduced will be beneficial. Note that the health benefits of vitamin C described here were seen with 2 g/day of vitamin C over 5 to 10 days—an amount much higher than the 110 to 125 mg/day recommended for smokers.

Although vitamin C can reduce some of the risks associated with cigarette smoking, the risk factors associated with regular cigarette smoking far outweigh vitamin C's ability to fight oxidation-related damage. It is encouraging, however, to know there are protective steps that smokers can take while "breaking the habit."

Vitamin C may also help prevent the metal ion–induced oxidation of low-density lipoproteins (LDL) (Polidori et al. 2004)—an important role, since LDL oxidation significantly increases the risk of atherosclerosis. The associations between antioxidants and cardiovascular disease are discussed in more detail later in this chapter.

Under certain circumstances, vitamin C can also act as a **prooxidant**—a substance that *increases* the production of free radicals and enhances oxidative damage. When administered at very low concentrations in vitro, vitamin C increased hydroperoxide lipid peroxidation (Lee et al. 2001). At amounts typical of supplementation (e.g., 500 mg), vitamin C also induced DNA damage in humans (Podmore et al. 1998). Herbert (1993a) asserted that vitamin C is a powerful prooxidant in the presence of high body iron stores. Approximately 1 in 200 people of Northern European descent are predisposed to the genetic disorder hemochromatosis, which causes enhanced iron absorption and high body iron stores (Higdon 2003). Increased serum concentrations of vitamin C augment the release of catalytic iron from ferritin; the released iron then accelerates oxidative damage. Thus, combining vitamin C supplements with iron supplements may be a poor, and possibly hazardous, choice for people with high iron stores or people at risk for hemochromatosis. "The Relationship Between Vitamin C and Iron" reviews the potentially dangerous prooxidant relationship between iron and vitamin C.

Methods of Assessment

The most commonly used measure of vitamin C status is **serum ascorbic acid concentrations** (Gibson 2005). Only fasting blood samples are used, since recent dietary intake of vitamin C influences serum levels (serum levels increase proportionally for small doses up to 150 mg). As with many other vitamins, serum ascorbic acid concentrations are not accurate indicators of vitamin C status in persons consuming chronically high levels of the vitamin. Serum levels do not increase proportionally above 400 mg/day of vitamin C. This is due to several factors, such as increased excretion, decreased absorption, and saturation of cells and tissues (Levine et al. 2002). Blood levels of vitamin C eventually peak and fail to increase even when greater amounts of vitamin

---

Highlight

The Relationship Between Vitamin C and Iron

Vitamin C promotes the absorption of iron from the digestive tract by capturing iron and keeping it in the ferrous form (Fe^{2+}), which is the form that is more readily absorbed. In addition, vitamin C can mobilize iron from body stores in situations in which people have high iron body stores; this can result in **iron-induced cardiac failure.** The death of three athletes from iron-induced cardiac failure may have resulted from taking megadoses of vitamin C (Herbert 1993b; also see chapter 12).

What is the mechanism by which iron and other metals form free radicals? When iron and other metals are in the free or unbound form, they are capable of forming free radicals through the "iron-catalyzed Haber-Weiss reaction" (McCord and Day 1978). The net reaction is

$$O_2 \cdot + H_2O_2 \rightarrow O_2 + OH \cdot + OH^-.$$

Iron catalyzes this reaction as follows:

$$Fe^{3+} + O_2 \cdot \rightarrow Fe^{2+} + O_2.$$
$$Fe^{2+} + H_2O_2 \rightarrow Fe^{3+} + OH \cdot + OH^-.$$

It is important to understand that depending on the body's chemistry, vitamin C and other "antioxidants" can also act as prooxidants. It is critical that people have their iron status assessed before taking supplemental iron and doses of vitamin C greater than 1 to 2 g/day. Herbert (1993b) stated that 12% of Americans have excess iron levels, and taking large doses of vitamin C can be harmful by increasing oxidative damage and causing other complications resulting from excessive circulating free iron.

C are consumed. However, serum vitamin C is an adequate indicator of chronically low vitamin C intakes. Several nonnutritional factors can lower serum vitamin C concentrations, including cigarette smoking, oral contraceptive use, acute stress, surgery, and chronic inflammatory diseases.

A more reliable indicator of tissue stores of vitamin C is **leukocyte ascorbic acid concentration,** since this measure is less affected by short-term fluctuations in dietary intake of vitamin C. The assay is technically difficult, however, and requires relatively large samples of blood (Gibson 2005). While **urinary excretion** of vitamin C reflects recent dietary intake, it is not a sensitive indicator of vitamin C status. Measurement of **capillary fragility** has also been used as a functional test of vitamin C status: A blood pressure cuff is applied to the upper arm, and the pressure at which hemorrhages appear on the skin is noted. This test is inconsistent, and other diseases can cause capillary fragility; thus, it is not a sensitive and reliable test of vitamin C status. The most reliable method of assessing vitamin C status is **isotope dilution** (Baker et al. 1971). An oral dose of ^{14}C- or ^{13}C-labeled ascorbic acid is administered, and the specific activity of blood or urine ascorbate is measured over 24 to 48 h. This method has been used to establish total body pool vitamin C levels.

Dietary Sources, Recommended Intakes, and Supplementation Products

Fruits and vegetables are the best sources of vitamin C. In particular, broccoli, oranges, strawberries, grapefruit juice, red bell peppers, and kiwi fruit are excellent sources. Raw fruits and vegetables usually have a higher density of vitamin C because vitamin C is destroyed by heat. Thus, reducing cooking time of vegetables assists in preserving the vitamin C content. It is also important to store produce in airtight, closed containers, as vitamin C is easily oxidized. Severe vitamin C deficiencies are rare in the United States due to the availability of food sources high in this nutrient. There is no evidence that active people consume inadequate amounts of vitamin C; in fact, individuals who consume fruits and vegetables on a regular basis have no difficulty consuming more than the RDA for vitamin C—90 mg/day and 75 mg/day for men and women, respectively. The median intake for adults is 102 mg/day (IOM 2000). Because smokers experience increased oxidative stress and greater turnover of vitamin C, the RDA is increased by 35 mg/day. The body's increased use of vitamin C to fight damage from smog and other environmental pollutants may also contribute to higher vitamin C needs (Atalay et al. 2006). Increasing oxygen consumption and free radical production with exercise may further burden the antioxidant systems, raising an active person's need for vitamin C above the current RDA. However, active people who regularly consume fruits and vegetables are most likely getting adequate vitamin C from dietary sources.

Vitamin C supplements are easily available and relatively inexpensive. As vitamin C is water soluble, it can be consumed in doses much higher than the RDA with minimal side effects. However, people taking more than 2 to 3 g/day may suffer from a variety of side effects including nausea, diarrhea, abdominal cramps, and erythrocyte hemolysis. An additional risk with **megadoses** of vitamin C is iron overload toxicity (see "The Relationship Between Vitamin C and Iron"). There is no conclusive evidence that consuming heavy doses (greater than 1 g/day or 1000 mg/day) of vitamin C prevents colds in healthy adults, although vitamin C has been shown to reduce blood histamine (Johnston et al. 1992). Since histamine can suppress the immune response, this is one possible mechanism by which vitamin C may affect immune system responses.

Other Functions Related to Exercise

Vitamin C has a variety of functions in the body besides its antioxidant properties:

- Is essential for collagen synthesis; collagen is the dominant protein of connective tissues and is the matrix on which teeth and bones are formed
- Plays a yet unidentified role in the stress response—possibly associated with vitamin C's role in production of norepinephrine and thyroxine and its role as an antioxidant during increased immune system activity
- Is required for the biosynthesis of carnitine
- Assists with amino acid metabolism
- Increases absorption of dietary iron (ferric iron) or non-heme iron
- Improves symptoms of upper respiratory infections in sedentary people and ultramarathon runners (Bucca et al. 1992; Peters et al. 1993)

These functions are important to maintaining the health of sedentary and active people. Supporters of supplementation insist that one can achieve adequate intakes of vitamin C only by taking dietary supplements. However, a person can consume more than four times the RDA by eating a combination of one medium orange; 1 cup of chopped, cooked broccoli (from fresh); and 1/2 cup of raw red bell pepper (or 1 cup of raw green bell pepper). The combined vitamin C from all these foods is approximately 265 mg, an intake level that is very achievable in the daily diet. Regularly consuming a diet containing only a few fruits and vegetables will result in lower than recommended vitamin C intakes and low serum concentrations of vitamin C.

β-Carotene and Vitamin A

β-Carotene is one of many compounds classified as **carotenoids**. Carotenoids are part of the red, orange, and yellow pigments found in many fruits and vegetables. They are fat soluble, transported in the blood by lipoproteins, and stored in the fatty tissues of the body. β-Carotene, the most widely researched carotenoid, is a precursor to vitamin A. This means that vitamin A can be produced in the body from β-carotene. Like vitamin A, β-carotene has antioxidant properties. There are actually over 600 carotenoids in nature, some of which do not convert to vitamin A. These non-provitamin A carotenoids include **lycopene** (found in tomatoes) and **lutein** (found in green leafy vegetables), which may have antioxidant properties more potent than β-carotene.

β-Carotene performs its functions in the lipid portion of cell membranes and in LDL particles. In addition to quenching singlet oxygen, β-carotene quenches hydroperoxyl radicals and protects against lipid peroxidation (Higdon 2007). β-Carotene is a relatively weak antioxidant in comparison to vitamin E. As previously mentioned, there are numerous other carotenoids that may be stronger antioxidants than β-carotene. More studies on these carotenoids need to be conducted to fully elucidate their role in antioxidant metabolism.

Vitamin A protects LDLs against oxidation and may reduce oxidative damage in infants who are vitamin A deficient (Livrea et al. 1995; Schwarz et al. 1997). Vitamin A is a much weaker antioxidant than β-carotene, and vitamin A supplementation in individuals without deficiency is highly toxic. In contrast, β-carotene can be taken in supplemental doses with very low risk of toxicity. One side effect of large doses of β-carotene is yellowing of the skin. This condition is called hypercarotenemia, or carotenosis, and appears to be reversible and harmless. Although β-carotene is converted to vitamin A in the body, high doses of β-carotene do not result in toxic levels of vitamin A. Thus, most of our discussion focuses on β-carotene's actions as an antioxidant.

Methods of Assessment

High-performance liquid chromatography (HPLC) is the predominant method used to assess serum carotenoid concentrations. However, it has been shown to reflect short-term dietary intake only. A newer method of carotenoid detection is currently being validated. Studies evaluating macular carotenoid levels have utilized resonance Raman spectroscopy. Raman spectroscopy is a noninvasive test in which a small laser is used to create vibrations in the retina (for macular carotenoid levels) or the palm of the hand (for skin carotenoid levels). The stretching vibrations of the single and double bonds of carotenoids are detected and measured. This method has shown high sensitivity and specificity as well as strong correlations with plasma carotenoid levels (Ermakov et al. 2005; Hata et al. 2000). Raman spectroscopy may be a promising noninvasive method of measuring long-term carotenoid intake.

Of the 600 carotenoids, only about 12 are commonly found in the diet. The six most common carotenoids identified in human blood are these (Crews et al. 2001):

- β-Carotene
- α-Carotene
- Lutein
- Zeaxanthin
- Cryptoxanthin
- Lycopene

Analyses of serum β-carotene concentrations in NHANES III showed that most people have levels ranging from 0.39 μmol/L (low vegetable intake) to 0.46 μmol/L (high vegetable intake) (Su and Arab 2006). Women in general, and men and women who consume fruits and vegetables, have higher concentrations. Smokers typically have lower concentrations than nonsmokers (Galan et al. 2005). Plasma carotenoid concentrations fluctuate throughout the menstrual cycle, with concentrations lowest at menses and significantly higher thereafter (Forman et al. 1996). β-Carotene concentrations appear to peak in the late follicular phase. These results emphasize the importance of tracking menstrual cycle status when measuring carotenoid concentrations in premenopausal women.

Dietary Sources, Recommended Intakes, and Supplementation Products

The best sources of β-carotene are dark green leafy vegetables such as spinach; deep orange fruits such as cantaloupe and apricots; and vegetables such as winter squash, carrots, sweet potatoes, and broccoli. People who eat recommended amounts of fruits and vegetables (five to nine servings per day) have a much higher intake of β-carotene than others, with values averaging 10 mg/day or more. A diet meeting the minimum requirement of five servings of fruits and vegetables per day provides approximately 5 or 6 mg/day of β-carotene (IOM 2000). At present, there is no RDA for β-carotene, but some researchers have recommended that an intake of 3 to 6 mg/day is sufficient to maintain serum levels of β-carotene at concentrations associated with reduced risk of chronic diseases such as cancer and heart disease (IOM 2000). These levels are achievable through the diet; table 10.2 lists foods rich in β-carotene.

β-Carotene supplements are commonly sold in combination with other antioxidant nutrients. Although intakes of 3 to 6 mg/day are associated with reduced risk for cancer and heart disease in epidemiological studies, clinical trials designed to study β-carotene's effects on disease status have supplemented with larger doses of 15 to 30 mg/day. These doses were shown to be harmful to heavy smokers and alcohol drinkers (Albanes et al. 1995; ABCPSG 1994; Omenn et al. 1996; Leppala et al. 2000). Skin yellowing, a common side effect of high β-carotene intakes, occurred in 20% to 25% of the participants in these trials. At this time, there are no definitive data suggesting that people benefit from β-carotene supplementation. It appears that consuming five to nine servings of fruits and vegetables per day will maintain healthy levels of β-carotene in the blood.

Selenium

Selenium is a trace mineral whose primary action is associated with the antioxidant enzyme GPX. Glutathione peroxidase is termed the "selenium-dependent enzyme." Remember that GPX removes hydrogen peroxide, reduces lipid hydroperoxides, and prevents damage to RNA and DNA, thus acting as an important protector against oxidative damage (Burk and Levander 2006). As GPX cannot carry out its function without adequate selenium, this mineral plays a critical role in antioxidant metabolism.

Methods of Assessment

Currently, the predominant measure of selenium is plasma or serum selenium levels. Both generally reflect short-term selenium status and are a measure of acute dietary changes in selenium. The best index of long-term selenium status is whole-blood selenium concentrations, since low blood

Table 10.2 Food Sources of β-Carotene

Foods	Serving size	β-Carotene (mg/serving)
Sweet potato, baked in skin	1 medium (146 g)	16.8
Kale, boiled and drained	1 cup (130 g)	10.6
Carrots, raw	1 medium (72 g)	6.0
Winter squash, baked	1 cup (205 g)	5.7
Cantaloupe, cubes	1 cup (160 g)	3.2
Spinach, raw	1 cup (30 g)	1.7
Mango, cubed	1 cup (165 g)	0.7
Broccoli, chopped, raw	1 cup (88 g)	0.4
Apricots, raw	1 medium (35 g)	0.4
Watermelon, cubes	1 cup (152 g)	0.5

Adapted from the *USDA national nutrient database for standard reference,* Release 20, Nutrient Lists. Available: http://www.nal.usda.gov/fnic/foodcomp/Data/SR20/nutrlist/sr20w321.pdf

levels reflect chronic deficiencies of selenium (Gibson 2005). Erythrocyte levels of selenium can also be used to indicate long-term status, as can hair and nails (Thomson 2004). However, using hair samples is not recommended; many shampoos contain selenium, making this an unreliable measure. Random urine samples are also unreliable measures due to their sensitivity to dilution and selenium content from a previous meal (Burk and Levander 2006). Urinary selenium levels over a 24 h period are associated with plasma levels and dietary intake (Thomson 2004). Glutathione peroxidase activity can be used as a functional index of selenium status in people with habitually low dietary intakes (Whanger et al. 1988).

Dietary Sources, Recommended Intakes, and Supplementation Products

Selenium intakes can vary considerably by geographic location. Areas known to have soil depleted of selenium include parts of China, New Zealand, and parts of Finland. Low intakes of selenium have also been reported in European countries (Rayman 2000). Low selenium intakes have been linked with various diseases in these areas, including Keshan disease, certain cancers, and cardiovascular disease (Boosalis 2008; Burk and Levander, 2006). Selenium content of soils in the United States varies considerably. However, selenium deficiencies are rare in the United States for two primary reasons: (1) Most people consume foods from various parts of the country; and (2) most Americans eat meat that comes from multiple geographic areas, and meat is an excellent source of selenium. The most important food sources of selenium are seafoods, meat (including muscle, liver, and kidney), and some grain products (depending on where they were grown).

Olson (1986) reported that the margin between selenium toxicity and deficiency is much narrower than for other trace minerals. Toxicity can easily result from supplementation. The RDA for selenium is 55 μg/day based on the amount needed for maximal synthesis of GPX. Most adults meet or exceed the RDA with intakes of approximately 105 μg/day (IOM 2000). Chronic doses of as little as 1 to 3 mg/day result in toxicity. A maximum safe dose for adults is considered to be 15 μg/kg of body weight (Rayman 2000). The UL of 400 μg/day is based on hair loss and high blood concentrations of selenium at this dose. Multivitamin-mineral supplements typically contain 25 to 250 μg/day of selenium per dose.

Other Nutrients With Antioxidant Properties

In addition to the nutrients already discussed, several others appear to play a role in antioxidant metabolism. Some of them are not antioxidants, but are important cofactors in reactions that protect the body against oxidative damage. These nutrients include the minerals listed in table 10.1.

One that has received considerable attention as an antioxidant is ubiquinone, or coenzyme Q_{10} (although not established as a vitamin, it is sometimes referred to as vitamin Q) (see "Coenzyme Q_{10} as an Antioxidant and Ergogenic Aid"). Table 10.3 lists other potential antioxidant compounds and their food sources. These substances are currently under study. Some of these compounds are called **bioflavonoids**—substances found in tea, red wine, and certain fruits and vegetables that may have antioxidant properties. The compounds listed in table 10.3 are generally referred to as **phytochemicals**—a term that in general simply means a chemical from a plant but that is often used more specifically to refer to compounds that may protect against diseases such as heart disease and cancer.

ASSESSMENT OF OXIDATIVE DAMAGE

It is difficult to assess oxidative damage within body tissues and cells. Free radicals are highly reactive and short-lived. Although techniques have been developed that *directly* measure free radical production or activity, these techniques are cost prohibitive for many. Most assays measure secondary by-products—in the blood, urine, or breath—that result from oxidative damage at the cellular level.

Measuring Free Radical Production

Two direct techniques to assess free radical production in humans are **electron spin resonance** and **paramagnetic resonance spectrometry.** Both detect superoxide radicals and can be used in vivo or in vitro. As the superoxide radicals spin, they emit a signal. These procedures measure the peak of the resonance signal as an indicator of superoxide radical production (Alessio 1993) and show great promise for enhancing our understanding of oxidative damage during exercise. The

Highlight

Coenzyme Q₁₀ as an Antioxidant and Ergogenic Aid

Coenzyme Q_{10}, or ubiquinone, is a naturally occurring lipid-soluble compound that is part of the electron transport chain, or ETC (refer to figure 10.1). It transfers electrons from NADH to the b-c_1 *enzyme complex* in the ETC. Coenzyme Q_{10} has been identified as the rate-limiting electron shuttle in the ETC. It is touted as an ergogenic aid, with claims that increasing coenzyme Q_{10} levels with supplementation will increase electron flux through the ETC—which will result in enhanced production of adenosine triphosphate and work output. Studies of coenzyme Q_{10} as an ergogenic aid are equivocal, with some showing benefits of supplementation (Amadio et al. 1991; Guerra et al. 1987; Zeppilli et al. 1991) and others showing no effect (Braun et al. 1991; Snider et al. 1992; Nielsen et al. 1999) or an adverse effect (Laaksonen et al. 1995; Malm et al. 1996).

It is also claimed that coenzyme Q_{10} scavenges free radicals and reduces lipid peroxidation (Greenberg and Frishman 1988; Karlsson 1987; Langsjoen and Folkers 1990). It is important to emphasize that these claims are derived from studies of people recovering from a heart attack and from in vitro studies of oxidative damage related to myocardial ischemia-reperfusion, cardiomyopathies, and muscular dystrophy. In vivo studies with healthy adults have not been performed to confirm coenzyme Q_{10}'s role as an antioxidant.

Table 10.3 Compounds in Our Food Sources to Which Antioxidant and Disease-Fighting Properties Have Been Attributed

Compound	Food source
Allylic sulfides	Garlic and onion
Carotenoids	Carrots, parsley, orange and green vegetables
Flavonoids	Berries, grapes, citrus, apples
Indoles	Broccoli, cabbage, brussels sprouts
Thiocyanates	Horseradish, radish
Lycopenes	Tomatoes, watermelon
Resveratrol	Strawberries, blueberries, red and purple grapes

Adapted from J. Higdon, 2007, *An evidenced-based approach to dietary phytochemicals* (New York, NY: Thieme Publishing).

invasiveness, the high cost, and the sophisticated equipment needed, however, limit the widespread use of these techniques at the present time.

Markers of Lipid Peroxidation

Tests available to assess lipid peroxidation are indirect, measuring the secondary reaction products of lipid peroxidation, and are not foolproof. Kneepkens and colleagues (1994) claimed that the sensitivity and specificity of most such tests are questionable. Standard procedures for these tests need to be established, and further studies of their validity are needed.

One test of lipid peroxidation is the assessment of **conjugated dienes.** Once the chain reaction of lipid peroxidation is initiated, dienes are immediately formed. While conjugated dienes have been measured in exercising humans (Duthie et al. 1990), these products are very difficult to determine in human blood and urine (Gutteridge and Halliwell 1990). The accuracy of the appearance of conjugated dienes as a marker of lipid peroxidation is also questionable, as these dienes can be derived from sources other than the peroxidation of lipids (Kneepkens et al. 1994).

Lipid hydroperoxides (LPOs) are the major initial products of lipid peroxidation (see "Definition of a Free Radical" on p. 304). Decomposition products of hydroperoxides can be measured in the blood as an indicator of lipid peroxidation. The decomposition product most commonly assessed is **malonaldehyde (MDA),** which is measured by its reaction with thiobarbituric acid (Gutteridge and Halliwell 1999). The products generated are referred to as **thiobarbituric acid reactive substances (TBARS).** This assay technique is relatively simple to perform, which most likely contributes to its widespread use. However, lipid peroxidation is not the only source of MDA, nor is TBARS specific to MDA. A preferred technique is the combination of TBARS with HPLC; however, this technique may underestimate MDA (Gutteridge and Halliwell 1999). Despite its widespread use, the reliability and validity of MDA as a marker of lipid peroxidation is questionable, and it should be used in conjunction with other markers (Halliwell 2000a).

Another commonly used marker of lipid peroxidation is **aliphatic hydrocarbons,** which are measured in a person's breath. While numerous aliphatic hydrocarbons are produced in the human body, the best markers of lipid peroxidation are **ethane** and **pentane.** Since other aliphatic hydrocarbons are produced in the colon, and since the concentration of hydrocarbons in ambient air is similar to that in breath, the mere presence of random hydrocarbons in the breath does not necessarily indicate lipid peroxidation. Ethane and pentane are considered specific markers of lipid peroxidation. However, ethane is the main product of the peroxidation of linolenic acid and other omega-3 fatty acids, while pentane is the main product of the peroxidation of linoleic and arachidonic acids (omega-6 fatty acids). Ethane and pentane are considered minor end products of lipid peroxidation, however, and their levels are sensitive to the rate at which peroxides are broken down. The accuracy of measuring these gases is also questionable, as levels detected have been inconsistent (Halliwell 2000b).

Recently, F_2-**isoprostanes** have become the "gold standard" for measuring lipid peroxidation. **Isoprostanes** are prostaglandin-like substances formed from free radical peroxidation of the PUFA arachidonic acid. Although there are other isoprostanes, the F_2-isoprostanes are the most stable and the most often used isoprostanes to detect lipid peroxidation. There are several advantages to measuring F_2-isoprostanes. Not only are they stable and specific to lipid peroxidation, but they are also found in detectable amounts in all tissues and are not susceptible to dietary intake. The reference method for measuring isoprostanes is with gas chromatography-mass spectroscopy. However, this method is expensive and time-consuming. Commercial immunoassays are available, but they vary in specificity and sensitivity (Montuschi et al. 2004).

Markers of DNA and Protein Damage

Free radicals target not only lipids, but DNA and protein as well. To assess oxidative DNA damage, most current assays measure urinary products of

DNA repair. The most commonly used index of free radical–induced DNA damage is 8-hydroxy-20-de-oxyguanosine (8OHdG). Urinary levels of 8OHdG have been used as a marker of whole-body DNA damage, but measurements appear susceptible to artifacts. Depending on the type of analysis—HPLC, gas chromatography-mass spectrometry, enzymatic assays—results can be highly variable (Halliwell 2000b). More studies are now using the Comet assay (single-cell gel electrophoresis) in leukocytes (white blood cells), which measures oxidative DNA base damage. This assay is more reproducible in exercise studies than 8OHdG (Hartmann et al. 1998; Niess et al. 1998). As with other oxidative biomarker measurements, there is a need to standardize and validate laboratory methods.

Protein carbonyls are the most common marker used to assess protein oxidation from free radicals. The carbonyl assay measures protein carbonyls that are generated from the free radical–induced oxidation of several amino acids (e.g., histidine, arginine, lysine, and proline). When oxidized, these amino acids produce protein carbonyls. Values should be used with caution, as carbonyls are not specific to oxidative damage (Halliwell and Gutteridge 1999; Urso et al. 2003).

Other Markers of Oxidative Stress

Changes in antioxidant enzymes can be used to assess the functional activity of the antioxidant system. For example, changes in the reduced form of glutathione (GSH) can be measured to indicate the activity of the GPX system. A decrease in GSH and an increase in GSSG (the oxidized form of glutathione) indicate an increase in the activity of the glutathione antioxidant defense system. The activity of specific antioxidant enzymes can also be measured. These enzymes include GPX, SOD, CAT, and GR (see p. 308 for definitions). Increases in these enzyme activities indicate an increase in the antioxidant activity of the body, suggesting that free radical production and oxidative damage have occurred.

Many researchers use antioxidant markers to assess changes in the antioxidant system. Plasma levels of tocopherol and vitamin C are the most commonly used. Unfortunately, results are highly variable and most likely related to differences in training status, age, gender, and timing of measurements (Vollaard et al. 2005).

Limitations to Markers of Oxidative Damage

A number of biomarkers are used to assess oxidative damage, all with some limitations. Whereas direct measures are costly and difficult, indirect measures often lack specificity and sensitivity. Further research needs to be conducted to validate methods of assessing biomarkers of lipid peroxidation, DNA, and protein oxidation. Not only are laboratory techniques limited, but studies differ in methodology, making study comparisons and interpretations difficult. Until these issues are resolved, the best recommendation is to use multiple measures of oxidative damage to provide a better estimate of free radical damage.

RATIONALE FOR INCREASED ANTIOXIDANT NEED AMONG ACTIVE INDIVIDUALS

Ken is a triathlete who has come to you for nutritional advice because soreness and fatigue have been interfering with his training sessions. He has also been plagued with numerous upper respiratory infections over the previous six months, coinciding with an increase in training volume and intensity. While he has sought medical treatment for the symptoms of the infections, the causes of the soreness, fatigue, and infections remain unidentified. Ken's fellow competitors suggested that he take antioxidant supplements to ward off the possible weakening of his cellular defense systems due to heavy training and to improve his ability to train and compete. Ken's questions to you include these:

- Will antioxidant supplements improve his health and performance?
- If yes, what are the best antioxidant supplements he can take?
- How much should he take if he decides to supplement?

This scenario highlights two very important questions: (1) Do athletes and highly active people have a higher requirement than others for antioxidants? (2) If so, why is their need increased? The suggestion that athletes have an increased need for antioxidants stems from three primary assumptions:

- Athletes generate excessive free radicals through heavy physical training as they consume more oxygen than sedentary individuals.
- The antioxidant systems in place are not sufficient to cope with the increased free radical production that accompanies heavy training.
- Athletes in urban areas may need even more antioxidants than those in rural areas since high levels of air pollution can increase free radical production.

As will be discussed in more detail later in this chapter, exercise also increases our ability to handle free radicals. Training adaptation includes enhanced endogenous defense systems (e.g., increased SOD). So, do athletes really need more dietary antioxidants?

Support for Increased Need

Research data suggest that acute exercise increases free radical production. Exercise also increases oxygen consumption ($\dot{V}O_2$), which increases the activity of cellular respiration. Increasing the rate of oxygen consumption and electron flux leads to increased free radical production and the leaking of reactive oxygen species out of the ETC. Other factors that may lead to increased free radical production during exercise include an increase in catecholamines (including epinephrine) that can produce free radicals. Tissue damage from intense exercise can also lead to lipid peroxidation of membranes and free radical production via the inflammation response. As mentioned on p. 307, other potential sources of exercise-induced free radical production include the xanthine oxidase pathway, ischemia-reperfusion, disruption of iron-containing proteins, and increased production of nitric oxide by the skeletal muscle (Powers et al. 2004; Finaud et al. 2006).

Two ways to assess the effects of exercise on free radical production are (1) measuring free radical production directly or measuring the secondary by-products of free radical production and (2) measuring changes in antioxidant enzyme systems. A number of excellent articles describe the effects of acute exercise and exercise training on free radicals and antioxidant enzyme systems in more detail (Finaud et al. 2006; Powers et al. 2004; Vollaard et al. 2005; Bloomer and Goldfarb 2004).

Effects of Acute Exercise on Antioxidant Systems

Much of the research conducted in the areas of exercise, free radical production, and antioxidant metabolism has used experimental animals. While the use of animal studies appears to be highly controversial in this area of research, experimental human studies are ideal for examining antioxidant activities during exercise. The discussion here focuses primarily on results from studies of humans during exercise.

As previously reviewed, a variety of methods can be used to quantify free radical production. Each method has its limitations, and no one best marker is available. The majority of studies in humans have used indirect markers of lipid peroxidation to indicate free radical production and consequent damage (e.g., MDA, TBARS, expired hydrocarbons). Newer studies use the "gold standard" method of F_2-isoprostanes, which accounts for some of the conflicting data to be discussed. In addition, the use of various forms and intensities of exercise, use of different markers of free radical production, and the assessment of various tissues have led to inconsistent results. These inconsistencies make it difficult to confirm with confidence the relationships among exercise, free radical damage, and lipid peroxidation. They also make it difficult to prescribe specific antioxidant nutrient recommendations to active people. Despite these limitations, there is evidence supporting an increase in free radical production and lipid peroxidation during exercise.

Three studies using the direct measures of electron spin resonance and electroparamagnetic resonance showed an increase in free radical production with exercise in animals (Davies et al. 1982; Jackson et al. 1985) and humans (Bailey et al. 2007). Measurement of lipid peroxidation using expired pentane and TBARS confirms that free radical production and subsequent lipid peroxidation may increase with acute exercise in humans. Early work by Dillard and colleagues (1978) showed that expired pentane increased with exercise intensity; obvious increases occurred at 75% $\dot{V}O_2$max. Leaf and colleagues (1997) also found significant increases in expired ethane and pentane at approximately 72% $\dot{V}O_2$max; the levels remained elevated to maximal exercise. Exposure to high altitude increases expired pentane production, and exercise at high altitude combined with poor energy intakes may exacerbate this condition (Simon-Schnass 1992). Many older studies reported increases in TBARS, MDA, or LPOs as a result of exercise in humans, as reviewed by Vollaard and colleagues (2005). More recent studies have shown significant increases in F_2-isoprostanes with a wide range of exercise protocols ranging from short, high-intensity cycling bouts to prolonged running (>2.5 h) (Waring et al. 2003; McAnulty et al. 2003; Steensberg et al. 2002).

Other studies have focused on DNA oxidative damage associated with exercise. Mastaloudis and colleagues (2004) found a significant increase in DNA damage during a 50 km (31-mile) ultramarathon. Davison and colleagues (2005) also noted an increase in DNA damage following a $\dot{V}O_2$max treadmill test.

Changes in antioxidant enzyme concentrations also occur as a result of acute exercise. Erythrocyte and blood levels of GSH appear to decrease with acute exercise, accompanied by an increase in GSSG in some instances (Duthie et al. 1990; Goldfarb 1993; Bryer and Goldfarb 2006). Increases in erythrocyte GR activity after moderate exercise have also been reported. These changes indicate an increase in the activity of the glutathione antioxidant enzyme system (refer to equations 10.3, 10.4, and 10.5 on p. 308) and suggest that exercise increases the production of hydrogen peroxide and lipid hydroperoxides.

Yet there is contradictory evidence. In the study by Leaf and colleagues (1997) previously mentioned, the researchers found no significant increase in MDA levels despite significant changes in expired hydrocarbons. Bloomer and colleagues (2006b) also reported conflicting measures. No significant changes were found in MDA following a 30 min run at 80% $\dot{V}O_2$max despite a significant increase in protein carbonyls. In yet another study, neither protein carbonyls nor MDA was affected by repeated squats or sprints (Bloomer et al. 2006a). These investigations illustrate the difficulty in comparing studies using different oxidative stress measures. None measured F_2-isoprostanes, the "gold standard" for lipid peroxidation. Further, numerous factors (e.g., diet) may influence the degree of lipid peroxidation and protein oxidation that occur with exercise, partly explaining the inconsistencies in these studies. When evaluating a research study, it is important to determine how well researchers controlled for some of the factors listed below, which can contribute to variability in results between studies.

- Exercise intensity: Intense, acute, maximal bouts may increase lipid peroxidation more than moderate exercise.
- Type of exercise: Eccentric contractions may increase free radical production and subsequent damage as compared to concentric muscle contractions (Dekkers et al. 1996).
- Training status of subjects: Untrained persons performing intense exercise may experience more lipid peroxidation than trained athletes.
- Different methods used: Methods are imperfect, and it is inappropriate to compare data from different assessment techniques; furthermore, the anatomical source of sampled tissue will affect results.
- Nutritional status of subjects: This strongly affects subjects' responses to exercise. Dietary and supplemental intakes of antioxidant nutrients should be controlled.
- Antioxidant status of the subjects: There are many *interrelated* antioxidant systems, and it is virtually impossible to control the levels of each before beginning an exercise test.

Effects of Chronic Exercise Training on Antioxidant Systems

As increases in mitochondrial enzymes and oxidative capacity occur with endurance training, the potential for oxidative damage is greater in the trained athlete. There is evidence that antioxidant enzyme activity increases with training; controversy exists, however, as to whether the increases in antioxidant activity are sufficient to protect the system from the increased oxidative damage that may accompany exercise training. Antioxidant nutrient pools within the body may also change with training. In animals, muscle levels of vitamin E have been shown to decrease with endurance training; these levels may also depend on initial vitamin E status. Exercise training may conserve vitamin E in a vitamin D deficient animal as compared to a vitamin E deficient animal that does not exercise. Cross-sectional data show a significant positive correlation between $\dot{V}O_2$max and activities of antioxidant enzymes; and trained athletes appear to have higher SOD, GPX, and CAT activities than untrained individuals (Powers et al. 1999; Knez et al. 2007). Results of training studies show a reduction in TBARS (i.e., lipid peroxidation) (Miyazaki et al. 2001) and increased

activities of CAT, SOD, and GPX (Elosua et al. 2003; Miyazaki et al. 2001). These changes indicate that the trained system adapts to increased oxygen consumption with complementary changes in the protective antioxidant enzymes. However, virtually all studies examining the effects of antioxidant supplementation and training on antioxidant defense systems have shown that although oxidative damage is attenuated, it is not eliminated (Powers et al. 1999; Vollaard et al. 2005). Whether or not this is harmful for the athlete is an area of continued debate.

Antioxidant Deficiencies and Exercise

Most studies of nutritional deficiencies and their effects on exercise performance have been conducted with animals. Studying nutrient deficiencies in humans is limited by ethical considerations and the length of time it takes to induce a nutrient deficiency. It is important to note that antioxidant nutrient deficiencies are rare in sedentary animals or in humans consuming a nutritionally adequate diet (Ji 1995). Since exercise increases utilization (Mastaloudis et al. 2001) and reduces stored levels of vitamin E (Bowles et al. 1991; Kumar et al. 1992; Packer 1986), it has been speculated (but not demonstrated) that highly active individuals may be predisposed to antioxidant nutrient deficiency if adequate dietary intakes are not achieved (Packer 1986).

What effects do antioxidant deficiencies have on oxidative damage and exercise performance? Selenium deficiency results in increased lipid peroxidation in the liver and muscle of rats (Ji et al. 1988) but appears to have no effect on acute exercise performance or endurance capacity (Ji et al. 1988; Lang et al. 1987). Vitamin E deficiency increases exercise-induced oxidative damage (Davies et al. 1982; Gohil et al. 1986; Goldfarb 1993; Quintanilha et al. 1982) and decreases endurance performance in animals (Davies et al. 1982; Coombes 2002). Few data exist regarding the effects of vitamin C deficiency on exercise-induced oxidative damage. However, Packer (1986) found that myocardial oxidative capacity and endurance time were reduced in animals deficient in vitamin C. Given the many functions of vitamin C, a deficiency would most likely result in impaired aerobic and anaerobic performance secondary to anemia, fatigue, and poor connective tissue (Keith 2006).

Deficiencies of vitamins E, C, and β-carotene are rare. Researchers who have measured the vitamin

A, C, or E status of athletes using blood samples have found no evidence of deficiencies (Fogelholm et al. 1992; Guilland et al. 1989; Weight et al. 1988). While many athletes exceed the RDA for these nutrients, it has been found that those with poor energy or dietary intakes and weight concerns, and those who eat few or no fruits or vegetables, consume inadequate antioxidant nutrients and may require supplementation (Keith 2006).

At the present time, there does not appear to be enough evidence to support the suggestion that active individuals are deficient in antioxidant nutrients. We need more research to assess the antioxidant nutrient status of the general population using objective measures. It is not known whether exercise training improves antioxidant protection to an extent sufficient to protect against increases in oxidative damage that may accompany regular, vigorous physical training. Further, emerging research suggests that some free radicals such as nitric oxide act as signaling molecules that may influence training adaptation (Sen 2001; Jackson et al. 2004). If this is the case, do we want to completely "turn off" free radical production? Are free radicals all bad? Until these questions are answered, it is unwise to make sweeping recommendations regarding antioxidant needs of active people.

Potential Risks Associated With Antioxidant Supplementation

While it appears that supplementing to address antioxidant deficiencies is beneficial in restoring cellular functions, there is controversy regarding whether supplementation is associated with a variety of health risks. The following risks may be associated with antioxidant supplementation:

- Vitamin E supplementation: hemorrhaging at high doses, increased mortality in those with chronic disease (Miller et al. 2005)
- Vitamin C supplementation (in combination with high iron intake): increased risk of iron-induced cardiac failure or of hemochromatosis (see "The Relationship Between Vitamin C and Iron" on p. 312)
- β-Carotene supplementation: increased rates of lung cancer in smokers and mortality due to cardiovascular disease (ABCPSG 1994; Omenn et al. 1996; Leppala et al. 2000)

Note that these risks are associated with supplemental intakes, not an increased intake of antioxidants from food. It is important for the reader to understand that the issues listed are controversial. A recent review by Hathcock and colleagues (2005) largely debunks these safety concerns but supports remaining below the UL for antioxidants. Since some evidence does exist to suggest that supplementation with antioxidant nutrients may be harmful in certain circumstances, consumers should exercise caution when considering supplementation.

ANTIOXIDANTS AND CHRONIC DISEASES

Antioxidant nutrients are purported to reduce the risk of many chronic diseases such as cardiovascular disease and diabetes. Contrary to popular opinion, there is no conclusive evidence that consuming antioxidant nutrients in amounts greater than recommended will prevent or cure certain chronic diseases. The purpose of this section is to familiarize the reader with known associations among specific antioxidant nutrients and chronic diseases and to review the mechanisms by which antioxidant nutrients may act to reduce risks for these diseases.

Cardiovascular Disease

The highly publicized results of epidemiological studies (Christen et al. 2000; Stampfer et al. 1992), showing significant relationships between intake of antioxidant nutrients and reduced incidence of cardiovascular events, has led the general public to assume that there is a cause-and-effect relationship between antioxidants and cardiovascular disease. It is important to stress that *associations* among variables in these studies do not prove cause and effect. At the present time, there are no published results from large experimental studies supporting a definitive role of antioxidant nutrients in the prevention of heart disease. (For a discussion of types of epidemiological studies, refer to "Different Types of Epidemiological Studies".) Indirect evidence and correlational findings, however, highlight the roles that antioxidant nutrients may play in the progression of heart disease. The following risk factors for heart disease have been associated with low intakes of antioxidant nutrients:

- Oxidation of LDLs
- Reduced serum levels of high-density lipoprotein (HDL)-cholesterol

- Hypertension
- Insulin resistance and type 2 diabetes
- Reperfusion injury associated with an ischemic event
- Impaired vasomotor tone as it relates to arterial stiffness and coronary artery spasm
- Increased platelet adhesiveness

One factor hypothesized to contribute significantly to atherosclerosis is the oxidation of LDLs (Wilcox et al. 2008). Atherosclerosis first appears as fatty streaks along the arterial wall; these fatty streaks are initiated from damage incurred to the endothelium. Oxidized LDLs attach to the dam-aged areas of the endothelium and contribute to the perpetual damage of the vascular wall over many years. This damage results in the formation of plaque and the development of atherosclerosis. Vitamin E has been shown to decrease the oxidation of LDLs in humans (Dieber-Rotheneder et al. 1991; Jialal and Grundy 1992), while vitamin C and β-carotene were found to inhibit LDL oxidation in vitro (or in cellular preparations).

Diabetes is a well-known risk factor for cardiovascular disease, and associations between elevated serum glucose and oxidative stress have been reported in humans with diabetes (Williamson et al. 1993). It is theorized that the altered glucose metabolism that accompanies diabetes

Highlight

Different Types of Epidemiological Studies

Can all epidemiological studies be defined as experimental? What determines whether an epidemiological study is an experimental research study? An experiment is a scientific project in which the investigator attempts to control all factors that affect the outcome of interest (Rothman 1986). In addition, conditions of interest are manipulated in an experiment. Rothman (1986) provides an excellent review of types of epidemiological studies that can be classified as experimental or nonexperimental. Experimental studies include randomized clinical trials and community intervention trials. Nonexperimental epidemiological studies include case-control and many cohort studies. Projects that are descriptive or observational are considered nonexperimental studies. Due to many ethical constraints, use of certain experimental designs is limited in much of epidemiological research. According to Rothman (1986), these constraints include

- the inability to limit the research subjects' exposure to potential preventives of disease and
- the inappropriateness of depriving subjects of the preferable form of treatment or of any preventive that is not included in the study.

Because of researchers' inability to control many confounding variables, it is critical that they report the results of nonexperimental epidemiological research in a way that emphasizes the limitations of the study. It is also important for readers to understand that an association between antioxidant nutrients and disease risks does not prove cause and effect. While nonexperimental epidemiological studies provide the scientific community with invaluable information, the results of these studies need to be distributed with a clear explanation of the implications for health and disease status. For example, an epidemiological study that looks at a large population in retrospect and finds a correlation between one lifestyle variable and a disease is a nonexperimental study that can provide important information on which to base future experimental studies, but it does not prove cause and effect. Merely observing a strong correlation between smoking and heart disease, for instance, does not prove that smoking is a causative factor. But, inspired by such nonexperimental data, one could design an experimental epidemiological study: identify a large group of smokers and follow them for 10 years, helping all who wish to kick the habit, then compare heart disease data between those who kept smoking and those who quit. If the latter group had significantly less heart disease, those data would be more persuasive for claiming a causal relationship.

may be related to peroxidation. Administration of 900 mg/day of vitamin E for four months resulted in improvements in glucose clearance and disposal in individuals with type 2 diabetes mellitus (Paolisso et al. 1993). Similar benefits of vitamin E supplementation were observed in elderly nondiabetic subjects (Paolisso et al. 1994). Vitamin E has also been found to improve retinal blood flow and endothelial-dependent blood vessel dilation in type 1 diabetics (Bursell et al. 1999; Skyrme-Jones et al. 2000). This has important implications for the role of vitamin E in preventing complications associated with diabetes.

Antioxidants may also play a role in reducing the damage from **reperfusion injury,** which results from an ischemic event such as a myocardial infarction or stroke. Once ischemia occurs, reoxygenation of the tissue is critical to slow the death of the cells. Restoring oxygen to cells results in oxidative stress and subsequent excessive production of free radicals. The consequent damage has been termed reoxygenation or reperfusion injury. Vitamin E supplementation has been shown to reduce oxidative damage resulting from the reperfusion associated with coronary artery bypass surgery (Cavarocchi et al. 1986; Ferriera et al. 1991). Other mechanisms through which antioxidants may reduce risk of cardiovascular disease include altering platelet adhesiveness and vasomotor tone. Supplementation with vitamins C and E may decrease the "stickiness," or aggregability, of platelets (Bordia and Verma 1985; Salonen et al. 1991; Steiner and Mower 1982); and vitamin C supplementation was found to improve endothelium-dependent arterial dilation in individuals with established coronary heart disease (Levine et al. 1996). Thus, antioxidant nutrients may play a role in altering the development of cardiovascular disease (see "Coenzyme Q$_{10}$ as an Antioxidant and Ergogenic Aid" p. 317).

Whether antioxidant supplements can prevent or cure cardiovascular disease has been the subject of a number of investigations. Several epidemiological studies have shown inverse relationships between intakes of vitamin E, vitamin C, and β-carotene and cardiovascular disease. Consistently, diets high in fruits, vegetables, and whole grains (i.e., diets high in antioxidants) are related to lower rates of chronic disease. As an example, cohort studies examining vitamin E intake have shown as much as a 40% decrease in coronary heart disease rates (Gaziano 2004). Several large clinical trials have been conducted,

and unfortunately none have shown an effect of supplementation of these vitamins on cardiovascular risk. The Heart Protection Study (2002) included evaluation of the cardiovascular effects of 600 mg vitamin E, 250 mg vitamin C, and 20 mg β-carotene or placebo on 20,000 adults for five years and showed no difference in heart attack rates between the treatment and placebo groups. The large-scale Women's Health Study looked at over 40,000 women for 10 years and showed that 600 IU of vitamin E had no effect on cardiovascular disease, stroke, total mortality, or cancer (Lee et al. 2005). Further, in the Heart Outcomes Protection Evaluation (HOPE) Study (2000), it was found that 400 IU of supplemental vitamin E had no effect on heart disease. Interestingly, the HOPE-TOO Study (2005), which enrolled study participants with heart disease or diabetes, showed a 13% increased risk of heart failure in those supplemented with vitamin E. These studies should be interpreted cautiously, as none used biomarkers—plasma vitamin E levels or oxidative stress measures—to evaluate the effectiveness of vitamin E supplementation (Traber 2007). Currently, the American Heart Association does not recommend routine antioxidant supplementation for the prevention or treatment of heart disease, but rather encourages a diet of colorful fruits and vegetables (Kris-Etherton et al. 2004).

Cancer

The process of transforming normal cells into cancerous cells occurs through multiple stages. While the exact functions of antioxidant nutrients in cancer prevention or reversal are unknown, these nutrients may play a role in preventing initiation by detoxifying carcinogens or blocking their actions; they may also affect the various stages of cancer development. The aim in most intervention studies has been to examine the effects of antioxidant supplements on precancerous lesions, which is controversial. It is imperative that when precancerous lesions are used as midpoint markers in intervention studies, the lesions be strongly linked with the eventual development of cancer. Studies showing a reduction in midpoint markers of cancer and heart disease are not equal to studies showing a reduction in the incidence of these diseases. Well-designed studies would ideally include midpoint markers of disease progression and documentation of disease incidence.

Epidemiological studies have shown that β-carotene and vitamins A, C, and E have significant associations with certain cancers. For example, high intakes of vitamin E were associated with decreased risk of colon cancer in the Iowa Woman's Health Study (Bostick et al. 1993). The study also demonstrated that high dietary intakes of β-carotene, vitamin C, and E were associated with lower rates of cancers of the upper digestive tract (Zheng et al. 1995). Vitamins C and E may reduce the risk of stomach cancer through their role in blocking the formation of nitrosamines and other carcinogenic agents in the stomach (Mirvish 1986). Vitamin A and β-carotene can also lead to remission of precancerous lesions of oral cancer (Stich et al. 1988). Conversely, low dietary intakes and serum levels of vitamin C and β-carotene are related to increased incidence of cervical dysplasia (a precancerous lesion of cervical cancer) (Harris et al. 1986; Wassertheil-Smoller et al. 1981; Wylie-Rosett et al. 1984). Erhardt and colleagues (1997) found that humans fed a diet high in dietary fat and meat and low in dietary fiber had a significant decrease in plasma levels of β-carotene and vitamin C. This diet also resulted in a significant production of hydroxyl radicals in the feces and a higher concentration of iron in the feces. In contrast, the same subjects fed a vegetarian diet, low in dietary fat and high in fiber, had higher serum concentrations of β-carotene and vitamin C and a lower serum MDA concentration, indicating less lipid peroxidation on this diet.

As with cardiovascular disease, results from large-scale intervention studies do not support benefits of antioxidant supplements in reducing cancer risk (Lee et al. 2005; HOPE and HOPE-TOO Trial Investigators 2005; Albanes et al. 1995; ABCPSG 1994; Blot et al. 1993, 1995; Hennekens et al. 1996; Omenn et al. 1996). The only study yielding positive results was the Linxian study (Blot et al. 1993, 1995), in which rates of stomach and esophageal cancers were reduced, as was overall mortality, in middle-aged Chinese men and women. The Physicians' Health Study (Hennekens et al. 1996) showed no effect of β-carotene supplementation on cancer, heart disease, or overall mortality. In contrast, the Alpha-Tocopherol Beta-Carotene (ATBC) Study (Albanes et al. 1995; ABCPSG 1994) and the β-Carotene and Retinol Efficacy Trial (CARET) (Omenn et al. 1996) obtained negative results for mixed antioxidant supplements. The ATBC Study showed an increase in lung cancer rates and overall mortality, with no effect on heart disease, while the CARET study was ended early due to a trend toward increased mortality and cancer rates associated with supplementation. Heavy smokers and drinkers seemed to be particularly vulnerable to the negative effects of supplementation in these studies. From the results of these investigations, it appears that more research needs to be conducted on the effects of antioxidants (from food and supplemental sources) on cancer before conclusive recommendations regarding intakes of these nutrients can be made. Currently, clinical trials are under way to investigate the role of other antioxidants such as lycopene and selenium on cancer.

Cataracts

Cataract is defined as "a dysfunction of the lens due to partial or complete opacification" (Taylor 1993). Cataracts are formed when proteins in the lens of the eye are damaged. As the lens proteins have an extremely long life, they are exposed to many damaging factors. These damaged proteins accumulate, aggregate, and precipitate, which causes opacification of the lens (Taylor 1993). Some have suggested that free radical damage resulting from repeated exposure to oxygen and ultraviolet light may contribute to development of cataracts (Harding and van Heyningen 1987).

With age, the blood levels of antioxidants and the activity of proteases (enzymes that remove damaged proteins) and antioxidant enzymes decline. Thus, the combination of increased oxidative damage and a reduced capacity to protect against this damage leads to lens opacification. Some studies have shown that individuals with cataracts have lower serum concentrations of vitamin E, vitamin C, and β-carotene (Lyle et al. 1999; Jacques and Chylack 1991; Jacques et al. 1988). Researchers noted a 50% reduction in cataracts in those with the highest antioxidant intake of vitamins E, C, and β-carotene (Jacques et al. 1988). Moreover, individuals taking vitamin C and E supplements (400 IU/day vitamin E and 300 to 600 mg/day vitamin C) had a significantly lower risk of cataracts than those not taking supplements (Robertson et al. 1989). Despite these positive findings, results have been mixed regarding the effects of antioxidant dietary intake and supplementation on cataracts (Wu and Leske 2000). Thus, antioxidant nutrients—particularly vitamins C and E—may reduce the risk of cataracts in older people by providing the

Highlight

Antioxidants and Aging

Can antioxidants slow the aging process? Can duration and quality of life be enhanced by the use of antioxidant supplements? These are very important questions, since the elderly are the fastest-growing age group in the United States. The free radical theory of aging suggests that free radicals are the primary cause of aging; if this assumption holds true, then reducing oxidative damage should reduce the progression of the aging process. Aging is associated with decreased activities of antioxidant enzymes in most body tissues (Ji 1995). Interestingly, the activities of antioxidant enzymes such as SOD, CAT, and GPX reportedly are enhanced in aging skeletal muscle. Despite this magnified activity in skeletal muscle, lipid peroxidation is higher in aging muscle than in young muscle (Ji et al. 1990). It has been speculated that antioxidant enzymes become less efficient in protecting the body with age.

Despite findings of decreased ability to fight free radical damage with age, no studies have shown prolonged life as a result of antioxidant supplementation. However, there is strong support for increasing the RDAs for many nutrients among the elderly due to the reduced food intake and impairment of nutrient absorption and metabolism with increasing age. In addition to the diseases discussed in this chapter, osteoporosis and impaired immune function are related to nutritional factors. Memory performance and cognitive function are also related to antioxidant and B vitamin intakes (La Rue et al. 1997; Perrig et al. 1997; Wengreen et al. 2007). It is possible that many elderly individuals would benefit from vitamin and mineral supplementation to improve nutritional status.

Because elderly people differ physiologically according to age, sex, health status, and physical activity status, Blumberg (1991) suggested separate RDAs for age brackets such as 51 to 60, 61 to 70, 71 to 80, and 81 to 90 years. He proposed that the recommendations for micronutrients need to be higher among the elderly if the goal of the RDAs is to maximize health. Unfortunately, when the new Dietary Reference Intakes (DRIs) for antioxidants were developed in 2000, not enough research was available to warrant recommendations for these nutrients based on these age groups (IOM 2000). Since antioxidants and other nutrients have been associated with reduced risks for chronic diseases, it may be that supplementation, while not increasing the *duration* of life, will enhance the *quality* of life. Studies focusing on the interactions among antioxidants, life span, and morbidity need to be conducted to determine the impact of antioxidant nutrients on the aging process.

lens of the eye with additional protection from oxidative damage, but more research is needed in this area. For further discussion of antioxidants and the aging process, see "Antioxidants and Aging."

ANTIOXIDANTS AND PERFORMANCE

The popularity of supplementation and prevalent use of performance-enhancing products emphasize the competitive athlete's strong desire to win at any cost. As discussed throughout this chapter, specific antioxidant nutrients may reduce free radical production and subsequent tissue damage, while exercise training may enhance the

protective capabilities of the antioxidant system. Although this information is interesting, the most important question for many athletes is, "Does the use of antioxidant supplements enhance performance?"

Antioxidant Supplementation and Performance

It is theorized that consuming antioxidant supplements will augment the antioxidant defenses even beyond the increases caused by regular training. It may also be that "weekend warriors," or occasional exercisers, may benefit from antioxidant supplements. In fact, it has been suggested that occasional exercisers will benefit even more from supplementation than the trained athlete because they have a less highly developed antioxidant defense system (Finaud et al. 2006; Vollaard et al. 2005).

Most studies investigating the effects of antioxidant supplementation on performance have focused on vitamins E, C, or a combination of antioxidants. Although many studies have shown that supplementation with vitamin E reduces markers of lipid peroxidation with exercise (Bryant et al. 2003; Sacheck et al. 2003; Kanter et al. 1993), others have shown no effect (Avery et al. 2003; Warren et al. 1992) or an increase in lipid peroxidation (Nieman et al. 2004). Most studies have assessed vitamin C supplementation in humans in combination with other antioxidant nutrients. However, Thompson and colleagues (2001) found no effect on MDA, muscle soreness, or creatine kinase (a marker of muscle damage) in runners following two weeks of supplementation with 400 mg of vitamin C. Conversely, Bryer and Goldfarb (2006) found a decrease in the oxidized glutathione/total glutathione ratio following supplementation with 3 g vitamin C before and after eccentric exercise, and Alessio and colleagues (1997) found an *increase* in TBARS with submaximal exercise following supplementation of 1 g of vitamin C for one day. Studies using a combination of vitamin E and C have shown a decrease in protein carbonyls (Bloomer et al. 2006b) and decreased GPX (Margaritis et al. 2003).

Although antioxidant supplementation seemed to reduce oxidative damage in some studies, the impact on performance does not appear to be significant. There is little evidence to support vitamin E as an ergogenic aid (Mastaloudis and Traber 2006). Studies of vitamin E supplementation in swimming, submaximal cycling, cycling to exhaustion, hockey, and marathon running have shown no effect on performance (Rokitzki et al. 1994; Tidus et al. 1995). Well-controlled studies of vitamin C supplementation also have shown no improvements in performance (Keith 2006). Selenium supplementation was found to have no effect on endurance exercise training (Tessier et al. 1995). Likewise, there is no evidence to support any relationship between vitamin A and exercise. The individual effects of β-carotene supplementation have not been studied in relation to exercise performance. Most recent studies have focused on the effects of an antioxidant cocktail (e.g. vitamins C, E, lipoic acid, coenzyme Q_{10}), and these studies have also shown little effect on exercise

performance. For example, Nielson and colleagues (1999) found no change in $\dot{V}O_2$max, muscle fatigue, or energy metabolism in triathletes following six weeks of supplementation with vitamins C, E, and coenzyme Q_{10}.

It should be noted that recent research on antioxidants has focused on the potential effects of these nutrients on the immunosuppression noted with prolonged, high-intensity exercise (Nieman 2001). Although research indicates that antioxidant supplementation may attenuate cortisol increases with such exercise, this does not necessarily translate to improved immune function (Davison et al. 2007). Carbohydrate has also been shown to attenuate the cortisol response to prolonged, high-intensity exercise *and* decrease immunosuppression (Nieman et al. 2001).

Two situations in which antioxidant supplementation may affect exercise performance are exposure to altitude and to conditions of extremely high ambient temperatures. In a study conducted on Pikes Peak, Colorado (elevation 4300 m or 14,100 ft), power output and time to exhaustion were improved following three weeks of antioxidant supplementation (Subudhi et al. 2006). Kotze and colleagues (1977) and Strydom and colleagues (1976) found that vitamin C supplementation in South African miners enhanced acclimatization to high ambient temperatures and reduced rectal temperature and total sweat output. It is possible that antioxidant supplementation is beneficial under extreme environmental conditions. Note also that nutritional status of people working in these extreme conditions may be compromised due to poor appetite and limited food availability, emphasizing the link between adequate nutritional status and exercise performance.

Recommendations for Antioxidant Intake

Is there sufficient evidence to warrant making recommendations for antioxidant nutrients? Since evidence arguing for supplementation appears inadequate at this time, recommendations appear premature. Recommendations for antioxidants were increased with the 2000 DRIs (IOM 2000); however, amounts are still below what some researchers in the area recommend. Table 10.4 lists the present RDAs and suggested optimal intakes of vitamins C, E, and selenium. The reader should note that table 10.4 is not provided as a definitive recommendation for antioxidant

Table 10.4 Current RDA, Proposed Recommended Intakes, and Upper Tolerable Limit (UL) of Selected Antioxidant Nutrients

Nutrient	RDA[1]	Recommended intake[2]	UL[1]
Vitamin C	60 mg/day (nonsmokers)	200 mg/day	2000 mg/day
Vitamin E	8 mg/day (women) 10 mg/day (men)	200 mg/day[3]	1000 mg/day
Selenium	55 μg/day	200 μg/day (men)[4]	400 μg/day

[1] Institute of Medicine (IOM), Food and Nutrition Board, 2005, *Dietary reference intakes for vitamin C, vitamin E, selenium, and carotenoids* (Washington, DC: National Academy Press).
[2] Higdon J, 2003, *An evidence-based approach to vitamins and minerals: health benefits and intake recommendations* (New York: Thieme).
[3] Natural source *d-* or *RRR*-α-tocopherol.
[4] Level recommended to decrease the risk of prostate cancer.

supplementation but rather as an illustration of how opinions differ regarding the adequacy of present RDAs. There are several concerns regarding the safety of antioxidant supplementation, including

- toxicity risks of certain nutrients,
- impact of long-term supplementation on health,
- bioavailability of supplement pills, and
- potential interactions among nutrients.

Although vitamin A is known to be highly toxic, higher doses of vitamins E, C, and β-carotene appear to be tolerable. Intakes of 200 to 600 mg/day, 1 to 2 g/day, and 30 to 90 mg/day for vitamin E, vitamin C, and β-carotene, respectively, have been reported with no side effects. Unfortunately, most studies of supplementation are short-term (four to eight weeks), and the impact of long-term supplementation in humans is not known. The effects of supplementation are dependent upon the supplement's bioavailability, which can change according to the nutritional status of the individual. Many environmental factors can affect a person's need for antioxidant nutrients, including environmental pollution, certain medications, smoking, disease status, and exposure to herbicides.

Finally, interactions among antioxidant nutrients are unknown. Does consuming these nutrients in combination have a synergistic effect? Does supplementation with these nutrients reduce absorption or activity of other nutrients? Does high-dose supplementation with antioxidants impair training adaptation? These questions need to be answered before definitive recommendations can be made. However, it is prudent for all people, including highly trained athletes and recreationally active individuals, to consume a diet that contains a wide variety of foods. Meeting the American Cancer Society's recommendation of eating five or more fruits or vegetables per day will result in many people's meeting and exceeding the RDA for antioxidant nutrients. Multivitamin and mineral supplements can also be used to safely supplement diets.

CHAPTER IN REVIEW

We started this chapter with questions regarding the role of antioxidants in health and performance. From the information discussed in this chapter, the following conclusions can be drawn:

- Antioxidant nutrients are important to minimize damage resulting from free radical formation.
- Deficiencies of antioxidant nutrients can result in increased oxidative damage and may increase the risk for various diseases. Furthermore, poor antioxidant status probably impairs physical performance.
- There is no evidence that antioxidant supplementation improves performance in well-fed, healthy adults who have good overall nutritional status and good antioxidant status.
- Epidemiological studies indicate that healthy individuals may benefit from antioxidant supplementation; however, more experimental clinical trials need to be performed to establish a cause-and-effect relationship between antioxidant nutrients and reduced disease risk.

While consuming two to three times the RDA for most antioxidant nutrients appears to cause little harm, people should discuss supplementation of these products with a qualified medical professional, as some individuals may respond adversely to supplementation.

Key Concepts

1. Define free radicals.

A free radical is a molecule with an unpaired electron in its outer orbit. Free radicals are highly reactive and can damage cells when produced in excess.

2. List the enzymes involved in antioxidant activities, and describe the reactions in which they participate.

The enzymatic antioxidant defense systems include (1) superoxide dismutase, which accelerates the conversion of the superoxide radical to hydrogen peroxide; (2) catalase, which removes hydrogen peroxide; (3) glutathione, which assists in the removal of hydrogen peroxide and reduction of lipid hydroperoxides; (4) glutathione peroxidase, which removes hydrogen peroxide and reduces lipid hydroperoxides; (5) glutathione reductase, which converts oxidized glutathione back to reduced glutathione; and (6) peroxidase, which rids the body of excess hydrogen peroxide.

3. Discuss the nutrients involved in antioxidant activities.

Vitamin E halts lipid peroxidation and protects polyunsaturated fatty acids. Vitamin C quenches singlet oxygen and regenerates the reduced form of vitamin E. β-Carotene quenches singlet oxygen. Selenium is part of the glutathione peroxidase enzyme system. Other nutrients that act as antioxidants include coenzyme Q_{10}, copper, zinc, iron, and manganese.

4. Describe the methods used to assess oxidative damage.

Electron spin resonance and paramagnetic resonance spectrometry are used to assess superoxide radical production. Markers of lipid peroxidation include conjugated dienes, lipid hydroperoxides, malonaldehyde (or TBARS), F_2-isoprostanes, and the aliphatic hydrocarbons ethane and pentane. Markers of DNA damage and protein oxidation are 8-hydroxy-20-deoxyguanosine (8OHdG) and protein carbonyls. Changes in antioxidant enzymes can also indicate the functional activity of the antioxidant system.

5. Describe the proposed rationale for increased antioxidant need among active people.

It is suggested that active people's higher oxygen consumption leads to excessive free radical production—and that such people need more antioxidants because their existing antioxidant systems are not sufficient to cope with the elevated levels of free radicals. Active people may also have higher exposure to environmental pollutants, which again can increase the need for antioxidants.

6. Discuss how antioxidants play a role in chronic diseases.

Heart disease risk factors—such as hypertension, oxidation of LDLs, type 2 diabetes, and reperfusion injury with an ischemic event—have been associated with low intakes of antioxidant nutrients. Low intakes of vitamin C and E have been associated with certain cancers, but recent studies have not indicated that supplementation prevents or reduces the risk for these cancers. Vitamins C and E may reduce the risk of cataracts in older individuals by providing the lens of the eye with additional protection from oxidative damage.

7. Discuss the relationship between antioxidants and athletic performance.

Although antioxidant supplementation is popular among many athletes and active people, there are no data to suggest that supplementing with antioxidants improves athletic performance in healthy individuals with good nutritional status. A nutritionally balanced diet is critical to optimal performance, and eating a combination of five servings of fruits and vegetables per day will result in most people's meeting or exceeding the RDA for antioxidants.

Key Terms

α-tocopherol 309
β-carotene 314
aliphatic hydrocarbon 318
antioxidant 304
ascorbate 311
bioflavonoid 316
breath pentane measurement 310
capillary fragility 313
carotenoid 314
catalase (CAT) 308
cataract 325
conjugated diene 317
cytochrome-c 304
electron spin resonance 316
electron transport chain (respiratory chain) 304
erythrocyte hemolysis test 310
ethane 318
F_2-isoprostane 318
free radical 304
glutathione 308
glutathione peroxidase (GPX) 308
glutathione reductase (GR) 308
gulonolactone oxidase 311
hydrogen peroxide 305
hydroperoxyl free radical 305
hydroxyl radical 305
iron-induced cardiac failure 312

isoprostane 318
isotope dilution 313
leukocyte ascorbic acid concentration 313
lipid hydroperoxides (LPOs) 317
lipid peroxidation 304
lutein 314
lycopene 314
malonaldehyde (MDA) 317
megadose 313
nitric oxide free radical 305
opacification 325
paramagnetic resonance spectrometry 316
pentane 318
peroxidase 308
phytochemical 316
prooxidant 312
protein carbonyl 318
reperfusion injury 324
serum ascorbic acid concentration 312
singlet oxygen 305
superoxide dismutase (SOD) 308
superoxide radical 305
thiobarbituric acid reactive substance (TBARS) 317
ubiquinone (coenzyme Q_{10}) 304
urinary excretion 313

Additional Information

Vollaard NBJ, Shearman JP, Cooper CE. Exercise-induced oxidative stress: myths, realities and physiological relevance. Sports Med 2005;35(12):1045-1062.

> This article reviews the evidence, mechanisms, and health and performance consequences of exercise-induced oxidative stress.

Peake JM, Suzuki K, Coombes JS. The influence of antioxidant supplementation on markers of inflammation and the relationship to oxidative stress after exercise. J Nutr Biochem 2007;18:357-371.

> This article reviews the role of antioxidants in exercise-induced inflammation and oxidative stress.

Wilcox BJ, Curb JD, Rodriguez BL. Antioxidants in cardiovascular health and disease: key lessons from epidemiologic studies. Am J Cardiol 2008;101(10A):75D-86D.

> This article reviews the mismatch between epidemiological and clinical intervention studies investigating the effects of antioxidants on cardiovascular health.

Lawenda BD, Kelly KM, Ladas EJ, Sagar SM, Vickers A, Blumberg JB. Should supplemental antioxidant administration be avoided during chemotherapy and radiation therapy? J Natl Cancer Inst 2008;100(11):773-783.

> This commentary reviews the controversial use of antioxidants for radiation and chemotherapy.

References

Albanes D, Heinonen OP, Huttunen JK et al. Effects of alpha-tocopherol and beta-carotene supplements on cancer incidence in the Alpha-Tocopherol Beta-Carotene Cancer Prevention Study. Am J Clin Nutr 1995;62(suppl):1427S-1430S.

Alberg A. The influence of cigarette smoking on circulating concentrations of antioxidant micronutrients. Toxicology 2002;180(2):121-137.

Alberts B, Bray D, Lewis J, Raff M, Roberts K, Watson JD. Molecular biology of the cell, 2nd ed. New York: Garland, 1989.

Alessio HM. Exercise-induced oxidative stress. Med Sci Sports Exerc 1993;25(2):218-224.

Alessio HM, Goldfarb AH, Cao G. Exercise-induced oxidative stress before and after vitamin C supplementation. Int J Sport Nutr 1997;7:1-9.

Alpha-Tocopherol, Beta-Carotene Cancer Prevention Study Group (ABCPSG). The effect of vitamin E and beta-carotene on the incidence of lung cancer and other cancers in male smokers. N Engl J Med 1994;330:1029-1035.

Amadio E, Palermo R, Peloni G, Littarru G. Effect of Co Q10 administration on $\dot{V}O_2$max and diastolic function in athletes. In: Folkers K, Littarru G eds. Biomedical and clinical aspects of coenzyme Q. Amsterdam: Elsevier, 1991;525-533.

Atalay M, Lappalainen J, Sen C. Dietary antioxidants for the athlete. Curr Sports Med Rep 2006;5:182-186.

Avery NG, Kaiser JL, Sharman MJ, Scheett TP, Barnes DM, Gómez AL, Kraemer WJ, Volek JS. Effects of vitamin E supplementation on recovery from repeated bouts of resistance exercise. J Strength Cond Res 2003;17:801-809.

Bailey DM, Lawrenson L, McEneny J, Young IS, James PE, Jackson SK et al. Electron paramagnetic spectroscopic evidence of exercise-induced free radical accumulation in human skeletal muscle. Free Radic Res 2007;41(2):182-190.

Baker EM, Hodges RE, Hood J, Sauberlich HE, March SC, Canham JE. Metabolism of ^{14}C and ^{3}H-labeled L-ascorbic acid in human scurvy. Am J Clin Nutr 1971;24:444-454.

Bloomer RJ, Falvo MJ, Fry AC, Schilling BK, Webb AS, Moore CA. Oxidative stress response in trained men following repeated squats or sprints. Med Sci Sports Exerc 2006a;38(8):1436-1442.

Bloomer RJ, Goldfarb AH. Anaerobic exercise and oxidative stress: a review. Can J Appl Physiol 2004;29(3):245-263.

Bloomer RJ, Goldfarb AH, McKenzie MJ. Oxidative stress response to aerobic exercise: comparison of antioxidant supplements. Med Sci Sports Exerc 2006b;38(6):1098-1105.

Blot WJ, Li JY, Taylor PR et al. Nutrition intervention trials in Linxian, China: supplementation with specific vitamin/mineral combinations, cancer incidence, and disease-specific mortality in the general population. J Natl Cancer Inst 1993;85:1483-1492.

Blot WJ, Li J, Taylor PR, Guo W, Dawsey SM, Li B. The Linxian trials: mortality rates by vitamin-mineral intervention group. Am J Clin Nutr 1995;62(suppl):1424S-1426S.

Blumberg JB. Considerations of the recommended dietary allowances for older adults. Clin Appl Nutr 1991;1(4):9-18.

Boosalis MG. The role of selenium in chronic disease. Nutr Clin Pract 2008; 23(2): 152-160.

Bordia AK, Verma SK. Effects of vitamin C on platelet adhesiveness and platelet aggregation in coronary artery disease patients. Clin Cardiol 1985;8:552-554.

Bostick RM, Potter JD, McKenzie DR, Sellers TA, Kushi LH, Steinmetz KA, Folsom AR. Reduced risk of colon cancer with high intake of vitamin E: the Iowa Women's Health Study. Cancer Res 1993;53(18):4230-4237.

Bowles DK, Torgan CE, Kehrer JP, Ivy JI, Starnes JW. Effects of acute, submaximal exercise on skeletal muscle vitamin E. Free Radic Res Comm 1991;14(2):139-143.

Braun B, Clarkson P, Freedson P, Kohl R. Effects of coenzyme Q10 supplementation on exercise performance, VO_2max, and lipid peroxidation in trained cyclists. Int J Sport Nutr 1991;1:353-365.

Bruno RS, Leonard SW, Atkinson J, Montine TJ, Ramakrishnan R, Bray TM, Traber MG. Faster plasma vitamin E disappearance in smokers is normalized by vitamin C supplementation. Free Radic Biol Med 2006;40(4):689-697.

Bruno RS, Ramakrishnan R, Montine TJ, Bray TM, Traber MG. α-Tocopherol disappearance is faster in cigarette smokers and is inversely related to their ascorbic acid status. Am J Clin Nutr 2005;81:95-103.

Bryant RJ, Ryder J, Martino P, Kim J, Craig BW. Effects of vitamin E and C supplementation either alone or in combination on exercise-induced lipid peroxidation in trained cyclists. J Strength Cond Res 2003;17:792-800.

Bryer SC, Goldfarb AH. Effect of high dose vitamin C supplementation on muscle soreness, damage, function, and oxidative stress to eccentric exercise. Inter J Sport Nutr Exerc Metab 2006;16:270-280.

Bucca C, Rolla G, Farina JC. Effect of vitamin C on transient increase of bronchial responsiveness in conditions affecting the airways. Ann NY Acad Sci 1992;669:175-186.

Burk RF, Levander OA. Selenium. In: Shils ME, Shike M, Ross AC, Caballero B, Cousins RJ eds. Modern nutrition in health and disease, 10th ed. Philadelphia: Lippincott Williams & Wilkins, 2006;312-325.

Bursell SE, Clermont AC, Aiello LP, Aiello LM, Schlossman DK, Feener EP, Laffel L, King GL. High-dose vitamin E supplementation normalizes retinal blood flow and creatinine clearance in patients with type 1 diabetes. Diabetes Care 1999;22:1245-1251.

Cavarocchi NC, England MD, O'Brien JF et al. Superoxide generation during cardiopulmonary bypass: is there a role for vitamin E? J Surg Res 1986;40:519-527.

Christen WG, Gaziano JM, Hennekens CH. Design of Physicians' Health Study II—a randomized trial of beta-carotene, vitamins E and C, and multivitamins, in prevention of cancer, cardiovascular disease and eye disease, and a review of results of completed trials. Ann Epidemiol 2000;10(2):125-134.

Coombes JS, Rowell B, Dodd SL, Demirel HA, Naito H, Shanely RA, Powers SK. Effects of vitamin E deficiency on fatigue and muscle contractile properties. Eur J Appl Physiol 2002;87(3):272-277.

Crews H, Alink G, Andersen R et al. A critical assessment of some biomarker approaches linked with dietary intake. Br J Nutr 2001;86:S5-S35.

Cutler RG. Antioxidants, aging, and longevity. In: Pryor WA, ed. Free Radicals in Biology. London: Academic Press, 1984:371-428.

Davies KJA, Quintanilha AT, Brooks GA, Packer L. Free radicals and tissue damage produced by exercise. Biochem Biophys Res Comm 1982;107:1198-1205.

Davison G, Gleeson M, Phillips S. Antioxidant supplementation and immunoendocrine responses to prolonged exercise. Med Sci Sports Exerc 2007;39(4):645-652.

Davison GW, Hughes CM, Bell RA. Exercise and mononuclear cell DNA damage: the effects of antioxidant supplementation. Int J Sport Nutr Exerc Metab 2005;15:480-492.

Dekkers C, van Doornen LJP, Kemper HCG. The role of antioxidant vitamins and enzymes in the prevention of exercise-induced muscle damage. Sports Med 1996;21(3):213-238.

Dieber-Rotheneder M, Puhl H, Waeg G, Striegl G, Esterbauer H. Effect of oral supplementation with D-alpha tocopherol on the vitamin E content of human LDL resistance to oxidation. J Lipid Res 1991;1325-1333.

Dietrich M, Block G, Benowitz NL, Morrow JD, Hudes M, Jacob P 3rd, Norkus EP, Packer L. Vitamin C supplementation decreases oxidative stress biomarker f_2-isoprostanes in plasma of nonsmokers exposed to environmental tobacco smoke. Nutr Cancer 2003;45(2):176-184.

Dillard CJ, Litov RE, Savin WM, Dumelin EE, Tappel AL. Effects of exercise, vitamin E, and ozone on pulmonary function and lipid peroxidation. J Appl Physiol Respir Environ Exerc Physiol 1978;45(6):927-932.

Duthie GG, Robertson JD, Maughan RJ, Morrice PC. Blood antioxidant status and erythrocyte lipid peroxidation following distance running. Arch Biochem Biophys 1990;282:78-83.

Elosua R, Molina L, Fito M et al. Response of oxidative stress biomarkers to a 16-week aerobic physical activity program and to acute physical activity in healthy young men and women. Atherosclerosis 2003;167:327-334.

Erhardt JG, Lim SS, Bode JC, Bode C. A diet rich in fat and poor in dietary fiber increases the in vitro formation of reactive oxygen species in human feces. J Nutr 1997;127:706-709.

Ermakov IV, Sharifzadeh M, Ermakova M, Gellermann W. Resonance Raman detection of carotenoid antioxidants in living human tissue. J Biomed Optics 2005;10(6):064028-1 to 064028-17.

Ferriera RF, Milei J, Liesuy S, Flecha BG et al. Antioxidant action of vitamins A and E in patients submitted to coronary artery bypass surgery. Vasc Surg 1991;25:191-195.

Finaud J, Lac G, Filaire E. Oxidative stress: relationship with exercise training. Sports Med 2006;36(4):327-358.

Fogelholm GM, Himberg J, Alopaeus K, Gref C, Laakso JT, Lehto JJ, Mussalo-Rauhamaa H. Dietary and biochemical indices of nutritional status in male athletes and control. J Am Coll Nutr 1992;11(2):181-191.

Forman MR, Beecher GR, Muesing R et al. The fluctuation of plasma carotenoid concentrations by phase of the menstrual cycle: a controlled diet study. Am J Clin Nutr 1996;64:559-565.

Galan P, Viteri FE, Bertrais S, Czernichow S, Faure H et al. Serum concentrations of beta-carotene, vitamins C and E, zinc and selenium are influenced by sex, age, diet, smoking status, alcohol consumption and corpulence in a general French adult population. Eur J Clin Nutr 2005;59(10):1181-1190.

Gaziano JM. Vitamin E and cardiovascular disease: observational studies. Ann NY Acad Sci Dec 2004;1031:280-291.

Gibson RS. Principles of nutritional assessment, 2nd ed. New York: Oxford University Press, 2005.

Gohil K, Packer L, deLumen B, Brooks GA, Terblanche SE. Vitamin E deficiency and vitamin C supplementation: exercise and mitochondrial oxidation. J Appl Physiol 1986;60:1986-1991.

Goldfarb AH. Antioxidants: role of supplementation to prevent exercise-induced oxidative stress. Med Sci Sports Exerc 1993;25:232-236.

Greenberg SM, Frishman WH. Coenzyme Q10: a new drug for myocardial ischemia? Med Clin North Am 1988;72(1):243-258.

Guerra G, Ballardini E, Lippa S, Oradei A, Littarru G. Effect of the administration of ubidecarenone over the maximum consumption of oxygen and on the physical performance in a group of young cyclists. Med Sport 1987;40:359-364.

Guilland JT, Penaranda C, Gallet V, Boggio F, Fuchs, Klepping J. Vitamin status of young athletes including the effects of supplementation. Med Sci Sports Exerc 1989;21:441-449.

Gutteridge JMC, Halliwell B. The measurement and mechanism of lipid peroxidation in biological systems. Trends Biochem Sci 1990;15:129-135.

Gutteridge JMC, Halliwell B. Antioxidants in nutrition, health, and disease. Oxford: Oxford University Press, 1994.

Halliwell B. Lipid peroxidation, antioxidants, and cardiovascular disease: how should we move forward? Cardiovasc Res 2000a;47:410-418.

Halliwell B. Why and how should we measure oxidative DNA damage in nutritional studies? How far have we come? Am J Clin Nutr 2000b;72:1082-1087.

Halliwell B, Gutteridge JMC. Free radicals in biology and medicine, 3rd ed. Oxford: Clarendon Press, 1999;351-425.

Harding JJ, van Heyningen R. Epidemiology and risk factors for cataract. Eye 1987;1:537-541.

Harris RWC, Forman D, Doll R, Vessey MP, Wald NJ. Cancer of the cervix uteri and vitamin A. Br J Cancer 1986;83:653-659.

Hartmann AS, Pfuhler S, Dennog C, Germadnik D, Pilger A, Speit G. Exercise-induced DNA effects in human leukocytes are not accompanied by increased formation of 8-hydroxy-2-deoxyguanosine or induction of micronuclei. Free Radic Biol Med 1998;24:245-241.

Hata TR, Scholz A, Ermakov A, McClane RW, Khachick F, Gellermann W, Pershing LK. Non-invasive Raman spectroscopic detection of carotenoids in human skin. J Invest Dermatol 2000;115:441-448.

Hathcock JN, Azzi A, Blumberg J, Bray T, Dickinson A et al. Vitamins E and C are safe across a broad range of intakes. Am J Clin Nutr 2000;81(4):736-745.

Heart Protection Study Collaborative Group. MRC/BHF Heart Protection Study of antioxidant vitamin supplementation in 20,536 high-risk individuals: a randomized placebo-controlled trial. Lancet 2002;360(9326):23-33.

Heitzer T, Just H, Münzel T. Antioxidant vitamin C improves endothelial dysfunction in chronic smokers. Circulation 1996;94:6-9.

Hennekens CH, Buring JE, Manson JE et al. Lack of effect of long-term supplementation with beta-carotene on the incidence of malignant neoplasms and cardiovascular disease. N Engl J Med 1996;334:1145-1149.

Herbert V. Dangers of iron and vitamin C supplements. J Am Diet Assoc 1993a;93:526-527.

Herbert V. Does mega-C do more good than harm, or more harm than good? Nutr Today 1993b;28(1):28-32.

Higdon J. An evidence-based approach to vitamins and minerals. New York: Thieme, 2003.

Higdon J. An evidence-based approach to dietary phytochemicals. New York: Thieme, 2007.

HOPE and HOPE-TOO Trial Investigators. Effects of long-term vitamin E supplementation on cardiovascular events and cancer. JAMA 2005;293:1338-1347.

HOPE Study Investigators. Vitamin E supplementation and cardiovascular events in high risk patients. N Engl J Med 2000;342:154-160.

Institute of Medicine (IOM), Food and Nutrition Board, National Academy of Science. Dietary reference intakes for vitamin C, vitamin E, selenium, and carotenoids. Washington, DC: National Academy Press, 2000.

Jackson MJ, Edwards RHT, Symons MCR. Electron spin resonance studies of intact mammalian skeletal muscle. Biochem Biophys Acta 1985;847:185-190.

Jackson MJ, Khassaf M, Vasilaki A, McArdle F, McArdle A. Vitamin E and the oxidative stress of exercise. Ann NY Acad Sci 2004;1031:158-168.

Jacques PF, Chylack LT Jr. Epidemiologic evidence of a role for the antioxidant vitamins and carotenoids in cataract prevention. Am J Clin Nutr 1991;53(suppl):352S-355S.

Jacques PF, Chylack LT Jr, McGandy RB, Hartz SC. Nutritional status in persons with and without senile cataract: blood vitamin and mineral levels. Am J Clin Nutr 1988;48:152-158.

Jenkins RR, Goldfarb A. Introduction: oxidant stress, aging, and exercise. Med Sci Sports Exerc 1993;25(2):210-212.

Ji LL. Oxidative stress during exercise: implications of antioxidant nutrients. Free Radic Biol Med 1995;18(6):1079-1086.

Ji LL, Dillon D, Wu E. Alteration of antioxidant enzymes with aging in rat skeletal muscle and liver. Am J Physiol 1990;258:R918-R923.

Ji LL, Stratmen FW, Lardy HA. Antioxidant enzyme systems in rat liver and skeletal muscle. Arch Biochem Biophys 1988;263:150-160.

Jialal I, Grundy SM. The effect of dietary supplementation with alpha-tocopherol on the oxidative modification of low density lipoprotein. J Lipid Res 1992;6:899-906.

Johnston CS, Martin LJ, Cai X. Antihistamine effect of supplemental ascorbic acid and neutrophil chemotaxis. J Am Coll Nutr 1992;11:172-176.

Kanter MM, Nolte LA, Holloszy JO. Effects of an antioxidant vitamin mixture on lipid peroxidation at rest and postexercise. J Appl Physiol 1993;74:965-969.

Karlsson J. Heart and skeletal muscle ubiquinone or CoQ10 as a protective agent against radical formation in man. Adv Myochem 1987;1:305-318.

Karlsson J. Antioxidants and exercise. Champaign, IL: Human Kinetics, 1997.

Keith RE. Vitamin C. In: Wolinsky I, Driskell JA eds. Sport nutrition: vitamins and trace minerals. Boca Raton, FL: CRC Press, 2006;29-46.

Kneepkens CMF, LePage G, Roy CC. The potential of the hydrocarbon breath test as a measure of lipid peroxidation. Free Radic Biol Med 1994;17(2):127-160.

Knez WL, Jenkins DG, Coombes JS. Oxidative stress in half and full ironman triathletes. Med Sci Sports Exerc 2007;39(2):283-288.

Kotze HF, van der Walt WH, Rogers GG, Strydom NB. Effects of plasma ascorbic acid levels on heat acclimatization in man. J Appl Physiol 1977;42:711-716.

Kris-Etherton PM, Lichtenstein AH, Howard BV, Steinberg D, Witztum J. Antioxidant vitamin supplements and cardiovascular disease. Circulation 2004;110:637-641.

Kumar CT, Reddy VK, Prasad M, Thyagaraju K, Redanna P. Dietary supplementation of vitamin E protects heart tissue from exercise-induced oxidant stress. Mol Cell Biochem 1992;111:109-15.

Laaksonen R, Fogelholm M, Himberg JJ, Laaksoc J, Salorinne Y. Ubiquinone supplementation and exercise capacity in trained young and older men. Eur J Appl Physiol 1995;72:95-100

Lang JK, Gohil K, Packer L, Burk RF. Selenium deficiency, endurance exercise capacity, and antioxidant status in rats. J Appl Physiol 1987;63:2532-2535.

Langsjoen PH, Folkers K. Long-term efficacy and safety of coenzyme Q10 therapy for idiopathic dilated cardiomyopathy. Am J Cardiol 1990;65:521-523.

La Rue A, Koehler KM, Wayne SJ, Chiulli SJ, Haaland KY, Garry PJ. Nutritional status and cognitive functioning in a normally aging sample: a 6-y reassessment. Am J Clin Nutr 1997;65:20-29.

Leaf DA, Kleinman MT, Hamilton M, Barstow TJ. The effect of exercise intensity on lipid peroxidation. Med Sci Sports Exerc 1997;29(8):1036-1039.

Lee IM, Cook NR, Gaziano JM, Gordon D, Ridker PM, Manson JE et al. Vitamin E in the primary prevention of cardiovascular disease and cancer. The Women's Health Study: a randomized controlled trial. JAMA 2005;294:56-65.

Lee SH, Oe T, Blair IA. Vitamin C-induced decomposition of lipid hydroperoxides to endogenous genotoxins. Science 2001;292:2083-2086.

Leppala JM, Virtamo J, Fogelholm R et al. Controlled trial of alpha-tocopherol and beta-carotene supplements on stroke incidence and mortality in male smokers. Arterioscler Thromb Vasc Biol 2000;20:230-235.

Levine GN, Frei B, Koulouris SN, Gerhard MD, Keaney JF, Vita JA. Ascorbic acid reverses endothelial vasomotor dysfunction in patients with coronary artery disease. Circulation 1996;93:1107-1113.

Levine GN, Katz A, Padayatty S. Vitamin C. In: Shils ME, Shike M, Ross AC, Caballero B, Cousins RJ eds. Modern nutrition in health and disease, 10th ed. Philadelphia: Lippincott Williams & Wilkins, 2006;507-524.

Levine GN, Wang Y, Padayatty SJ. Vitamin C pharmacokinetics in healthy men and women. In: Packer L, Traber MG, Kraemer K, Frei B eds. The antioxidant vitamins C and E. Champaign, IL: AOCS Press, 2002;17-31.

Livrea MA, Tesoriere L, Bongiorno A, Pintaudi AM, Ciaccio M, Riccio A. Contribution of vitamin A to the oxidation resistance of human low density lipoproteins. Free Radic Biol Med 1995;18(3):401-409.

Lyle BJ, Mares-Perlman JA, Klein BE et al. Antioxidant intake and risk of incident age-related nuclear cataracts in the Beaver Dam Eye Study. Am J Epidemiol 1999;149:801-809.

Makhija N, Sendasgupta C, Kiran U, Lakshmy R, Hote MP, Choudhary SK, Airan B, Abraham R. The role of oral coenzyme Q10 in patients undergoing coronary artery bypass graft surgery. J Cardiothorac Vasc Anesth 2008; 22(6): 832-839.

Malm C, Svensson M, Sjoberg B, Ekblom B, Sjodin S. Supplementation with ubiquinone-10 causes cellular damage during intense exercise. Acta Physiol Scand 1996;157:511-512.

Maras JE, Bermudez OI, Qiao N, Bakun PJ, Boody-Alter EL, Tucker KL. Intake of alpha-tocopherol is limited among US adults. J Am Diet Assoc 2004;104:567-575.

Margaritis I, Palazzetti S, Rousseau AS, Richard MJ, Favier A. Antioxidant supplementation and tapering exercise improve exercise-induced antioxidant response. J Am Coll Nutr 2003;22(2):147-156.

Mastaloudis A, Leonard S, Traber M. Oxidative stress in athletes during extreme endurance exercise. Free Radic Biol Med 2001;31:911-922.

Mastaloudis A, Yu TW, O'Donnell RP, Frei B, Dashwood RH, Traber MG. Endurance exercise results in DNA damage as detected by the comet assay. Free Radic Bio Med 2004;36(8):966-975.

Mastaloudis M, Traber MG. Vitamin E. In: Wolinsky I, Driskell JA eds. Sport nutrition: vitamins and trace minerals. Boca Raton, FL: CRC Press, 2006;183-200.

McAnulty SR, McAnulty LS, Nieman DC et al. Influence of carbohydrate ingestion on oxidative stress and plasma antioxidant potential following a 3h run. Free Radic Res 2003;37(8):835-840.

McCord JM, Day ED Jr. Superoxide dependent production of hydroxyl radical catalyzed by iron-EDTA complex. FEBS Lett 1978;86:139-142.

Miller ER, Pastor-Barriuso RP, Dalal D, Riemersma RA, Appel LJ, Guallar E. Meta-analysis: high dosage vitamin E supplementation may increase all-cause mortality. Ann Intern Med 2005;142:37-46.

Mirvish SS. Effects of vitamins C and E on N-nitroso compound formation, carcinogenesis and cancer. Cancer 1986;58:1842-1850.

Miyazaki H, Oh-ishi S, Okawara T et al. Strenuous endurance training in humans reduces oxidative stress following exhaustive exercise. Eur J Appl Physiol 2001;84:1-6.

Montuschi P, Barnes PJ, Roberts J. Isoprostanes: markers and mediators of oxidative stress. FASEB J 2004;18:1791-1800.

Nielson AN, Mizuno M, Ratkevicius A, Mohr T, Rohde M, Mortensen SA, Quistorff B. No effect of antioxidant supplementation in triathletes on maximal oxygen uptake, 31P-NMRS detected muscle energy metabolism and muscle fatigue. Int J Sports Med 1999;20:154-158.

Nieman DC. Exercise immunology: nutritional considerations. Can J Appl Physiol 2001;26:S45-55.

Nieman DC, Henson DA, McAnulty SR, McAnulty LS, Morrow JD, Ahmed A, Heward CB. Vitamin E and immunity after the Kona Triathlon World Championship. Med Sci Sports Exerc 2004;36(8):1328-1335.

Niess AM, Baumann M, Roecker K, Horstmann T, Mayer F, Dickhuth HH. Effects of intensive endurance exercise on DNA damage in leucocytes. J Sports Med Phys Fit 1998;38:111-115.

Olson OE. Selenium toxicity with emphasis on man. J Am Coll Toxicol 1986;5:45-70.

Omenn GS, Goodman GE, Thornquist MD et al. Effects of a combination of beta-carotene and vitamin A on lung cancer and cardiovascular disease. N Engl J Med 1996;334:1150-1155.

Packer L. Oxygen radicals and antioxidants in endurance training. In: Benzi G, Packer L, Siliprandi N eds. Biochemical aspects of physical exercise. New York: Elsevier, 1986;73-92.

Paolisso G, D'Amore A, Giugliano D, Ceriello A, Varricchio M, D'Onofrio F. Pharmacologic doses of vitamin E improve insulin action in healthy subjects and non-insulin-dependent diabetic patients. Am J Clin Nutr 1993;57:650-656.

Paolisso G, Di Maro G, Galzerano D, Cacciapuoti F, Varricchio G, Varricchio M, D'Onofrio F. Pharmacological doses of vitamin E and insulin action in elderly subjects. Am J Clin Nutr 1994;59:1291-1296.

Perrig WJ, Perrig P, Stähelin HB. The relation between antioxidants and memory performance in the old and very old. J Am Geriatr Soc 1997;45:718-724.

Peters EM, Goetzsche JM, Grobbelaar B, Noakes TD. Vitamin C supplementation reduces the incidence of postrace symptoms of upper-respiratory-tract infection in ultramarathon runners. Am J Clin Nutr 1993;57:170-174.

Podmore ID, Griffiths HR, Herbert KE, Mistry N, Mistry P, Lunec J. Vitamin C exhibits pro-oxidant properties. Nature 1998;392(9):559.

Polidori MC, Mecocci P, Levine M, Frei B. Short-term and long-term vitamin C supplementation in humans dose-dependently increases the resistance of plasma to ex vivo lipid peroxidation. Arch Biochem Biophys 2004;423(1):109-115.

Powers SK, DeRuisseau KC, Quindry J, Hamilton KL. Dietary antioxidants and exercise. J Sports Sci 2004;22:81-94.

Powers SK, Ji LL, Leeuwenburgh C. Exercise training-induced alterations in skeletal muscle antioxidant capacity: a brief review. Med Sci Sports Exerc 1999;31(7):987-997.

Quintanilha AT, Packer L, Davies JMS, Racanelli T, Davies KJA. Membrane effects of vitamin E deficiency: bioenergetics and surface charge density studies of skeletal muscle and liver mitochondria. Ann NY Acad Sci 1982;399:32-47.

Rayman MP. The importance of selenium to human health. Lancet 2000;356:233-241.

Robertson JM, Donner AP, Trevithick JR. Vitamin E intakes and risk of cataract in humans. Ann NY Acad Sci 1989;570:372-382.

Rokitzki L, Logemann E, Huber G et al. Alpha-tocopherol supplementation in racing cyclists during extreme endurance training. Int J Sport Nutr 1994;4:253-264.

Rothman KJ. Modern epidemiology. Boston: Little, Brown, 1986;51-76.

Sacheck JM, Milbury PE, Cannon JG, Roubenoff R, Blumberg JB. Effect of vitamin E and eccentric exercise on selected biomarkers of oxidative stress in young and elderly men. Free Radic Biol Med 2003;34:1575-1588.

Salonen JT, Salonen R, Seppaenen K et al. Effects of antioxidant supplementation on platelet function: a randomized pair-matched, placebo-controlled, double-blind trial in men with low antioxidant status. Am J Clin Nutr 1991;53:1222-1229.

Schwarz KB, Cox JM, Sharma S et al. Possible antioxidant effect of vitamin A supplementation in premature infants. J Pediatr Gastroenterol Nutr 1997;25(4):408-414.

Sen CK. Antioxidant and redox regulation of cellular signaling: introduction. Med Sci Sports Exerc 2001;33(3):368-370.

Simon-Schnass IM. Nutrition at high altitude. J Nutr 1992;122:778-781.

Skyrme-Jones RA, O'Brien RC, Berry KL, Meredith IT. Vitamin E supplementation improves endothelial function in type I diabetes mellitus: a randomized, placebo-controlled study. J Am Coll Cardiol 2000;36:94-102.

Snider I, Bazzarre T, Murdoch S, Goldfarb A. Effects of coenzyme athletic performance system as an ergogenic aid on endurance performance to exhaustion. Int J Sport Nutr 1992;2:272-286.

Stampfer MJ, Manson JAE, Colditz GA, Speizer FE, Willett WC, Hennekens CH. A prospective study of vitamin E supplementation and risk of coronary disease in women. Circulation 1992;86(suppl 4):I-463.

Steensberg A, Morrow J, Toft AD et al. Prolonged exercise, lymphocyte apoptosis and F2-isoprostanes. Eur J Appl Physiol 2002;87(1):38-42.

Steiner M, Mower R. Mechanism of action of vitamin E on platelet function. Ann NY Acad Sci 1982;393:289-299.

Stich HF, Rosin MP, Hornby AP, Mathew B, Sankaranarayanan R, Nair MK. Remission of oral leukoplakias and micronuclei in tobacco/betel quid chewers treated with beta carotene and with beta carotene plus vitamin A. Int J Cancer 1988;42:195-199.

Strydom NB, Kotze HF, van der Walt WH, Rogers GG. Effect of ascorbic acid on rate of heat acclimatization. J Appl Physiol 1976;41:202-205.

Su LJ, Arab L. Salad and raw vegetable consumption and nutritional status in the adult US population: results from the

Third National Health and Nutrition Examination Survey. J Am Diet Assoc 2006;106:1394-1404.

Subudhi AW, Jacobs KA, Hagobian TA, Fattor JA, Stephen RM, Fulco CS, Allen C, Friedlander AL. Effects of antioxidants on ventilatory threshold at high altitude. Med Sci Sports Exerc 2006;38:1425-1431.

Tate RM, Repine JE. Phagocytes, oxygen radicals, and lung injury. In: Pryor WA ed. Free radicals in biology. London: Academic Press, 1984;199-209.

Taylor A. Cataract: relationships between nutrition and oxidation. J Am Coll Nutr 1993;12(2):138-146.

Tessier F, Margaritis I, Richard MJ, Moynot C, Marconnet P. Selenium and training effects on the glutathione system and aerobic performance. Med Sci Sports Exerc 1995;27(3):390-396.

Thompson D, Williams C, McGregor SJ, Nicholas CW, McArdle F, Jackson MJ, Powell JR. Prolonged vitamin C supplementation and recovery from demanding exercise. Int J Sport Nutr Exerc Metab 2001;11(4):466-481.

Thomson CD. Assessment of requirements for selenium and adequacy of selenium status: a review. Eur J Clin Nutr 2004;58:391-401.

Tidus PM, Houston ME. Vitamin E status and response to exercise training. Sports Med. 1995;18:1079-86.

Traber MG. Vitamin E. In: Shils ME, Shike M, Ross AC, Caballero B, Cousins RJ eds. Modern nutrition in health and disease, 10th ed. Philadelphia: Lippincott Williams & Wilkins, 2006;396-411.

Traber MG. Heart disease and single-vitamin supplementation. Am J Clin Nutr 2007;85:293S-299S.

Traber MG, Blatt DB. Vitamin E: evidence for the 2:1 preference for *RRR-* compared with *all-rac*-alpha-tocopherols. In: Packer L, Traber MG, Kraemer K, Frei B eds. The antioxidant vitamins C and E. Champaign, IL: AOCS Press, 2002;161-170.

Urso ML, Clarkson PM. Oxidative stress, exercise, and antioxidant supplementation. Toxicology 2003;189:41-54.

Vollaard NBJ, Shearman JP, Cooper CE. Exercise-induced oxidative stress: myths, realities and physiological relevance. Sports Med 2005;35(12):1045-1062.

Waring WS, Convery A, Mishra V et al. Uric acid reduces exercise-induced oxidative stress in healthy adults. Clin Sci (Lond) 2003;105(4):425-430.

Warren JA, Jenkins RR, Packer L, Witt EH, Armstrong RB. Elevated muscle vitamin E does not attenuate eccentric exercise-induced muscle injury. J Appl Physiol 1992;72:2168-2175.

Wassertheil-Smoller S, Romney SL, Wylie- Rosett J et al. Dietary vitamin C and uterine cervical dysplasia. Am J Epidemiol 1981;114:714-724.

Weber C, Erl W, Weber K, Weber PC. Increased adhesiveness of isolated monocytes to endothelium is prevented by vitamin C intake in smokers. Circulation 1996;93:1488-1492.

Weight LM, Noakes TD, Labadarios D, Graves J, Jacobs P, Berman PA. Vitamin and mineral status of trained athletes including the effects of supplementation. Am J Clin Nutr 1988;47:186-191.

Wengreen HJ, Munger RG, Corcoran CD, Zandi P, Hayden KM et al. Antioxidant intake and cognitive function of elderly men and women: the Cache County Study. J Nutr Health Aging 2007;11(3):230-237.

Whanger PD, Beilstein MA, Thomson CD, Robinson MF, Howe M. Blood selenium and glutathione peroxidase activity of populations in New Zealand, Oregon, and South Dakota. FASEB J 1988;2:2996-3002.

Wilcox BJ, Curb JD, Rodriguez BL. Antioxidants in cardiovascular health and disease: key lessons from epidemiologic studies. Am J Cardiol 2008;101(10A):75D-86D.

Williamson JR, Chang K, Frangos M et al. Hyperglycemic pseudohypoxia and diabetic complications. Diabetes 1993;42(6):801-813.

Wu SY, Leske MC. Antioxidants and cataract formation: a summary review. Int Ophthamol Clin 2000;40(4):71-81.

Wylie-Rosett JA, Romney SL, Slagle S et al. Influence of vitamin A on cervical dysplasia and carcinoma in situ. Nutr Cancer 1984;6:49-57.

Zeppilli P, Merlino B, DeLuca A et al. Influence of coenzyme Q10 in physical work capacity in athletes, sedentary people, and patients with mitochondrial disease. In: Folkers K, Littarru G, Yamagimi T eds. Biomedical and clinical aspects of coenzyme Q. Amsterdam: Elsevier, 1991;541-545.

Zheng W, Sellers TA, Doyle TJ, Kushi LH, Ptter JD, Folsom AR. Retinol, antioxidant vitamins, and cancers of the upper digestive tract in a prospective cohort study of postmenopausal women. Am J Epidemiol. 1995;142(9):955-960.

CHAPTER 11

Minerals and Exercise

Chapter Objectives

After reading this chapter you should be able to

- identify the exercise-related functions, dietary requirements, and food sources of zinc, magnesium and chromium,
- explain the rationale and scientific support for the hypothesized increased need for certain minerals in active people and athletes,
- understand the assessment methods for zinc, magnesium, and chromium,
- discuss the zinc, magnesium, and chromium status of active people, and
- describe if and when athletes might need to supplement with zinc, magnesium, chromium, or more than one of these.

Athletes and active individuals alike are bombarded with advice and inundated with advertisements about supplements that supposedly enhance athletic performance. Minerals such as calcium (Ca) and iron (Fe) are often identified as nutrients that athletes (particularly female athletes) may not be getting enough of, and not surprisingly are two of the most frequently consumed mineral supplements among athletes. But what about other minerals that are known to be involved in energy metabolism and muscle function (and thus likely affect athletic performance)—minerals such as zinc (Zn), magnesium (Mg), and chromium (Cr)? Should athletes and active individuals be concerned about these as well? Because minerals are different from vitamins in a number of ways, the decision to supplement with minerals involves different decision-making criteria.

This chapter addresses these questions, specifically examining the role of zinc, magnesium, and chromium with respect to exercise; the requirements for these minerals; and risk for deficiency in athletes and active individuals. Because these minerals are especially important for the metabolism of macronutrients and the production of energy, they are grouped together in one chapter. Chapter 12 discusses the blood-building minerals (such as iron and copper) in detail; here we discuss only their role in energy metabolism. Chapter 13 covers the minerals that help build bone, especially magnesium and calcium. In this chapter we discuss magnesium only as it relates to energy metabolism and exercise-associated functions unrelated to bones. Chapter 10 covers selenium in its role as an antioxidant.

We first review the metabolic and exercise-related functions and the dietary requirements and sources of each mineral. Then we briefly examine the rationale and scientific support for increased need for these minerals in active people. Next we discuss how minerals differ from vitamins in their bioavailability, homeostatic mechanisms, and use by the body. We review the methods for assessing mineral status, including the biochemical assessment parameters that are measured. Then we review the mineral intakes of active people and address the impact of mineral deficiency or marginal mineral status on exercise performance. Finally, we examine whether exercise increases the mineral requirements of active people and whether mineral supplementation in healthy individuals enhances exercise performance.

EXERCISE-RELATED FUNCTIONS, DIETARY REQUIREMENTS, AND FOOD SOURCES

In order to determine whether exercise might increase a person's need for minerals, we must first examine the role of minerals in energy metabolism, their exercise-related functions, and their role in the maintenance of good health. Table 11.1 lists each mineral discussed in this chapter, the various metabolic pathways that require the mineral, and some of the specific enzymes that utilize the mineral as a cofactor. Zinc, magnesium, iron, and copper are especially important for the metabolic pathways involved in energy metabolism and for the maintenance, building, and repair of

muscle tissues. Chromium is important for glucose metabolism and optimal insulin action. The following section briefly discusses the specific metabolic and exercise-related functions of each of these minerals. Since chapter 12 reviews iron and copper in detail, only a brief description of their role in energy metabolism is provided here.

Iron

One of the primary functions of iron is the transport of oxygen in red blood cells, but iron is also important for energy metabolism during exercise. Approximately 74% of the body's iron is found in hemoglobin and myoglobin, while only 1% is found in oxidative enzymes (Gropper et al. 2009)—yet this 1% is vital to energy metabolism and is as important in energy production during exercise as is the delivery of oxygen via hemoglobin (table 11.1). Chapter 12 describes the dietary requirements for iron and its food sources.

Copper

Although copper is important for proper iron metabolism (see chapter 12) and hemoglobin production, like iron it is also important for energy metabolism. Copper is an important cofactor for the enzymes of the electron transport pathway (and therefore for energy production). Copper is also required for **superoxide dismutase (SOD)**, an antioxidant enzyme that helps protect cells against oxidative damage. Finally, copper is important for the synthesis and maintenance of collagen (Gropper et al. 2009). Chapter 12 describes the dietary requirements for copper and its food sources.

Zinc

Zinc is ubiquitous in human physiology and metabolism. Zinc is required for the structure and function of more than 300 enzymes in the human body (McCall et al. 2000), many of which are involved in macronutrient metabolism and thus energy production during exercise (Lukaski 2004; King and Cousins 2006). For example, the zinc-containing enzyme lactate dehydrogenase is essential in carbohydrate metabolism, while carbonic anhydrase regulates the elimination of carbon dioxide from cells. Superoxide dismutase, another zinc-dependent metalloenzyme, is a powerful endogenous antioxidant enzyme that scavenges free radicals and may protect against oxidative damage during exercise (Lukaski 2004). Tables 11.1 and 11.2 list some of the zinc-containing

Table 11.1 Exercise and Energy-Related Metabolic Functions of Minerals (Zinc, Magnesium, Iron, Copper, and Chromium)

Mineral	Common form	RDA or AI	UL	Functions related to exercise	Major enzymes or pathways that require the mineral as a cofactor
Zinc (Zn)	Zn^{2+}	Males: 11 mg/day Females: 8 mg/day	40 mg/day	Zn-containing enzymes function in carbohydrate, lipid, protein, alcohol, and nucleic acid metabolism.	Lactate dehydrogenase, carbonic anhydrase, malate dehydrogenase, carboxypeptidase, alkaline phosphatase, alcohol dehydrogenase, glutamate dehydrogenase, superoxide dismutase
Magnesium (Mg)	Mg^{2+}	Males: 400-420 mg/day Females: 320 mg/day	350 mg/day from supplements	Mg-containing enzymes are involved in the glycolytic pathway, β-oxidation of fat, protein synthesis, ATP hydrolysis, electrolyte balance, muscle contractions, and second-messenger systems.	Hexokinase, phosphofructokinase, pyruvate kinase, pyruvate dehydrogenase complex, acyl-CoA synthase
Iron (Fe)	Ferric (Fe^{3+}—oxidized form); ferrous iron (Fe^{2+}—reduced iron)	Males: 8 mg/day Females: 18 mg/day	45 mg/day	Fe is required for numerous enzymes involved in energy production during exercise; required for the synthesis of hemoglobin and myoglobin.	Pyruvate oxidase, mitochondrial cytochromes, cytochrome P-450, ribonucleotide reductase, tyrosine and proline hydrolase, monoamine oxidase, catalase, glucose-6-phosphatase, 6-phosphogluconate dehydrogenase
Copper (Cu)	Cu^0, Cu^{1+}, Cu^{2+}	Males: 900 μg/day Females: 900 μg/day	10,000 μg/day	Cu is an important component of hemoglobin and myoglobin and is required for the proper utilization of iron. Important for electron transport enzymes, enzymes involved in collagen synthesis, and synthesis of norepinephrine. Cu is also required to protect cells against oxidative damage.	Cytochrome-c oxidase, superoxide dismutase, protein-lysine 6-oxidase, dopamine-β-monooxygenase
Chromium (Cr)	Cr^{3+} as part of glucose tolerance factor	Males: 30-35 μg/day Females: 20-25 μg/day	–	Potentiates the effect of insulin.	No chromium-dependent enzymes identified

RDA = Recommended Dietary Intake; AI = Adequate Intake; UL = Tolerable Upper Intake Level. For more information on mineral-specific enzymes for zinc and copper see Grider 2006; for magnesium see Rude and Shils 2006; and for iron see Beard 2006.

enzymes and their related functions. In addition to its role in enzyme structure and activity, zinc is required for nucleic acid and protein synthesis, cellular differentiation and replication, and muscle function (Lukaski 2004; King and Cousins 2006). Zinc exerts regulatory actions in the production, storage, and secretion of various hormones including growth hormone, thyroid hormones, gonadotropins, sex hormones, prolactin, insulin, and corticosteroids (Lukaski 2006b). Finally, zinc is important for wound healing and skin integrity,

skeletal and brain development, proper taste acuity, reproduction, and immune and gastrointestinal function (King and Cousins 2006).

Zinc is found in almost all body tissues but is concentrated in muscle, kidney, liver, bone, and skin, with 95% being found intracellularly. The amount of zinc in muscle tissue is somewhat variable, but generally, the highest concentrations are found in slow-twitch oxidative skeletal muscle fibers. Zinc is also found in high concentrations within bone tissue. Bone zinc levels appear to be

Table 11.2 Zinc-Dependent Enzymes and Their Functions

Specific enzyme	Function	Tissue
Carboxypeptidase	Digestion of dietary protein	Pancreas
Carbonic anhydrase	Acid–base balance	Numerous tissues
Alkaline dehydrogenase	Phosphate hydrolysis	Numerous tissues
Alcohol dehydrogenase	Metabolism of alcohol	Liver, kidney
Lactate dehydrogenase	Conversion of lactate to pyruvate	Liver, muscle cells
Malate dehydrogenase	Metabolism of macronutrients	TCA cycle of the cells
Glutamate dehydrogenase	Transamination of amino acids	Numerous tissues and cells

See McCall and colleagues 2000 for more information on zinc-requiring enzymes. TCA = trycarboxylic acid

Adapted from K.A. McCall, C. Huang, and C.A. Fierke, 2000, "Function and mechanism of zinc metalloenzymes," *Journal of Nutrition* 130: 1437S-1446S.

the most responsive to changes in dietary intake and may reflect a gradual decline in total body zinc when zinc intake is poor (Lukaski 2006b). The distribution of zinc within blood heavily favors the red blood cells, with 75% to 88% of blood zinc found in the erythrocyte, 12% to 20% in the plasma, and ≤3% in the leukocyte.

It has been estimated that the body needs to absorb approximately 5 mg zinc per day to maintain the required total body zinc pool of ~1.5 to 2.5 g. Since maximal zinc absorption is only about 40% (range: 10-40%) under controlled conditions (King and Cousins 2006), dietary zinc recommendations need to be higher than the actual amount ingested. The current Recommended Dietary Allowance (RDA) for zinc is 11 mg/day for adult men and 8 mg/day for women aged 19 years and older (Institute of Medicine 2001). Zinc requirements are slightly elevated during pregnancy (11 mg/day) and lactation (12 mg/day). Symptoms of zinc deficiency include growth retardation, delayed wound healing, impaired immune function, decreased taste acuity, anorexia, and a variety of skin ailments and lesions (Gropper et al. 2009; Shay and Mangian 2000).

In 2001, the U.S. Institute of Medicine (IOM), Food and Nutrition Board set the Tolerable Upper Intake Level (UL) for zinc for adults at 40 mg/day, including dietary sources as well as supplements (IOM 2001). High zinc intake can reduce copper status; thus the point at which high zinc intake negatively affects copper status was used to set the UL for zinc (IOM 2001). Indeed, zinc intakes of 60 mg/day (50 mg supplemental and 10 mg dietary zinc) have resulted in signs of copper deficiency (IOM 2001). Gastrointestinal distress has been reported at doses of 50 to 150 mg/day of supplemental zinc. Although rare, isolated outbreaks of

acute zinc toxicity have occurred as a result of the consumption of food or beverages contaminated with zinc released from galvanized containers (IOM 2001). Signs of acute zinc toxicity are abdominal pain, diarrhea, nausea, and vomiting. Single doses of 225 to 450 mg of zinc usually induce vomiting (IOM 2001). Recently, zinc-containing cold lozenges (~13 mg zinc per lozenge, dose = six lozenges a day) have been marketed as a way of reducing the severity of colds. Using the lozenges as recommended would result in ~80 mg of zinc per day (King and Cousins 2006). People should use caution when supplementing with zinc, especially with regard to chronically high intakes.

Protein-rich foods are generally the best sources of zinc. Shellfish, beef, and other red meats are particularly high in zinc content and provide nearly 70% of the dietary zinc intake in the United States (King and Cousins 2006; IOM 2001) (see table 11.3). In fact, oysters have the highest zinc content by weight (25 mg in three medium oysters). By comparison, 3 oz (85 g) of ground beef contains just 5.4 mg, while white meats including chicken and turkey have less than half that much. Nuts and legumes are among the best plant sources of zinc. Grains, including breads, cereals, rice, and pasta, contain very little zinc, and much of it is lost during processing or is not particularly bioavailable. For example, most of the zinc in cereal grains is in the bran and germ portions of the kernel; and if these are removed with milling, then a significant portion of the zinc is lost. This explains why whole wheat bread provides 0.7 mg of zinc per slice while white bread provides less than half that amount (0.3 mg per slice). The zinc in whole grain products (and many other plant proteins) is less bioavailable due to their relatively high content of phytic acid, a compound that inhibits zinc absorption (King and Cousins 2006). The enzymatic action of yeast reduces the level of phytic acid in foods. Therefore, leavened whole grain breads have more bioavailable zinc than unleavened whole grain breads. Fruits, vegetables (with the exception of beans), fats and oils, soft drinks, candies, and other highly refined carbohydrates are generally poor sources of zinc. Likewise, drinking water is also typically low in zinc. Although some breakfast cereals are fortified with zinc and can provide 25% to 100% of the RDA in one serving, the bioavailability of this zinc may be low due to the cooking process used in making these products. This cooking process, called extrusion cooking, inhibits the degradation of phytic acid in the gut and causes less efficient absorption of zinc (King and Cousins 2006). Other dietary factors that may reduce the bioavailability of dietary zinc are high supplemental intakes of iron, calcium, or tin; the tannic acid in tea and coffee; and caffeine (King and Cousins 2006).

Magnesium

Like zinc, magnesium functions as a cofactor for over 300 enzymes. Many of these enzymes catalyze reactions in cellular energy production and storage, protein synthesis, DNA and RNA synthesis, cell growth and reproduction, maintenance of electrolyte balance, and stabilization of mitochondrial membranes (Bohl and Volpe 2004; Rude and Shils 2006) (see table 11.1). Magnesium is required for the glycolytic pathway; the synthesis and oxidation of fatty acids and proteins; adenosine triphosphate (ATP) hydrolysis; and the formation of cyclic adenosine monophosphate (cAMP), a second-messenger system within cells (Lukaski 1995; Rude and Shils 2006). Several key enzymes in the glycolytic pathway require magnesium (e.g., hexokinase, phosphofructokinase, and pyruvate kinase); in the tricarbolic acid (TCA) cycle, pyruvate dehydrogenase requires magnesium. The first step in β-oxidation of fatty acids also requires magnesium for the acyl-CoA synthase complex (Rude and Shils 2006). In addition, magnesium plays a central role in the control of neuromuscular transmission, cardiac excitability, vasomotor tone, and blood pressure (Bohl and Volpe 2004; IOM 1997). It is clear that magnesium plays a vital role in substrate metabolism and in the production of energy for exercise.

The adult human body contains about 25 g of magnesium. Over 60% of all the magnesium in the body is found in the skeleton; about 27% is found in muscle, while 6% to 7% is within various other cells and less than 1% is found extracellularly (Volpe 2006; IOM 1997). The body maintains magnesium homeostasis through both fecal and urinary excretion. With free-living diets containing 234 to 323 mg/day of magnesium, absorption ranges from 21% to 27% (Rude and Shils 2006). Magnesium absorption varies with dietary intake. When magnesium intake is low (~7-36 mg/day), absorption increases (~65-77% of intake is absorbed); with high intakes of magnesium (~960-1000 mg/day), absorption decreases (~11-14% of magnesium absorbed) (Rude and Shils 2006). The kidneys further regulate magnesium homeostasis through urinary magnesium excretion by either increasing or decreasing output, depending on intake, while maintaining blood magnesium concentrations.

The current RDA for magnesium is 400 mg/day for men ages 19 to 30 years and 420 mg/day for men ages 31 to 70 years. For women, the RDA is 310 mg/day for ages 19 to 30 years and 320 mg/day for ages 31 to 70 years (IOM 1997). The slight increase in the RDA for magnesium with age is attributed to more instances of negative balance in older subjects. It is recommended that pregnant women consume 360 to 400 mg/day of magnesium and that nursing mothers consume 320 to 360 mg/day (IOM 1997). The specific amount of magnesium recommended during pregnancy or lactation depends on age, with younger women (14-18 years) requiring higher amounts. Magnesium deficiency in healthy individuals consuming a balanced diet is quite rare because magnesium is abundant in both plant and animal foods and because the kidneys are able to limit urinary excretion of magnesium when intake is low (IOM 1997). Indeed, overt deficiencies generally occur only secondary to disease states (e.g., gastrointestinal or renal disorders, alcoholism, chronic diarrhea). Symptoms of magnesium deficiency include decreased serum magnesium levels (hypomagnesemia), decreased serum calcium levels (hypocalcemia; due to alterations in parathyroid hormone), low serum potassium levels (hypokalemia), retention of sodium, neurological and muscular symptoms (tremor, muscle spasms, tetany), loss of appetite, nausea, vomiting, and personality changes (Rude and Shils 2006).

Because no adverse effects of excess magnesium consumption from food have been documented, a UL has been set only for supplemental magnesium, at 350 mg/day for > 8 years of age. The initial symptom of excess magnesium supplementation is diarrhea—a well-known side effect of

Table 11.3 Zinc and Magnesium Content of Commonly Consumed Foods

Food	Serving size	Zinc (mg/serving)	Magnesium (mg/serving)
Meat and Fish			
Pacific oysters, steamed	3 medium (~75 g)	25	33
Ground beef (20% fat), pan broiled	3 oz (85 g)	5.4	19
Beef chuck roast, choice, cooked	3 oz (85 g)	5.8	17
Pork chop, center cut, fried	3 oz (85 g)	1.7	15
Chicken, boneless, roasted	3 oz (85 g)	1.8	20
Turkey, white meat, cooked	3 oz (85 g)	1.7	24
Tuna, canned in water	3 oz (85 g)	0.5	24
Shrimp, steamed	3 oz (85 g)	1.3	29
Beans, legumes, nuts, and seeds			
Black beans, cooked	1/2 cup (86 g)	1.0	60
Hummus	1/2 cup (125 g)	2.3	89
Almonds, dry roasted	1 oz (28 g)	0.9	78
Peanut butter, chunky	2 tbsp	0.9	52
Sunflower seeds	1/4 cup	1.8	43
Dairy products			
Milk (2%)	1 cup (244 g)	1.0	27
Yogurt, low-fat	1 cup (244 g)	2.2	42
Cereals, grains, and pasta			
Cheerios	1 cup (30 g)	4.6	39
Oatmeal, cooked	1 cup (234 g)	1.1	54
Shredded Wheat	1 cup (43 g)	1.3	57
Whole grain Total cereal	1 cup (40 g)	23.3	52
Barley, cooked	1 cup (184 g)	5.1	245
Whole wheat bread	1 slice (28 g)	0.7	33
White bread	1 slice (28 g)	0.3	8.0
Pasta (spaghetti), cooked	1 cup (115 g)	0.7	42
Rice, long grain, brown, cooked	1 cup (195 g)	1.2	84
Fruit			
Apple, with peel, medium	1 each (188 g)	0.1	7.0
Avocado, slices	1 cup (146 g)	0.1	42
Banana, medium	1 each (118 g)	0.2	32
Blueberries, fresh	1 cup (145 g)	0.2	9.0
Orange, large	1 each (146 g)	0.1	18
Vegetables			
Artichoke, medium, cooked	1 each (120 g)	0.6	72
Broccoli, cooked	1 cup (156 g)	0.7	33
Green beans, cooked	1 cup (125 g)	0.3	23
Green peas, cooked	1 cup (125 g)	2.0	62
Lima beans, cooked	1 cup (130 g)	1.3	126
Potato, with skin, baked	1 small (138 g)	0.5	62
Tomato, whole	1 each (123 g)	0.2	14
Spinach, cooked	1 cup (180 g)	1.4	157

Data from Food Processor SQL Edition, Version 9.9.l, 2006. ESHA Research, Salem, OR.

magnesium, which is frequently used therapeutically as a laxative. Chronically elevated serum levels of magnesium (hypermagnesemia) may result in a fall in blood pressure (hypotension), which appears to underlie many of the other symptoms of chronically high magnesium intake including lethargy, confusion, disturbances in normal cardiac rhythm, and deterioration of kidney function. As hypermagnesemia progresses, muscle weakness and difficulty breathing may occur. Severe hypermagnesemia may result in cardiac arrest (Rude and Shils 2006; IOM 1997). Because magnesium is part of chlorophyll, the green pigment in plants, green leafy vegetables are rich in magnesium. Unrefined grains, seeds, and legumes also have high magnesium content. (See table 11.3 for magnesium content of various foods and food groups.) Since >80% of the magnesium in cereal grains is in the germ and bran, processed cereal products lose much of their magnesium content. A slice of whole wheat bread contains 33 mg of magnesium, while white bread contains only 8 mg per slice. Thus, diets high in processed and convenience foods may be low in magnesium. Based on U.S. dietary survey data, ~45% of the dietary magnesium comes from vegetables, fruits, grains, and nuts, while only 29% comes from dairy, meat, and eggs (IOM 1997). Water is a variable source of intake; harder water usually has a higher concentration of magnesium salts (IOM 1997).

As with zinc, the bioavailability of magnesium may be affected by a number of dietary factors. Large increases in the intake of dietary fiber have been found to decrease magnesium absorption in experimental studies. However, the extent to which dietary fiber affects magnesium status in individuals with a varied diet outside the laboratory is not clear (IOM 1997). Moreover, fiber-rich foods, such as fruits, vegetables, and whole grains, are also rich sources of magnesium, and thus the decreased absorption due to the fiber content is balanced out (Bohl and Volpe 2004). Other factors that have been shown to decrease magnesium absorption include phytates, unabsorbed fatty acids, and large intakes of supplemental zinc, calcium, and phosphorus. Inhibiting or promoting other dietary components can also influence magnesium absorption. Conversely, vitamin D and its metabolites 25-hydroxy vitamin D and 1, 25-dihydroxy vitamin D_3 have been found to enhance intestinal magnesium absorption (Rude and Shils 2006). Simple sugars, including lactose and fructose, may also enhance magnesium absorption (Gropper et al. 2009).

Chromium

The role of chromium in exercise is less well defined than the roles of the other minerals discussed thus far. According to current research, chromium's primary biological role is to potentiate the effect of insulin, thereby enhancing the uptake and utilization of carbohydrate, protein, and fat (Vincent 2003; IOM 2001). Chromium is a constituent of a complex known as **glucose tolerance factor (GTF),** which also contains nicotinic acid and various amino acids (Stoecker 2006a, 2006b). Although the exact physiological function of GTF is not known, one suggestion is that it facilitates the binding of insulin to its cellular receptor, increases the insulin receptor number, and improves insulin internalization and sensitivity (Anderson 1997; IOM 2001). This in turn would lower glucose levels and increase amino acid and fatty acid uptake after a meal. The amino acids would be used for tissue building and repair, and the fat and carbohydrate for either energy or storage. The role chromium plays in glucose uptake and metabolism has been confirmed in several small studies examining chromium supplementation in chromium-deficient individuals. For example, Anderson (1995) described patients on total parenteral nutrition who had symptoms suggestive of adult onset diabetes; the symptoms were reversed by chromium supplementation but not insulin administration. A recent meta-analysis examining the effect of chromium on glucose utilization in healthy individuals and those with diabetes showed no effect in healthy individuals, while the results in persons with diabetes were inconclusive (Althuis et al. 2002). In addition to its role in macronutrient metabolism, chromium has been shown to be important for growth, synthesis of DNA and RNA, and proper immune function (Stoecker 2006b).

Chromium is widely distributed throughout the body; tissues with particularly high concentrations include the kidney, liver, muscle, spleen, heart, pancreas, and bone. Chromium is often stored in tissues along with ferric iron, supposedly because of its transport by the iron-binding protein transferrin (Stoecker 2006b). In 2001, an Adequate Intake (AI) was set for chromium based on estimated mean dietary intakes. Because of insufficient evidence, an Estimated Average Requirement (EAR) for chromium was not set. The AI for chromium is 35 μg/day and 25 μg/day for adult men and women (19-50 years), respectively (IOM 2001). Pregnancy and lactation appear to increase chromium losses, and thus requirements are slightly higher during these times (30 μg/day and 45 μg/day, respectively). As discussed later in the chapter, some research suggests that exercise increases urinary chromium losses, which might imply a negative chromium balance and increased requirement in physically active individuals. Few serious adverse effects have been associated with excess intake of chromium from food; therefore, a UL was not established (IOM 2001).

The amount of chromium in foods appears to be quite variable and has been measured accurately in relatively few foods (IOM 2001). Thus, there is presently no large database for the chromium content of foods. Processed meats, whole grain products, wheat germ, ready-to-eat bran cereals, green beans, broccoli, mushrooms, and spices are believed to be relatively rich in chromium. Foods high in simple sugars, such as sucrose and fructose, not only are low in chromium but also have been found to promote chromium loss (IOM 2001). The chromium content of some foods is listed in table 11.4. Because chromium content in different batches of the same food has been found to vary significantly, the information in the table should serve only as a guide (Anderson et al. 1992). Beer and wine can also contain chromium due to processing. Cabrera-Vique and coworkers (1997) estimated that wine provides ~4.1 μg/day of chromium per resident in France, red wines having the highest chromium concentrations. Processing appears to have a variable effect on the chromium content of foods. Offenbacher and Pi-Sunyer (1983) documented the accumulation of chromium in foods that were heated in stainless steel containers (particularly those foods that are acidic). This leaching of chromium from steel containers also appears to explain why some foods, such as beers, contain significant amounts of chromium (Stoecker 2006a, 2006b).

Intestinal absorption of chromium is low (~0.5-3%), and absorption increases or decreases within this range depending on the chromium status and dietary chromium intake (Stoecker 2006a). A number of dietary factors appear to alter the availability of dietary chromium. For example, starch and ascorbic acid (vitamin C) increase absorption, while oxalates and phytates may either increase or decrease absorption depending on their concentration in the diet (Stoecker 2006a). High simple sugar intakes increase the loss of chromium in urine and decrease chromium absorption, while high iron intakes may alter chromium transport in the blood. Both chromium and iron are transported on transferrin. If transferrin is saturated

Table 11.4 Chromium Content of Selected Foods

Food	Serving size	Chromium (μg/serving)
Cheese, Edam	1 slice (24 g)	0.5
Milk, whole	1 cup (244 g)	2.4
Oysters, raw	3 oz (90 g)	13
Beef, ground, cooked	3 oz (85 g)	2.0
Turkey, boneless, breast, cooked	3 oz (85 g)	1.7
Turkey, boneless, leg, cooked	3 oz (85 g)	10.4
Corn Flakes	1 cup (25 g)	1.8
Brown rice (raw)	1/2 cup (198 g)	6.0
Apple, with peel, medium	1 each (150 g)	7.5
Banana, medium	1 each (118 g)	1.0
Orange juice	8 fl oz (249 g)	2.2
Broccoli, cooked	1 cup (156 g)	22.0
Green beans, cooked	1 cup (125 g)	2.2
Mushrooms, white	1/2 cup (35 g)	16
Potatoes, mashed with whole milk	1 cup (210)	2.7
Brewer's yeast	1 tbsp (8 g)	3.3
Bagel, plain, small	1 each	2.5
Cocoa	1 tbsp (5 g)	0.7
White wine	3.5 fl oz (102 g)	8
Beer	12 fl oz (360 g)	3.2

Adapted from R.A. Anderson, N.A. Bryden, and M.N. Polansky, 1992, "Dietary chromium intake. Freely chosen diets, institutional diets and individual foods," *Biological Trace Element Research* 32: 117-121.

with iron, then the ability to transport chromium is reduced and chromium must be transported on an alternative protein like albumin. The reverse also appears to be true. High intakes of chromium (>200 mg/day) apparently decrease iron absorption and transport and appear to negatively affect iron status (Lukaski, Bolonchuk et al. 1996). The impact of chromium supplementation on iron status may depend on the level of chromium and iron in the diet, initial iron status, and the length of chromium supplementation. Short-term chromium supplementation (<12 weeks) did not negatively affect iron status in older men engaged in a strength training program (Campbell et al. 1997).

ASSESSMENT OF MINERAL STATUS

Assessment of mineral status is different from the assessment of vitamin status in a number of ways:

- Bioavailability of dietary minerals is generally less than that of vitamins since a number of dietary factors can inhibit the absorption and the transport of minerals in the system. **Bioavailability** is defined as the proportion of any nutrient in food that is absorbed, transported, and utilized.

- For many minerals, total body homeostasis is regulated, in part, by limiting absorption of the mineral in the gut, thereby increasing the loss of excess mineral in the feces. In contrast, for most water-soluble vitamins, total body homeostasis is regulated largely through urinary excretion of the excess vitamin.

- To protect the body from toxic levels of minerals, absorption decreases as intake increases. The mineral may be absorbed into the intestinal mucosal cell but not transported into the system. In this way, the mineral is lost in the feces when the mucosal cell turns over. Although vitamin absorption also decreases as intake increases, for many (although not all) vitamins, the amounts absorbed in excess are readily excreted in the urine.

- Many minerals are found in trace amounts or in very specific foods in the diet. It is difficult to overload with diet alone; toxic levels are generally achieved only through supplementation or contamination.

- High mineral intakes (many times the RDA) are generally much more toxic than high vitamin intakes.

- Some trace minerals, like chromium, occur in quantities so small or are so highly variable in the food supply that it is difficult to accurately predict dietary intake as well as body-wide status.

- Many minerals compete with other minerals for absorption and transport. For example, high zinc intake can inhibit copper absorption when the two minerals are taken simultaneously. This nutrient–nutrient interaction occurs to a lesser extent with vitamins.

- Forms of minerals in food may vary, making minerals more or less bioavailable depending on their dietary source. Although vitamins also come in many different forms, bioavailability is generally less an issue than with minerals.

- Unlike vitamins, many minerals are lost in the sweat. The loss of minerals via sweat may be a contributing factor in total body mineral balance and may increase mineral requirements.

While dietary intake of a mineral can serve as a red flag for potential nutritional risk, alone it is insufficient to assess mineral status. Accurate assessment of an individual's mineral status generally requires biochemical measures of body fluids or tissues (or both) that reflect the body's stores of the mineral (see table 11.5). The amount of the mineral lost from the body in urine, blood, feces, sweat, or some combination of these should also be determined. If available, functional measurements of mineral status should also be included (Lukaski 2002; Lukaski and Penland 1996)—that is, measurements of the *availability* of the mineral to perform a particular physiological function within the body. For example, one might measure the activity of a specific mineral-dependent enzyme to determine if the body contains adequate levels of the mineral to support the enzymatic activity. Finally, a typical dietary intake of the mineral should be determined. Dietary factors that may increase or decrease bioavailability of the mineral should be identified, including supplemental vitamins and minerals, drugs, or food supplements.

The ideal mineral status measure would be specific to the mineral of interest and sensitive enough to distinguish not only sufficient from deficient status but also graded degrees of deficiency within those two distinct endpoints. It would reflect body stores of the mineral as well as adequacy of function and would respond proportionally to changes in dietary intake. It should also be practical, economical, and minimally invasive (Lukaski 2002). Unfortunately, at the present time, status measures of zinc, magnesium, and chromium that meet all of these requirements are not available. The most frequently utilized status measures for these minerals are discussed next. For a more thorough review on the topic, the reader is urged to consult Lukaski 2002 and Gibson 2005.

Table 11.5 Experimental Approaches for Assessment of Human Mineral Status

Approach	Variable	Standard
Diet records: 7 consecutive days of weighed (single common measure) food intake preferable; typical week (including exercise)	Assessment of daily absolute mineral intake (mg/day) and relative mineral intake (mg/1000 kcal); assessment of all supplemental mineral intake and all dietary factors that may influence mineral bioavailability	Average intake of a group compared against the Estimated Average Requirement believed to meet the needs of 50% of individuals in a specific life stage or gender group; average intake of an individual compared against the Recommended Dietary Allowance or Adequate Intake
Biochemical assessment—static test	Measurement of the amount or concentration of a given mineral in plasma, serum, erythrocyte, whole blood, tissues, or some combination of these	Within range of values for nutritionally adequate, gender-matched, control subjects or published standards
Biochemical assessment—functional measurement	Measurement of a mineral-specific function within a specific tissue or cell, for example, mineral-specific enzyme activity in erythrocytes, platelets, or leukocytes	Perturbation of response to a challenge that affects the performance of an integrated biological system or subsystem
Biochemical assessment—excretion losses	Measurement of urinary, fecal, blood, or sweat losses of minerals; includes basal excretion rates and excretion after a "load" (oral, IV) of a mineral	Alterations (increase or decrease) in absolute (mg/day) or relative (% of daily intake) amounts over some designated time period
Clinical measures	Assessment of overt signs and symptoms associated with mineral status (e.g., lips, gums, skin, eyes, hair, musculature and fat mass, etc.)	Comparison to nutritionally adequate; gender- and age-matched control subjects

Adapted from H.C. Lukaski ,1995, "Micronutrients (magnesium, zinc, and copper): Are mineral supplements needed for athletes?" *International Journal of Sport Nutrition* 5:S74-S83; H.C. Lukaski and J.G. Penland, 1996, "Functional changes appropriate for determining mineral element requirements," *Journal of Nutrition* 126: 2354S-2364S.

Zinc

Accurate assessment of zinc status is hampered by the lack of a single specific and sensitive biochemical or functional test in humans (King et al. 2000; King and Cousins 2006; Wood 2000). The most common method of assessing zinc status is to measure fasting levels of zinc in the plasma or serum (or both), even though these appear to be relatively insensitive to modest changes in dietary zinc intake or to changes in the total body zinc pool (Lukaski 2002; Wood 2000). As zinc deficiency occurs (e.g., low dietary zinc intakes), the body conserves zinc, making serum zinc unreliable as a measure of zinc status. In addition, serum zinc concentrations do not decrease unless dietary zinc intake is so low that the total zinc pool is decreased and homeostasis cannot be maintained (Gropper et al. 2005). Thus, serum zinc can be thought of as a labile pool of zinc that is part of the total body zinc pool. The body draws on this pool when intake is low; thus, low serum zinc is

an indication that the body's labile zinc pool is low and that dietary zinc intake is probably low also. Another problem with using serum or plasma zinc as a measure of zinc status is that a number of other factors, unrelated to poor zinc intake, can alter serum zinc concentrations (see "What Is the Difference Between Serum and Plasma?"). Exercise, stress, acute infection or inflammation, short-term fasting, or hormonal status can alter the distribution of zinc within the body, thus influencing the amount of zinc in the serum (Lukaski 2002, 2006b).

Erythrocyte zinc, while specific, is not particularly sensitive to marginal zinc deficiency (IOM 2001). Similarly, urinary zinc remains fairly constant over a range of intakes, diminishing only with severe zinc deficiency (Gropper et al. 2009). Recently, hair analysis has gained attention as a method of assessing zinc status. It should be noted that this method, while appealing because it is noninvasive, is indicative only of chronic zinc intake; thus, it is not sufficiently sensitive. Moreover, the concentration of zinc in hair will depend not only on the delivery of zinc to the hair root but also on the rate of hair growth, which is readily affected by a number of other factors, including energy balance and protein status. Contamination (e.g. shampoos, perms, and coloring) can also confound interpretation of zinc hair analysis (Gropper et al. 2009).

Zinc status can also be assessed via measurement of the activity of one or more zinc-dependent enzymes. The procedure involves measuring either the basal activity of the enzyme or the ratio of basal enzyme activity to stimulated enzyme activity—that is, the difference between the enzyme activity before and after a zinc load. If enzyme activity is low at baseline but increases with the addition of zinc, then the assumption is that zinc status was inadequate or poor. Given the large number of zinc-dependent enzymes that have been identified, it is somewhat surprising that no single enzyme has found broad acceptance as an indicator of zinc status. Part of the problem is the lack of enzyme specificity; that is, for many of the zinc-dependent enzymes, zinc deficiency is not the only factor that can alter enzymatic activity. In addition, there are likely homeostatic processes in place that maintain zinc occupancy of the catalytic sites of these enzymes. Other factors include a lack of sensitivity, the inaccessibility of optimal tissues to assay, and inadequate research to determine normative values. Given these limitations, the activities of zinc-dependent enzymes, including alkaline phosphatase, carbonic anhydrase, nucleoside phosphorylase, and ribonuclease, can

at most serve as supportive indicators of dietary zinc status (Lukaski 2002).

As previously mentioned, zinc is essential for the integrity of the immune system, and thus inadequate zinc intake would be expected to have many adverse effects (Gleeson et al. 2004; Wintergerst et al. 2006, 2007). Unfortunately, while changes in immune function are sensitive to even mild zinc deficiency, the effects on functional indices of zinc status are not specific. At this time, therefore, changes in indices of immune status with manipulation of dietary zinc can serve only as a limited indicator for dietary zinc requirements. Other suggested functional measures for zinc are resting metabolic rate, ethanol metabolism, and cognitive performance measures (Lukaski and Penland 1996). Again, the lack of specificity of these measures, as well as the lack of normative values, limits their usefulness for measuring zinc status. Finally, a zinc tolerance test based on the plasma zinc increase after an oral zinc "load" of 25 to 50 mg has been described in the literature, although it has not attained widespread use as a status measure (King and Cousins 2006).

In summary, because there is no single assessment parameter for zinc that is optimally specific, sensitive, and valid, clinicians and researchers often use a combination of biochemical and functional measures to assess status. These assessment parameters should always be accompanied by the measurement of dietary zinc intakes and evaluated with respect to dietary and physiological factors that could potentially confound zinc bioavailability.

Highlight

What Is the Difference Between Serum and Plasma?

Plasma is the noncellular portion of the circulating blood; serum is the noncellular portion of the blood that is obtained after coagulation of the blood. To obtain plasma, blood is drawn in a tube containing an anticoagulant and then centrifuged (spun). The cells of the blood settle to the bottom of the tube, and the plasma is left on top. To obtain serum, blood is drawn in a tube that does not contain an anticoagulant. The clotting factors in the blood settle to the bottom of the tube, with the cells, when the tube is centrifuged; what remains on top is serum. Depending on the biochemical assay being done, you may need serum or plasma. Sometimes either is acceptable. In general, minerals are usually measured in serum to avoid any mineral contamination that might occur due to the additives used as anticoagulants. For example, with zinc and magnesium, it is usually serum that is measured, but plasma is also acceptable as long as the anticoagulant is free of mineral contamination.

Magnesium

As with zinc, there is no single, specific, reliable biochemical marker for magnesium status (Rude and Shils 2006; Lukaski 2002). Assessment of magnesium status is complicated by the fact that only ~1% of total body magnesium is found extracellularly and it is tightly homeostatically regulated (Gropper et al. 2009). Moreover, the concentration of magnesium in serum has not been shown to correlate with the concentration in any other tissue pools except, perhaps, interstitial fluid (Lukaski 2002). Nonetheless, total serum magnesium remains the most commonly used index for determining magnesium status, despite its low sensitivity and specificity (e.g., serum levels may remain normal despite intracellular deficiencies). One reason for this is that better indices are not readily available. In addition, there does appear to be a correlation between serum magnesium and magnesium intake such that serum magnesium declines when dietary magnesium is low. This point is illustrated in figure 11.1, which shows that both serum and urinary magnesium concentrations decrease when magnesium is removed from the diet. However, a number of other factors—such as various diseases and stressors, artificial factors (e.g., dehydration, medications, or drugs being used), and diurnal variations—can also alter serum magnesium concentration; thus, it is not an ideal indicator of status. As mentioned earlier, serum represents only a small portion of the body's total magnesium pool (<1%) (Gibson 2005). Normal serum magnesium ranges from 0.8 to 1.2 mmol/L (Lukaski 1995) and comprises three general components: ionized or unbound magnesium (55% of serum magnesium), complexed magnesium (13%), and bound magnesium (32%) (Gibson 2005; Rude and Shils 2006). Magnesium that is bound to

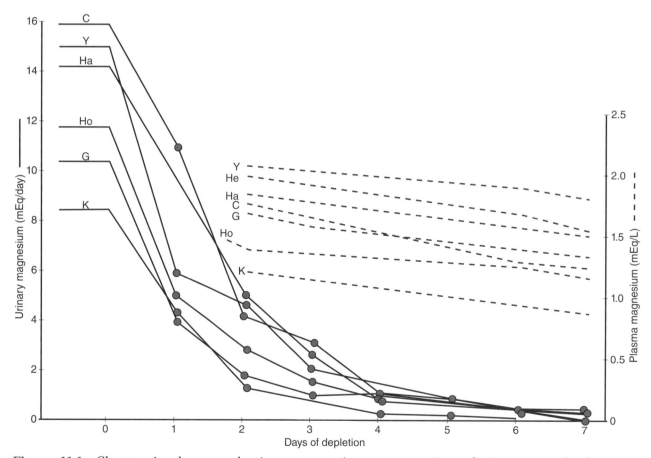

Figure 11.1 Changes in plasma and urinary magnesium concentrations during one week of a zero-magnesium diet. The rapid decrease in magnesium excretion is depicted in six subjects. By the 10th day, all plasma values except that of Y were more than two standard deviations below the normal mean. Letters indicate individual subjects.

Reprinted, by permission, from M.E. Shils, 1994, Magnesium. In *Modern nutrition in health and disease,* 8th ed., edited by M.E. Shils, J.A. Olson, and M. Shike (Philadelphia, PA: Lippincott, Williams, and Wilkins), 172.

transport proteins (e.g., albumin or globulin), or complexed with other substances in the blood (e.g., citrate or phosphate), seems to vary with changes in the concentrations of such ligands and acid–base conditions. It has thus been suggested that the level of ionized magnesium may be a more reliable clinical measure of magnesium status (Lukaski 2002), yet work still needs to be done to validate this as a reliable status marker.

Erythrocyte magnesium concentrations are frequently measured and appear to reflect chronic magnesium status, since the half-life of the red cell is 120 days and concentrations decrease only after several weeks of poor magnesium intake (Gibson 2005). However, as with serum magnesium, erythrocyte magnesium has not been shown to be a significant predictor of tissue magnesium concentrations, and a number of factors unrelated to dietary magnesium may influence erythrocyte magnesium concentrations (e.g., hormonal status, hypertension) (Lukaski 2002). More recently, magnesium concentrations of the mononucleated white cell have been examined as a possible indicator of cellular magnesium status (Lukaski 2002). While the magnesium concentration of mononucleated white cells does not correlate with serum or erythrocyte magnesium, data from both human and animal models suggest that these values reflect cardiac and muscle tissue magnesium content (Gibson 2005; Lukaski 2002). Unfortunately, current clinical data have not been supportive of this hypothesis (Rude and Shils 2006).

Urinary magnesium excretion, in combination with dietary magnesium intake, can provide some insight into magnesium status (Gibson 2005). In someone with normal renal function, excretion of >80% of an intravenous magnesium load within 24 h is considered normal (Gibson 2005). In contrast, when magnesium intake (or absorption) is inadequate, there is a fairly rapid and significant reduction in urinary magnesium excretion (Rude and Shils 2006).

Currently, there are no good functional measures of magnesium status. In fact, the only viable functional test is the magnesium load test (Lukaski 2002; Rude and Shils 2006). This test involves first the IV infusion (or oral consumption) of a large dose of magnesium and then the collection of urinary magnesium for at least 24 h. Individuals retaining more than 20% to 25% of the magnesium load are considered to have some body depletion (Rude and Shils 2006). Unfortunately, this test is not standardized and is expensive, invasive, and time-consuming; it also requires hospitalization (or other close supervision) for the full 24 h urine collection and thus is not practical outside a research setting (Rude and Shils 2006).

Like zinc, magnesium is lost in sweat; thus, active individuals with high sweat rates may have increased magnesium losses. Sweat losses of magnesium are estimated to be ~1.5 to 7 mg/L, with estimates of 15 to 18 mg of magnesium lost per day in hot environments (Montain et al. 2007; Lukaski 1995). The amount of magnesium lost in the sweat represents approximately 10% to 15% of total daily magnesium losses (feces, urine, and sweat losses combined), including 4% to 5% of the daily requirement for men and 5% to 6% of the requirement for women (Bohl and Volpe 2004; DeRuisseau et al. 2002; Lukaski 1995). Since no single reliable assessment measure is available, most clinicians use a combination of static biochemical measures and determination of dietary magnesium intake to assess magnesium status.

Chromium

Currently, no reliable indicator of chromium status exists. Although chromium concentrations can be measured in a number of biological fluids and tissues, none is specific enough to serve as a good marker of chromium status. In addition, chromium is present in such trace amounts that it is difficult to measure accurately, and contamination can easily occur. Blood or serum chromium concentrations do not appear to reflect tissue concentrations in periods of marginal chromium depletion (Gropper et al. 2009), although serum chromium concentrations have been shown to be low in individuals with chromium deficiency and high serum concentrations may indicate excessive environmental exposure to chromium (Stoecker 2006b).

Assessment of hair chromium may reflect endogenous chromium available to the hair, but the samples need to be carefully prepared to prevent chromium contamination from other sources (no bleaches or dyes). In addition, a number of other factors appear to influence hair chromium concentrations, such as age, hair growth rate, pregnancy, and diabetes. Thus, hair chromium does not reflect solely dietary chromium intake (Gibson 2005). Urinary chromium is frequently used as an index of chromium status because the kidneys appear to regulate chromium homeostasis (Gibson 2005; Stoecker 2006b). Unfortunately, changes in urinary chromium better reflect increases in total body chromium (induced by excessive chromium intakes or exposure) than deficiencies. Urinary chromium can be used to determine if chromium supplements are being used or if an individual has been exposed to high environmental chromium levels. However, no data are available demonstrating that decreased urinary chromium excretion indicates moderate chromium deficiency (Gibson 2005). A number of confounding factors also affect urinary chromium concentrations, such as diurnal variations, industrial exposure, dietary glucose or sucrose intake, recent dietary intake of chromium, acute strenuous exercise, trauma, medications (e.g. aspirin, antacids, corticosteroids), and diabetes (Gibson 2005).

Currently, the best method for diagnosing chromium deficiency is to observe whether chromium supplementation improves glucose tolerance (Gibson 2005). This method requires the administration of two **oral glucose tolerance tests (OGTTs).** The first OGTT determines the baseline response to a glucose load (75 g glucose, or 1 g glucose per kilogram body weight); the second test is done after supplementation with physiological levels of chromium. After each OGTT, the total area under the curve is determined. If the area under the curve decreases with chromium supplementation, then poor chromium status is indicated. This test is very time-consuming, is expensive, requires numerous blood samples, and is not practical for clinical diagnosis.

RATIONALE FOR INCREASED NEED FOR ACTIVE INDIVIDUALS

Because minerals are cofactors for many energy-producing metabolic reactions, it is only natural to hypothesize that exercise could increase the need for these nutrients. Minerals are also necessary for other biological functions important for exercise, such as the synthesis and repair of muscle tissues, a healthy immune function, and cell reproduction. Finally, by increasing mineral loss in urine or sweat, exercise may alter the body's overall mineral balance and increase the intakes required to maintain good status. Despite the soundness of the hypothesis, there is currently little direct evidence to suggest that exercise negatively affects mineral status, thereby increasing mineral requirements. As discussed previously in the chapter, research on the specific impact of exercise on mineral status is hampered by

the lack of specific, sensitive, accurate, and valid measures of status as well as the inability to accurately interpret the measures currently available (i.e., lack of good "norms"). Nonetheless, dietary intake data as well as some limited biochemical evidence suggest that some athletes may be at risk for mineral deficiency.

As people become more physically active, it is logical to assume that they will increase their energy intake and thus their dietary intakes of minerals—so that there should be no need for mineral supplements. Unfortunately, this is not always the case. If individuals make poor dietary choices, their mineral intake may not increase in parallel with their higher energy intake. And, if people increase physical activity but fail to increase their energy intake (to cover the additional energy expenditure), the overall need for minerals may increase. This is especially true for active individuals or athletes who are restricting energy intake for weight loss. One might speculate that an easy fix to the problem would be to supplement with minerals; yet there are problems with casually adding mineral supplements to the diet. High supplements of one mineral may change the bioavailability and status of another. Moreover, as discussed earlier, some minerals can be toxic even at doses only slightly above the RDA. For these reasons, it is important to examine a person's overall mineral intake and status before making dietary and supplemental mineral recommendations.

The following section briefly reviews the dietary intakes of active individuals for zinc, magnesium, and chromium. Dietary intakes of these minerals are compared to the typical American diet as well as the respective DRIs and EARs. In 1997, a new RDA for magnesium was determined; the new RDAs for zinc and chromium were published in 2001 (IOM 1997, 2001). Because many studies examining the intakes of these minerals in active people were done before the new RDAs were published, in some cases intakes are compared to the 1989 RDA (FNB 1989). Chapter 12 reviews the dietary intakes of iron and copper in active people.

Zinc

Results of two national surveys, the National Health and Nutrition Examination Survey (NHANES III 1988-1994) (IOM 2001) and the Continuing Survey of Food Intakes of Individuals (1994 CSFII) (Interagency Board for Nutrition Monitoring and Related Research 1995), indicate that most infants, children, and adults consume the recommended amounts of zinc.

Self-reported dietary zinc intakes of active males and male athletes are usually well above the current EAR (9.4 mg/day) and at or above the current RDA (11 mg/day). Table 11.6 gives the dietary zinc intakes of active men who did not take zinc supplements: No study indicated mean intakes in men to be less than the EAR, and most reported mean intakes were above the current RDA. As is true in the general female population, female athletes are more likely than their male counterparts to have inadequate zinc intakes. The lower zinc intakes of active women are usually attributed to their overall lower energy intake and lower intakes of zinc-rich foods (i.e., protein-rich animal products). Nonetheless, interpretation of zinc intakes among active women is complicated by the fact that many of the data were collected before the new (2001) RDA for zinc was published. Using the old RDA (12 mg/day), only one study listed in table 11.6 showed mean zinc intakes for active women above the RDA. Conversely, using the new EAR (6.8 mg/day) or RDA (8.0 mg/day), none of the studies indicated that mean intakes were inadequate. As highlighted in the table, athletes participating in sports that emphasize leanness (e.g., long-distance running, gymnastics, ballet) generally have lower mean zinc intakes than athletes participating in sports that do not (basketball, handball).

Magnesium

Dietary survey data indicate that magnesium intakes of Americans average about 329 mg/day (94% of the EAR; 78% of the 1997 RDA) for men

Table 11.6 Incidence of Low or Marginal Zinc (Zn) and Magnesium (Mg) Status in Nonsupplemented Active People

Study	Assessment indices	Subjects	Low status (%)	Mean dietary intake (mg/day)
Zinc				
Beals and Manore 1998	Serum Zn, 7-day weighed food record[1]	24 control female athletes 24 SCED female athletes	0% 0%	10.4 9.7
Couzy et al. 1990	Serum Zn	6 male middle-distance runners	0%	–
Dressendorfer et al. 2002	Serum Zn, maintained typical diets; no Zn supplements	9 male cyclists	0%	–
Deuster et al. 1989	Plasma and RBC Zn, 24 h urinary Zn, oral Zn load, 3-day food record	13 female runners	100%	10.3
Fogelholm, Rehunen et al. 1992	Serum Zn, 28-day food record	5 male elite Nordic skiers 7 female elite Nordic skiers	0% 0%	21.9 15.8
Fogelholm, Himberg et al. 1992	Serum Zn, FFQ	418 male athletes	1%	17.5
Fogelholm et al. 1991	Serum Zn, RBC Zn, FFQ	114 male endurance athletes	0%	17.7
Koury et al. 2004	Plasma Zn, RBC Zn, 2 to 24 h recalls	44 male triathletes, runners, swimmers	0%	14.0[3]
Lukaski et al. 1990	Plasma Zn, 7-day food record	13 male swimmers 16 female swimmers	0% 0%	15.6 10.4
Lukaski, Siders et al. 1996	Plasma Zn, 3-day food record	5 male swimmers 5 female swimmers	0% 0%	17.6 10.5
Lukaski et al. 2001	Plasma, urine, fecal Zn; metabolic diet for 28 days (55% energy CHO)	3 male cyclists	0%	23.9

(continued)

Table 11.6   (continued)

Study	Assessment indices	Subjects	Low status (%)	Mean dietary intake (mg/day)
Manore et al. 1993	Serum Zn, 9-day weighed food record	34 trained males	0%	10.8*
Nuviala et al. 1999	Serum Zn, urinary Zn 7-day weighed food record	65 female nonathletic controls	1.5%	8.5
		19 female basketball players	0%	11.9
		20 female handball players	0%	10.0
		16 female karate participants	0%	9.0
		23 female runners	0%	9.2
Singh, Moses and Deuster 1992	Plasma, RBC, urinary Zn,[2] 4-day food record	11 active males	0%	10.8*
Telford et al. 1992	Serum Zn	44 male and female athletes[2]	2%	–
Weight et al. 1988	Serum Zn, 5-day food record	30 male runners	0%	13.2
Magnesium				
Beals and Manore 1998	Serum Mg, 7-day weighed food record	24 control female athletes	0%	351
		24 SCED female athletes	0%	283*
Dressendorfer et al. 2002	Serum Mg, maintained typical diets; no Mg supplements	9 male cyclists	0%	–
Fogelholm, Himberg et al. 1992	Serum Mg, FFQ	418 male athletes	0%	510
Fogelholm et al. 1991	Serum Mg, RBC Mg, FFQ	114 male endurance athletes	0%	548
Lukaski, Siders et al. 1996	Serum Mg, 3-day food record	5 male swimmers	0%	393*
		5 female swimmers	0%	269*
Lukaski et al. 2001	Plasma, urine, fecal Mg; metabolic diet for 28 days (55% energy CHO)	3 male cyclists	0%	518
Manore et al. 1995	Serum Mg, RBC Mg, urinary Mg, 9-day weighed food record	34 males in a 12-week exercise program	0%	330*
Nuviala et al. 1999	Serum Mg, urinary Mg, 7-day weighed food record	65 female nonathletic controls	4.6%	213*+
		19 female basketball players	0%	258*+
		20 female handball players	10%	244*+
		16 female karate participants	18.7%	218*+
		23 female runners	0%	259*+
Singh, Moses and Deuster 1992	Plasma, RBC, and urinary Mg, 4-day food record	11 active males	0%	355*
Telford et al. 1992	Serum Mg	44 male and female athletes	0%	–
Weight et al. 1988	Serum Mg, 5-day food record	30 male runners	0%	372*

FFQ = food frequency questionnaire; CHO = carbohydrate; RBC = red blood cell; SCED = subclinical eating disorder.

[1] 25% of subjects supplemented with some type of vitamin or mineral supplement.

[2] Data from placebo group (no supplements).

[3] 27% of athletes had zinc intakes <11 mg/day.

* Mean value is less than the Recommended Dietary Allowance (RDA). RDA for zinc is 8 mg/day for women and 11 mg/day for men (IOM 2001); RDA for magnesium is 310 mg/day for women 1 to 30 years, 320 mg/day for women 31 to 70 years, 410 mg/day for men 19 to 30 years, and 420 mg/day for men 31 to 70 years (IOM 1997).

+ Mean value is less than the Estimated Average Requirement (EAR). EAR for zinc is 6.8 for women and 9.4 for men (IOM 2001); EAR for magnesium is 265 mg/day for women and 350 mg/day for men.

and 207 mg/day for women (78% of the EAR; 65% of the 1997 RDA) (IOM 1997). The 1982-1991 Total Diet Studies indicated that for males aged 14 to 16 years and 25 to 30 years, magnesium intake was 75% and 86% of the 1989 RDA (FNB 1989), respectively (Pennington 1996). For females of the same age groups, magnesium intake was 65% and 70% of the 1989 RDA (FNB 1989), respectively (Pennington 1996). Similarly, data from the CSFII indicated average magnesium intakes of 323 mg/day for men and 228 mg/day for women. Intakes were even lower for men and women over 70 years of age (Alaimo 1994). According to the new RDA for magnesium, these intakes are ~65% to 85% of the EAR and 53% to 73% of the RDA, suggesting that most American adults consume at least 66% of the 1997 RDA for magnesium; however, the magnesium intakes of younger females, aged 14 to 16 years, appear to be low (IOM 1997).

The magnesium density of the typical American diet is ~120 mg of magnesium per 1000 kcal (IOM 1997). On the basis of this nutrient density, the typical man would need to consume 3500 kcal/day and the typical woman would need to consume 2666 kcal/day to meet the 1997 RDA for magnesium. These estimates demonstrate the importance of total energy intake in relation to dietary magnesium intake. People who reduce energy intake without increasing the magnesium density of the diet (mg/1000 kcal) will consume inadequate levels of magnesium.

The magnesium intake of active people appears to be similar to that reported for the typical adult in the United States. Most studies published before release of the new RDAs showed mean magnesium intakes of athletes or active individuals at or above two-thirds of the 1989 RDA (FNB 1989), which was 350 mg/day for men and 280 mg/day for women (Clarkson and Haymes 1995; Jensen et al. 1992). As mentioned earlier, in 1997 the RDA for magnesium increased for both men (to 410-420 mg/day) and women (to 310-320 mg/day). Table 11.6 shows that mean magnesium intakes of male athletes are usually well above both the 1989 RDA and the 1997 EAR (350 mg/day and 265 mg/day for men and women, respectively) but below the 1997 RDA. The lowest reported levels for men (Manore et al. 1995) were for males participating in fitness-type exercise, whose mean intakes were 80% of the 1997 RDA. No studies have reported mean intakes for magnesium less than two-thirds of the RDA among male athletes. The high magnesium intake of male athletes is frequently attributed to their high energy intakes. Table 11.6 shows that mean magnesium intakes of female athletes also appear to be at or near the new EAR but below the new RDA for magnesium.

Researchers examining the magnesium intakes of female athletes often find that they are below the RDA (Hinton et al. 2004; Jonnalagadda et al. 2004; Nuviala et al. 1999; Papadopoulou et al. 2002). For example, Nuviala and colleagues (1999) found that the magnesium intakes among 78 women competing in a variety of sports, including karate, handball, basketball, and running, were well below the current RDA as well as the EAR. One needs to consider two issues when looking at these data: (1) whether athletes underreported their energy intake while self-reporting weight stability and (2) whether the athletes were trying to lose weight, therefore, were not eating as much as expected. As mentioned earlier, if energy intake is restricted, magnesium intakes can be low. For example, Beals and Manore (1998) reported that mean intakes of magnesium among athletes with subclinical eating disorders (283 mg/day) were less than the current RDA, while 54% were consuming less than the old RDA. In contrast, mean intakes among the control athletes exceeded the current RDA, and only 17% of the control athletes consumed less than the old RDA. In this study, the athletes with subclinical eating disorders reported consuming only 1989 kcal/day, while the control athletes consumed 2293 kcal/day—closer to the energy requirement needed to meet the RDA for magnesium.

Three other studies dramatically demonstrate the effect of low energy intakes on dietary magnesium in female athletes. Baer and Tapper (1992) reported that eumenorrheic runners consuming 1644 kcal/day took in only 148 mg/day of magnesium (~56% of the EAR), while amenorrheic runners consuming 1912 kcal/day obtained 224 mg/day (84% of the EAR). Kaiserauer and colleagues (1989) also reported that among female runners who consumed less than 1582 kcal/day, 55% had magnesium intakes less than 280 mg/day. Finally, Clark and colleagues (2003) examined the diets of National Collegiate Athletic Association female soccer players at the beginning and end of their season. During the preseason, mean energy intakes were 2290 kcal/day and mean magnesium intake was low, at 178 mg/day (RDA = 320 mg/day; 56% of RDA). By postseason, energy intakes had decreased to 1865 kcal/day, with an even further decrease in magnesium intake (127 mg/day; 40% of RDA and 48% of EAR). From these data it is easy to see that as energy intakes decrease, intake of magnesium decreases unless food is selected carefully to keep micronutrient intake high. This was demonstrated by Beshgetoor and Nichols (2003), who examined the diets of master female cyclists and runners (mean age = 50.4 years) using four-day diet records. They compared the diets of those who supplemented and those who did not (mean energy intake = 2079 kcal/day and 2001 kcal/day, respectively). They found that the mean magnesium intakes of both groups (supplements = 601 ± 58 mg/day; no supplements = 366 ± 45 mg/day) met the RDA for magnesium. Thus, it is possible to meet the dietary requirements if careful food selections are made.

Chromium

Since there are no reliable nutrient databases for chromium, determining chromium intake is difficult, and few researchers have attempted it. Anderson and Kozlovsky (1985) examined the typical chromium intakes of 10 men and 22 women for seven days using duplicate meal analyses. Average intake for male subjects was 33 µg/day (range: 22-48 µg/day), which is below the current AI, while females consumed on average the AI of 25 µg/day (range: 13-36 µg/day). Additional information supporting low chromium intakes among adults in the United States comes from chromium supplement studies, which indicate that approximately 50% of the subjects show improvement in glucose tolerance with chromium supplementation (Anderson 1995, 1997). These data suggest that the current chromium intake in the United States is not optimal. To date, no study has addressed dietary chromium intake in active people. However, if we use the chromium data reported for the typical American diet, it is safe to assume that unless active people are making good dietary choices, chromium intake may be inadequate.

NUTRITIONAL STATUS OF ACTIVE PEOPLE

Attempts to determine the effects of exercise on the metabolism of and requirements for zinc, magnesium, and chromium have been hampered by the lack of biochemical indices of mineral status that are sensitive, specific, and reliable, as well as by the use of varied experimental designs, which make comparing studies difficult (Lukaski 2004). This section briefly reviews the limited available research documenting the impact of exercise (acute, chronic, or both) on zinc, magnesium, and

chromium status in active individuals. For a more in-depth review, see the work of Bohl and Volpe (2004), Lukaski (2004), and Nielsen and Lukaski (2006).

Zinc

Both acute and chronic exercise appear to significantly affect zinc metabolism. Research indicates that serum zinc increases immediately after acute strenuous exercise (Anderson et al. 1995; Deuster et al. 1991; Hetland et al. 1975; Lukaski et al. 1984). For example, Deuster and colleagues (1991) measured serum zinc concentrations before and after the first women's Olympic marathon trials in May 1984. Immediately after exercise, serum zinc concentrations were 10% above prerace values, but they returned to baseline or below baseline concentrations within 30 min to 24 h postexercise. Similarly, serum zinc levels were 19% higher than prerace values immediately following a 70 km (43-mile) cross-country ski race, but returned to prerace values the day after the race (Hetland et al. 1975). Interestingly, erythrocyte zinc levels, which are typically 10 times higher than serum levels, were not altered by the acute exercise bout. This phenomenon does not appear to be restricted to endurance exercise. Mundie and Hare (2001) examined the effects of resistance exercise on plasma, erythrocyte, and urinary zinc levels in 12 male cadets. Plasma zinc levels were elevated at 5 and 30 min postexercise (by as much as 225%) but returned to baseline levels by 24 h postexercise. Moreover, the increases in plasma zinc levels in this study were significantly greater than those seen in studies employing endurance exercise protocols.

The magnitude of the increase in serum zinc immediately postexercise cannot be explained by hemoconcentration alone. It has been hypothesized that the increase in serum zinc results from leakage of zinc from damaged muscle tissue into the extracellular fluid or from a redistribution of zinc from other tissues to the serum (Cordova and Alvarez-Mon 1995; Lukaski 2006b; Ohno et al. 1985). This point was demonstrated by Mundie and Hare (2001), who found that plasma zinc increased dramatically after moderate and heavy resistance exercise but returned to baseline levels within 24 h postexercise. The return of serum zinc concentrations to preexercise levels (and occasionally below) during the recovery period may be due to increased loss of zinc in the urine, or possibly to the uptake of zinc by other tissues (e.g., liver or muscles) or reuptake by the erythrocytes. If exercise causes an increase in urinary zinc losses, then overall zinc balance could be negatively affected. Research examining the effect of exercise on urinary zinc losses has been equivocal. For example, Anderson and colleagues (1984) observed a 50% increase in runners' urinary zinc 1 h after a 10-mile (16 km) race, but others have reported no changes in urinary zinc excretion after exercise (Anderson et al. 1995; Buchman et al. 1998; Mundie and Hare 2001; Singh, Moses et al. 1992). These inconsistencies may result in part from differences in exercise duration and intensity, in the fitness levels of the subjects, and in dietary zinc intakes.

In contrast to acute exercise, chronic exercise may result in a decrease in plasma zinc levels that may or may not be indicative of compromised status; however, the data are equivocal. For example, Couzy and colleagues (1990) found that serum zinc levels were significantly decreased after five months of intensive training among six highly trained athletes, an effect that was independent of dietary intake. Similarly, Ohno and colleagues (1990) reported that 10 weeks of endurance training (running more than 5 km [3 miles], six times a week) in previously sedentary men resulted in a reduction of circulating exchangeable zinc. Dressendorfer and Sockolov (1980) observed that runners ($n = 77$) had significantly lower serum zinc concentrations than controls ($n = 21$). Eighteen of the runners (23% of the group) had serum zinc concentrations <11.5 mmol/L. These investigators also reported that serum zinc concentrations were inversely related to weekly training distance. These data have been supported by subsequent observations of low resting serum zinc concentrations in athletes (Deuster et al. 1989; Haralambie 1981; Miyamura et al. 1987; Singh et al. 1991). However, not all data are supportive. Dressendorfer and colleagues (2002) observed that male cyclists participating in a high-volume training program (six weeks) did not show a drop in resting serum zinc. The cyclists consumed their typical diet and did not supplement; however, energy intake could have increased during the training period, which may have increased zinc intake naturally.

For those studies showing decreases in serum zinc with training, it is possible that the findings are due to one or more of the following factors:

- Endurance athletes have low dietary zinc intakes because their diets are high in carbohydrate and lower in meat.
- Endurance athletes have higher zinc losses in sweat.
- Skeletal muscle breakdown in endurance athletes may increase urinary zinc losses.

Indeed, sweat and urinary zinc losses have often been implicated in the lower serum zinc levels seen in endurance athletes. Sweat zinc losses appear to depend on the location from which the sweat is collected, on exercise intensity and duration, and on environmental conditions (Lukaski 1995, 2006b; Montain et al. 2007). Losses of trace minerals in sweat are hard to measure because of their low concentration, the technical problems of measuring total sweat losses, and the high probability of sample contamination from body cells and handling techniques. Given these problems with zinc sweat measurements, Tipton and colleagues (1993) measured arm sweat rates in male and female athletes exercising at 50% $\dot{V}O_2$max for 1 h in a neutral and in a hot environment. Sweat zinc concentrations ranged from 0.35 to 1.5 mg/mL. These figures imply that the zinc lost in 1 L of sweat would range from 0.35 to 1.5 mg, or from 2% to 13% of total daily recommended zinc intakes. The impact that zinc sweat losses have on total zinc balance depends on total sweat losses, zinc lost through other routes, and total zinc intake. Montain and colleagues (2007) measured zinc losses in six males and one female during exercise in the heat (27° and 35° C) for 5 h. They found that zinc sweat rates declined 42% to 45% after the first hour of exercise, regardless of the level of sweat rate; zinc sweat rates ranged from 0.66 mg/mL during the first hour to 0.36 mg/mL during the last hour of exercise.

It should be noted that not all studies have shown low serum zinc concentrations in athletes. Moreover, even in studies documenting a reduction in serum zinc, levels often do not drop below "normal" values. Table 11.6 lists studies of serum zinc concentrations in active people. It is noteworthy that few of these papers indicate mean serum zinc concentrations below normal or lower than levels in controls (see the "Low status" column). Among the researchers listed, only Deuster and colleagues (1989) observed poor zinc status, in 13 female runners who averaged 57 miles (92 km) a week. Their mean dietary zinc intake was 10.3 mg/day, and mean serum zinc concentration was 10.1 mmol/L (<12 mmol/L is considered low). In addition, the runners had significantly higher 24 h urinary zinc concentrations than sedentary controls with similar dietary zinc intake. In this study, the lower dietary zinc intakes and the higher urinary zinc losses could have contributed to the lower serum zinc concentrations observed. Sweat zinc, which was not measured, could also have contributed to total zinc losses. Earlier studies also indicated that intense exercise training depresses serum zinc concentrations, with or without altering urinary zinc losses. Singh and colleagues (1991) observed a 33% decrease in serum zinc concentrations in 66 men participating in the U.S. Navy Seal Hell Week. During this five-day period, the subjects participated in strenuous physical exercise and endured psychological stress and were allowed only 5 h of sleep. Energy and zinc intakes were high (5830 kcal/day; 23.6 mg/day of zinc), but urinary zinc losses did not increase during the five-day period. Miyamura and colleagues (1987) monitored 30 U.S. Army male soldiers during a 34-day intensive training camp in Hawaii. Subjects consumed approximately 17.3 mg/day of zinc (157% of the current RDA). By the end of the training period, serum zinc had decreased 14%, and 24 h urinary zinc had increased 171%. These results suggest that severe exercise training can affect zinc metabolism and could compromise zinc status if continued for an extended period of time, especially if zinc intake is low.

Another explanation for depressed serum zinc concentrations in some active people may be that the low levels are only transient, due to the body's response to changes in exercise intensity or duration. Manore and colleagues (1993) measured serum and urinary zinc changes in men participating in either a 12-week aerobic or a 12-week aerobic-anaerobic training program. Serum zinc concentrations had significantly decreased by week 6 of the aerobic training program but returned to baseline concentrations by week 12. The opposite occurred in the aerobic-anaerobic exercise program; serum zinc concentrations had significantly increased by week 6 but returned to baseline by week 12. These results may help explain the inconsistencies in data regarding changes in plasma or serum zinc levels with different exercise programs (Couzy et al. 1990; Dressendorfer and Sockolov 1980; Lukaski et al. 1990; Singh et al. 1991) and differences between athletes and controls (Fogelholm et al. 1991; Fogelholm, Himberg et al. 1992). When athletes change either the intensity or duration of their exercise, they may undergo a period of adaptation during which zinc homeostasis is altered. If blood samples are taken during this period of adaptation, the values may be abnormal compared to norms or compared to values in control groups.

What are the health and performance consequences of low serum zinc? Can low levels affect health and exercise performance? Theoretically, yes, although research supporting this hypothesis is somewhat scarce. Low serum zinc has been associated with muscular fatigue (Cordova and Alvarez-Mon 1995). Moreover, some limited research suggests that zinc supplementation can enhance muscle strength and endurance. Using an animal model, Richardson and Drake (1974) found that zinc supplementation enhanced in vitro muscle contraction. Similarly, in a crossover, placebo-controlled, double-blind study, muscle strength and endurance were improved in middle-aged women supplemented with 30 mg/day of zinc for 14 days (Krotkiewski et al. 1982). The authors hypothesized that zinc supplementation enhanced the activity of lactate dehydrogenase, a zinc-dependent enzyme.

However, other researchers have questioned this metabolic rationale. Lukaski (2004) has proposed that the observed effects of zinc on performance are due to zinc's role as a cofactor for carbonic anhydrase, an enzyme that regulates the elimination of carbon dioxide from cells. In a recently published study, Lukaski (2005) examined the effects of low zinc intake on carbonic anhydrase activity in red blood cells and cardiorespiratory function during exercise. In this double-blind, randomized crossover study, 14 men (20-31 years) were fed low-zinc (3.8 mg/day) and supplemented-zinc (18.7 mg/day) diets for nine weeks with a six-week washout period between diets. During the low dietary zinc regimen, serum and erythrocyte zinc concentrations, zinc retention, and total carbonic anhydrase and isoform activities in red blood cells were all significantly reduced. On the low zinc intake diet, peak oxygen uptake, carbon dioxide output, and respiratory exchange ratio were significantly lower ($P < 0.05$), while ventilatory equivalents for metabolic responses during exercise were significantly higher ($P < 0.05$), than with the high-zinc diets. Similar functional responses were observed during prolonged submaximal exercise (70% peak intensity for 45 min). These data show that marginal zinc intake is associated with significant reductions in zinc status and impaired metabolic responses during exercise. Until we have better markers for zinc status, it will be difficult to determine the prevalence of low status in active individuals and the impact of poor status on exercise performance.

Because chronic participation in intense or prolonged exercise may result in reduced serum zinc concentrations, and also because of the limited existing research suggesting that compromised zinc status can negatively affect performance, active individuals should be careful to ensure adequate zinc intakes and to avoid dietary or drug factors that decrease zinc availability. There is currently no evidence to suggest that supplemental zinc improves exercise performance in individuals with good zinc status. If an athlete has poor zinc status, then supplemental zinc may be warranted. However, before beginning supplementation, people should make every effort to increase their dietary zinc intake. People who decide to use supplements should use amounts close to the RDA unless there are medical or health reasons to use more, as excessive intakes of zinc can be toxic and may interfere with the bioavailability of other vitamins and minerals.

Magnesium

As with zinc, acute exercise that is intense or prolonged appears to result in a significant decrease in serum magnesium levels (Deuster et al. 1987; Deuster and Singh 1993; Lijnen et al. 1988; Stendig-Lindberg 1987). Buchman and colleagues (1998) measured serum magnesium concentrations in 26 male and female runners before and after the 1996 Houston-Tenneco Marathon. They observed a 15% decrease in serum magnesium immediately after exercise as compared to baseline concentrations measured two weeks before the marathon. Other researchers have observed decreases in serum magnesium of 2% to 14% after strenuous exercise (Deuster et al. 1987; Lijnen et al. 1988; Stendig-Lindberg et al. 1987; Joburn et al. 1985; Cordova 1992; Cordova and Alvarez-Mon 1996).

As with zinc, serum magnesium concentrations appear to return to baseline concentrations within 2 to 24 h after acute exercise (Deuster et al. 1987; Cordova and Alvarez-Mon 1996; Lijnen et al. 1988). For example, Cordova and Alvarez-Mon (1996) studied the effects on serum magnesium levels of a series of daily high-intensity exercise bouts on a cycle ergometer for one week. After each exercise session, total serum magnesium concentrations increased by 5% to 7% but returned to baseline the following day. This transient increase in serum magnesium postexercise does not appear to be exclusive to athletes. Cordova (1992) reported a significant increase in serum magnesium levels postexercise in both athletes (9% increase) and healthy subjects (12% increase). Interestingly, in both of the studies by Cordova and colleagues (1992, 1996), plasma volume decreased sig-

nificantly postexercise but returned to baseline values within 24 h (i.e., prior to the subsequent testing session). Thus, the transient increase in serum magnesium concentrations seen with acute exercise could very well be an artifact of the decrease in plasma volume. Other researchers have attributed the changes in serum magnesium to a transient redistribution of magnesium in the body, losses of magnesium in urine and sweat, or both (Deuster et al. 1987; Lijnen et al. 1988). The effect of acute exercise on urinary magnesium concentrations varies depending on when the urine samples are collected. Urinary magnesium concentrations appear to decrease during and immediately following strenuous exercise (Buchman et al. 1998) but to increase 21% to 35% over the next 12 to 24 h (Deuster et al. 1987; Lijnen et al. 1988). As indicated earlier, exercise also induces magnesium sweat losses, which represent another way in which active people lose magnesium (Lukaski 1995).

It should be noted that not all studies have shown an increase in serum magnesium concentrations with acute exercise or intense exercise training. Indeed, researchers examining the effect of prolonged endurance exercise (e.g., cross-country skiing, distance running) have consistently reported significant mean *decreases* in serum magnesium. For example, Casoni and colleagues (1990) observed a significant decrease in serum magnesium among 11 trained athletes after a 25 km (15.5-mile) running race. The decrease in serum magnesium was accompanied by an increase in erythrocyte magnesium, prompting the authors to speculate that redistribution of magnesium from serum to erythrocytes was occurring. However, other studies have failed to show an increase in erythrocyte magnesium concomitant with serum magnesium. Laires and Alves (1991) examined erythrocyte, plasma, and urinary magnesium in a group of eight well-trained swimmers and a group of 10 untrained subjects before, 2 min after, and 30 min after a swimming test. Plasma magnesium decreased significantly in both groups; however, neither erythrocyte nor urinary levels were significantly altered. The impact of intense exercise training on serum and urinary magnesium has also been examined. Dressendorfer and colleagues (2002) put nine competitive male cyclists through a six-week high-intensity training program and found no significant changes in plasma or urinary magnesium across the training period. They concluded that male endurance cyclists can maintain healthy mineral status while doing hard volume training if they do not restrict their diets or attempt to lose weight.

More recently it has been suggested that the adipocytes are involved in the redistribution of magnesium from serum. More specifically, it is hypothesized that magnesium is taken up by adipocytes during lipolysis, which is often increased during the later stages of endurance exercise (when muscle glycogen has become significantly depleted) (Lukaski 2006a). A transient shift of magnesium from extracellular fluid to skeletal muscle is another proposed mechanism for the decrease in serum magnesium seen with endurance exercise (Lukaski 2006a). Support for this hypothesis comes from research indicating that the magnesium concentration of skeletal muscle increases in almost direct correlation with the loss of magnesium from serum (Resina et al. 1995). It appears that the degree of the translocation of extracellular magnesium into these sites is modulated by the level of aerobic energy production or use (Lukaski 2006a). Following aerobic exercise, a redistribution of magnesium from the tissues (e.g., adipocytes and skeletal muscle) into circulation occurs, restoring plasma magnesium concentrations (and thereby explaining the reestablishment of normal or baseline serum magnesium levels within 24 h postexercise seen in most studies) (Lukaski 2006a).

There is no doubt that exercise alters magnesium homeostasis; however, the direction, locations, and implications of the observed magnesium "shifts" are currently not well understood. Although some researchers have maintained that the transient redistribution of magnesium between body tissues is of little consequence, others have argued that over time (as a result of chronic exercise) these shifts in body-wide magnesium distribution could result in compromised magnesium status. This argument is largely prompted by reports that exercise can result in significant sweat and urinary losses of magnesium (Lukaski 2006a). To be sure, significant sweat losses of magnesium have been seen in individuals exercising in hot or humid environments; and both prolonged and short-term high-intensity exercise have been found to increase urinary magnesium excretion (Lukaski 2006a).

The ability of the body to adjust to these losses and reestablish homeostasis depends on the amount of exercise and the dietary magnesium intake. Table 11.6 reviews research studies assessing magnesium status in active people. Only one study showed magnesium intakes below the current EAR for magnesium (Nuviala et al. 1999), and none showed serum magnesium concentrations to be low. These data indicate that active people appear to maintain good magnesium status as long as magnesium intakes are adequate. If a person is performing hard physical activity and has poor magnesium intake, magnesium status could suffer.

Few studies have specifically addressed the effect of magnesium deficiency on exercise performance. Nonetheless, findings in experimental animals and in humans with secondary hypomagnesemia (induced by drugs or disease states) indicate that magnesium deficiency results in muscle weakness, neuromuscular dysfunction, and muscle cramping, all of which would most certainly negatively affect athletic performance. In animals, marginal magnesium deficiency appears to impair exercise performance. For example, marginally magnesium-deficit rats exhibited reduced exercise capacity as measured by endurance on a treadmill (McDonald and Keen 1988). Limited evidence in humans seems to support these findings. Lukaski and Nielsen (2002) observed that marginal magnesium deficiency resulted in impaired exercise capacity among a group of untrained postmenopausal women.

Currently, there is no indication that magnesium supplementation improves serum magnesium concentrations in active people with good magnesium status (Manore et al. 1995; Nielsen and Lukaski 2006; Singh, Moses, and Deuster 1992). No researchers have observed improved exercise performance or time to exhaustion with magnesium supplements (Finstad et al. 2001). Brilla and Haley (1992) suggested that magnesium supplementation might improve muscle strength and power; unfortunately, they did not assess magnesium status in this project, making it impossible to determine why muscle strength improved. Was the improvement due to better magnesium status in people who had poor status initially? Although magnesium supplementation does not appear to benefit active people with good magnesium status, exercise can increase magnesium losses and thereby increase the risk of poor magnesium status if dietary magnesium intake is not maintained.

Chromium

Since there is no accurate way to assess chromium status, it is not surprising that we know little about the effect of exercise on chromium status of active people. Exercise appears to increase serum chromium concentrations (Anderson et al. 1982, 1984; Gatteschi et al. 1995). This increase may indicate that chromium is being mobilized from body stores in order to improve insulin's effectiveness and enhance glucose uptake during exercise (Clarkson and Haymes 1994). Once chromium is in the blood, it cannot be reabsorbed by the kidneys and therefore is lost in the urine. Indeed, research consistently shows that urinary chromium excretion is significantly increased 2 to 24 h postexercise (Anderson et al. 1982, 1984, 1988, 1991). For example, Anderson and colleagues (1984) examined the effect of an acute strenuous exercise (running) bout on serum and urinary chromium levels in trained athletes. Serum chromium concentrations increased significantly immediately following the run and remained elevated for an additional 2 h, while urinary chromium losses doubled on the day of the run (compared to the nonrunning day).

It is unknown whether the urinary losses seen with acute exercise persist with chronic training or whether, over time, the body is able to better conserve chromium. If we assume that the losses persist, then athletes who exercise strenuously on a regular basis could be at risk for poor chromium status. Anderson and colleagues (1988) observed that trained individuals had lower baseline 24 h chromium losses on nonexercise days than untrained individuals even when carbohydrate and chromium intakes were controlled. These data could be interpreted in two ways. (1) Low baseline urinary chromium excretion could mean that trained people have adapted to the chromium losses induced by exercise and are conserving their total body chromium by reducing urinary losses when they are not exercising. (2) It could also mean that trained individuals have low chromium stores and that the low baseline chromium excretion on nonexercise days indicates marginal chromium status. As noted earlier, high carbohydrate intakes, especially from simple carbohydrates, also increase urinary chromium losses and decrease chromium absorption (Anderson 1997). Since many athletes (especially endurance athletes) consume high-carbohydrate diets and sport drinks, their levels of exercise added to their high-carbohydrate diets may be compromising their bodies' chromium balance. To examine more closely the function of chromium release during exercise, Anderson and colleagues (1990) fed five different carbohydrate drinks (glucose, uncooked starch, glucose and fructose, uncooked starch and fructose, water and fructose) during exercise. The drink containing only glucose produced the highest insulin response and the greatest

urinary chromium losses. These results support the hypothesis that chromium is released during exercise to enhance insulin's action and the uptake of glucose. They also further support the notion that exercise combined with the consumption of refined carbohydrates can increase urinary chromium losses and may place athletes at risk for poor chromium status.

Interestingly, the idea of supplementing with chromium in athletes arose not out of concerns about chromium losses during exercise, but rather because of claims that supplemental chromium could provide a "natural" way to increase lean body mass and decrease body fat. The stimulus behind this supplement craze was two reports by Evans (1989) suggesting that chromium supplements improved lean body mass in football players and weightlifters compared to those receiving a placebo. Unfortunately, these studies did not adequately control diet, did not assess chromium status, used inappropriate measures to assess changes in lean body mass, and used small sample sizes. Although these studies were not well controlled, manufacturers have sold millions of chromium supplements using this research to support their claims. Attempts to replicate these studies in active people have failed.

A number of researchers have now examined chromium supplements in football players and in people participating in weight control programs and have found no effect on lean body mass (Campbell et al. 2002; Clancy et al. 1994; Hasten et al. 1992; Hallmark et al. 1996; Lukaski, Bolonchuk et al. 1996; Trent and Thieding-Cancel 1995; Volpe et al. 2001). In one of the best well-controlled studies to date, Lukaski and colleagues (1996) examined the effects of chromium supplementation and resistance training on body composition, muscle strength, and trace element status in young men. Thirty-six physically active men were randomly assigned to one of three groups: placebo (n = 12), chromium chloride supplements (n = 12), and chromium picolinate supplements (n = 12). All subjects participated in a monitored resistance training program five days a week, 60 min/day, for eight weeks. Diets were monitored at the beginning and end of the training program, and body composition was measured using the skinfold technique and dual-energy X-ray absorptiometry. Finally, blood and urine were collected for measurement of chromium concentrations. The results showed that chromium supplementation had no effect on body composition or strength gains in these men. Chromium supplementation did increase serum chromium concentrations and urinary chromium excretion regardless of the form of chromium ingested. According to these data, there appears to be no scientific evidence that chromium supplementation improves lean body mass over a placebo. Finally, a recent review by Vincent (2003) was an effort to summarize the research literature related to the role that chromium may play in weight loss and lean tissue development. Based on this review of the literature covering more than a decade of research, it appears that there is no evidence to support an effect of chromium picolinate on body composition.

CHAPTER IN REVIEW

This chapter began with two general questions: (1) Does exercise alter the metabolism of zinc, magnesium, or chromium, thereby increasing the requirements for these minerals among athletes? (2) Does supplementation with these particular minerals enhance athletic performance? With respect to the first question, current research suggests that exercise *does* alter the metabolism of zinc, magnesium, and chromium and may increase mineral losses from the body in sweat and urine; active individuals have greater losses of minerals from the body than sedentary people. This observation might seem to imply that active individuals have increased requirements for these minerals; yet it appears that if energy intake is adequate and diets contain a variety of foods, any exercise-induced mineral losses can be met through the diet. Current research indicates that few athletes exhibit poor mineral status while consuming free-living diets. For active people who restrict energy intake, avoid meat products, or eat a lot of processed foods, mineral intakes may not be adequate. If you have such clients, carefully examine their diets and recommend appropriate and achievable dietary changes and mineral supplements when necessary. If you recommend supplements, be sure to avoid mineral–mineral interactions. If an athlete or active individual wants to use a mineral supplement containing zinc, magnesium, or chromium, make sure that he or she uses a multiple mineral supplement that contains these minerals in concentrations close to those reflected in the RDAs. This will help avoid mineral–mineral interactions and the chance of toxic intakes.

Does supplementation with zinc, magnesium, or chromium or some combination of these enhance athletic performance? The answer to this question appears to be much more straightforward. According to current research, there is no evidence that supplementation with these minerals improves exercise performance or muscle strength in a person who already has good mineral status. For people whose mineral status is poor, supplementation may improve status and therefore exercise performance.

Key Concepts

1. Identify the exercise-related functions, dietary requirements, and food sources of minerals.

Zinc, magnesium, iron, and copper are important for the metabolic pathways involved in energy metabolism and for the maintenance, building, and repair of muscle tissue. Chromium is important for glucose metabolism and optimal insulin action. Chapter 12 discusses iron and copper in more detail. The RDA for magnesium for men and women 19 to 70 years and older is 400 to 420 mg/day and 310 to 320 mg/day, respectively (IOM 1997). The RDA for zinc for adult men and women is 11 mg/day and 8 mg/day, respectively (IOM 2001), while the RDA for iron is 8 mg/day for adult men and postmenopausal women and 18 mg/day for premenopausal women (IOM 2001). The RDA for copper is 900 μg/day for men and women (IOM 2001). There is no RDA for chromium, but the AI is 30 to 35 μg/day and 20 to 25 μg/day for adult men and women ages 19 to 70 years and older, respectively (IOM 2001). Zinc is especially high in animal products, which provide 70% of the dietary zinc in the United States. As with zinc, available iron is high in meat, fish, and poultry. Magnesium is widespread in foods, especially whole grain cereals, seeds, and legumes. The chromium content of food depends on where the food is grown and the processing techniques used. The best sources of chromium are whole grains, some ready-to-eat cereals, mushrooms, and processed meats.

2. **Explain the rationale for increased need of certain minerals in active people.**

Minerals are cofactors for many metabolic reactions that produce energy. Minerals are also necessary for the building and repair of muscle tissue, healthy immune function, and cell reproduction. Exercise may increase the loss of minerals in the sweat and urine, thus altering the body's overall mineral balance and increasing the need for the minerals.

3. **Understand the assessment methods for zinc, magnesium and chromium.**

There are no single good measures of zinc or magnesium status and no good functional tests in humans; status is determined through measurement of a number of static biochemical parameters (urine, blood, sweat), measurement of the activity of a mineral-dependent enzyme, use of a mineral load test, or some combination of these. There are no good biochemical or clinical methods for assessing chromium status. Currently, the best way to diagnose chromium deficiency is to observe whether chromium supplementation improves glucose tolerance.

4. **Discuss the zinc, magnesium, and chromium status of active people.**

Self-reported dietary zinc intake data indicate that active men usually have zinc intakes at or above the current RDA while active women have intakes less than the RDA. Likewise, magnesium intakes in active men are typically near the RDA, while women consume less than the RDA, especially if they restrict energy intake. There are no data on the chromium intake of active people. Low intakes of these nutrients usually can be attributed to poor energy intakes or to the elimination of food groups high in these nutrients.

5. **Discuss when an active individual might need to supplement with zinc, magnesium, or chromium.**

Biochemical assessments for zinc, magnesium and chromium status are not readily available. Thus, we rely more on dietary intake data to determine if an individual might be low in these nutrients, especially zinc and magnesium. Assessment of dietary chromium is difficult because the chromium content of food can change depending on where the food is grown. If an individual eliminates foods from the diet that are high in these nutrients, supplementation may be warranted; however, a complete assessment of the diet should be done first. If supplements are recommended, be sure to avoid mineral–mineral interactions by using a multiple mineral supplement that contains these minerals in concentrations close to those reflected in the RDAs.

Key Terms

bioavailability 345

glucose tolerance factor (GTF) 343

oral glucose tolerance test (OGTT) 350

superoxide dismutase (SOD) 338

Additional Information

Bohl CH, Volpe SL. Magnesium and exercise. Crit Rev Food Sci Nutr 2004;42:533-563.
An update on the research related to magnesium and exercise.

King JC, Shames DM, Woodhouse LR. Zinc homeostasis in humans. J Nutr 2000;130:1260S-1355S.
A complete review of the issues of measuring zinc status in humans and of how the body maintains homeostasis.

Lukaski HC. Vitamin and mineral status: effects on physical performance. Nutrition 2004;20:632-644.
Overview of the effect of physical activity on vitamin and mineral status.

References

Alaimo K. Dietary intake of vitamins, minerals and fiber of persons ages 2 months and over in the United States: Third National Health and Nutrition Examination Survey, phase I 1988-1991. Advance data from vital and health statistics. Hyattsville, MD: National Center for Health Statistics, 1994.

Althuis MD, Jordan NE, Ludington EA, Wittes JT. Glucose and insulin responses to dietary chromium supplements: a meta-analysis. Am J Clin Nutr 2002;76:148-155.

Anderson RA. Chromium in parenteral nutrition. Nutrition 1995;11(suppl):83-86.

Anderson RA. Nutritional factors influencing the glucose/insulin system: chromium. J Am Coll Nutr 1997;16(5):404-410.

Anderson RA, Bryden NA, Polansky MM. Dietary chromium intake—freely chosen diets, institutional diets and individual foods. Biol Trace Elem Res 1992;32:117-121.

Anderson RA, Bryden NA, Polansky MM, Deuster PA. Exercise effects on chromium excretion of trained and untrained men consuming a constant diet. J Appl Physiol 1988;64(1):249-252.

Anderson RA, Bryden NA, Polansky MM, Deuster PA. Acute exercise effects on urinary losses and serum concentrations of copper and zinc of moderately trained and untrained men consuming a controlled diet. Analyst 1995;120(3):867-875.

Anderson RA, Bryden NA, Polansky MM, Reiser S. Urinary chromium excretion and insulinogenic properties of carbohydrate. Am J Clin Nutr 1990;51:864-868.

Anderson RA, Kozlovsky AS. Chromium intake, absorption and excretion of subjects consuming self-selected diets. Am J Clin Nutr 1985;41:1177-1183.

Anderson RA, Polansky MM, Bryden NA. Strenuous running: acute effects on chromium, copper, zinc, and selected clinical variables in urine and serum of male runners. Biol Trace Elem Res 1984;6:327-336.

Anderson RA, Polansky MM, Bryden NA, Canary JJ. Supplemental-chromium effects on glucose, insulin, glucagon, and urinary chromium losses in subjects consuming controlled low-chromium diets. Am J Clin Nutr 1991;54:909-916.

Anderson RA, Polansky MM, Bryden NA, Roginski EE, Patterson KY, Reamer DC. Effect of exercise (running) on serum glucose, insulin, glucagon, and chromium excretion. Diabetes 1982;31(3):212-216.

Baer JT, Taper LJ. Amenorrheic and eumenorrheic adolescent runners: dietary intake and exercise training status. J Am Diet Assoc 1992;92:89-91.

Beals KA, Manore MM. Nutritional status of female athletes with subclinical eating disorders. J Am Diet Assoc 1998;98:419-425.

Beard J. Iron. In: In: Bowman BA, Russell RM eds. Present knowledge in nutrition, 9th ed. Washington, DC: ILSI Press, 2006;430-444.

Beshgetoor D, Nichols JF. Dietary intake and supplement use in female master cyclists and runners. Int J Sport Nutr Exerc Metab 2003;13:166-172.

Bohl CH, Volpe SL. Magnesium and exercise. Crit Rev Food Sci Nutr 2004;42:533-563.

Brilla LR, Haley TF. Effect of magnesium supplementation on strength training in humans. J Am Coll Nutr 1992;11(3):326-329.

Buchman AL, Keen C, Commisso J et al. The effects of a marathon run on plasma and urine mineral and metal concentrations. J Am Coll Nutr 1998;17(2):124-127.

Cabrera-Vique C, Teissedre PL, Cabanis MT, Cabanis JC. Determination and levels of chromium in French wine and grapes by graphite furnace atomic absorption spectrometry. J Agric Food Chem 1997;45:1808-1811.

Campbell WW, Beard JL, Joseph LJ, Davey SL, Evans WJ. Chromium picolinate supplementation and resistive training by older men: effects on iron-status and hematologic indexes. Am J Clin Nutr 1997;66:944-949.

Campbell WW, Joseph LJO, Anderson RA, Davey SL, Hinton J, Evans WJ. Effects of resistive training and chromicum picoliante on body composition and skeletal muscle size in older women. Int J Sport Nutr Exerc Metab 2002;12:125-135.

Casoni I, Guglielmini C, Graziano L, Reali MG, Mazzotta D, Abbasciano V. Changes of magnesium concentration in endurance athletes. Int J Sports Med 1990;11:234-237.

Clancy SP, Clarkson PM, DeCheke ME et al. Effects of chromium picolinate supplementation on body composition, strength and urinary chromium loss in football players. Int J Sport Nutr 1994;4:142-153.

Clark M, Reed DB, Crouse SF, Armstrong RB. Pre- and postseason dietary intake, body composition, and performance indices of NCAA Division I female soccer players. Int J Sport Nutr Exerc Metab 2003;13:303-319.

Clarkson PM, Haymes EM. Trace mineral requirements of athletes. Int J Sport Nutr Exerc Metab 1994;4:104-119.

Clarkson PM, Haymes EM. Exercise and mineral status of athletes: calcium, magnesium, phosphorus, and iron. Med Sci Sports Exerc 1995;27:831-843.

Cordova A. Changes in plasmatic and erythrocyte magnesium levels after high intensity exercise in man. Physiol Behav 1992;52:819-821.

Cordova A, Alvarez-Mon M. Behaviour of zinc in physical activity: a special reference to immunity and fatigue. Neurosci Biobehav Rev 1995;19(3):439-445.

Cordova A, Alvarez-Mon M. Serum magnesium and immune parameters after maximal exercise in sportsmen. Magnesium Bull 1996;18:66-70.

Couzy F, Lafargue P, Guezennec CY. Zinc metabolism in the athlete: influence of training, nutrition and other factors. Int J Sports Med 1990;11(4):263-266.

DeRuisseau KC, Cheuvront SN, Haymes EM, Sharp RG. Sweat iron and zinc losses during prolonged exercise. Int J Sport Nutr Exerc Metab 2002;12:428-437.

Deuster PA, Day BA, Singh A, Douglass L, Moser-Veillon PB. Zinc status of highly trained women runners and untrained women. Am J Clin Nutr 1989;49:1295-1301.

Deuster PA, Dolev E, Kyle SB, Anderson RA, Schoomaker EB. Magnesium homeostasis during high-intensity aerobic exercise in men. J Appl Physiol 1987;62(2):545-550.

Deuster PA, Kyle SB, Singh A et al. Exercise-induced changes in blood minerals, associated proteins and hormones in women athletes. J Sports Med Phys Fit 1991;31:552-560.

Deuster PA, Singh A. Responses of plasma magnesium and other cations to fluid replacement during exercise. J Am Coll Nutr 1993;12(2):286-293.

Dressendorfer RH, Peterson ST, Lovshin SEM, Keen CL. Mineral metabolism in male cyclists during high-intensity endurance training. Int J Sport Nutr Exerc Metab 2002;12:63-72.

Dressendorfer RH, Sockolov R. Hypozincemia in runners. Phys Sportsmed 1980;8(4):97-100.

Evans GW. The effect of chromium picolinate on insulin controlled parameters in humans. Int J Biosocial Med Res 1989;11:163-180.

Finstad EW, Newhouse IJ, Lukaski HC, Mcauliffe JE, Stewart CR. The effects of magnesium supplementation on exercise performance. Med Sci Sports Exerc 2001;33(3):493-498.

Fogelholm GM, Himberg JJ, Alopaeus K et al. Dietary and biochemical indices of nutritional status in male athletes and controls. J Am Coll Nutr 1992;11:181-191.

Fogelholm GM, Laakso J, Lehto J, Ruokonen I. Dietary intake and indictors of magnesium and zinc status in male athletes. Nutr Res 1991;11:1111-1118.

Fogelholm M, Rehunen S, Gref C et al. Dietary intake and thiamin, iron, and zinc status in elite nordic skiers during different training periods. Int J Sport Nutr 1992;2:351-365.

Food and Nutrition Board (FNB), Institute of Medicine. Recommended dietary allowances, 10th ed. Washington, DC: National Academy Press, 1989.

Gatteschi L, Castellani W, Galvan P, Parise G, Resina A, Rubenni MG. Effects of aerobic exercise on plasma chromium concentrations. In: Kies CV, Driskell JA eds. Sports nutrition: minerals and electrolytes. Boca Raton, FL: CRC Press, 1995;199-203.

Gibson RS. Principles of nutritional assessment, 2nd ed. New York: Oxford University Press, 2005.

Gleeson M, Nieman DC, Pedersen BK. Exercise, nutrition and immune function. J Sports Sci 2004;22(1):115-125.

Grider A. Zinc, copper and manganese. In: Stipanuk MH ed. Biochemical, physiological, molecular aspects of human nutrition, 2nd ed. St. Louis: Saunders Elsevier, 2006;1043-1067.

Gropper SS, Smith JL, Groff JL. Advanced nutrition and human metabolism, 5th ed. Thomson, Wadworth, Belmont, CA.2009; 429-532.

Hallmark MA, Reynolds TH, DeSouza CA, Dotson CO, Anderson RA, Rogers MA. Effects of chromium and resistive training on muscle strength and body composition. Med Sci Sports Exerc 1996;28(1):139-144.

Haralambie G. Serum zinc in athletes in training. Int J Sports Med 1981;2(3):135-138.

Hasten DL, Rome EP, Franks BD, Hegsted M. Effect of chromium picolinate on beginning weight training students. Int J Sport Nutr 1992;2:343-350.

Hetland O, Brubak EA, Refsum HE, Stromme SB. Serum and erythrocyte zinc concentrations after prolonged exercise. In: Howard H, Poortmans J eds. Metabolic adaptation to prolonged exercise. Basel: Birkhausen, 1975;367-370.

Hinton PS, Sanford TC, Davidson M, Yakushko OF, Beck NC. Nutrition intakes and dietary behaviors of male and female collegiate athletes. Int J Sport Nutr Exerc Metab 2004;14:389-405.

Institute of Medicine (IOM), Food and Nutrition Board. Dietary reference intakes for calcium, phosphorus, magnesium, vitamin D, and fluoride. Washington, DC: National Academy Press, 1997.

Institute of Medicine (IOM), Food and Nutrition Board. Dietary reference intakes for vitamin A, vitamin K, arsenic, boron, chromium, copper, iodine, iron, manganese, molybdenum, nickel, silicon, vanadium, and zinc. Washington, DC: National Academy Press, 2001.

Interagency Board for Nutrition Monitoring and Related Research. Third report on nutrition monitoring in the United States. Washington, DC: U.S. Government Printing Office, 1995.

Jensen CD, Zaltas ES, Whittam JH. Dietary intakes of male endurance cyclists during training and racing. J Am Diet Assoc 1992;92:986-988.

Joburn H, Akerstrom G, Ljunghall S. Effects of exogenous catecholamines and exercise on plasma magnesium concentrations. Clin Endocrinol (Oxford) 1985;23:219-226.

Jonnalagadda SS, Ziegler PJ, Nelson JA. Food preferences, dieting behaviors, and body image perception of elite figure skaters. Int J Sport Nutr Exerc Metab 2004;14:594-606.

Kaiserauer S, Snyder AC, Sleeper M, Zierath J. Nutritional, physiological and menstrual status of distance runners. Med Sci Sports Exerc 1989;21(2):120-125.

King JC, Cousins RJ. Zinc. In: Shils ME, Shike M, Ross AC, Caballero B, Cousins RJ eds. Modern nutrition in health and disease, 10th ed. Baltimore: Lippincott Williams & Wilkins, 2006;271-285.

King JC, Shames DM, Woodhouse LR. Zinc homeostasis in humans. J Nutr 2000;130:1260S-1355S.

Koury JC, de Oliveira AV, Portella ES, de Oliveira CF, Lopes GC, Donangleo CM. Zinc and copper biochemical indices of antioxidant status in elite athletes in different modalities. Int J Sport Nutr Exerc Metab 2004;14:364-378.

Krotkiewski M, Gudnmundsson P, Backstrom P, Mandroukas K. Zinc and muscle strength and endurance. Acta Physiol Scand 1982;116:309-311.

Laires MJ, Alves F. Changes in plasma, erythrocyte, and urinary magnesium with prolonged swimming exercise. Magnesium Res 1991;4(2):119-122.

Lijnen P, Hespel P, Fagard R, Lysens R, Eynde EV, Amery A. Erythrocyte, plasma and urinary magnesium in men before and after a marathon. Eur J Appl Physiol 1988;58:252-256.

Lukaski HC. Micronutrients (magnesium, zinc, and copper): are mineral supplements needed for athletes? Int J Sport Nutr 1995;5:S74-S83.

Lukaski HC. Assessment of mineral status in athletes. In: Driskel JA, Wolinsky I eds. Nutritional assessment of athletes. Boca Raton, FL: CRC Press, 2002;339-372.

Lukaski HC. Vitamin and mineral status: Effects on physical performance. Nutrition 2004;20:632-644.

Lukaski HC. Low dietary zinc decreases erythrocyte carbonic anhydrase activities and impairs cardiorespiratory function in men during exercise. Am J Clin Nutr 2005;81:1045-1051.

Lukaski HC. Update on the relationship between magnesium and exercise. Magnesium Res 2006a;19:180-189.

Lukaski HC. Zinc. In: Driskell JA, Wolinsky I eds. Sports nutrition. Vitamins and trace elements, 2nd ed. Boca Raton, FL: CRC Press, 2006b;217-234.

Lukaski HC, Bolonchuk WW, Klevay LM, Milne DB, Sandstead HH. Changes in plasma zinc content after exercise in men fed a low-zinc diet. Am J Physiol 1984;247(10):E88-E93.

Lukaski HC, Bolonchuk WW, Klevay LM, Milne DB, Sandstead HH. Interactions among dietary fat, mineral status, and performance in endurance athletes: a case study. Int J Sport Nutr Exerc Metab 2001;11:186-198.

Lukaski HC, Bolonchuk WW, Siders WA, Milne DB. Chromium supplementation and resistance training: effects of body composition, strength, and trace elements status of men. Am J Clin Nutr 1996;63:954-965.

Lukaski HC, Hoverson BS, Gallagher SK, Bolonchuk WW. Physical training and copper, iron and zinc status of swimmers. Am J Clin Nutr 1990;51:1093-1099.

Lukaski HC, Nielsen FH. Dietary magnesium depletion affects metabolic responses during submax exercise in postmenopausal women. J Nutr 2002;132(5):930-935.

Lukaski HC, Penland JG. Functional changes appropriate for determining mineral element requirements. J Nutr 1996;126:2354S-2364S.

Lukaski HC, Siders WA, Hoverson BS, Gallagher SK. Iron, copper, magnesium and zinc status as predictors of swimming performance. Int J Sports Med 1996;17:535-540.

Manore MM, Helleksen JM, Merkel J, Skinner JS. Longitudinal change in zinc status in untrained men: effect of two different 12-week exercise training programs and zinc supplementation. J Am Diet Assoc 1993;93:1165-1168.

Manore MM, Merkel J, Helleksen JM, Skinner JS, Carroll SC. Longitudinal changes in magnesium status in untrained males: effect of two different 12-week exercise training programs and magnesium supplementation. In: Kies CV, Driskell JA eds. Sports nutrition: minerals and electrolytes. Boca Raton, FL: CRC Press, 1995;179-187.

McCall KA, Huang C, Fierke CA. Function and mechanism of zinc metalloenzymes. J Nutr 2000;130:1437S-1446S.

McDonald R, Keen C. Iron, zinc, and magnesium nutrition and athletic performance. Sports Med 1988;5:171-184.

Miyamura JB, McNutt SW, Lichton IJ, Wenkam NS. Altered zinc status of soldiers under field conditions. J Am Diet Assoc 1987;87:595-597.

Montain SJ, Cheauvront SN, Lukaski HC. Sweat mineral-element responses during 7 h of exercise-heat stress. Int J Sport Nutr Exerc Metab 2007;17:574-582.

Mundie TG, Hare B. Effects of resistance exercise on plasma, erythrocyte, and urine zinc. Biol Trace Elem Res 2001;79(1):23-28.

Nielson FH, Lukaski HC. Update on the relationship between magnesium and exercise. Magnesium Res 2006;19(3):180-189.

Nuviala RJ, Lapieza MG, Bernal E. Magnesium, zinc and copper status in women involved in different sports. Int J Sport Nutr 1999;9(3):295-309.

Offenbacher EG, Pi-Sunyer FX. Temperature and pH effects on the release of chromium from stainless steel into water and fruit juices. J Agric Food Chem 1983;31:89-92.

Ohno H, Sato Y, Ishikawa M. Training effects on blood zinc levels in humans. J Sports Med Phys Fit 1990;30(30):247-253.

Ohno H, Yamashita K, Doi R, Yamamura K, Kondo T, Taniguchi N. Exercise-induced changes in blood zinc and related proteins. J Appl Physiol 1985;58(5):1453-1458.

Papadopoulou SK, Papadopoulou SD, Gallos GK. Macro- and micro-nutrient intake of adolescent Greek female volleyball players. Int J Sport Nutr Exerc Metab 2002;12:73-80.

Pennington JAT. Intakes of minerals from diets and foods: is there a need for concern? J Nutr 1996;126:2304S-2308S.

Resina A, Gatteschi L, Rubenni MG, Galvan P, Parise G, Tjouroudis N, Virol L. Changes in serum and erythrocyte magnesium after training and physical exercise. In: L Viecchiet ed. Magnesium and physical activity. London: Parthenon, 1995;199-210.

Richardson JH, Drake PD. The effect of zinc on fatigue of striated muscle. J Sports Med Phys Fit 1979;19:133-138.

Rude RK, Shils ME. Magnesium. In: Shils ME, Shike M, Ross AC, Caballero B, Cousins RJ eds. Modern nutrition in health and disease, 10th ed. Baltimore: Lippincott Williams & Wilkins, 2006;223-247.

Shay NF, Mangian HF. Neurobiology of zinc-influenced eating behavior. J Nutr 2000;130:1493S-1499S.

Shils ME. Magnesium. In: Shils ME, Olson JA, Shike M eds. Modern nutrition in health and disease, 8th ed. Baltimore: Lippincott Williams & Wilkins, 1994;172.

Singh A, Moses FM, Deuster PA. Vitamin and mineral status in physically active men: effects of a high-potency supplement. Am J Clin Nutr 1992;55:1-7.

Singh A, Moses FM, Smoak BL, Deuster PA. Plasma zinc uptake from a supplement during submaximal exercise. Med Sci Sports Exerc 1992;24(4):442-446.

Singh A, Smoak BL, Patterson KY, LeMay LG, Veillon C, Deuster PA. Biochemical indices of selected trace minerals in men: effect of stress. Am J Clin Nutr 1991;53:126-131.

Stendig-Lindberg G, Shapiro Y, Epstein Y et al. Changes in serum magnesium concentrations after strenuous exercise. J Am Coll Nutr 1987;6(1):35-40.

Stoecker BJ. Chromium. In: Bowman BA, Russell RM eds. Present knowledge in nutrition, 9th ed. Washington, DC: ILSI Press, 2006a;498-505.

Stoecker BJ. Chromium. In: Shils ME, Shike M, Ross AC, Caballero B, Cousins RJ eds. Modern nutrition in health and disease, 10th ed. Baltimore: Lippincott Williams & Wilkins, 2006b;332-337.

Telford RD, Catchpole EA, Deakin V, McLeay AC, Plank AW. The effect of 7 to 8 months of vitamin/mineral supplementation on the vitamin and mineral status of athletes. Int J Sport Nutr 1992;2:123-134.

Tipton K, Green NR, Haymes EM, Waller M. Zinc loss in sweat of athletes exercising in hot and neutral temperatures. Int J Sport Nutr 1993;3:261-271.

Trent JK, Thieding-Cancel D. Effects of chromium picolinate on body composition. J Sports Med Phys Fit 1995;35:272-280.

Vincent JB. The potential value and toxicity of chromium picolinate as a nutritional supplement, weight loss agent and muscle development agent. Sports Med 2003;33:213-230.

Volpe SL. Magnesium. In: Bowman BA, Russell RM eds. Present knowledge in nutrition, 9th ed. Washington, DC: ILSI Press, 2006;400-408.

Volpe SL, Huang HW, Larpadisorn K, Lesser II. Effect of chromium supplementation and exercise on body composition, resting metabolic rate and selected biochemical param-eters in moderately obese women following an exercise program. J Am Coll Nutr 2001 Aug;20(4):293-306.

Weight LM, Noakes TD, Labadarios D, Graves J, Jacobs P, Berman PA. Vitamin and mineral status of trained athletes including the effects of supplementation. Am J Clin Nutr 1988;47:186-191.

Wintergerst ES, Maggini S, Horning DH. Immune-enhancing role of vitamin C and zinc and effect on clinical conditions. Ann Nutr Metab 2006;50(2):85-94.

Wintergerst ES, Maggini S, Horning DH. Contribution of selected vitamins and trace elements to immune function. Ann Nutr Metab 2007;51(4):301-323.

Wood RJ. Assessment of marginal zinc status in humans. J Nutr 2000;130:1350S-1354S.

CHAPTER 12

Micronutrients Important in Blood Formation

Chapter Objectives

After reading this chapter you should be able to

- identify the exercise-related functions, dietary requirements, and food sources of the blood-forming nutrients (iron, copper, folate, and vitamin B_{12}),
- explain the rationale for increased need for the blood-building nutrients in active individuals,
- understand the nutrition assessment methods for iron, copper, folate, and vitamin B_{12}, and
- discuss the iron, copper, folate, and vitamin B_{12} status of active individuals.

Without adequate oxygen, the metabolic pathways that produce energy cannot maintain a constant supply of energy to the muscles. The **red blood cells (RBCs)** deliver oxygen to the muscles and transport carbon dioxide back to the lungs. Since the oxygen-carrying capacity of the blood is proportional to the hemoglobin concentration within RBCs, it is important that athletes have an adequate number of RBCs and adequate hemoglobin within each of these cells. If adequate hemoglobin is not available, the athlete's exercise performance can suffer since the ability to deliver oxygen to the tissues during exercise is impaired.

In order for the body to synthesize hemoglobin and produce the red cells that contain hemoglobin, the diet must provide certain micronutrients. Four micronutrients are especially important in hemoglobin synthesis and RBC production; two are minerals (iron and copper), and two are B-complex vitamins (folate and vitamin B_{12}). If the diet is deficient in any of these nutrients, or if the absorption, utilization, or turnover of the nutrients is altered to decrease status, hemoglobin synthesis and red cell production will be impaired. Because these four nutrients are so interrelated in their roles for the production of hemoglobin and RBCs, we discuss them together in this chapter.

EXERCISE-RELATED FUNCTIONS, DIETARY REQUIREMENTS, AND FOOD SOURCES

To understand how exercise might increase the need for these nutrients, we must first understand their role in the formation of hemoglobin and healthy red cells. Table 12.1 outlines how iron, copper, folate, and vitamin B_{12} each play a role in the formation of red cells or the production of hemoglobin. For the most part, these micronutrients are cofactors or coenzymes for enzymes required for hemoglobin synthesis or cell formation. Folate and vitamin B_{12}, for example, help catalyze reactions related to the production of new cells, including red cells. But there are also nonenzymatic functions—iron is part of the structure of heme in hemoglobin, while copper is required for normal iron transport within the body. Some of these micronutrients are also required for other metabolic pathways or functions associated with exercise (table 12.1). In the following section, we briefly discuss the specific roles each of these nutrients plays in the formation of hemoglobin and red cells and in other functions related to exercise; we also cover dietary requirements and food sources.

Iron

Of all the nutrients related to RBC formation, iron is probably the most familiar to athletes. The reason is that iron plays a primary role in the formation of two iron-containing proteins: hemoglobin and myoglobin. **Hemoglobin** is the principal

Table 12.1 Exercise-Related Metabolic Functions That Require Iron, Copper, Folate, or Vitamin B_{12}

Vitamin or mineral	Forms of the vitamin or mineral in food and body	Functions related to exercise	Major enzymes or pathways that require the nutrient as a cofactor
Iron (Fe)	Ferric iron (Fe^{3+})—oxidized iron Ferrous iron (Fe^{2+})—reduced iron	Required for hemoglobin and myoglobin production and for numerous enzymes involved in energy production during exercise	Pyruvate oxidase, mitochondrial cytochromes, cytochrome P-450, ribonucleotide reductase, tyrosine and proline hydrolase, monoamine oxidase, catalase, glucose 6-phosphatase, 6-phosphogluconate dehydrogenase
Copper (Cu)	Found in three oxidation states, Cu^0, Cu^{1+}, and Cu^{2+}; Cu^{2+} is the most common in nature.	Required for ceruloplasmin, or ferroxidate I, a plasma protein having ferroxidase activity; important for electron transport enzymes, enzymes involved in collagen synthesis, and synthesis of norepinephrine	Cytochrome-*c* oxidase, superoxide dismutase, protein-lysine 6-oxidase, dopamine-β-monooxygenase
Folate	*Folate* typically refers to food folate; the term *folic acid* is used to identify supplemental folic acid in foods or supplements. Tetrahydrofolate is the source of active folate coenzymes in the body.	Important for cellular division and cell regeneration, especially of the red blood cells, which turn over every 120 days	Folate coenzymes required for the synthesis of purines and pyrimidines, including thymidylate, which is incorporated into DNA
Vitamin B_{12}	Cobalamin	Important for single-carbon metabolism required for normal cell division, especially in the methylation of homocysteine to produce methionine; important for red blood cell production	Methylmalonyl coenzyme A-mutase, leucine mutase, methionine synthetase

protein constituent of the RBC (**erythrocyte**) and gives blood its red color. A protein synthesized in the bone marrow, hemoglobin comprises four globulin units and four heme units. Hemoglobin is responsible for the red cell's ability to transport oxygen to the muscles and carry carbon dioxide away from the muscles to the lungs. **Heme,** an iron-containing molecule at the center of the hemoglobin unit (figure 12.1), binds oxygen and carbon dioxide reversibly. Hemoglobin contains four of these oxygen-binding heme units (porphyrin rings). **Myoglobin,** a heme protein found in skeletal muscle, increases the rate of oxygen diffusion from the blood to the cells. During iron deficiency, the amount of myoglobin in the muscle is reduced, decreasing the diffusion of oxygen from the RBCs to the mitochondria. Iron has other metabolic functions related to energy production during exercise (table 12.1). For example, it is a cofactor for enzymes in the electron transport pathway and for enzymes related to carbohydrate and protein metabolism.

Because of the role iron plays in hemoglobin, getting adequate dietary iron is very important, especially for physically active people. Without adequate iron, iron deficiency anemia can develop since there is not enough iron for hemoglobin production (see "Types of Anemia," p. 370). This results in a person's feeling tired, weak, and fatigued and can impair exercise performance. Low or poor dietary iron intake is only one factor

that can contribute to the development of anemia in active people. Any condition that increases blood loss, and therefore loss of iron from the body, can also cause anemia (see "Case Studies of Iron Deficiency Anemia," p. 381). For example, iron loss due to blood donations, excessive menstrual blood losses, exercise-induced hemoglobinuria or hematuria (increased loss of blood in urine), gastritis (inflammation of the stomach lining, often due to the use of anti-inflammatory drugs), hemorrhoids, or peptic ulcer disease (bleeding of the gastrointestinal tract) can cause or contribute to anemia. Determining the cause of anemia is not always easy, and anemia cannot always be attributed to poor dietary iron intakes. The current Recommended Dietary Allowance (RDA) for iron is 18 mg/day for premenopausal women and 8 mg/day for men and postmenopausal women (Institute of Medicine [IOM] 2001). This dietary recommendation is based on an overall estimated daily iron turnover of 1.5 mg/day for sedentary menstruating women and 1 mg/day for sedentary men. However, the iron turnover rate appears to rise in active individuals (Haymes 2006; Nielson and Nachitigal 1998). Figure 12.2 outlines the various ways in which exercise can alter iron losses and turnover in the body. For example, data collected from endurance-trained athletes indicated

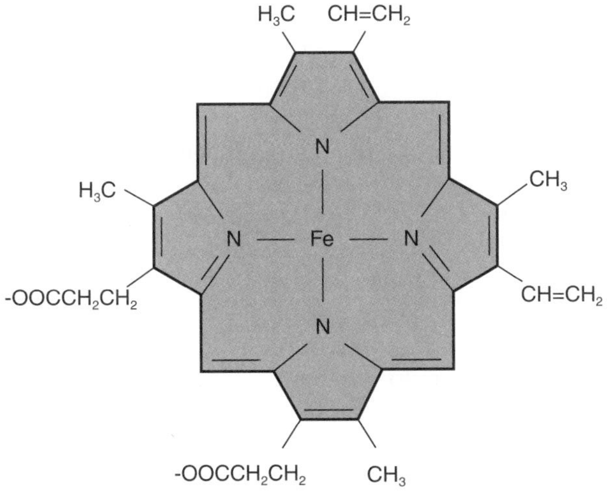

Figure 12.1 Structure of heme, an organometallic complex of protoporphyrin IX and Fe²⁺.

From *Clinical chemistry,* L.A. Kaplan, A.I. Pesce, and S.C. Kazmierczak, editors. Iron, porphyrin, and bilirubin metabolism, W.E. Schreiber, pgs. 196-509, Copyright 1989, with permission from Elsevier.

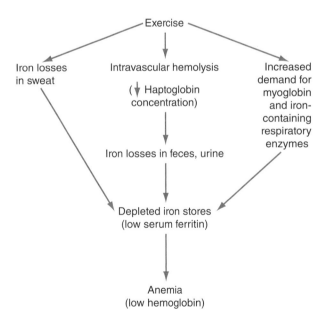

Figure 12.2 Possible mechanisms for exercise-induced iron deficiency.

JOURNAL OF NUTRITION, ONLINE by C.M. Weaver and S. Rajaram. Copyright 1992 by American Society for Nutrition. Reproduced with permission of American Society for Nutrition in the format Textbook via Copyright Clearance Center.

Highlight

Types of Anemia

Anemia is a general term for any condition in which hemoglobin is low. In fact, the word anemia literally means "without blood." Anemia is characterized by too few RBCs or by RBCs that are ill formed so that they cannot properly transport oxygen. Ill-formed RBCs are usually immature (too small), or they contain too little hemoglobin. Either way, the RBCs cannot carry the normal amount of oxygen. There are many different types of anemia caused by a variety of factors, including nutrient deficiencies, bleeding, increased RBC destruction, or defective formation of red cells. The following are the major anemias associated with iron, copper, folate, and vitamin B_{12} deficiencies.

Pernicious Anemia

Pernicious anemia is caused by vitamin B_{12} deficiency that arises through lack of intrinsic factor. **Intrinsic factor** is a glycoprotein made in the stomach that aids in the absorption of vitamin B_{12}. Without intrinsic factor, vitamin B_{12} absorption decreases dramatically. Some people naturally produce less intrinsic factor than others, and some produce less intrinsic factor as they get older. Elderly people have elevated risk for vitamin B_{12} deficiency and for development of macrocytic anemia.

Iron Deficiency Anemia

Iron deficiency anemia is caused by too little iron in the diet, poor iron absorption, or increased loss of iron from the body. In iron deficiency anemia, the body stores are exhausted; the amount of circulating iron has declined; and the person exhibits frank microcytic, hypochromic anemia (small RBCs with inadequate hemoglobin concentration). Diagnosis of iron deficiency anemia is usually based on decreases in the following: blood concentrations of ferritin, transferrin saturation, serum iron levels, hemoglobin, RBC count, mean cell volume (MCV), and hematocrit.

Megaloblastic Anemia

Megaloblastic anemia is associated with a dietary folate deficiency that impairs DNA synthesis. This results in larger than normal red cells (macrocytosis) with increased MCV. Folate deficiency is primarily due to poor dietary folate intake or to drugs that alter intestinal absorption or metabolism of folate.

---

that iron losses in feces, urine, and sweat were ~1.75 mg/day for men and ~2.3 mg/day for women (Weaver and Rajaram 1992). Females lose more iron than males because of monthly menses; iron losses decrease in cases of amenorrhea. Because of their higher iron turnover, highly active people may have increased risk for iron deficiency, especially if they are

- female athletes,
- long-distance runners, or
- vegetarian athletes.

These groups are at risk for iron deficiency due to decreased iron intake; decreased bioavailability of iron in their diet; or increased iron losses in sweat, blood, urine, or feces.

Dietary iron comes in two forms: heme iron and non-heme iron. Heme iron is the iron bound to hemoglobin or myoglobin in meat, fish, or poultry.

This type of iron is much more bioavailable and has a much higher absorption rate (5-35%) than non-heme iron (2-25%). The iron found in animal foods is about 40% heme and 60% non-heme iron. Non-heme iron is the iron found in plant foods, such as breads, grains, legumes, vegetables, and fruit. All the iron found in plant foods is non-heme iron. In general, the typical Western diet has an iron density of about 6 mg iron per 1000 kcal consumed. If a diet has a higher iron density, the individual probably consumes iron-fortified foods or eats large amounts of meat, fish, or poultry. Table 12.2 gives some specific examples of dietary sources of heme and non-heme iron and the amount of iron per typical serving. The bioavailability of iron for absorption from a particular meal depends on several factors that either inhibit or enhance iron absorption; it also depends on current body stores, the amount of iron in the meal, and the chemical nature of the iron (table 12.3). Because so

Table 12.2 Dietary Sources of Heme and Non-Heme Iron

	Iron content (mg)
Animal sources (~40% heme iron, ~60% non-heme iron)	
Beef (all types) (3 oz cooked)	2.5-3.5
Chicken, white meat (3 oz cooked)	1
Chicken, dark meet (3 oz cooked)	1
Chicken, livers (3 oz cooked)	7
Fish (swordfish) (3 oz cooked)	1
Pork chops, center cut and boneless (3 oz cooked)	1
Ham, boneless (3 oz cooked)	1
Plant sources (100% non-heme iron)	
Breads (whole wheat, bagels, English muffins) (1 slice)	1
Beans (pinto, navy, kidney) (1/2 cup cooked)	1.5-2.5
Cereals, ready to eat, fortified (1 oz)	5-9
Cereals, ready to eat, total fortification (1 oz)	10-15
Hummus (1/2 cup)	2
Pasta (all types) (1 cup cooked)	2
Rice (white) (1 cup cooked)	2
Raisins (1/4 cup)	1
Spinach (1/2 cup cooked)	3
Tortilla (10 in. flour)	2.5

many factors can inhibit iron absorption, dietary iron is much less bioavailable than water-soluble vitamins, which means that improving iron status takes much longer than reversing deficiency in a water-soluble vitamin. Since too much iron can be toxic, the body regulates its total iron stores by regulating iron absorption. If dietary iron intake is high or iron status is good, total iron absorption will decrease to prevent too much iron from being absorbed. Because some people are at risk for hemochromatosis, iron supplementation should be done with caution (see "Hemochromatosis: Iron Overload Disease," p. 372).

Copper

Copper plays an indirect role in hemoglobin synthesis since it has ferroxidase activity—that is, it helps convert ferrous iron (Fe^{2+}) to ferric iron (Fe^{3+}). In order for iron to be transported in the blood by **transferrin,** an iron transport protein, iron must be in the ferric (Fe^{3+}) form. **Ferroxidase I,** also called **ceruloplasmin,** a plasma protein containing most of the copper in the body, is responsible for this conversion (Milne 1998). Ceruloplasmin also plays a role in the transfer of iron from storage to the blood so that it is available for hemoglobin synthesis. Thus, without adequate copper to synthesize ceruloplasmin, iron cannot be made available for transport within the body, and hemoglobin synthesis does not occur. Anemia can develop if the diet is low in copper, even if dietary iron is adequate. In addition to its role in iron metabolism, copper is required for several enzymes important for exercise (table 12.1). It is

Table 12.3 Factors That Either Enhance or Inhibit Iron Absorption

Enhance iron absorption	Inhibit iron absorption
Heme iron in the diet: • Meat, fish, or poultry in the diet increases absorption of non-heme iron	Decreased iron demand: • Good iron status
Increased demand for iron in the body: • Pregnancy • Low iron stores • High altitude • High blood loss • High exercise training	Factors in the meal that complex with iron and decrease availability for absorption: • Phytates and polyphenols (tea and coffee) • Oxalic acid • Fiber • Soy
Vitamin C in the meal: • Vitamin C promotes absorption of non-heme iron in a meal	Mineral–mineral interaction, which causes minerals to compete for transport into the intestinal cell: • Calcium
High gastric acid production, which results in a low stomach pH	High antacid use, which results in higher stomach pH and mineral–mineral interactions

Highlight

Hereditary Hemochromatosis: Iron Overload Disease

Since hemochromatosis is the most prevalent genetic disorder in the United States, iron supplements should be avoided if iron status is good and the diet provides adequate iron. **Hemochromatosis (iron toxicity)** results in an increase in iron absorption. The excess iron accumulates in the body, especially in the liver, heart, and pancreas, causing organ damage. If left untreated, hemochromatosis can cause severe health problems such as heart disease, cirrhosis of the liver, or liver cancer. Hemochromatosis was once thought to be a rare disease affecting only white males; however, we now know that it affects four in every 1000 people (Yip 2001). These individuals, who have two copies of the recessive gene (homozygous), absorb about twice as much iron as unaffected individuals, with storage iron levels reaching 10 times the normal level. About one in 8 to 10 people carries one copy of the gene (heterozygous); these individuals also have increased iron absorption but to a lesser extent, and iron overload is less of an issue (Yip 2001). Before taking iron supplements, people should have their iron status checked to make sure they are not at risk for hereditary hemochromatosis. Diagnosis of hemochromatosis is usually based on clinically high serum concentrations of ferritin and serum iron and on a high percentage of transferrin saturation (>60% for men and >50% for women) (Yip 2001).

an essential cofactor for cytochrome-*c* oxidase, the rate-limiting enzyme in the electron transport chain. In addition, superoxide dismutase, a copper-requiring enzyme, acts as an antioxidant and helps protect the body against free radicals (see chapter 10).

The current RDA for copper is 900 μg/day for adult men and women (IOM 2001). Most of the copper consumed in the American diet is from meat, seafood, vegetables, legumes, peanut butter, nuts, and seeds, with the highest concentrations found in cooked organ meats (~3.8 mg/3 oz or 85 g serving) and oysters (2.3 mg/3 oz serving) (Reeves and Cooper 1997). Some ready-to-eat cereals are fortified with copper, and wheat bran cereals and whole grain products can also be good sources of copper (IOM 2001). As with iron, however, a number of factors can influence copper bioavailability from the diet (Wapnir 1998). For example, vegetables are a major source of copper in the human diet, but compared to the copper found in animal foods they require more extensive digestive enzymatic attack in order for the copper to be released and made available for absorption. In addition, the milling of grains, the canning of vegetables, or the addition of salt or other chemicals for preservation of foods can decrease the copper content of food or its bioavailability. As with iron, fiber and mineral–mineral interactions— especially zinc–copper competitive binding—can decrease copper bioavailability, while vitamin

C and protein can increase copper absorption (Reeves and Cooper 1997; Wapnir 1998).

Median copper intakes from food in the United States are reported to be slightly more than 1.0 mg/day—about 1.2 to 1.6 mg/day for men and 1.0 or 1.1 mg/day for women (IOM 2001). One study that chemically assessed copper intake from the diets of 849 North Americans and Europeans showed that more than 30% of the diets contained less than 1.0 mg/day of copper (Klevay et al. 1993). These data suggest that many individuals may have marginal copper intakes.

Folate

Adequate folate intake is very important for athletes because of its roles in RBC production and in tissue repair and maintenance. Specifically, folate functions as a donor or acceptor of one-carbon units in reactions involving nucleotide and amino acid metabolism (Shane 1995) (see table 12.1). Through this role, folate plays a significant part in cell division, especially in tissues with rapid turnover (such as RBCs). Thus, a primary function of folate that directly relates to exercise is the formation of red cells. Folate deficiency leads to **megaloblastic anemia,** which is caused by the failure of the red cell precursors, **megaloblasts,** to replicate into functional red cells (Wagner 1995) (see "Types of Anemia," p. 370). The result is abnormally large, **macrocytic red cells** in the blood that cannot effectively transport oxygen or remove carbon dioxide.

Tetrahydrofolate (THF) serves as the source of active folate coenzyme forms required for numerous biological reactions in the body, including red cell formation (Savage and Lindenbaum 1995). Both vitamin B_6 and vitamin B_{12} are required for the conversion of folate to THF (Herbert 1996). A deficiency of folate or of vitamin B_{12} causes a failure of THF synthesis and of folate enzyme production, which leads to impaired DNA synthesis and to development of macrocytic red cells (Savage and Lindenbaum 1995). Because of its role in DNA synthesis, folate is involved in the building and repairing of body tissues, including those damaged due to physical activity. Thus, adequate folate intake ensures that the cells of the body can be replaced or repaired when necessary. Finally, low folate intakes have been associated with elevated plasma homocysteine concentrations, which are an important risk factor for developing premature coronary artery disease and cerebral vascular disease (Scott et al. 1995).

In 1998, the RDA for folate was revised; the new RDA is 400 μg/day for men and women >19 years of age (IOM 1998). The 1989 RDA for folate was 200 μg/day for adult men and 180 μg/day for adult women (Food and Nutrition Board 1989). The new RDA was derived using a combination of blood indices (IOM 1998). Although not used as criteria for setting the new folate RDA, high blood homocysteine concentrations and increased risk of neural tube defects are now recognized as associated with low folate intake (IOM 1998; Scott et al. 1995). It is now recommended that to reduce the risk of neural tube defects in newborn babies, women in their childbearing years obtain an additional 400 μg/day of synthetic folic acid from fortified foods or supplements, or both, in addition to the folate in their food (IOM 1998).

Folate is found in many foods but is especially high in leafy green vegetables (spinach, asparagus, mustard and turnip greens, broccoli), nuts, legumes (peanuts; black-eyed peas; navy, pinto, and kidney beans), and liver. Brewer's yeast is especially high in folate, with 1 tbsp containing 300 μg. Thus, 1 tbsp of brewer's yeast provides 75% of the 1998 RDA for folate (400 μg/day). The bioavailability of folate in food is approximately 50% (IOM 1998), but the availability can be further reduced by various cooking procedures. Similar to other water-soluble vitamins, folate can be lost or destroyed by prolonged cooking or canning procedures and acid environments. Today many foods are fortified with synthetic folic acid. For example, most fortified breakfast cereals contain 50% to 100% of the 1998 RDA for folate. In addition, in 1998 the U.S. Department of Agriculture (USDA) mandated the fortification of folic acid in enriched breads, flours, corn meals, rice, noodles, macaroni, and other grain products. This synthetic folic acid appears to be highly available for absorption (85% bioavailable). Because our diets contain a mixture of food folate and synthetic folic acid, and because the bioavailability is different between these two types of folate, you need to use a calculation, **dietary folate equivalents (DFEs),** to determine the amount of folate available for absorption. See "Calculating Dietary Folate Equivalents."

Highlight

Calculating Dietary Folate Equivalents

Dietary folate has only half the bioavailability of synthetic folic acid. The definition of dietary folate equivalent is 1 μg of DFE = 1 μg of food folate = 0.5 μg of folic acid taken on an empty stomach or 0.6 μg of folic acid with meals (IOM 1998). To calculate the total intake of DFEs in a person's diet, use the following calculation:

μg of DFE provided = μg of food folate per day + 1.7 (μg synthetic folic acid per day).

Here is an example of a calculation for total DFEs, for a diet containing 1500 kcal/day:

Assume food folate = 70 μg/day; synthetic folic acid = 224 μg/day.

DFEs = 70 μg/day + 1.7 (224 μg/day) = 451 μg/day.

Of this person's ~451 μg of DFE per day, 84% is from fortified foods (breakfast cereals).

Vitamin B$_{12}$

As with folate, the importance of vitamin B$_{12}$ for active people is primarily related to its role in RBC production. Vitamin B$_{12}$, or **cobalamin,** functions in two primary reactions within the body. First, methylcobalamin is required for the methylation of **homocysteine** to re-form the amino acid methionine. Vitamin B$_{12}$ and folate participate in this reaction since one of the substrates for the reaction is a methylated form of THF (figure 12.3) (Herbert 1996). This is the reason either folate or vitamin B$_{12}$ deficiency can cause **macrocytic anemia** (see "Types of Anemia," p. 370): Without vitamin B$_{12}$, THF cannot be produced, and without THF, normal red cell production does not occur. Second, cobalamin is required as a cofactor for methylmalonyl-CoA mutase, which converts methylmalonyl-CoA to succinyl-CoA—a reaction required for degradation of some amino acids and fatty acids. As with folate, the primary function of vitamin B$_{12}$ as it relates to exercise is its role in red cell formation. A deficiency of vitamin B$_{12}$ results in **pernicious anemia,** characterized by macrocytic red cells and large megaloblasts (Savage and Lindenbaum 1995) (again, see "Types of Anemia," p. 370). Thus, either a folate or vitamin B$_{12}$ deficiency can limit the synthesis of healthy red cells required for the transport of oxygen during exercise.

The RDA for vitamin B$_{12}$ was revised in 1998 and set at 2.4 µg/day for adults aged 19 to 50 years (IOM 1998); the old (1989) RDA had been set at 2.0 µg/day (Food and Nutrition Board 1989). The increase is due, in part, to the new method of deriving the RDA and new information about the bioavailability of dietary vitamin B$_{12}$. The new RDA is based on a 50% absorption rate for dietary

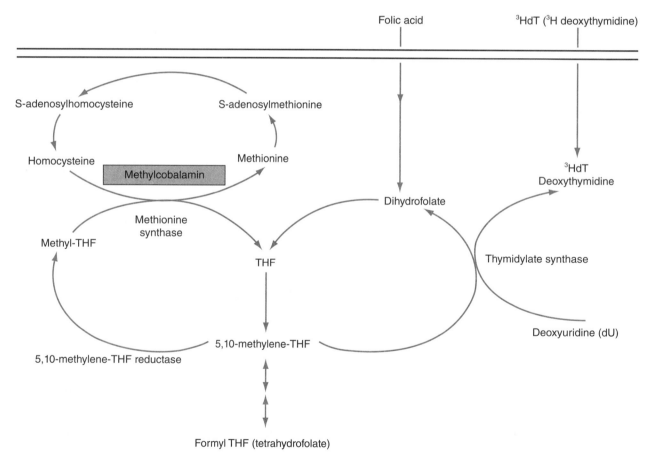

Figure 12.3 The methionine synthase reaction, which is dependent on both vitamin B$_{12}$ (cobalamin) and folate. In the deoxyuridine suppression test (dUST), preincubation of normal bone marrow with deoxyuridine (dU) suppresses the incorporation of 3HdT (tritiated deoxythymidine) into DNA; dU suppression is reduced when vitamin B$_{12}$ and folate are deficient. THF = tetrahydrofolate.

vitamin B_{12}. Because vitamin B_{12} absorption may change with age, it is recommended that adults 50 years or older obtain their daily vitamin B_{12} intake from fortified foods (e.g., fortified breakfast cereals or bars, sport foods) or from supplements (IOM 1998). Vitamin B_{12} absorption depends on a number of intestinal conditions, including the production of intrinsic factor, which can decrease with age. There are few data on the effects of cooking on vitamin B_{12} content; however, it is known that the boiling or cooking of milk reduces vitamin B_{12} content by 50% to 75% (IOM 1998).

Vitamin B_{12} is different from the other B-complex vitamins in that it is found only in animal foods such as milk and dairy products, meat, eggs, fish, and poultry. Vegetarians who avoid all animal products (vegans) need to obtain vitamin B_{12} through fortified foods or supplements. Foods highest in vitamin B_{12} are shellfish (clams, oysters, mussels, crab, and lobster), fin fish (herring, sardines, trout, mackerel, salmon, and canned tuna), and organ meats (liver, kidney, heart, brains, and tongue). However, these foods are usually limited in the typical American diet. Foods that contribute the most vitamin B_{12} to American diets are dairy (especially milk and yogurt), mixed foods containing meat (sandwiches containing meat and mixed meat dishes), beef, and fortified cereals (IOM 1998).

Other Nutrients (Vitamin B_6, Protein)

Several other nutrients, such as vitamin B_6 and protein, are required for formation of hemoglobin and RBCs. Vitamin B_6 is important in the formation of the porphyrin ring, which is at the center of the hemoglobin molecule (figure 12.1). Vitamin B_6 deficits impair hemoglobin synthesis by diminishing heme production. Protein is also important for hemoglobin synthesis. Since both hemoglobin and myoglobin are proteins synthesized in the body, adequate dietary protein is required to provide the amino acids necessary to make these proteins.

RATIONALE FOR INCREASED NEED FOR ACTIVE INDIVIDUALS

Because exercise requires delivery of oxygen to and removal of carbon dioxide from working cells, it has been suggested that exercise may increase the need for micronutrients required to make hemoglobin and RBCs. Exercise may also increase the loss of these nutrients. Additionally, active people may require more folate and vitamin B_{12} to build and repair muscle cells on a daily basis, and they may need more iron because of the increased iron losses associated with exercise (see figure 12.2). Theoretically, exercise could increase the need for any of these nutrients in the following ways:

- By altering absorption of the nutrient due to decreased transit time
- By increasing the turnover, metabolism, or loss of the nutrient in urine, feces, or sweat
- By increasing the need due to the biochemical adaptations (e.g., increased concentrations of enzymes that require the nutrient as a cofactor) associated with training
- By increasing the need for the nutrient for tissue maintenance and repair
- By altering RBC fragility or turnover, which decreases the half-life of the RBC and increases the need for new RBC formation

In fact, there is some biochemical evidence of poor micronutrient status for these nutrients in active people, although the data for folate, vitamin B_{12}, and copper are limited and equivocal. Some active people may exhibit poor nutritional status due to long-term marginal dietary intakes associated with either poor dietary choices or reduced energy intake. Inconsistencies in these studies may be related to differences in the experimental design. Studies can differ in a number of factors:

- Degree of dietary control
- Type and intensity of exercise used
- Type and number of status indices measured
- Level of regular physical activity in which subjects engage
- Type of subjects included
- Whether or not a control group was included

In summary, exercise may increase the turnover of RBCs, which may in turn increase the total daily needs of iron, copper, folate, and vitamin B_{12} in active people. Even more vitamin B_{12} and folate may be required to help repair and maintain muscle tissue damaged with regular exercise. Finally, exercise appears to increase the losses of iron (figure 12.2). Ideally, if energy intake is adequate to cover energy expenditure, dietary intakes of these micronutrients should be adequate unless dietary food choices are poor or limited.

ASSESSMENT OF VITAMIN AND MINERAL STATUS

As mentioned in chapter 11, minerals are different from vitamins in their bioavailability, the length of time required for nutritional status to change, toxicity level, and their storage and turnover within the body. Changing a person's iron or copper status may take much longer and require a different dietary approach than changing the nutritional status of folate or vitamin B_{12}. The following section discusses the most common assessment parameters—including biochemical, dietary intake, and food source data—for iron, copper, folate, and vitamin B_{12}.

Biochemical Assessment of Status

As discussed in chapters 9 and 11, a number of parameters must be measured in order to assess a person's status for a particular vitamin or min-

eral. These parameters usually include biochemical measures that reflect the body's stores of the nutrient and the amount of the nutrient lost from the body in urine, blood, feces, or sweat. If available, functional measurements should be included—that is, measurements that determine the availability of the nutrient to function as a coenzyme within the body. Biochemical measurements can be either direct (measurement of blood, urine, or fecal concentration of the nutrient or its metabolite) or indirect (measurement of an enzyme that requires the nutrient as a cofactor or measurement of that enzyme's functional activity). Finally, the typical dietary intake of the vitamin or mineral should be determined. Since minerals often exhibit poor bioavailability, the form of the dietary mineral needs to be ascertained, as well as any dietary factors that may alter bioavailability.

Iron

Determination of iron status, done routinely in clinical settings, requires the assessment of blood

---

Highlight

How Do You Measure Iron Status in an Active Individual?

At the present time, assessment of iron status is not routinely done with active individuals. Currently, only about 50% of National Collegiate Athletic Association (NCAA) schools screen for iron status in their female athletes (Cowell et al. 2003). Until we have established guidelines from sports governing bodies for assessing iron status in active individuals, follow these steps to determine iron status and the best method of treatment.

1. Measure blood iron status parameters and determine stage of iron deficiency as outlined in table 12.4. Measure at least one parameter for each stage of iron deficiency. A typical routine blood test for iron status usually measures serum ferritin, transferrin receptor, serum iron, serum total iron-binding capacity (TIBC), hemoglobin, hematocrit, MCV, and RBC count.

2. Assess total dietary iron intake, and roughly determine intake of heme versus non-heme iron. Is the individual a vegetarian who consumes no heme iron?

3. Assess inhibitors of dietary iron absorption (high tea or coffee consumption, high fiber intake, low vitamin C intake, mineral supplementation, gastrointestinal distress).

4. Determine if there is excess iron loss (fecal, urine, blood losses; blood donations).

5. Determine level and type of physical activity. Has the individual just begun a fitness program, or has he or she been exercising for a long time?

6. Find out if the person has been diagnosed with iron deficiency in the past. Is there a history of iron deficiency in the family?

7. Determine the individual's prior use of iron supplements and whether iron supplements cause gastrointestinal distress. People who do not tolerate iron supplements may need to use small doses more frequently during the day and with meals, or increase their intake of heme iron sources, in order to reverse anemia.

and hematological parameters (see "How Do You Measure Iron Status in an Active Individual?"), dietary iron intake, other dietary factors that may alter iron absorption, and any factors that may increase iron loss from the body (Gibson 2005). Figure 12.4 outlines the various iron pools within the body and the routes for iron recycling and loss. The body carefully recycles the iron in hemoglobin from old RBCs and uses it to make new RBCs. However, if the loss of iron exceeds the ability to recycle iron or to absorb iron from the diet, iron deficiency can develop.

Table 12.4 describes the stages of iron deficiency and the blood and hematological parameters traditionally assessed. **Iron depletion (stage I)** is characterized by poor serum ferritin concentrations, which indicate that iron stores within the body are depleted. In addition, iron absorption, serum **soluble transferrin receptors (sTfR),** and TIBC (the available sites on transferrin for binding are high) will begin to increase. A classification of **iron deficiency erythropoiesis (stage II)** is used if serum ferritin and iron concentrations are low, saturation of transferrin with iron is low, serum transferrin receptors are increased, and TIBC is high. Finally, **iron deficiency anemia (stage III)** is diagnosed by low hemoglobin concentrations, low RBC count, and low hematocrit (the ratio, by volume, of packed red cells and whole blood). It is not unusual for a person (especially an athletic woman) to stabilize at either stage I or II iron deficiency without progressing to stage III iron deficiency anemia. As table 12.4 demonstrates, the development of iron deficiency is slow and progresses through each of the stages. As iron deficiency progresses, the effect on physical activity becomes more dramatic. The specific effects of stage I or stage II iron deficiency on exercise performance and the ability to do work are just now being examined, and some mixed results have been produced. Recent research (Hinton et al. 2000; Brownlie et al. 2004) shows that iron supplementation in untrained women with low ferritin concentrations who were put through a training program, even when serum iron and hemoglobin levels

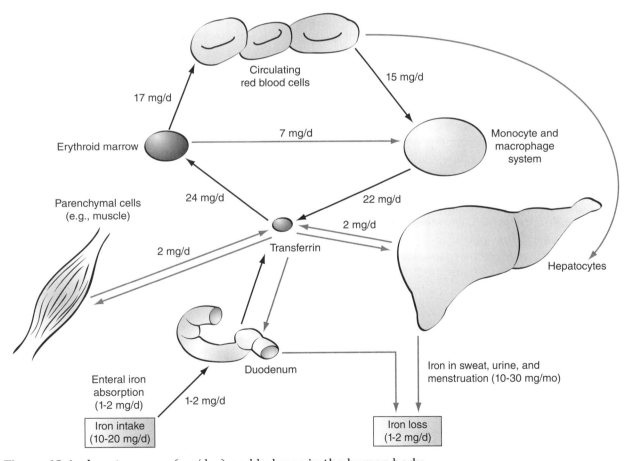

Figure 12.4 Iron turnover (mg/day) and balance in the human body.

Reprinted, by permission, from P. Nielson and D. Nachtigal, 1998, "Iron supplementation in athletes. Current recommendations," *Sports Medicine* 26(4): 207-216.

Table 12.4 Stages of Iron Deficiency

Stage of deficiency	Clinical parameter altered	Effect on exercise performance
I. Iron deficiency: Iron stores are low.	• Plasma ferritin <12 μg/L (<12 ng/ml)	• Enzymes requiring Fe may be inhibited, causing glucose oxidation and lactic acid production to increase.
II. Iron deficiency erythropoiesis: Ability to synthesize new RBCs is decreased.	• Plasma ferritin <12 μg/L (<12 ng/ml) • Serum soluble transferrin receptor (sTfR) (mg/L) >8.5 mg/L • Total iron-binding capacity (TIBC) >4000 μg/L (>400 μg/dL) • Transferrin saturation <16% • Plasma iron <500 μg/L (<50 μg/dL)	• Iron available for hemoglobin synthesis is now decreased and new RBCs will not be made. Delivery of oxygen to the cells may be inhibited, especially in high-intensity exercise.

III. Iron deficiency anemia: Number of red cells is decreased because iron is not available.	• Plasma ferritin <12 μg/L (<12 ng/ml)
	• sTfR (mg/L) >8.5 mg/L
	• TIBC >4000 μg/L (>400 μg/dL)
	• Transferrin saturation <16%
	• Plasma iron <500 μg/L (<50 μg/dL)
	• Hemoglobin <120 g/L (<12 mg/dL)
	• Hematocrit <36%
	• RBCs decreased in number; microcytic and hypochromic
		• Ability to do exercise is decreased, especially the ability to do high-intensity exercise. The following physiological parameters may change:
		  • ↓Oxygen delivery
		  • ↓$\dot{V}O_2$max
		  • ↓Endurance exercise
		  • ↓Oxidative capacity
		  • ↓Respiratory quotient, glucose oxidation, and lactic acid production

Adapted from R.S. Gibson, 2005, *Principles of nutritional assessment*, 2nd ed. (New York: Oxford University Press); Institute of Medicine, 2001, *Food and nutrition board. Dietary reference intakes: Vitamin A, vitamin K, arsenic, boron, chromium, copper, iodine, iron, manganese, molybdenum, nickel, silicon, vanadium and zinc* (Washington, DC: National Academy Press).

were normal, significantly decreased 15 km running times and improved endurance capacity compared to values in controls who were not supplementing. Thus, individuals in stage I iron depletion may have reduced cellular oxidative capacity, which decreases their aerobic capacity, endurance, energetic efficiency, voluntary activity, and work productivity (Haas and Brownlie 2001). So, people with good iron status, or those who improve their iron status, may find that their hours of training result in a greater training effect and improved exercise performance compared to what occurs in people who continue to have low ferritin and serum transferrin receptor values.

Helping athletes improve iron status takes time, but the time required to return a person to good iron status from stage I depletion is much shorter than it would be if the person had progressed to stage III iron deficiency anemia. For this reason, active people, especially females who limit their intake of heme iron, should be routinely assessed for iron status, including measurement of *all* assessment parameters (see "How Do You Measure Iron Status in an Active Individual?"). "Iron Status Assessment Parameters: What Do They Measure? What Do They Mean?" explains each of the iron status assessment parameters in more detail.

Highlight

Iron Status Assessment Parameters: What Do They Measure? What Do They Mean?

Body iron can be divided into two categories: storage iron and functional iron. Storage iron is that which is stored in the liver, spleen, and bone marrow; functional iron is that found in hemoglobin, myoglobin, and the iron-requiring enzymes of the body. Storage iron represents the balance between the amount of iron taken in or recycled and the amount of iron lost each day. In the United States, males typically have 1000 mg of stored iron while females have 300 mg. Iron can be stored as either **ferritin** or **hemosiderin.** One can estimate the amount of stored iron by measuring serum ferritin concentrations.

Ferritin

Ferritin is a protein that binds iron and stores it within the cells, especially in the liver. A small amount of ferritin circulates in the blood. Since circulating ferritin reflects the amount of stored iron within the body, measurement of serum ferritin can be used to estimate iron stores. To estimate iron stores using serum ferritin concentrations, assume that 1 μg ferritin per liter = 8 mg stored iron.

Hemosiderin

Hemosiderin is an insoluble form of stored iron that forms large concentrated clusters within the cell.

Soluble Transferrin Receptor

The measurement of soluble serum transferrin receptor (sTfR) has recently been proposed as a new sensitive indicator of iron deficiency. The sTfR is an iron-related protein that regulates the uptake of iron into body cells. When the cells need more iron, the expression of sTfR increases, thus allowing more uptake of iron by the cells. A soluble form of sTfR circulates in the blood and is a good indicator of the total body mass of cellular sTfR (Gibson 2005). The circulating levels of sTfR are a good indicator of the degree of iron within the tissues. As iron status decreases, the expression of sTfR increases, which allows cells to compete more effectively for the circulating transferrin-bound iron. Thus, sTfR is a good method for assessing functional iron deficiency without anemia. In addition, the sTfR is not affected by the acute-phase response as ferritin is (Rocker et al. 2002). Some researchers report the concentration of sTfR (mg/L), while others report the ratio of sTfR concentration and the logarithm of the ferritin concentration: TfR/logFerr index. When either the sTfR or the sTfR/logFerr index increases, iron status is decreasing. The actual cutoff values considered high will depend on the assays used. Usually sTfR values >8.5 mg/L are considered high (IOM 2001), while a sTfR/logFerr value >1.8 is considered high.

Serum Iron

Serum iron represents the total amount of iron in the serum, both free iron (usually very little) and iron bound to transferrin (a transport protein in the blood).

Transferrin Saturation

Transferrin is a blood protein that transports minerals, including iron, to the cells. Normally about one third of transferrin is saturated with iron; normal saturation ranges are from 16% to 50%.

Total Iron-Binding Capacity

Total iron-binding capacity (TIBC) represents the total capacity for transferrin to bind and carry iron to the cells. If little iron is available, TIBC is high, for the reason that transferrin has a strong ability to bind iron but none is available to bind. With increasing iron deficiency, TIBC concentration increases while other iron status assessment parameters decrease.

Hemoglobin

Whole-blood hemoglobin concentration is a quantitative measure of the amount of hemoglobin in the blood. If this value is low, then the body has insufficient hemoglobin available to make normal RBCs.

Hematocrit

Hematocrit is a proportional measure of the actual volume of red cells in whole blood compared to the total blood volume. A lowered hematocrit means that there are fewer red cells in the blood.

People who have progressed to stage III iron deficiency anemia have the classic symptoms of fatigue, lethargy, and inability to exercise at previous levels of intensity. Reversing iron deficiency anemia (stage III) usually requires supplemental iron, changes in dietary habits, and reduction of iron losses if they are present. Because iron absorption is low (~5-10% of dietary iron), it usually takes four to six months or longer before hemoglobin levels are normal. People in stage I or stage II deficiency may see improvement in iron status in three or four months if they follow dietary recommendations and minimize iron losses. "Case Studies of Iron Deficiency Anemia" describes one case of deficiency caused by blood loss and another that resulted from poor dietary iron intake and increased iron losses.

Copper

Currently, there is no generally acknowledged index of copper status similar to that used for iron (Milne 1998). One reason it is difficult to identify a consistent assessment marker for copper is that the body has strong homeostatic control over copper and maintains tissue copper within a constant range (Gibson 2005). Assessment of copper status usually involves measuring serum copper and ceruloplasmin concentrations, hair concentrations, and the activities of certain copper enzymes in the blood (superoxide dismutase or cytochrome-c oxidase). Serum copper concentrations are the most routinely measured clinical assessment of severe copper deficiency but are not sensitive enough to use as an index of copper status in healthy people (Gibson 2005; Milne 1998). Serum copper and ceruloplasmin can be artificially increased by many factors such as oral contraceptives, infection, inflammation, stress, and various diseases (leukemia, Hodgkin's disease, collagen disorders, hemochromatosis, inflammation, and myocardial infarctions). Conversely, a number of factors—such as protein-energy malnutrition, malabsorption syndromes, and ulcerative colitis—can decrease serum copper concentrations independent of copper intake. Because numerous factors appear to influence serum copper and ceruloplasmin concentrations, copper-containing enzymes in blood cells, such as RBC superoxide dismutase and platelet cytochrome-c oxidase, may be better indicators of copper status (Milne 1998).

Folate

Assessment of folate status has been well characterized and developed into a four-stage model,

similar to the three-stage model used for assessing iron status (Herbert and Das 1994; Gibson 2005) (see table 12.5). **Negative folate balance (stage I)** is determined by poor folate concentrations, which indicate that folate stores within the body are becoming depleted. Low serum folate concentrations and a decrease in erythrocyte folate concentrations characterize **folate depletion (stage II)**. A classification of **folate deficiency erythropoiesis (stage III)** is used if serum folate and RBC folate concentrations are low and if DNA synthesis is impaired as determined by the deoxyuridine (dU) suppression test. In this test, normal folate must be present for the methylation of dU to thymidine (Gibson 2005). Thus, in stage III folate deficiency, the ability to make RBCs has become impaired, and the signs of anemia will begin to develop if folate intake does not increase. Finally, clinical **folate deficiency anemia (stage IV)** is characterized by the classic anemia symptoms and elevated mean corpuscular volume (MCV) (Herbert and Das 1994). As you can see from table 12.5, the development of folate deficiency is similar to that discussed for iron. As folate intake decreases and less folate is available for metabolic functions, one slowly progresses through each of the stages.

Vitamin B_{12}

Assessment of vitamin B_{12} status has also been characterized as a four-stage process (Herbert and Das 1994; Gibson 2005) (table 12.6). **Negative vitamin B_{12} balance (stage I)** is marked by a decrease in vitamin B_{12} absorption such that the level of vitamin B_{12} transported on serum transcobalamin II (TC II) is decreased. Transcobalamin II is a transport protein for vitamin B_{12}. When vitamin B_{12} (cobalamin) is attached to TC II, it is termed holoTC II. **Vitamin B_{12} depletion (stage II)** is characterized in part by a decrease in the percent saturation of the transport protein (TC II) with vitamin B_{12} and a decrease in the absolute amount of holoTC II. Approximately 20% of serum vitamin B_{12} is attached to TC II, and the remaining 80% is bound to other glycoproteins collectively called haptocorrins (Gibson 2005). When vitamin B_{12} is attached to these transport proteins they are called holohaptocorrins (holohap). Stage II, then, is characterized by (1) low serum holoTC II concentrations, (2) decreased saturation of TC II, *and* (3) decreased holohap levels.

A classification of **vitamin B_{12} deficiency erythropoiesis (stage III)** is used if (1) all these characteristics are present, (2) RBC folate and serum vitamin B_{12} are low (<100 pg/ml), *and* (3)

Case Studies of Iron Deficiency Anemia

A number of factors may contribute to the development of iron deficiency anemia in an active person. These two case studies provide you with two very different examples of how an individual might have developed poor iron status. In the male hockey player, iron deficiency anemia is related to another health problem, while in the female athlete the iron deficiency anemia is due to poor diet.

Case Study 1: Male Hockey Player With Gastrointestinal Bleeding

A 25-year-old minor league hockey player had been diagnosed with iron deficiency anemia the year before while playing for another team. At that time, his iron deficiency was determined by blood work, and he was started on supplemental iron therapy. No further investigation was done to determine the cause of the deficiency. The player said that he took the supplemental iron whenever he felt fatigued. He could relate no obvious sources of blood loss. He admitted having dark stools but attributed them to the iron therapy. He reported no history of peptic ulcer disease or chronic use of nonsteroidal anti-inflammatory drugs (NSAIDs). The player reported occasional bouts of cramping in the lower abdomen but said they were not severe enough to prevent him from playing. He attributed some of his abdominal pain to the iron therapy. He had no family history of inflammatory bowel disease or anemias.

Although the physical exam did not show abdominal tenderness or palpable masses, the rectal exam revealed dark stools that were positive for blood. Blood work indicated significant iron deficiency as evidenced by low iron, percent transferrin saturation, and ferritin.

Iron Status Assessment Parameters for Male Hockey Player With Anemia

	Patient values	Normal for men[a]
Hemoglobin (g/dL)	13.1	14.0-18.0
Hematocrit (%)	41.0	42.0-52.0
Mean corpuscular volume (MCV) (mm^3)	80.6	80-100
Serum iron (mg/dL)	20	76-198
Total iron-binding capacity (mg/dL)	312	213-521
Transferrin saturation (%)	6	20-50
Ferritin (ng/ml)[b]	28	30-300

[a] Normal values will depend on the laboratory assessing the parameters.
[b] Ferritin level increases with inflammation, cancer, and liver disease.

The player was referred to a gastroenterologist. Colonoscopy revealed extensive ulceration in the small intestine and deformity of the ileocecal valve. Pathology reports confirmed diagnosis of Crohn's disease. Drugs were used to help control the disease and to stop the gastrointestinal bleeding. After a month of convalescence, the player was able to finish the last month of the hockey season. The player was informed of the seriousness of his disease and the risk of increased exacerbations if he continued his hockey career.

Summary: In this case study, the athlete had iron deficiency anemia due to excessive blood loss from the bowel. Although iron supplements helped replace iron lost in the blood, the source of the blood loss needed to be identified before appropriate treatment could begin.

(continued)

Reprinted from R.J. Browne, 1996, "Evaluating and treating active patients for anemia," *Physician Sportsmedicine* 24(9): 79-84.

Case Studies of Iron Deficiency Anemia *(continued)*

Case Study 2: Female Athlete With Poor Dietary Iron Intake

A 21-year-old female athlete and personal trainer complained of fatigue, inability to perform high-intensity workouts, and a decrease in exercise performance. She participated in 23 to 25 h of exercise per week (running, cycling, strength training, and stair climbing) and competed in local road races and duathlons. Assessment of body composition indicated body fat at 16.6% and a body mass index of 19.1 kg/m². Examination of the athlete's diet showed a total energy intake of 2234 kcal/day, iron intake of 10.9 mg/day, calcium intake of 936 mg/day, and zinc intake of 9.1 mg/day. This person generally avoided flesh foods (meat, fish, and poultry) but would occasionally consume tuna or chicken. Most of her dietary iron came from plant foods (whole grains, spinach, and beans) and fortified breakfast cereals (bran cereals).

Iron Status Assessment Parameters for Female Athlete With Anemia

	Patient values	Normal for women[a]
Hemoglobin (g/dL)	11.3	11.5-15.0
Hematocrit (%)	32	34-43
Mean corpuscular volume (MCV) (mm³)	93	80-100
Serum iron (mg/dL)	40	60-160
Total iron-binding capacity (mg/dL)	480	250-400
Transferrin saturation (%)	10	20-50
Ferritin (ng/ml)[b]	<5	12-120

[a] Normal values will depend on the laboratory assessing the blood parameters.
[b] Ferritin level increases with inflammation, cancer, and liver disease.

The athlete had never had her iron status measured. She reported no donation of blood or excessive blood losses. Menstrual blood flow was regular and normal. However, she had been limiting her intake of flesh foods over the past five years in order to reduce her total fat intake. She agreed to increase daily intake of heme iron (fish and chicken), to add orange juice to meals with cereal or meals high in non-heme iron, and to begin taking an iron supplement daily. Reevaluation of status would be done in four to six months.

Summary: In this case study, the athlete had iron deficiency anemia due to poor iron intake over the last five years. She agreed to increase daily intake of heme iron foods (tuna and chicken) and take a daily iron supplement to improve overall iron intake. No sources of the blood loss were identified.

DNA synthesis is impaired as determined by the dU suppression test (Gibson 2005). Thus, in stage III vitamin B_{12} deficiency, the biochemical function of vitamin B_{12} is impaired, making folate unavailable for RBC synthesis. At this stage of deficiency, the classic signs of anemia will begin to develop if vitamin B_{12} intake does not increase.

Finally, the classic anemia symptoms, along with elevated MCV and low hemoglobin (Herbert and Das 1994), characterize clinical **vitamin B_{12} deficiency anemia (stage IV)**. As you can see from table 12.6, the development of vitamin B_{12} deficiency is similar to the process described for both iron and folate.

Table 12.5 Stages of Folate Deficiency

Stage of deficiency	Clinical parameter altered	Effect on exercise performance
I. Negative folate balance: Folate stores are low.	• Serum folate <3 ng/ml	Enzymes requiring folate may be inhibited.
II. Folate depletion: Folate stores are depleted.	• Serum folate <3 ng/ml • RBC folate <160 ng/ml • Serum homocysteine may be elevated	Enzymes requiring folate may be inhibited.
III. Folate deficiency erythropoiesis: Ability to synthesize new RBCs is decreased due to defective DNA synthesis.	• Serum folate <3 ng/ml • RBC folate <160 ng/ml • Deoxyuridine (dU) suppression test abnormal • Liver folate <1.2 μg/g	Ability to produced RBCs is inhibited, and new RBCs will not be made. Delivery of oxygen to the cells may be inhibited, especially in high-intensity exercise.
IV. Folate deficiency anemia: Number of red cells is decreased because folate is not available for DNA synthesis.	• Serum folate <3 ng/ml • RBC folate <110 ng/ml • dU suppression test abnormal • Liver folate <1.2 μg/g • MCV = elevated and RBCs are macrocytic • Hemoglobin <120 g/L (<12 g/dL) • RBCs low	Ability to do (especially high-intensity) exercise is decreased. RBCs are larger than normal, with poor ability to transport oxygen. The following physiological parameters may change: • ↓Oxygen delivery • ↓$\dot{V}O_2$max • ↓Endurance exercise • ↓Oxidative capacity

RBC = red blood cells; MCV = mean cell volume.

Adapted from R.S. Gibson, 2005, *Principles of nutritional assessment,* 2nd ed. (New York: Oxford University Press); V. Herbert, K.C. Das, 1994, Folic acid and vitamin B-12. In *Modern nutrition in health and disease,* edited by M.E. Shils, J.A. Olson, and M. Shike (Philadelphia, PA: Lippincott, Williams, and Wilkins), 402-425; J. Lindenbaum and R.H. Allen, 1995, Clinical spectrum and diagnosis of folate deficiency. In *Folate in health and disease,* edited by L.B. Bailey (New York: Marcel Dekker), 43-73.

Dietary Intakes of Active Individuals

As discussed in chapters 9 and 14, determination of accurate and typical dietary intakes of micronutrients can be difficult. If you use dietary records, you must rely on clients' abilities to accurately record portion sizes, remember foods consumed, and save and record information from labels and restaurant menus. (Remember also, as you read research articles, to pay close attention to how the authors collected the nutrient intake data they reported—shaky data lead to shaky conclusions!) Most active individuals, especially athletes, have a weekly training schedule, which may affect their eating behaviors. For these individuals, collection of food records over this training period will give you a much better idea of their typical eating patterns than records for one or two days during the week. Thus, if you use diet records, have your clients report data for a minimum of three days, making sure these three days represent typical days within their week. And always consider carefully the energy intake that is required for a given client to maintain his or her current activity level.

Iron

Iron depletion (low serum concentrations of ferritin) is one of the most prevalent nutrient deficiencies in the world as well as in the United States (Yip 2001). It is estimated that 6% to 11% of females of reproductive age are iron depleted. The number is higher in some subgroups—about 14% of females aged 15 to 19 years, and 25% of pregnant women (Tobin and Beard 1997). This poor iron status is usually attributed to poor total and heme iron intakes, habitual dieting, or smoking (Houston et al. 1997).

Examination of dietary iron intakes of active people who do not supplement with iron indicates that for males, iron intakes are usually well above the RDA of 8 mg/day (IOM 2001) (table 12.7). This high iron intake is typically due to the higher energy intakes of male athletes since the iron density of their diets is similar to that seen in female athletes and in the typical Western diet (6 mg iron per 1000 kcal). The iron intake of female athletes is more variable (table 12.7). Studies published in the late 1980s and early 1990s typically showed that the dietary iron intakes of female athletes were less than the RDA of 18 mg/day (Haymes

Table 12.6   Stages of Vitamin B$_{12}$ Deficiency

Stage of deficiency	Clinical parameter altered	Effect on exercise performance
I. Negative vitamin B$_{12}$ balance: Vitamin B$_{12}$ absorption is decreased.	• Serum holoTC II <40 pg/ml • TC II% saturation <4%	Enzymes requiring vitamin B$_{12}$ may be inhibited.
II. Vitamin B$_{12}$ depletion: Vitamin B$_{12}$ stores are depleted.	• Serum holoTC II <40 pg/ml • TC II% saturation <4% • Holohap <150 pg/ml	Enzymes requiring vitamin B$_{12}$ may be inhibited.
III. Vitamin B$_{12}$ deficiency erythropoiesis: Ability to synthesize new RBCs is decreased due to defective DNA synthesis.	• Serum holoTC II <40 pg/ml • TC II% saturation <4% • Holohap <100 pg/ml • Serum B$_{12}$ <100 pg/ml • Deoxyuridine (dU) suppression test abnormal • TBBC % sat <15%	Ability to produce RBCs is inhibited, and new RBCs will not be made. Delivery of oxygen to the cells may be inhibited, especially in high-intensity exercise.
IV. Vitamin B$_{12}$ deficiency anemia: Number of red cells is decreased because vitamin B$_{12}$ is deficient.	• Serum holoTC II <40 pg/ml • TC II% saturation <4% • Holohap <100 pg/ml • Serum B$_{12}$ <100 pg/ml • dU suppression test abnormal • MCV = elevated and RBCs are macrocytic • Hemoglobin <120 g/L • Serum homocysteine elevated • Serum methylmalonic acid elevated	Ability to do (especially high-intensity) exercise is decreased. RBCs are larger than normal, with poor ability to transport oxygen. The following physiological parameters may change: • ↓Oxygen delivery • ↓$\dot{V}O_2$max • ↓Endurance exercise • ↓Oxidative capacity

RBC = red blood cells; MCV = mean cell volume; holoTC II = holotranscobalamin II (transcobalamin II with attached cobalamin); TC II% = percentage of total TC II with attached cobalamin; holohap = holohaptocorrin with attached cobalamin; TBBC % sat = percentage of total B$_{12}$-binding capacity of plasma with attached B$_{12}$.

Adapted from R.S. Gibson, 2005, *Principles of nutritional assessment,* 2nd ed. (New York: Oxford University Press); V. Herbert, K.C. Das, 1994, Folic acid and vitamin B-12. In *Modern nutrition in health and disease,* edited by M.E. Shils, J.A. Olson, and M. Shike (Philadelphia, PA: Lippincott, Williams, and Wilkins), 402-425; J. Lindenbaum and R.H. Allen, 1995, Clinical spectrum and diagnosis of folate deficiency. In *Folate in health and disease,* edited by L.B. Bailey (New York: Marcel Dekker), 43-73.

and Clarkson 1998). However, more recent studies show higher iron intakes in female athletes from diet alone. For example, Beals and Manore (1998) examined the diets of 24 female athletes classified with subclinical eating disorders and 24 female athlete controls. Although 20% to 30% of the athletes had low plasma ferritin concentrations (indicating stage I iron depletion), they had mean dietary iron intakes between 17 and 22 mg/day, levels similar to the current RDA of 18 mg/day. However, much of this iron in the diets of these athletes is from non-heme–fortified foods such as breakfast cereal, energy and breakfast bars, and fat-free or low-fat snacks. Unfortunately, this type of iron is less bioavailable. The increased prevalence of fortified foods in the typical American diet, and particularly in the diets of athletes, has increased the intake of many micronutrients, including iron. However, this increased intake of iron has not eliminated the iron deficiency in these athletes.

Copper

Determination of copper intake in active people is limited since most current nutrient databases have poor or limited copper data. For the six studies that have reported copper intake in active individuals (see table 12.8), mean intakes were 1.3 to 2.7 mg/day. Only Gropper and colleagues (2003) reported lower copper intakes, in their female softball and soccer players who did not supplement with copper (~0.6 mg/day). The current RDA for copper is 900 µg/day or 0.9 mg/day (IOM 2001).

Folate and Vitamin B$_{12}$

According to large population surveys done in the United States (NHANES III), mean dietary folate intake is reported to be 313 to 322 µg/day for males and 254 to 269 µg/day for women 19 to 70 years— below the recommended 400 µg/day (IOM 1998). These intake data may underestimate the intake of folate and folic acid in the United States, partially

Table 12.7 Incidence of Low or Marginal Iron Status in Active Individuals

Study	Assessment indices	No. of subjects	Type of subjects	Low status (%)	Mean dietary intake (mg/day)[1]	(mg/1000 kcal)	Type of diet record
Aguilo et al. 2004	Ferritin[3,6]	18	Male endurance athletes	0%	28	6.5-7.0	3 day
Beals and Manore 1998	Ferritin[3,6]	24	Female athletes	21%	21.8	9.1	7 day
		24	SCED female athletes	29%	17.6	8.7	7 day
Choe et al. 2001	Ferritin[3,6]	148 M	High school athletes	3.4% (M)	–	–	24 h recall
		72 F		37.5% (F)	–	–	
Choi et al. 2001	Ferritin[2]	16	Male long-distance runners	31%	–	–	None
Constantini et al. 2000	Ferritin[2,6]	42 M	Elite young athletes (12-18 years)	9% (M)	–	–	None
		25 F		33% (F)			
Dubnov and Constantini 2004	Ferritin[2,6]	66 M	National-level basketball players (14-35 years)	M[7]: 5% ID, 3% anemia	–	–	None
		37 F		F[7]: 25% ID, 14% anemia			
Fogelholm et al. 1992	Ferritin[2]	427	Male athletes	3%	21.6	7.1	FFQ
Gray et al. 1993	Ferritin[2,6]	10	Male triathletes	0%	–	–	None
Landahl et al. 2005	Ferritin[3,6]	28	Female elite soccer players	57% ID,[7] 29% anemia	–	–	None
Malczewska et al. 2000	Ferritin[2,6]	126	Female endurance athletes (16-20 years)	26%	14.5-15.0	5.4-5.5	24 h recall
Malczewska et al. 2001	Ferritin and sTfR index[7]	131 M	Athletes (all sports)	11% (M)	–	–	None
		121 F		26% (F)			
Manore et al. 1989	Ferritin[2,6]	10	Female runners	50-60%	11.6	5.7	9 day
Matter et al. 1987	Ferritin[2]	85	Female runners	16%	–	–	None
Newhouse et al. 1989	Ferritin[2,6]	155	Female recreational runners	25%	80% of those with low ferritin reported consuming <14 mg/day of iron		None
Nuviala and Lapieza 1997	Ferritin[3]	78	Female athletes	18%	13.5-14.1	6.1-6.4	7 day
Rocker et al. 2002	Ferritin[2,6] sTfR index[7]	12	Female endurance triathlon participants	42% ferritin 33% TR	–	–	None
Sinclair and Hinton 2005	Ferritin[3,6] sTfR index[7]	49 M	Recreationally trained individuals (11 h/week)	4-6% (M)	–	–	–
		72 F		29-36% (F)			
Singh et al. 1992	Ferritin[5]	11	Active males	0%	23.2	8.3	4 day
Weight et al. 1988	Ferritin[6]	30	Male runners	0%	14.9	6.0	5 day
Wilkinson et al. 2002	Ferritin[2]	11	Elite male cyclists	0%	–	–	None

[1] Mean ± SD or range of intakes; [2] ferritin <20 µg/L used to indicate poor status, except that Matter and colleagues used <40 µg/L to indicate poor status; [3] <12 to 16 µg/L used to indicate poor status; [4] included both male and females; [5] data from placebo group only (no supplements); [6] measured all iron status parameters (ferritin, serum iron, total iron-binding capacity [TIBC], hemoglobin, hematocrit); [7] sTfR index = serum soluble transferrin receptor index; ID = iron deficiency (low ferritin); anemia = iron deficiency anemia (low hemoglobin). FFQ = food frequency questionnaire; SCED = athletes with subclinical eating disorders.

Note: The use of iron supplements was not always indicated, especially when diets records were not collected. Thus, some of the athletes in these studies were probably using supplements. No study was used in this table if the authors specifically indicated that athletes were supplementing with iron.

because people underestimate what they eat and also because there are analysis problems with measuring the folate content of food (IOM 1998). Thus, it is difficult to estimate the actual intake of folate in the U.S. population. The median intake of vitamin B_{12} from food in the United States is estimated to be 5 μg/day for men and 3.5 μg/day for women (IOM 1998).

Research on the folate and vitamin B_{12} intakes of recreationally active adults is limited, with most of the data reflecting the dietary intakes of competitive athletes. In general, studies examining dietary intakes of active males (using at least three-day diet records and published since 1988) show adequate mean intakes of folate and vitamin B_{12} (Faber and Benade 1991; Jensen et al. 1992; Niekamp and Baer 1995; Rico-Sanz et al. 1998). These adequate intakes can be attributed to the relatively high-energy diets of these subjects. However, others (Nieman et al. 1989; Rankinen et al. 1998; Rousseau et al. 2005; Weight et al. 1988; Worme et al. 1990) reported mean folate intakes in their male athletes to be less than the RDA, ranging from 264 to 386 μg/day. Some of these low folate intakes may be attributed to reduced energy intake during times of high training or for maintenance of low body weights. For example, Rankinen and colleagues (1998) reported that their elite male ski jumpers consumed only 286 μg/day of folate (four-day diet records), but their energy intake was 1816 kcal/day—very low for an active male. No study has shown low vitamin B_{12} intakes in male athletes. In summary, it appears that the high energy intake of active males keeps dietary intakes of folate and vitamin B_{12} high, usually 1.5 to 2.0 times the RDA.

As expected, dietary intakes of folate and vitamin B_{12} are lower in active females than in active males. Folate is the one B vitamin that appears to be consistently low in the diets of active females. The current RDA for folate is 400 μg/day for adult women (IOM 1998). It is also recommended that to prevent fetal neural tube defects, women of childbearing age consume 400 μg/day of synthetic folic acid over and above that present in the diet (IOM 1998; O'Keefe et al. 1995; Scott et al. 1995).

Currently, only one study in active females shows mean folate intakes >400 μg/day. Beshgetoor and Nichols (2003) found that female master athletes (mean age = 50 years) had a mean folate intake of 402 μg/day (four-day records). Typically the mean folate intakes reported for active young females range from 189 to 306 mg/day when at least three-day diet records are used (Beals and Manore 1998;

Clark et al. 2003; Faber and Benade 1991; Kaiser-auer et al. 1989; Keith et al. 1989; Kopp-Woodroffe et al. 1999; Manore et al. 1989; Nieman et al. 1989; Worme et al. 1990). Recent studies by Beals and Manore (1998) and Clark and colleagues (2003) showed that 47% to 68% of their female athletes consumed less than 400 μg/day of folate. These data suggest that many active women do not have adequate folate intakes even when they use fortified foods. Two factors may contribute to the low folate intake values in active women as reported in the literature. First, early studies on folate intake may have underreported the actual amount of folate in the diet since the folate databases for many foods were incomplete. Second, if the active women surveyed restricted energy intake or made poor food choices, then folate intakes would be low. However, in January 1998, the USDA mandated the fortification of bread, flour, cornmeal, pasta, and rice with folic acid. If female athletes consume these foods, then folate intake should increase above the levels observed before mandated fortification. However, only one study published after fortification has shown adequate mean intakes for folate (Beshgetoor and Nichols 2003). These higher intakes were observed in older women (master athletes) who may pay more attention to their diets. Thus, getting adequate folate into the diets of active women, especially young women, still appears to be a problem. No studies show low mean vitamin B_{12} intakes in active females (Woolf and Manore 2006). See the studies by Woolf and Manore (2006, 2005) for additional reading on the B vitamin intakes of active women.

NUTRITIONAL STATUS OF ACTIVE INDIVIDUALS

The following section deals with the incidence of poor status of iron, folate, and vitamin B_{12} in active people.

Iron

There are three primary reasons to examine iron status in active people:

1. Iron deficiency is one of the most prevalent deficiency problems in the United States, especially in adolescent girls and premeno-pausal women.

2. Active females appear to have a higher incidence of iron deficiency than is typically found in the general female population. This

Table 12.8 Incidence of Low or Marginal Copper (Cu), Folate, and Vitamin B$_{12}$ Status in Active Indviduals

Study	Assessment indices	No. of sub-jects	Type of subjects	Low status (%)	Mean dietary intake[1]		Type of diet record
Copper					**mg/day**	**mg/1000 kcal**	
Bazzarre et al. 1993	Serum Cu	16	Male athletes[2]	0%	2.7 ± 1.1	1.2	7 day
Dressendorfer et al. 2002	Serum Cu Urine Cu	9	Male competitive cyclists	0%	–	–	–
Gropper et al. 2003	Serum Cu and Ceruloplasmin	21	Female athletes (softball and soccer only)[2]	0%	0.6 ± 0.3	0.3	3 day
Koury et al. 2004	Plasma Cu and Ceruloplasmin	44	Male athletes	0%	1-2 median	0.3-0.6 median	24 h recall
Lukaski et al. 1990	Serum Cu	13	Male swimmers	0%	1.6 ± 0.1	0.5	7 day
		16	Female swimmers	0%	1.3 ± 0.1	0.6	7 day
Lukaski et al. 1996	Serum Cu	5	Male swimmers	0%	1.8 ± 0.2	0.5	3 day
		5	Female swimmers	0%	1.3 ± 0.2	0.6	3 day
Weight et al. 1988	Serum Cu	30	Male runners	0%	2.2 ± 0.6	0.9	5 day
Folate					**μg/day**	**μg/1000 kcal**	
Beals and Manore 1998	Serum folate	24	Female athletes	8%	364 ± 99	152	7 day
		24	SCED athletes	8%	306 ± 157	122	
Herrmann et al. 2005	Serum folate	72	Endurance athletes[3]	0%	–	–	None
Konig et al. 2003	Plasma folate	42	Male triathletes	0%	–	–	None
Matter et al. 1987	Serum folate	85	Female marathoners	33%	–	–	None
Real et al. 2005	Plasma folate	22	Male marathoners	0%	–	–	None
Singh et al. 1992	Serum folate	11	Active males	0%	399 ± 90	143	4 day
Telford et al. 1992	Serum folate	44	Athletes[3]	11%	–	–	None
Weight et al. 1988	Serum and RBC folate	30	Male runners	0%	264 ± 100	107	5 day
Vitamin B$_{12}$					**μg/day**	**μg/1000 kcal**	
Beals and Manore 1998	Serum B$_{12}$	24	Female athletes	0%	3.9 ± 2.6	1.79	7 day
		24	SCED athletes	0%	4.3 ± 1.9	1.55	
Herrmann et al. 2005	Serum B$_{12}$	72	Endurance athletes[3]	0%	–	–	None
Konig et al. 2003	Plasma B$_{12}$	42	Male triathletes	0%	–	–	None
Real et al. 2005	Plasma B$_{12}$	22	Male marathoners	0%	–	–	None
Singh et al. 1992	Whole-blood B$_{12}$	11	Active males	0%[4]	4.5 ± 0.9	1.61	4 day
Telford et al. 1992	Serum B$_{12}$	44	Athletes[3]	5%	–	–	None
Weight et al. 1988	Serum B$_{12}$	30	Male runners	0%	4.9 ± 3.2	2.01	5 day

[1] Mean ± SD or range of intakes; [2] data from groups with no supplements; [3] men and women combined; [4] data from placebo group only (no supplements). RBC = red blood cells; SCED = Subclinical eating disorders.

may be due to weight and health issues since this population frequently avoids foods high in heme iron, such as meat, fish, and poultry. Many female athletes follow vegetarian diets (which provide no heme iron) or are dieting for weight loss—or may be doing both. If energy intake is restricted, total daily iron intake will decrease unless the individual is supplementing. Finally, the low serum ferritin values observed in active females may represent a mere shift in the iron pools rather than a true iron deficiency (See "What Is Sports Anemia?").

3. Iron plays an essential role in hemoglobin formation, and active people need adequate RBCs to transport oxygen to working muscles. Moreover, active individuals may have greater iron losses than their sedentary counterparts (figure 12.2).

Iron status is typically determined via measurement of blood iron parameters for each of the stages of iron deficiency; however, ferritin is the most common iron assessment index reported. In active males, iron status is typically good, with most studies indicating 0% to 13% of subjects with low ferritin concentrations (table 12.7) (Haymes and Clarkson 1998). Although iron deficiency anemia is reported in some male athletes (Browne 1996), the incidence is similar to the 2% seen in the general U.S. male population. Only Fogelholm and colleagues (1993) examined the effect of gradual or rapid weight loss in male athletes on iron status. They found that neither gradual weight loss (5% of body weight lost over a three-week period) nor rapid weight loss (6% of body weight lost over a 59 h period) changed serum ferritin concentrations. However, most of the subjects had been supplementing before participating in the study and, even while dieting, were consuming more than the RDA for iron.

Incidence of poor iron status in active females is much more variable and often depends on the type of athlete examined. However, if ferritin concentrations are used as the assessment criterion (either <12 or <20 mg/L is typically used), 15% to 60% of female athletes are reported to have poor iron stores (table 12.7) (Haymes 2006; Haymes and Clarkson 1998). This number is somewhat higher than the incidence of iron depletion (~20%) in the general U.S. adolescent and female population (Haymes 2006; Haymes and Clarkson 1998). The number of female athletes with stage III iron deficiency anemia is much lower than the number with stage I depletion, and the percentage is similar to that seen in the general female U.S. population (5-6%). Thus, the incidence of stage I iron depletion, which is indicative of poor iron stores, is much higher in active females than active males. Because of this, assessment of iron status, including dietary iron intakes, should be routinely done for active females. Care should also be taken to determine if changes in iron status reflect changes in iron stores and are not artificial changes due to the alterations in plasma volume that occur with training.

Copper

Assessment of copper status in active people has been limited. Only a few laboratories have reported both dietary copper intake and serum copper concentrations (table 12.8). According to these studies, copper status, based on blood levels of copper, appears to be adequate. Dietary intakes are more variable, but dietary assessment of copper is more difficult.

Folate and Vitamin B$_{12}$

According to national surveys in the United States (NHANES III), ~10% to 15% of the population have low folate stores, based on low serum folate concentrations (<3 ng/ml) (IOM 1998). Those at highest risk for poor folate status are women aged 19 to 50 years: 15% of this subpopulation have low serum folate concentrations (stage I folate deficiency), and 13% have low RBC folate (<140 ng/ml) (stage II folate deficiency) (Sauberlich 1995). High levels of homocysteine can also be a marker of poor folate status; but other B vitamins can affect homocysteine levels as well, so homocysteine is not highly specific just for folate. Based on NHANES III values for homocysteine, ~10% of individuals have high homocysteine values (>12 μmol/L) (IOM 1998). These data were all collected prior to fortification of folate in grain and cereal products. Data collected after fortification indicate that folate status (both dietary intakes and blood levels of folate) has improved, with fortification increasing folate intake in women ages 20 to 59 years by 70 to 77 μg/day and in men in the same age group ~95 μg/day (Dietrich et al. 2005). Unfortunately, mean folate intakes in the women after fortification (~300 μg/day) were still below the recommended level of 400 μg/day, while the men achieved the recommended level. Current data, collected after fortification, also indicate that individuals who use B vitamin–fortified breakfast

What Is Sports Anemia?

In the 1960s and 1970s, the term "sports anemia" was coined to refer to the increased red cell destruction reported in active people and to reflect the widespread belief that active people were deficient in iron (Weight 1993). More recently, researchers have reported changes in iron status in athletes who increase their training programs and in sedentary people who begin an exercise program. It was unclear whether the observed changes were signs of iron deficiency or were merely transient changes that occurred with the initiation of a strenuous exercise program. Follow-up research indicated that some individuals with low iron status did not respond to iron supplementation, which implied that their poor iron status was due not to poor iron intake but to other metabolic factors such as increased plasma volume or incorporation of iron into muscle. Not everyone who presents with low iron status indices has an iron deficiency. It appears that exercise—especially in people who are increasing exercise training or who are initiating an exercise program—can cause transient changes in iron status parameters.

If your client has poor iron status, how do you know whether this is an artifact due to change in exercise training or intensity or a real change in iron status? Here are some questions to help you make this determination:

- Is there a history of iron deficiency?
- Does the individual have low iron intakes, especially heme iron?
- Are there dietary factors that decrease iron absorption?
- Has the person just increased his or her exercise training, or initiated an exercise program?
- Was iron status normal before exercise training was increased or initiated?
- Does the person respond to iron supplementation or to increased iron in the diet?
- Are there increased blood losses?

If people respond to iron supplementation, then their low iron status was most likely due to inadequate iron. If they do not respond, low hemoglobin may be due to other dietary factors or may be a transient change due to physical activity. In the studies reviewed by Haymes and Clarkson (1998) on iron supplementation (18-300 mg/day) in active individuals, only 6 of 16 papers reported increases in hemoglobin concentrations with supplementation, while 11 of 12 studies showed increases in ferritin concentrations. Whether improvement in ferritin concentrations improves exercise performance is equivocal and probably depends on whether the subject's serum ferritin concentrations are low initially (Lamanca and Haymes 1992). For example, Zhu and Haas (1997) reported a significantly lower $\dot{V}O_2$max in active women with serum ferritin concentrations <12 ng/ml (stage I iron depletion) compared with active women who had serum ferritin concentrations indicating adequate status. Finally, iron status measurements usually improve as people adapt to exercise programs or if exercise training is decreased.

The degree to which exercise may influence iron status assessment parameters depends on the following factors:

- Type of sport engaged in (endurance sports appear to change iron status assessment parameters more than other sports)
- Intensity and duration (hours per week) of the sport
- Adaptation to training
- Gender (females involved in endurance sports or aesthetic sports, which require a low body weight, are at much greater risk for iron deficiency than females in strength sports)
- Effect of exercise on menstrual blood losses

cereals have significantly lower homocysteine concentrations than people who do not use breakfast cereals (Song et al. 2005). People who smoke have a greater risk of low folate than nonsmokers.

The determination of folate and vitamin B_{12} status in active individuals is presented in table 12.8. Although a handful of researchers have examined folate in active individuals, assessment of supplementation was not always done. Even fewer studies have examined both blood biochemical variables and dietary intake data. Singh and colleagues (1992) and Weight and colleagues (1988) examined the folate status of active men and reported that all subjects had good status, although folate intakes were below the current RDA of 400 μg/day. In general, studies done in active men show good status based on blood folate levels even if the diet is not given. Matter and colleagues (1987) reported that 33% of their female marathon runners (n = 85) had poor folate status, while Telford and coworkers (1992) reported poor status in 11% of their active male and female subjects. Telford and colleagues also reported that 5% of their subjects had poor vitamin B_{12} status. Unfortunately, neither of these reports provided information on dietary folate or vitamin B_{12} intakes. Beals and Manore (1998) examined folate and vitamin B_{12} status in female athletes (~50% reported supplementing) and found 8% of the athletes to be in negative folate balance (plasma folate ≤1.8 nmol/L, or ≤3 ng/ml); none had poor vitamin B_{12} status. These data suggest that active women are at greater risk of poor folate status than active men, primarily due to their low folate intakes. However, the data also suggest that the prevalence of poor folate status is low. Based on the limited data available, the risk of poor vitamin B_{12} status is low in active people unless they consume no animal products and do not use supplements or vitamin B_{12}-fortified foods (see table 12.8).

CHAPTER IN REVIEW

We started this chapter by discussing the roles that iron, copper, folate, and vitamin B_{12} play in the synthesis of hemoglobin and production of RBCs, as well as other metabolic pathways related to exercise. We wanted to find out whether exercise increased the need for these micronutrients. In addition, we wanted to know if supplementation with these nutrients would improve exercise performance. This section summarizes the research available to answer these questions.

Does Exercise Increase the Need for Blood-Building Micronutrients in Active Healthy Individuals and Athletes?

Research on the need for these micronutrients in active people and athletes is still limited, most of the work having been done on iron metabolism. It appears that iron requirements increase with strenuous exercise, especially for endurance athletes. This increase in iron requirements appears to be due to increased losses of iron from the body. However, most male athletes consume more than adequate amounts of iron to cover any increased iron losses. Conversely, female athletes are at much greater risk for iron deficiency due to their increased iron losses with menstruation and exercise, their decreased iron intakes, and their decreased intake of heme iron. Since many active women restrict energy intake for weight loss, their intake of dietary iron will also decrease unless they take supplements or eat iron-dense foods. Because active females are at risk for iron deficiency, they should routinely have their iron status assessed. Performance of anemic athletes will improve when they reestablish normal iron status or correct the underlying cause of the anemia.

Our knowledge of the effect of exercise on folate and vitamin B_{12} metabolism is limited. There is not enough information to determine whether exercise increases the need for these vitamins. Available data suggest that although active men have good folate and vitamin B_{12} status due to their high energy intakes, reported mean folate intakes are still less than recommended (400 μg/day). Active women have a greater risk for folate deficiency because of their low dietary folate intakes. There are few data on vitamin B_{12} status in either men or women. No one has specifically examined whether being physically active increases the need for either folate or vitamin B_{12}. There also are few data on the effect of exercise on copper status. If athletes are anemic due to folate, vitamin B_{12}, or copper deficiency, their exercise performance will improve when they reestablish normal status through diet or supplementation. Little research has been done on the effect of combined diet and exercise for weight loss on iron, copper, folate, or vitamin B_{12} status. If active people restrict energy intake for weight loss or make poor dietary choices, their intakes of these nutrients will probably be low, and they will increase their risk of poor status.

Does Supplementation With Blood-Building Nutrients Improve Exercise Performance?

In active people who already have good nutritional status, there are no data to demonstrate that vitamin or mineral supplementation improves exercise performance. However, if a person has marginal or poor nutritional status, supplementation may improve performance by providing sufficient cofactors or coenzymes for the synthesis of hemoglobin, for production of new RBCs, and for activation of enzymes within the energy metabolism pathways.

Key Concepts

1. **Identify the exercise-related functions, dietary requirements, and food sources of the blood-forming nutrients (iron, copper, folate, and vitamin B_{12}).**

   The red blood cells (RBCs) deliver oxygen to the working muscles and transport carbon dioxide back to the lungs. Thus, these four nutrients are important to any active person. Iron is required as part of the structural formation of heme in hemoglobin; copper is required for normal iron transport; folate and vitamin B_{12} are important for new red cell production. The RDA for iron is 8 mg/day for adult men and 18 mg/day for premenopausal women. The RDAs for folate and vitamin B_{12} are 400 μg/day and 2 mg/day, respectively, for adults. The RDA for copper is 900 μg/day. The most bioavailable form of iron is heme iron, which is found only in meat, fish, and poultry. The highest concentrations of copper are found in cooked organ meats and oysters; but meat, seafood, vegetables, and legumes are good sources. Folate is found in many foods but is especially high in brewer's yeast, leafy green vegetables, legumes, and nuts. Since January 1998 in the United States, breads, cereals, pasta, and rice have been fortified with folate. Vitamin B_{12} occurs only in animal proteins such as milk and dairy products, meat, eggs, fish, and poultry.

2. **Explain the rationale for increased need for the blood-building nutrients in active individuals.**

   Theoretically, exercise could increase the need for any of these nutrients in the following ways:

   • By altering absorption of the nutrient due to decreased transit time

   • By increasing the turnover, metabolism, or loss of the nutrient in urine, feces, or sweat

   • By increasing the need due to the biochemical adaptations (e.g., increased concentrations of enzymes that require the nutrient as a cofactor) associated with training

   • By increasing the need for the nutrient for tissue maintenance and repair

   • By altering RBC fragility or turnover, which decreases the half-life of the RBCs and increases the need for new RBC formation

3. **Understand the nutrition assessment methods for iron, copper, folate, and vitamin B_{12}.**

   Determination of iron status requires the assessment of blood and hematological parameters, dietary iron intake, and other dietary factors that may alter iron absorption; it also requires determination of any factors that may increase iron loss from the body. Poor iron status can be classified into one of three stages: iron depletion, iron deficiency erythropoiesis, and iron deficiency anemia. Since there is no standardized assessment method for copper, assessment is done via measurement of copper concentrations in the blood and the activity of copper-dependent enzymes. Assessment of folate and vitamin B_{12} requires measurement of blood concentrations of the vitamins and of red cell characteristics. Poor folate or vitamin B_{12} status can be classified into one of four stages, similar to those for iron assessment.

4. Discuss the iron, copper, folate, and vitamin B_{12} status of active individuals.

The incidence of iron deficiency anemia (low hemoglobin concentrations) in active men and women is similar to that seen in the general population. However, active women have an increased incidence of iron depletion (low ferritin and transferrin receptor concentrations) compared to the general female population. Data on copper and vitamin B_{12} status in active individuals are limited, but the information available indicates good status. In addition, folate status appears to be good in active people, but current data also suggest that active women are at the highest risk of poor folate status.

Key Terms

ceruloplasmin 371

cobalamin 374

dietary folate equivalent (DFE) 373

erythrocyte 369

ferritin 379

ferroxidase I 371

folate deficiency anemia (stage IV) 380

folate deficiency erythropoiesis (stage III) 380

folate depletion (stage II) 380

heme 369

hemochromatosis (iron toxicity) 372

hemoglobin 368

hemosiderin 379

homocysteine 374

intrinsic factor 370

iron deficiency anemia (stage III) 377

iron deficiency erythropoiesis (stage II) 377

iron depletion (stage I) 377

macrocytic anemia 374

macrocytic red cell 372

megaloblast 372

megaloblastic anemia 372

myoglobin 369

negative folate balance (stage I) 380

negative vitamin B_{12} balance (stage I) 380

pernicious anemia 374

red blood cell (RBC) 367

soluble transferrin receptor (sTfR) 377

tetrahydrofolate (THF) 373

transferrin 371

vitamin B_{12} deficiency anemia (stage IV) 382

vitamin B_{12} deficiency erythropoiesis (stage III) 380

vitamin B_{12} depletion (stage II) 380

Additional Information

Joubert LM, Manore MM. Exercise, nutrition, and homocysteine. Int J Sport Nutr Exerc Metab Aug 2006;16(4):341-361.

> Physical activity may increase homocysteine, an independent cardiovascular disease risk factor. This review examines the influence of nutrition (B vitamins) and exercise on blood homocysteine levels.

Penry JT, Manore MM. Choline: an important micronutrient for maximal endurance-exercise performance? Int J Sport Nutr Exerc Metab Apr 2008;18(2):191-203.

> Choline is considered a B vitamin that may affect exercise performance. This paper reviews the role of choline in exercise performance.

Suedekum NA, Dimeff RJ. Iron and the athlete. Curr Sports Med Rep Aug 2005;4(4):199-202.

Provides an overview of iron assessment in active individuals.

Woolf K, Manore MM. B-vitamins and exercise: does exercise alter requirements? Int J Sport Nutr Exerc Metab Oct 2006;16(5):453-484.

Provides an in-depth review of the current literature on the B vitamins, including folate and vitamin B12, and exercise. The paper specifically addresses how physical activity may increase the needs for these vitamins.

References

Aguilo A, Tauler P, Fuentesprina E, Villa G, Cordova A, Tur JA, Pons A. Antioxidant diet supplementation influences blood iron status in endurance athletes. Int J Sport Nutr Exerc Metab 2004;14:147-160.

Bazzarre TL, Scarpino A, Sigmon R, Marquart LF, Wu SL, Izurieta M. Vitamin-mineral supplement use and nutritional status of athletes. J Am Coll Nutr 1993;12(2):162-169.

Beals KA, Manore MM. Nutritional status of female athletes with subclinical eating disorders. J Am Diet Assoc 1998;98:419-425.

Beshgetoor D, Nichols JF. Dietary intake and supplement use in female master cyclists and runners. Int J Sport Nutr Exerc Metab 2003;13:166-172.

Browne RJ. Evaluating and treating active patients for anemia. Phys Sportsmed 1996;24(9):79-84.

Brownlie T, Utermohlem V, Hinton PS, Haas JD. Tissue iron deficiency without anemia impairs adaptation in endurance capacity after aerobic training in previously untrained women. Am J Clin Nutr 2004;79:437-443.

Choe YH, Kwon YS, Jung MK, Kan KS, Hwang TS, Hong YC. *Heliobacter pylori*–associated iron-deficiency anemia in adolescent female athletes. J Pediatr 2001;139:100-104.

Choi SC, Choi SJ, Kim JA, Kim TH, Nah Y, Yazaki E, Evans DF. The role of gastrointestinal endoscopy in long-distance runners with gastrointestinal symptoms. Eur J Gastroenterol Hepatol 2001;13:1089-1094.

Clark M, Reed DB, Crouse SF, Armstrong RB. Pre- and postseason dietary intake, body composition, and performance indices of NCAA Division I female soccer players. Int J Sport Nutr Exerc Metab 2003;13:303-319.

Constantini NW, Eliakim A, Zigel L, Yaaron M, Falk B. Iron status in highly active adolescents: evidence of depleted iron stores in gymnasts. Int J Sport Nutr Exerc Metab 2000;10:62-70.

Cowell BS, Rosenbloom CA, Skinner R, Summers SH. Policies on screening female athletes for iron deficiency in NCAA Division I-A institutions. Int J Sport Nutr Exerc Metab 2003;13:277-285.

Dietrich M, Brown CJP, Block G. The effect of folate fortification of cereal-grain products on blood folate status, dietary folate intake, and the dietary folate sources among adult non-supplement users in the United States. J Am Coll Nutr 2005;24(4):266-274.

Dressendorfer RH, Petersen SR, Lovshin SEM, Keen CL. Mineral metabolism in male cyclists during high-intensity endurance training. Int J Sport Nutr Exerc Metab 2002;12:63-72.

Dubnov G, Constantini NW. Prevalence of iron depletion and anemia in top-level basketball players. Int J Sport Nutr Exerc Metab 2004;14:30-37.

Faber M, Benade AJ. Mineral and vitamin intake in field athletes (discus-, hammer-, javelin-throwers and shotputters). Int J Sports Med Jun 1991;12(3):324-327.

Fischbach F. A manual of laboratory and diagnostic tests, 6th ed. Baltimore: Lippincott, 2000.

Fogelholm GM, Himberg JJ, Alopaeus K et al. Dietary and biochemical indices of nutritional status in male athletes and controls. J Am Coll Nutr 1992;11(2):181-191.

Fogelholm GM, Koskinen R, Laakso J, Rankinen T, Ruokonen I. Gradual and rapid weight loss: effects on nutrition and performance in male athletes. Med Sci Sports Exerc 1993;25(7):371-377.

Food and Nutrition Board, Institute of Medicine. Recommended dietary allowances, 10th ed. Washington, DC: National Academy Press, 1989.

Gibson RS. Principles of nutritional assessment, 2nd ed. New York: Oxford University Press, 2005.

Gray AB, Telford RD, Weidemann MJ. The effect of intense interval exercise on iron status parameters in trained men. Med Sci Sports Exerc 1993;25(7):778-782.

Gropper SS, Sorrels LM, Blessing D. Copper status of collegiate female athletes involved in different sports. Int J Sport Nutr Exerc Metab 2003;13:343-357.

Haas JD, Brownlie T. Iron deficiency and reduced work capacity: a critical review of the research to determine a causal relationship. J Nutr 2001;131:676S-690S.

Haymes EM. Iron. In: Driskell JA, Wolinsky I eds. Nutrition in exercise and sport, 2nd ed. Boca Raton, FL: CRC Press, 2006;203-216.

Haymes EM, Clarkson PM. Minerals and trace minerals. In: Berning JR, Steen SN eds. Nutrition for sport and exercise. Gaithersburg, MD: Aspen, 1998;77-107.

Herbert V. Vitamin B-12. In: Ziegler EE, Filer LJ eds. Present knowledge in nutrition. Washington, DC: ILSI Press, 1996;191-205.

Herbert V, Das KC. Folic acid and vitamin B-12. In: Shils ME, Olson JA, Shike M eds. Modern nutrition in health and disease. Philadelphia: Lea & Febiger, 1994;402-425.

Herrmann M, Obeid R, Scharhag J, Kindermann W, Herrmann W. Altered vitamin B12 status in recreational endurance athletes. Int J Sport Nutr Exerc Metab 2005;15:433-441.

Hinton PA, Giordano C, Brownlie T, Haas JD. Iron supplementation improves endurance after training in iron-depleted, nonanemic women. J Appl Physiol 2000;88:1103-1111.

Houston MS, Summers SL, Soltesz KS. Lifestyle and dietary practices influencing iron status in university women. Nutr Res 1997;17(1):9-22.

Institute of Medicine (IOM), Food and Nutrition Board. Dietary reference intakes: thiamin, riboflavin, niacin, vitamin B6, folate, vitamin B-12, pantothenic acid, biotin, and choline. Washington, DC: National Academy Press, 1998.

Institute of Medicine (IOM), Food and Nutrition Board. Dietary reference intakes: vitamin A, vitamin K, arsenic, boron, chromium, copper, iodine, iron, manganese, molybdenum, nickel, silicon, vanadium and zinc. Washington, DC: National Academy Press, 2001.

Jensen CD, Zaltas ES, Whittam JH. Dietary intakes of male endurance cyclists during training and racing. J Am Diet Assoc 1992;92(8):986-988.

Kaiserauer S, Snyder AC, Sleeper M, Zierath J. Nutritional, physiological, and menstrual status of distance runners. Med Sci Sports Exerc 1989;21(2):120-125.

Keith RE, O'Keeffe KA, Alt LA, Young KL. Dietary status of trained female cyclists. J Am Diet Assoc 1989;89:1620-1623.

Klevay LM, Buchet JP, Bunker VW. Copper in the Western diet. In: Anke M, Meissner D, Mills CF eds. Trace elements in man and animals. TEMA-8. Gersdorf, Germany: Verlag Media Touristik, 1993;207-210.

Konig D, Bisse E, Deibert P, Muller HM, Wieland H, Berg A. Influence of training volume and acute physical exercise on the homocysteine levels in endurance-trained men: interactions with plasma folate and vitamin B12. Ann Nutr Metab 2003;47:114-118.

Kopp-Woodroffe SA, Manore MM, Dueck CA, Skinner JS, Matt KS. Energy and nutrient status of amenorrheic athletes participating in a diet and exercise training intervention program. Int J Sport Nutr 1999;9:70-88.

Koury JC, de Oliveira AV, Portella ES, de Oliveira CF, Lopes GC, Donangelo CM. Zinc and copper biochemical indices of antioxidant status in elite athletes of different modalities. Int J Sport Nutr Exerc Metab 2004;14:364-378.

Lamanca JJ, Haymes EM. Effects of low ferritin concentration on endurance performance. Int J Sport Nutr 1992;2:376-385.

Landahl G, Adolfsson P, Borjesson M, Mannheimer C, Rodjer S. Iron deficiency and anemia: a common problem in female elite soccer players. Int J Sport Nutr Exerc Metab 2005;15:689-694.

Lindenbaum J, Allen RH. Clinical spectrum and diagnosis of folate deficiency. In: Bailey LB ed. Folate in health and disease. New York: Marcel Dekker, 1995;43-73.

Lukaski HC, Hoverson BS, Gallagher SK, Bolonchuk WW. Physical training and copper, iron and zinc status of swimmers. Am J Clin Nutr 1990;51:1093-1099.

Lukaski HC, Siders WA, Hoverson BS, Gallagher SK. Iron, copper, magnesium and zinc status as predictors of swimming performance. Int J Sports Med 1996;17(7):534-540.

Malczewska J, Raczynski G, Stupnicki R. Iron status in female endurance athletes and in non-athletes. Int J Sport Nutr Exerc Metab 2000;10:260-276.

Malczewska J, Szczepanska B, Stupnicki R, Sendecki W. The assessment of frequency of iron deficiency in athletes from the transferrin receptor-ferritin index. Int J Sport Nutr Exerc Metab 2001;11:42-52.

Manore MM, Besenfelder PD, Wells CL, Carroll SS, Hooker SP. Nutrient intakes and iron status in female long-distance runners during training. J Am Diet Assoc 1989;89:257-259.

Matter M, Stittfall T, Graves J, Myburgh K, Adams B, Jacobs P, Noakes TD. The effect of iron and folate therapy on maximal exercise performance in female marathon runners with iron and folate deficiency. Clin Sci 1987;72:415-22.

Milne DB. Copper intake and assessment of copper status. Am J Clin Nutr 1998(suppl);67:1041S-1045S.

Newhouse IJ, Clement DB, Taunton JE, McKenzie DC. The effects of prelatent/latent iron deficiency on physical work capacity. Med Sci Sports Exerc 1989;21(3):263-268.

Niekamp RA, Baer JT. In-season dietary adequacy of trained male cross-country runners. Int J Sport Nutr 1995;5:45-55.

Nielsen R, Nachtigal D. Iron supplementation in athletes: current recommendations. Sports Med 1998;26(4):207-216.

Nieman DC, Butler JV, Pollett LM, Dietrich SJ, Lutz RD. Nutrient intake of marathon runners. J Am Diet Assoc 1989;89:1273-1278.

Nuviala RJ, Lapieza MG. Disparity between diet and serum ferritin in elite sportswomen. Nutr Res 1997;17(3):451-461.

O'Keefe CA, Bailey LB, Thomas EA. Controlled dietary folate affects folate status in nonpregnant women. J Nutr 1995;125:2717-2725.

Rankinen T, Lyytikainen S, Vanninen E, Penttila I, Rauramaa R, Uusitupa M. Nutritional status of the Finnish elite ski jumpers. Med Sci Sports Exerc 1998;30(11):1592-1597.

Real JT, Merchante A, Gomez JL, Chaves FJ, Ascaso JF, Carmena R. Effects of marathon running on plasma total homocysteine concentrations. Nutr Metab Cardiovasc Dis 2005;15:134-139.

Reeves PG. Copper. In: Wolinsky I, Driskell JA eds. Sport nutrition: vitamins and trace elements. Boca Raton, FL: CRC Press, 1997;175-187.

Rico-Sanz J, Frontera WR, Molé PA, Rivera MA, Rivera-Brown A, Meredith CN. Dietary and performance assessment of elite soccer players during a period of intense training. Int J Sport Nutr 1998;8(3):230-240.

Rocker L, Hinz K, Holland K, Gunga H, Vogelgesang J, Kiesewetter H. Influence of endurance exercise (triathlon) on circulating transferrin receptors and other indicators of iron status in female athletes. Clin Lab 2002;48:307-312.

Rousseau AS, Robin S, Roussel AM, Ducros V, Margaritis I. Plasma homocysteine is related to folate intake but not training status. Nutr Metab Cardiovasc Dis 2005;15:125-133.

Sauberlich HE. Folate status of U.S. population and groups. In: Bailey LB ed. Folate in health and disease. New York: Marcel Dekker, 1995;171-194.

Savage DG, Lindenbaum J. Folate-cobalamin interactions. In: Bailey LB ed. Folate in health and disease. New York: Marcel Dekker, 1995;237-285.

Schreiber WE. Iron, porphyrin, and bilirubin metabolism. In: Kaplan LA, Pesce AJ eds. Clinical chemistry. St. Louis: Mosby, 1989;496-509.

Scott JM, Weir DG, Kirke PN. Folate and neural tube defects. In: Bailey LB ed. Folate in health and disease. New York: Marcel Dekker, 1995;329-360.

Shane B. Folate chemistry and metabolism. In: Bailey LB ed. Folate in health and disease. New York: Marcel Dekker, 1995;1-22.

Sinclair LM, Hinton PS. Prevalence of iron deficiency with and without anemia in recreationally active men and women. J Am Diet Assoc 2005;105:975-978.

Singh A, Moses FM, Deuster PA. Vitamin and mineral status in physically active men: effects of a high-potency supplement. Am J Clin Nutr 1992;55(1):1-7.

Song WO, Chung C, Chun OK, Cho S. Serum homocysteine concentration of US adults associated with fortified cereal consumption. J Am Coll Nutr 2005;24(6):503-509.

Telford RD, Catchpole EA, Deakin V, McLeay AC, Plank AW. The effect of 7 to 8 months of vitamin/mineral supplementation on the vitamin and mineral status of athletes. Int J Sport Nutr 1992;2:123-134.

Tobin BW, Beard JL. Iron. In: Wolinsky I, Driskell JA eds. Sport nutrition: vitamins and trace elements. Boca Raton, FL: CRC Press, 1997;137-156.

Wagner C. Biochemical role of folate in cellular metabolism. In: Bailey LB ed. Folate in health and disease. New York: Marcel Dekker, 1995;23-42.

Wapnir RA. Copper absorption and bioavailability. Am J Clin Nutr 1998(suppl);67:1054S-1060S.

Weaver CM, Rajaram S. Exercise and iron status. J Nutr 1992;122:782-787.

Weight LM. Sports anemia: does it exist? Sports Med 1993;16:1-4.

Weight LM, Noakes TD, Labadarios D, Graves J, Jacobs P, Berman PA. Vitamin and mineral status of trained athletes including the effects of supplementation. Am J Clin Nutr 1988;47:186-191.

Wilkinson JG, Martin DT, Adams AA, Liebman M. Iron status in cyclists during high-intensity interval training and recovery. Int J Sports Med 2002;23:544-548.

Woolf K, Manore MM. Nutritional concerns of the female athlete. In: Ransdell L, Petlichkoff L eds. Ensuring the health of active and athletic girls and women. Waldorf, MD: National Association for Girls and Women in Sport, American Alliance for Health, Physical Education, Recreation and Dance, 2005;167-203.

Woolf K, Manore MM. B-vitamins and exercise: does exercise alter requirements? Int J Sport Nutr Exerc Metab 2006;16(5):453-484.

Worme JD, Doubt TJ, Singh A, Ryan CJ, Moses FM, Deuster PA. Dietary patterns, gastrointestinal complaints, and nutrition knowledge of recreational triathletes. Am J Clin Nutr 1990;51:690-697.

Yip R. Iron. In: Bowman BA, Russell RM eds. Present knowledge in nutrition. Washington, DC: ILSI Press, 2001;311-328.

Zhu YI, Haas JD. Iron depletion without anemia and physical performance in young women. Am J Clin Nutr 1997;66:334-341.

CHAPTER 13

Nutrients for Bone Health

Chapter Objectives

After reading this chapter you should be able to

- identify the primary nutrients associated with bone health,
- describe the five stages of the bone remodeling process and which stages involve osteoclasts and osteoblasts,
- discuss the methods used to assess calcium status, identify calcium requirements and intakes of athletes, and recognize sources of calcium and related supplementation products,
- describe the methods of assessment, the requirements, and the dietary sources of phosphorus,
- discuss magnesium's role in bone health,
- explain the methods of assessment, the requirements, dietary sources, and supplementation products of vitamin D, and
- describe how fluoride, energy, and protein play a role in bone metabolism.

Although we tend to think of bone as a rigid tissue that supports the body, bone is in fact a dynamic tissue that actively participates in serum calcium regulation. A number of nutrients play a critical role in bone metabolism, including calcium, phosphorus, magnesium, fluoride, and vitamin D. Adequate bone development during youth is necessary to achieve a healthy adult skeleton. While it is recognized that early bone development is critical to health, this chapter focuses primarily on the interactions of exercise, certain nutrients, and the skeleton in adults. We provide a brief review of bone metabolism prior to discussing the specific nutrients related to bone health.

REVIEW OF BONE METABOLISM

There are three stages of bone development (Heaney 2006):

1. Growth
2. Modeling
3. Remodeling

The *size* of a bone is determined during its years of growth; however, the *shape* of the bone is determined during modeling. **Remodeling,** also referred to as bone turnover, is a normal, healthy process of replacing existing bone matrix (Ander-

son 1991). Growth, modeling, and remodeling occur in a developing skeleton during youth and young adulthood, while remodeling alone occurs in adults. Remodeling maintains the mineral homeostasis of bone by preventing an accumulation of microfractures (Heaney 2006).

Figure 13.1 reviews the bone remodeling process, which has several distinct stages: activation, **resorption,** reversal, **formation,** and resting. The entire remodeling cycle takes three to six months and is driven by the need to repair microscopic structural imperfections. **Osteoblasts** and **osteoclasts** are cells involved in this process. During remodeling, osteoclasts perform resorption by eroding existing bone surfaces, forming cavities in

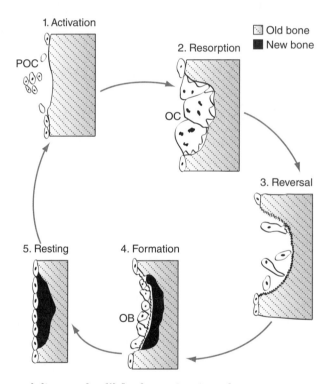

Figure 13.1   The bone remodeling cycle. (1) In the activation phase, precursor cells to osteoclasts (POC) respond to a stimulus and are recruited to the area of bone needing to be remodeled. (2) During the resorption phase, osteoclasts (OC) act to erode bone. (3) In the reversal stage, a cement line is formed that marks the end of resorption and acts to fuse together old and new bone. (4) During the formation phase, osteoblasts (OB) fill in the cavity with osteoid, which then becomes mineralized, forming new bone. (5) In the resting phase, the bone is covered by a layer of bone-lining cells. Completion of the five stages of the remodeling cycle takes three to six months. During formation, osteoblasts act to replace as much bone as was removed. In healthy adults, the amount of new bone formed is equal to the amount of bone resorbed. With aging, the amount of new bone formed may be less than the amount resorbed and a net bone loss will result, which over time can lead to osteoporosis.

Adapted from R.E. Baron, 1999, Anatomy and ultrastructure of bone. In *Primer on metabolic bone diseases and disorders of mineral metabolism*, 4th ed., edited by J. Murray, and M.D. Favus (Washington, DC: American Society for Bone and Mineral Research), 99-106.

the bone. Osteoblasts act at the site of the cavities to synthesize new bone matrix, a process called formation. The new matrix is subsequently mineralized, resulting in new bone tissue. Appropriate coupling of resorption and formation results in the maintenance of bone tissue. Bone loss results when the rate of resorption exceeds that of formation.

Many factors regulate bone remodeling, including

- hormones such as estrogen, parathyroid hormone (PTH), calcitonin, and vitamin D;

- nutrient status, particularly calcium bioavailability;

- exercise, especially weight-bearing activity; and

- hormonal status.

We discuss each of these factors in detail in subsequent sections of this chapter.

Adult bone comprises two major types of tissue: cortical and trabecular tissue. **Trabecular bone** (figure 13.2a) makes up approximately 20% of the entire skeleton and has a faster turnover rate than cortical bone. No more than 20% of adult trabecular bone is in active remodeling at one time (Frost 1989). **Cortical bone** (figure 13.2b) comprises the remaining 80% of the skeleton, has a slower turnover rate than trabecular bone, and has only 5% of its surface in active remodeling at one time. Cortical bone is found primarily in the shaft of long bones, while much of trabecular bone is found in the axial skeleton, the flat bones, and the ends of long bones (Baylink and Jennings 1994). Due to the faster remodeling rate of trabecular bone, it is more sensitive to changes in hormonal status, and bone loss at these sites is more easily detected than at sites with predominantly cortical bone (Heaney 2006). This helps explain why fractures commonly occur in the vertebrae, distal radius, and proximal femur; that is, these bones are mainly composed of trabecular tissue. A comparison between figures 13.2a and 13.3 displays the difference between healthy trabecular bone and osteoporotic bone.

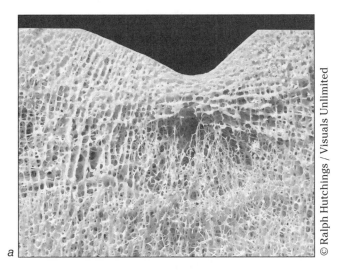

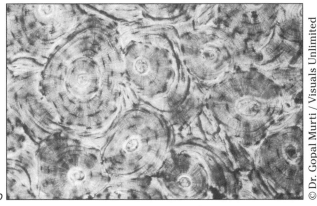

Figure 13.2 A microscopic view of *(a)* trabecular and *(b)* cortical bone. Trabecular bone can be found in the head of the femur, in the wrist, and in the spinal vertebrae. Cortical bone makes up the shaft of long bones.

© Ralph Hutchings / Visuals Unlimited

© Dr. Gopal Murti / Visuals Unlimited

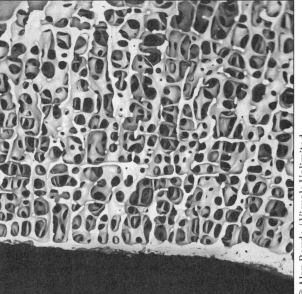

© Alan Boyde / Visuals Unlimited

Figure 13.3 Osteoporosis is a condition characterized by porous weak bones leading to an increased risk of fracture. Notice the difference in architecture between the healthy trabecular bone (shown in figure 13.2a) and the osteoporotic bone shown here.

Osteoporosis

Osteoporosis is a disease characterized by low bone mass that predisposes someone to an increased risk of fracture (National Institutes of Health [NIH] 2001). This disease affects over 44 million Americans, 80% of whom are women. In 2005, osteoporosis was responsible for more than 2 million fractures, with an estimated 297,000 hip fractures and 547,000 vertebral fractures, costing our health care system over $15 billion (NIH 2001). About half of all women and a quarter of all men over the age of 50 will have an osteoporosis-related fracture in their lifetime.

A primary strategy to prevent osteoporosis is to optimize peak bone mass development in youth and young adulthood. Figure 13.4 is a curve demonstrating **bone mineral density (BMD)** development throughout the life span. People who can optimize BMD during youth by following a healthy lifestyle can reduce their risk of developing osteoporosis later in life. Peak bone mass is generally achieved after adult height has been reached and the bones have gone through a consolidation phase. Research demonstrates that on average, females achieve peak BMD at the hip in late adolescence, while a peak is not reached at the spine or for the whole body until the third decade of life (Lin et al. 2003; Teegarden et al. 1995). Table 13.1 shows the ages at which peak BMD and peak bone mineral content occur at different bone sites.

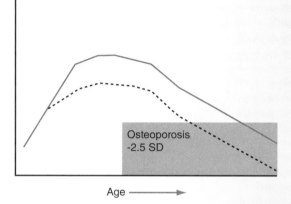

Figure 13.4 Someone who has ample intake of bone nutrients, such as those discussed in this chapter, and who participates in weight-bearing physical activity during the teenage and early adult years might develop a curve like the solid one. A person who avoids calcium-rich foods and leads a sedentary lifestyle might develop a curve like the dotted one. This would put the individual at an increased risk for fracture later in life.
JOURNAL OF THE AMERICAN COLLEGE OF NUTRITION. ONLINE by J.X. Ilich and J.E. Kerstetter. Copyright 2000 by American College of Nutrition. Adapted with permission of American College of Nutrition in the format Textbook via Copyright Clearance Center.

Bone mineral content (BMC) is a measurement of the grams of mineral in a bone. It is important to note that individual bones attain peak bone mass at different ages. Osteoporosis is defined as a BMD score 2.5 standard deviations below that of a young, healthy person (NIH 2001). **Osteopenia** is a condition of reduced bone mass and is diagnosed at BMD scores 1.0 to 2.4 standard deviations below that of a young, healthy person. If unaddressed, osteopenia may develop into osteoporosis. People who do not optimize peak bone mass can develop osteoporosis even without experiencing accelerated bone loss (NIH 2001). The risk factors for developing osteoporosis are listed in "Female Athlete Triad and Osteoporosis" p. 416.

Table 13.1 Estimates of Age at Which Females Achieve 99% of Peak Bone Mineral Content (BMC in g) and Bone Mineral Density (BMD in g/cm²)

Spine BMD (g/cm²)	Femoral neck BMD (g/cm²)	Femoral neck BMC (g)	Whole-body BMD (g/cm²)	Whole-body BMC (g)
23.0 ± 1.4 years	18.5 ± 1.6 years	18.3 ± 0.9 years	22.1 ± 2.5 years	26.2 ± 3.7 years

Adapted from Y.C. Lin et al., 1995, "Peak spine and femoral neck bone mass in young women," *Bone* 32: 546-553; D. Teegarden et al., 1995, "Peak bone mass in young women," *Journal of Bone and Mineral Research* 10: 711-715.

As a person ages, the rate of bone resorption exceeds that of bone formation, which results in a net loss of bone. Bone loss is accelerated during periods of prolonged inactivity or bed rest, following menopause in women, and when calcium or vitamin D nutrition is poor. As discussed in chapter 15, amenorrheic athletes may also experience bone loss due to estrogen deficiency. See "Osteoporosis" for an explanation of this syndrome and its prevention.

CALCIUM

Calcium is a unique nutrient in that its storage serves an important functional role, as 99% of this mineral resides in the skeleton. Calcium is the predominant component of bone: It is the largest constituent of the **hydroxyapatite** crystals, or solid particles, of bone. Other minerals present in bone are phosphorus and magnesium, with 88% and 60% of these minerals residing in the skeleton,

respectively (Gibson 2005). Although calcium is recognized primarily for its role in bone health, it has other important functions related to exercise, including

- enzyme activation,
- nerve transmission,
- muscle contraction,
- hormone function, and
- membrane transport.

The body prioritizes maintenance of blood calcium levels over bone tissue levels. When calcium intake is inadequate, blood calcium levels are maintained via the withdrawal of more calcium from bone, increase in the intestinal absorption of calcium, and increase in renal uptake of calcium. These adaptations occur through the actions of select hormones, such as PTH and vitamin D. The hormones associated with calcium metabolism are reviewed on this page.

Hormones Associated With Bone Metabolism, and Their Actions

Parathyroid Hormone

- Increases resorption of calcium from bone into blood to maintain blood calcium levels
- Stimulates conversion of the inactive form of vitamin D to its active form (1,25(OH)$_2$ vitamin D)
- Conserves calcium by causing the kidney to increase calcium reuptake

Thyroid Hormone

- Normal levels—critical to maintaining healthy bone metabolism
- Hyperthyroidism—results in significant increase in bone resorption, leading to bone loss
- Hypothyroidism—results in slowing of bone turnover and diminishes the bone calcium pool

Insulin-Like Growth Factor 1

- Regulates bone growth and remodeling through its action on osteoblast formation
- Enhances collagen synthesis
- Inhibits bone collagen degradation, preserving the bone

Estrogen

- Decreases bone resorption, possibly by lowering the responsiveness of osteoclasts to PTH

- In the absence of estrogen, osteoclasts are allowed to proliferate in number and increase in activity

Vitamin D

- Increases intestinal absorption of calcium and phosphorus
- Promotes bone resorption by increasing osteoclast number
- Increases reabsorption of calcium in the distal tubule of the kidney

Calcitonin

- Conserves bone tissue by inhibiting osteoclast activity
- Works to maintain normal serum calcium levels

Corticosteroids

- Modulate osteoclastic activity
- In excess levels, can inhibit bone formation by impairing synthesis of bone matrix
- In excess levels, stimulate bone resorption
- In excess levels, inhibit active calcium transport in the intestine

Methods of Assessment

There is no satisfactory direct method for assessing calcium status. Serum calcium levels cannot be used to indicate calcium status since these levels are tightly controlled and remain constant under most conditions. Approximately 50% of the serum calcium concentration is ionized and under hormonal control, while the remaining 50% is bound to plasma proteins, primarily albumin. Only the ionized form of serum calcium is physiologically active and capable of being used for muscular contractions, transmission of nerve impulses, and blood clotting (Gibson 2005). Normal adult values for ionized calcium in the serum are 4.65 to 5.28 mg/dL (1.16 to 1.32 mmol/L), while normal adult values for total serum calcium are 8.4 to 10.2 mg/dL (2.1 to 2.55 mmol/L) (Fischbach 2004). Conditions that could potentially affect serum measurements of calcium are consumption of a recent meal, high levels of magnesium or sodium, changes in pH, and the presence of trypsin or heparin.

Under certain conditions, measurements of urinary calcium are used to assess changes in calcium metabolism. Because urinary calcium levels have a significant, but low, correlation with calcium intake (Weaver 1990), they are of limited use as an indicator of adequate dietary calcium intake. Urinary calcium is affected by recent calcium intake, calcium requirement, urinary output, and dietary protein, making it more variable than plasma calcium. Expressing urinary calcium as a calcium-to-creatinine ratio normalizes calcium excretion values. This ratio corrects for differences among people in lean body mass and also corrects for errors in the timing of urine collections (Weaver 1990). It is important to interpret urinary calcium values in conjunction with assessments of dietary intake.

The assessment of bone health is crucial to evaluating long-term calcium status. Note that although poor calcium nutrition over one's lifetime is thought to have a negative impact on bone, many factors in addition to dietary calcium intake play a role in bone health, including hormonal status, genetic factors, and levels of physical activity. Bone measurements do not reflect recent dietary calcium intakes but may reflect long-term dietary patterns. See "Bone Measurement Methods" for more details about measurements. For a complete description of methods used to assess calcium status and metabolism, refer to Weaver 1990.

Requirements

Dietary calcium intake, intestinal absorption, urinary excretion, sweat losses, and fecal losses play an important role in calcium balance and affect individual calcium requirements. While calcium absorption from food is typically 25% to 35% (Heaney and Recker 1986), several factors can influence absorption and retention (see "Factors That May Affect Calcium Homeostasis," p. 404). The impact of many of these factors on bone health is controversial, and their effect on bone in healthy individuals may be minimal (Anderson 1991).

Determining calcium requirements is a process fraught with difficulty. Epidemiological studies have been used to estimate calcium intake by healthy people. While data from these types of projects can indicate patterns of dietary calcium intake, they do not clearly define calcium requirements. The use of typical intakes of Americans to set recommendations is not appropriate for calcium and other bone nutrients given the high incidence of osteoporosis in our population (Weaver 2003). Calcium balance and retention studies have been used to determine the dietary calcium intake required for maintaining calcium balance—with the assumption that negative calcium balance indicates bone loss. Calcium is considered a threshold nutrient in that its absorption improves in a linear manner with calcium intake below a threshold level (400-500 mg); however, retention is unrelated to intakes greater than the threshold amount (figure 13.5). In other words, the body can absorb only about 400 to 500 mg of calcium at one time, and consuming more than this will not increase absorption. Despite research limitations, dietary calcium requirements have been established for men and women across the life span using the threshold intake level for maximal retention. Table 13.2 includes Dietary Reference Intake (DRI) values for calcium, phosphorus, magnesium, vitamin D, and fluoride for various age groups. If no definitive data are available on which to base an RDA, the Adequate Intake (AI) is a useful goal for individual nutrient intakes (Institute of Medicine [IOM] 1997).

Intakes of Athletes

Results from the 1999-2000 National Health and Nutrition Examination Survey (Ervin et al. 2004) showed that average calcium intake for all people in the United States was 863 mg/day, which is lower than the present AI for calcium (1000 mg/day

Bone Measurement Methods

A common strategy to evaluate bone health is to measure BMD. While bone strength is of primary concern in predicting fracture risk, bone strength can really be measured only in vivo. Bone mineral density is often used as an alternative measure and accounts for about 70% of bone strength (NIH 2001). Although the correlation between BMD and bone strength is not perfect, BMD is a good predictor of fracture risk. The World Health Organization has defined osteoporosis as a BMD value 2.5 standard deviations below that of a healthy young subject (NIH 2001). Dual-energy X-ray absorptiometry (DXA; see figure 7.3 on p. 211) has become the most popular method for measuring BMD because of its good resolution, adequate precision, rapid scan time, and low radiation exposure (Weaver 1990). The DXA uses low-dose radiation to detect differences in bone and soft tissue. Common sites assessed using DXA are bones that are at risk for osteoporotic fracture, like the hip, spine, and wrist.

A number of biochemical markers in blood and urine can be used to assess bone turnover. The rate of bone formation or resorption can be evaluated through measurement of substances produced by bone cells (osteoblasts or osteoclasts) or of bone matrix components (collagen). Formation markers are produced by osteoblasts and are released into the blood during the formation phase. Bone resorption markers are breakdown products of collagen, the main protein in bone, and can be analyzed in blood or urine (Rosen and Tenenhouse 1998). Bone markers cannot detect changes in specific bone (trabecular vs. cortical or arm vs. leg) but rather reflect bone metabolism changes of the whole body. The following is a list some of the biochemical markers of bone turnover and the fluids in which they are found (Heaney 2006).

Formation (Blood)

Osteocalcin

Total alkaline phosphatase

Bone-specific alkaline phosphatase

N- and C-terminal procollagen peptides

Resorption (Blood)

Tartrate-resistant acid phosphatase

Pyridinoline and pyridinoline-containing peptides

N- and C-telopeptides

Resorption (Urine)

Hydroxyproline

Pyridinoline

Deoxypyridinoline (collagen cross-links)

N- and C-telopeptides

Although bone turnover markers are frequently used to assess skeletal status, they appear to be better markers when used to assess values for groups rather than for individuals (Lunar Corporation 1994). Variation in measurement results is large and could be due to the timing and accuracy of collection because of seasonal and diurnal variation. In general, serum markers of formation are less variable but are not as sensitive as urinary markers of resorption for detecting changes in bone metabolism (Rosen and Tenenhouse 1998). While research indicates that an increase in bone turnover markers in postmenopausal women is associated with an increased fracture risk, the markers alone cannot predict fracture (Szulac and Delmas 2008). In addition, bone turnover markers cannot be used to assess peak bone mass or current BMD. Therefore, it is recommended that biochemical markers be used in combination with bone density measures (via DXA) to define a person's skeletal status and to monitor therapy.

Factors That May Affect Calcium Homeostasis

Increase Absorption

Optimal vitamin D levels

Dietary fat

Acidic environment in intestines

Lactose (with normal lactase activity)

Dietary protein

Calcium deficiency

Consumption of calcium with a meal

Decrease Absorption

Vitamin D deficiency

Phytates and oxalates

High pH in intestines

Lactose (with lactase deficiency)

High dietary phosphate

Dietary fiber

Aging (low stomach acid)

Low-protein diet (≤0.7 g/kg)

Increase Excretion

High dietary sodium

High dietary animal protein

Caffeine

for ages 19-50 years; 1200 mg/day for ages 51-70 years). Data from 1999-2002 show that women 20 to 39 years of age have a lower average intake (801 mg/day) than men of similar age (1055 mg/day) and that average intakes decrease with increasing age for both genders (Forshee at al. 2006). Calcium consumption seems to be greatest for people living in the western United States, for non-Hispanic whites, and for those with the highest income (Fleming and Heimbach 1994). The lowest per capita intake measured was for people living in the southern United States, for non-Hispanic blacks, and for those with the lowest income. Milk and milk products supplied over 50% of the total calcium intake; milk as an ingredient in other foods (e.g., cheese on pizza, beef stroganoff) provided approximately 20% of total calcium intake, and grain products provided 12%. Although dietary calcium intake has increased in women between the ages of 12 and 59 over the last decade, data show that the U.S. population on average is consuming less than the 1997 AI for calcium (Forshee et al. 2006).

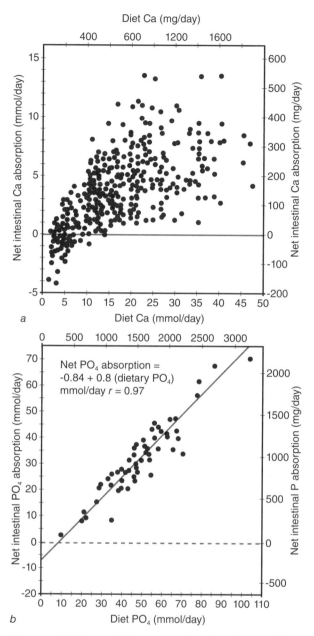

Figure 13.5 (a) Net intestinal calcium (Ca) absorption as measured by the metabolic balance method in relation to dietary Ca intake among healthy adults (top panel); (b) net intestinal phosphate (PO_4) absorption in relation to dietary PO_4 intake among healthy adults. Calcium is considered a threshold nutrient in that its absorption improves in a linear manner with calcium intake below a threshold level (400-500 mg); however, retention is unrelated to intakes greater than the threshold level. Phosphate absorption increases in a linear fashion with intake.

Table 13.2   **Dietary Reference Intakes: Recommended Levels for Individuals[a]**

Age group (years)	Calcium AI (mg/day)	Phosphorus RDA (mg/day)	Magnesium RDA (mg/day)	Vitamin D[b,c] AI (μg/day; IU)	Fluoride AI (mg/day)
Males					
14-18	1300	1250	410	5 (200)	3
19-30	1000	700	400	5 (200)	4
31-50	1000	700	420	5 (200)	4
51-70	1200	700	420	10 (400)	4
>70	1200	700	420	15 (600)	4
Females					
14-18	1300	1250	360	5 (200)	3
19-30	1000	700	310	5 (200)	3
31-50	1000	700	320	5 (200)	3
51-70	1200	700	320	10 (400)	3
>70	1200	700	320	15 (600)	3

[a] Values are those of the Institute of Medicine (IOM), Food and Nutrition Board (1997). RDA = Recommended Dietary Allowance; AI = Adequate Intake. RDAs and AIs may both be used as goals for individual intake. RDAs are set to meet the needs of almost all (97%) individuals in the group. The AI is believed to cover needs of most individuals in the group, but lack of data or uncertainty in the data does not allow specifying with confidence the percentage of persons covered by this intake.
[b] As cholecalciferol (previtamin D); 1 mg cholecalciferol = 40 IU vitamin D.
[c] In the absence of adequate exposure to sunlight.

Adapted from *Journal of the American Dietetic Association*, Vol 98, A.A. Yates, S.A. Schlicker, and C.W. Suitor, "Dietary reference intakes: the new basis for recommendations for calcium and related nutrients, B vitamins, and cholin," pgs. 699-706, Copyright 1998, with permission from Elsevier.

Similar inadequacies in dietary intake of calcium are found among athletes. Self-reported dietary records of female athletes show intakes of calcium that are less than the 1997 AI—particularly among participants in aesthetic sports and among distance runners (Benardot et al. 1989; Wiita and Stombaugh 1996). Slawson and colleagues (2001) found that female collegiate athletes were consuming an average of 898 mg of calcium per day while their male counterparts consumed 1354 mg/day. Female cross country runners had the lowest intake in this investigation at 605 mg/day. The difference between the reported calcium intakes of male and female athletes is probably due to the lower energy intakes of female athletes and to female athletes' tendency to avoid dairy products because they view them as high in dietary fat (Manore 1996, 1999). There are many calcium sources available in the U.S. diet. However, it may be necessary for many people, including athletes, to take supplemental calcium because they are unable or unwilling to consume adequate calcium from dietary sources. An investigation of female master athletes showed that those who supplemented reached the DRI for all nutrients, including calcium, while those who chose not to supplement consumed only 79% of the DRI for calcium (791 mg/day) (Beshgetoor and Nichols 2003).

Athletes in particular need to pay close attention to achieving optimal calcium intakes because of additional calcium loss via sweat. Research indicates that sweat losses of calcium can vary considerably depending on physical activity and environmental temperature. At normal temperatures (18° C or 64° F) and without exercise-induced sweating, we lose only small amounts of calcium (35 mg) via the skin each day (Rianon et al. 2003). However, Klesges and colleagues (1996) reported a dermal calcium loss in collegiate male basketball players of 247 mg per training session. Therefore, exercising in conditions that increase sweat rates could increase losses of calcium through the skin.

Dietary Sources and Supplementation Products

Dairy products are the most regularly consumed sources of calcium in the American diet. Yet these products are often avoided by physically active people for two reasons. First, about 30% of adults in the United States (and up to 75% of adults around the world) are lactose intolerant, and consumption of milk products causes gastrointestinal distress. Second, since dairy products are often thought of as high in dietary fat, people attempting to reduce fat in their diet tend to avoid these products (Manore 1996, 1999). For these reasons, it is important to stress to active populations that nonfat and low-fat dairy sources have calcium contents similar to those of the regular-fat products. Many people mistakenly assume that reducing the fat in dairy products also lowers the calcium content. Moreover, research shows that people with lactose maldigestion can often consume small amounts of dairy without adverse effects (Suarez et al. 1998). There are now many lactose-free dairy products in the dairy sections of grocery stores, in addition to many nondairy foods supplemented with calcium. Ready-to-eat breakfast cereals and calcium-fortified orange juice are cost-effective, nondairy sources of calcium at about $0.31 and $0.65 per 300 mg of calcium, respectively (Keller et al. 2002). Table 13.3 lists the calcium and phosphorus content of various foods.

The preferable source of calcium is from food because bone health is not a single-nutrient issue (Heaney and Weaver 2003). Foods that are high in calcium are often high in other nutrients important for bone health like phosphorus, magnesium, potassium, vitamin D, and protein. As table 13.3 reveals, dairy products, as well as calcium-fortified foods such as tofu and fruit juices, have the highest calcium contents per serving. Although spinach contains a relatively high amount of calcium, absorption may be limited by the oxalic acid present in spinach; only 5% of the calcium in spinach is absorbed, compared to 27% of the calcium in milk, when equal calcium loads are consumed (Weaver and Heaney 2006). The calcium absorption from kale is similar to that from milk products, but 10 cups would be necessary to meet the current calcium recommendations, which is not practical for most people. Meeting the current calcium recommendations through dietary means is difficult for people who do not regularly consume dairy products or calcium-containing vegetable products; it is also difficult for people with relatively low energy intakes. Thus, supplementing with calcium may be necessary. Recent evidence suggests that high calcium intakes and dairy consumption in particular may be related to weight loss and maintenance of a healthy body weight. Please see "Calcium, Dairy, and Weight Loss" on p. 409 for further discussion.

Hundreds of calcium supplements are available. How can one know which supplement to take? Unfortunately, it is difficult for average consumers to determine which supplement is best for their particular calcium needs. Important factors to consider when choosing a calcium supplement are convenience, cost, tolerability, safety, and absorbability. The percentage of calcium in various supplements and preparations is shown in table 13.4. Although there is a significant difference in cost among many supplemental forms of calcium, there is little evidence that one chemical compound of calcium is superior to another in maintaining bone health. Heaney and colleagues (2001) found that calcium carbonate and calcium citrate taken at similar doses have equal bioavailability in healthy persons when consumed with a meal. Considering that the two types of calcium supplements are equally absorbed, the calcium carbonate supplements have a more favorable cost-to-benefit relationship because they are typically cheaper. According to Keller and colleagues (2002), name-brand Tums (Glaxo-Smith Kline) or the generic equivalent is the cheapest source of supplemental calcium. Also, the greater volume of calcium in carbonate-based supplements means that fewer pills are needed to reach a desired intake. Even though the carbonate supplement has the highest percentage of calcium, it is relatively insoluble at a neutral pH. Individuals with a condition of low stomach acid content, or **achlorhydria** (common among older adults), cannot absorb this form of calcium very well. Such people more easily absorb the citrate form of calcium. Since calcium citrate does not require an acidic environment to be absorbed it can be taken at any time, in contrast to calcium carbonate, which should be taken with meals.

In addition to the factors listed previously that affect calcium absorption (see "Factors That May Affect Calcium Homeostasis" on p. 404), the amount of calcium consumed in one dose affects absorption. Absorption of calcium plateaus at about 400 to 500 mg (see figure 13.5); therefore supplemental doses divided over time appear to be better absorbed. Individuals supplementing with calcium should limit individual doses to <500 mg, with the doses spaced throughout the day, like one at breakfast and one at dinner (Levenson and Bockman 1994). Although the different calcium salts may be equally absorbed, some pharmaceutical formulations may not be. Some

Table 13.3 Food Sources of Calcium, Phosphorus, and Their Corresponding Levels of Fat and Energy (kcal)

Food	Serving size	Calcium (mg)	Phosphorus (mg)	Fat (g)	kcal/serving
Dairy					
Milk, 2% fat	8 fl oz	286	230	5	122
Milk, 1% fat	8 fl oz	291	232	2	102
Milk, nonfat	8 fl oz	306	248	0	83
Cheese, American	1 oz slice	156	145	9	106
Cheese, cottage, 2% fat	1 cup	156	341	4	203
Cheese, Monterey Jack	1 oz slice	193	126	8	103
Cheese, cream	1 oz	23	29	10	99
Cheese, cheddar	1 oz slice	204	145	9	114
Yogurt, low-fat (plain)	8 oz	300	200	3	130
Yogurt, nonfat with sweetener (strawberry)	8 oz	215	154	0	120
Desserts					
Ice cream, vanilla	1 cup	169	139	15	265
Ice milk, vanilla	1 cup	141	111	5	136
Yogurt, frozen soft-serve, vanilla	8 oz	324	293	13	370
Yogurt, frozen nonfat, strawberry or vanilla	8 oz	393	309	0	224
Vegetables					
Broccoli, steamed	1 cup	75	103	<1	44
Kale, fresh, chopped	1 cup	91	38	0	34
Kidney beans, canned	1 cup	87	333	2	215
Tofu, regular	3 oz	39	62	7	99
Tofu, with calcium sulfate	3 oz	1045	62	7	99
Spinach, cooked	1 cup	245	101	0	41
Beverages					
Apple-banana juice, with calcium added	8 fl oz	159	23	0	130
Orange juice (fresh)	8 fl oz	27	42	<1	111
Orange juice, with calcium added	8 fl oz	350	27	<1	110
Pepsi-Cola, regular	8 fl oz	0	35	0	100
Pepsi-Cola, diet	8 fl oz	0	27	0	1
Cereals					
Cheerios	1 cup	100	100	2	110
Corn Flakes	1 cup	1	10	0	101
Oatmeal (cooked)	1 cup	19	178	2	147

Values obtained from ESHA Research, Food Processor, Version 10.0, 2006.

Table 13.4 Percent Calcium in Various Food or Supplement Preparations

Preparation	Percent calcium	Comments
Carbonate	40	Insoluble at neutral pH
Tricalcium phosphate*	38	Phosphorus source
Dicalcium phosphate*	31	Insoluble; phosphorus source
Bone meal	31	May contain contaminating metals
Calcium-fortified orange juice	30	Food supplement
Oyster shell	28	May contain contaminating metals
Citrate	21	More soluble at neutral pH

*Formulated for medical use in enteral formulas.
Adapted from D.I. Levenson and R.S. Bockman, 1994, "A review of calcium preparations," *Nutrition Reviews* 52(7): 221-232.

products available on the market may not dissolve when consumed, limiting their absorption. If a calcium supplement does not dissolve, it will literally pass through the body without breaking down. To test the dissolution of a calcium supplement, place one tablet in 6 oz (180 mL) of white vinegar at room temperature and stir occasionally. The tablet should dissolve in about 30 min (Gossel 1991). The supplement industry has adopted some disintegration and dissolution standards for calcium supplements. Manufacturers' compliance with these standards is voluntary and is indicated with the USP (United States Pharmacopoeia) symbol on the label.

While supplementing with calcium may be a necessary consideration for vegans, lactose-intolerant individuals, and those trying to reduce energy intake, supplementation does have its disadvantages. Very high calcium intakes, from either supplements or calcium-fortified foods, can affect the nutrient status of other minerals in the body. For example, it has been suggested that calcium supplements decrease the absorption of dietary iron and zinc (Minihane and Fairweather-Tait 1998; Wood and Zheng 1997). However, Minihane and Fairweather-Tait (1998) found that long-term calcium supplementation did not reduce plasma

ferritin concentrations (a measure of iron status) in iron-replete people who consumed a typical Western diet. Although a high calcium intake can reduce zinc absorption, no one has investigated the effect on long-term zinc status. Calcium supplementation can also result in exposure to contaminants (e.g., lead). Consumers should also beware of possible lead contamination of calcium supplements. An analysis of 21 calcium supplements available in the market showed that eight had detectable amounts of lead (Ross et al. 2000). The current maximal accepted dietary lead intake is 6 μg/day for at-risk populations (such as children). The supplements in this study were found to contain lead at levels less than 2 μg/day per 800 mg of calcium. There is no indication that natural sources of calcium, such as oyster shell or bone meal, are superior to other sources. In fact, these natural sources are more likely to contain lead contaminants than refined sources of calcium carbonate (Ross et al. 2000). In addition, calcium supplements when taken in large amounts can cause constipation, bloating, and excess gas in some people. In conclusion, it is advisable for consumers to purchase supplements from reputable manufacturers that display the USP symbol and specific labeling indicating that the supplement has been tested for lead content (Ross et al. 2000).

While research supports the idea that high intakes of calcium, and dairy foods in particular, can contribute to weight loss, the data are still equivocal since an equal body of research shows no benefit of calcium on weight loss (Barr 2003; Thompson et al. 2005). The contradictory findings may be due to the health status of subjects being studied (obese vs. healthy weight), baseline calcium intake (deficient vs. adequate), and energy consumption (restriction vs. adding dairy to regular diet).

PHOSPHORUS

Phosphorus occurs in bone primarily as calcium phosphate and hydroxyapatite. Hydroxyapatite is a complex phosphate of calcium, $Ca_5(PO_4)_3OH$, that occurs as a mineral and is the primary structural element of bone. Approximately 88% of the phosphorus in the human body is found in the skeleton (Gibson 2005). Apart from that in bone, phosphorus is found primarily as inorganic phosphate. In relation to exercise, inorganic phosphate has important roles as a part of nucleic acids, proteins, adenosine triphosphate (ATP), and lipids. Phosphorus salts act as buf-

Highlight

Calcium, Dairy, and Weight Loss

There has recently been an increase of information in the media regarding calcium and dairy and their potential benefits for body weight. Many epidemiological investigations have shown a modest inverse relationship between fat mass and calcium intake (Parikh and Yanovski 2003). This means that when we examine large populations, people with higher calcium intakes also seem to have lower body weight or lower body fat.

Zemel and colleagues (2004) conducted a weight loss study in obese women, comparing

- a low-calcium diet (500 mg/day from food),
- a calcium-supplemented diet (500 mg/day from food + 800 mg/day supplement), and
- a high-dairy diet (1300 mg/day).

Each participant was randomized to follow one of the prescribed energy restriction diets (500 kcal/day deficit) for 24 weeks. The subjects following the low-calcium diet lost the least amount of weight (about 6 lb or 2.7 kg), while those following the calcium-supplemented diet lost significantly more (about 9 lb or 4 kg) and those following the high-dairy diet lost the most (about 11 lb or 5 kg). This suggests that calcium alone may play a role in weight loss but that calcium and dairy together may act synergistically in lowering body weight. The research suggests four possible mechanisms for the relationship between calcium or dairy intake and weight loss.

1. A high calcium intake can increase fat loss in the feces. Large loads of calcium, over 2000 mg/day, can result in a modest increase in fecal fat loss of 6% to 7% of total fat intake (Denke et al. 1993). This may not be a substantial fat loss alone, but in combination with other effects of calcium or dairy the amount could become noteworthy. Also, over long periods of time, a 6% to 7% increase in fecal fat loss could help contribute to maintenance of body weight.

2. A high dietary calcium intake can lower circulating levels of vitamin D_3 and PTH. Together the inhibition of these hormones leads to a decrease of intracellular calcium concentrations, which will stimulate lipolysis and decrease lipogenesis (Parikh and Yanovski 2003).

3. Whey protein, found in dairy foods, is a significant source of branched-chain amino acids, which may have an anabolic effect in skeletal muscle (Layman 2003). These amino acids may contribute to improved muscle maintenance during a weight loss diet.

4. Whey protein also contains bioactive compounds that may inhibit the angiotensin-converting enzyme (ACE). Conversion of angiotensin I to angiotensin II is controlled by ACE, and lipogenesis is regulated in part by angiotensin II (Pihlanto-Leppala et al. 2000). Therefore, ACE inhibition from dairy-based proteins could decrease amounts of angiotensin II and contribute to fat and weight loss.

fers that maintain acid–base balance and are also important as electrolytes in fluid balance. Additionally, inorganic phosphate is a component of **2,3-diphosphoglycerate (DPG)**, which affects the hemoglobin–oxygen dissociation curve. The highlight "Phosphorus and Sport Performance" (p. 410) reviews the practice of "phosphate loading" among athletes. Unlike calcium, phosphorus is readily absorbed at an efficiency of 60% to 70%. While calcium absorption plateaus at an intake of approximately 500 mg, absorption of phosphorus increases linearly with dietary intake (figure 13.5). Calcium and phosphorus absorption are coupled, such that low phosphorus absorption is linked with reduced calcium absorption. Following a meal, calcium and phosphorus appear to complex and are subsequently transported via passive mechanisms and then taken up by soft and bone tissues (Anderson 1991). Phosphorus regulation appears to be less tightly controlled than that of calcium, with phosphorus loss occurring through the urine, skin, and secretions into the gut.

Highlight

Phosphorus and Sport Performance

Phosphorus supplementation, or **phosphate loading,** involves consuming phosphate salts at doses five or six times the RDA (about 4 g/day) for several days before competition. Some research has shown that this practice can increase serum phosphorus, 2,3-DPG levels, $\dot{V}O_2$max, and anaerobic threshold and improve performance time and ratings of perceived exertion (Bremner et al. 2002; Goss et al. 2001; Kreider et al. 1992). Although the underlying physiological mechanism is unclear, the practice may

- increase the potential for ATP phosphorylation by increasing intracellular and extracellular phosphate levels;

- enhance 2,3-DPG synthesis, which results in better oxygen delivery to the exercising muscle;

- improve the body's respiratory and metabolic buffering capacity; and

- improve myocardial and cardiovascular capacity during exercise.

Despite sound theoretical rationale, benefits of phosphate loading have not consistently emerged. In their review of the practice, Clarkson and Haymes (1995) concluded that it may enhance performance, while others report no effects (Galloway 1996). Since phosphorus is widespread in foods, supplementation with phosphorus is unnecessary in healthy individuals. Clarkson and Haymes (1995) caution against using high amounts of phosphorus on a regular basis, as this practice can curb production of the active form of vitamin D and increase PTH, which together will reduce absorption of calcium and lead to bone resorption.

Methods of Assessment

Phosphorus status is usually determined through measurement of serum phosphorus levels. The predominant forms of phosphorus in serum are inorganic phosphates, particularly the divalent HPO_4^{2-} and monovalent $H_2PO_4^-$ anions (Gibson 2005). Children have higher serum phosphorus concentrations than adults, with normal values reached by the third decade of life. While the serum phosphorus levels of males decrease with age after the third decade, the levels for women generally decrease between the ages of 20 and 35 years and increase after 40 years of age. People with insulin-dependent diabetes mellitus have fluctuating serum phosphorus levels, as insulin decreases serum phosphorus. Normal serum phosphorus values for adults are 2.7 to 4.5 mg/dL (0.87-1.45 mmol/L) (Fischbach 2004). Serum phosphorus values can be falsely elevated by hemolysis of red blood cells, and laxatives containing large amounts of sodium phosphate can increase serum phosphorus levels (Fischbach 2004).

Requirements

The RDA for phosphorus is 700 mg/day for both men and women (table 13.2). In the typical Ameri-

can diet, phosphorus deficiencies are rare, as phosphorus is readily absorbed and is highly abundant in virtually all foods. Deficiencies can occur in people who consume large amounts of aluminum hydroxide antacids or in patients with diabetic ketoacidosis who are treated with insulin and without supplemental phosphorus. A more significant concern than phosphorus deficiency is the potential for bone loss with high dietary phosphorus intakes. Achievement of peak bone mass and the healthy maintenance of bone depend on a proper calcium–phosphorus balance. Teegarden and colleagues (1998) reported optimal BMC and BMD measurements in young women consuming 1000 to 1400 mg/day of calcium while receiving 1000 mg/day of phosphorus. It seems that at low calcium intakes (<600 mg/day), phosphorus has a positive influence on BMD. However, as calcium intake increases (up to 1400 mg/day), a high phosphorus intake (1800 mg/day) may be harmful to bone. An imbalance between phosphorus and calcium intake can cause **secondary hyperparathyroidism** and will also increase blood levels of $1,25(OH)_2$ vitamin D. Since these conditions can cause removal of calcium and phosphorus from bone, it is possible that over long time periods of time overconsumption of phosphorus may result in bone loss (Anderson and Barrett 1994). The effect of a high phosphorus intake on bone status in humans is controversial, and the long-term implications of a diet with a low calcium-to-phosphorus ratio have yet to be definitively determined (Calvo 1993; IOM 1997).

Dietary Sources and Supplementation Products

Although it is found in most food sources, phosphorus is particularly abundant in dairy foods. Common sources of phosphorus in the U.S. diet include milk products, meats, grains, soda, and phosphorus additives to foods (mostly in the form of phosphates). The phosphorus intake of humans appears to be more than adequate; the U.S. average intake is reported to be 136% to 150% of the RDA (IOM 1997; Ervin et al. 2004). In fact, it has been proposed that the phosphorus intake of Americans is even greater than that estimated, since the nutrient databases used to evaluate phosphorus intakes have not been updated with the levels of phosphorus in food additives. Consuming carbonated beverages high in phosphorus (like sodas) may be a poor nutritional choice since these beverages have a low calcium-to-phosphorus ratio. Table 13.3 lists the phosphorus content of selected foods. In light of the normally high intake of phosphorus from food sources, supplementation of phosphorus is not recommended.

MAGNESIUM

Since chapter 11 thoroughly reviewed magnesium, we include here only a brief description of this mineral as it relates to bone. Magnesium is the third most common mineral in bone, with 60% of the body's magnesium found in the skeleton (Gibson 2005). Magnesium is involved in the bone mineralization process, and the magnesium in bone can act as a reservoir to ensure that adequate magnesium is available for bodily functions. Magnesium also holds calcium in tooth enamel, which assists in preventing dental caries. Magnesium is critical to adult bone health, as serum magnesium and dietary intakes of magnesium are positively correlated with a higher BMC (Angus et al. 1988). Moreover, postmenopausal osteoporotic women tend to have low dietary intakes and serum levels of magnesium (Reginster et al. 1989; Tranquilli et al. 1994). Magnesium supplements have beneficial effects in reducing fracture risk and bone loss in

postmenopausal women (Sojka and Weaver 1995). Magnesium also plays an important role in substrate metabolism and energy production. Chapter 11 contains further details on magnesium's role in energy metabolism, the methods of assessment and requirements for magnesium, dietary sources of magnesium, and the magnesium status of athletes. Due to the abundance of magnesium in foods, deficiency in active and inactive individuals is rare; and although magnesium losses increase with exercise, the dietary intake and status of magnesium in athletes are adequate and do not appear to be nutritional concerns. However, magnesium intakes could be jeopardized in athletes with very low energy intakes, and postmenopausal female athletes need to be aware of the critical role that adequate magnesium plays in bone health.

VITAMIN D

Many recent publications have increased our knowledge in the area of vitamin D and bone health. Vitamin D is a *nutrient* involved in regulating serum calcium. In addition to being classified as a vitamin, vitamin D also functions as a hormone (Holick 2006a). The two primary sources of vitamin D are from its synthesis in skin tissue (stimulated by ultraviolet light) and from vitamin D–fortified food products (primarily milk). Figure 13.6 illustrates the conversion of **7-dehydrocholesterol** to previtamin D, also known as **cholecalciferol,** in the skin and subsequent conversion to the biologically active form of vitamin D **($1,25(OH)_2$ vitamin D,** or **calcitriol).** The primary role of vitamin D is to maintain skeletal calcium balance. Vitamin D meets this role by

- promoting absorption of calcium from the intestines,
- promoting bone resorption,
- maintaining adequate quantities of calcium and phosphorus for bone formation by its actions on the kidney and intestines, and
- allowing proper functioning of PTH to maintain serum calcium at proper levels.

With respect to all the nutrients important for bone health, the most new information has become available for vitamin D since the 1997 publication of DRIs. Recent research indicates that vitamin D may affect other systems of the body besides the skeleton, such as immune responses, cell proliferation, cell differentiation, inflammation, and **apoptosis.** Vitamin D receptors have

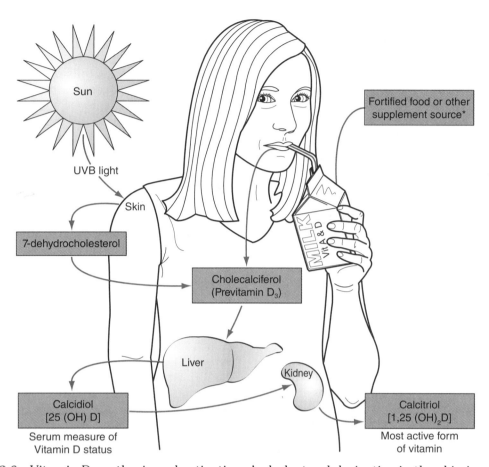

Figure 13.6 Vitamin D synthesis and activation. A cholesterol derivative in the skin is converted to previtamin D in the presence of ultraviolet light. Inactive forms of vitamin D, from both the skin and the diet, are activated via two sequential hydroxylation reactions, one in the liver and one in the kidneys, to create the active form of vitamin D (1,25(OH) vitamin D).

*Note: Dietary intake of ergocalciferol (vitamin D_2) is directly converted by the liver to calcidiol, although it is not as potent as cholecalciferol sources.

Adapted from C.A. Nowson and C. Margerison, 2002, "Vitamin D intake and vitamin D status of Australians," *Medical Journal of Australia* 177: 149-152.

been identified in the brain, breast, colon, pancreas, gonads, and skin. It is possible that cellular processes, not involving bone, are impaired at low circulating levels of **25(OH) vitamin D (25(OH)D or calcidiol)**, which are still higher than levels associated with rickets or osteomalacia. Vitamin D **insufficiency** may be associated with an increased risk of many chronic diseases like type 1 diabetes, cardiovascular disease, some cancers, multiple sclerosis, and arthritis (Holick 2004a, 2004b). In fact, experts believe that the link between vitamin D insufficiency and increased mortality due to breast, colon, lung, or prostate cancer is now well established (Hollick 2006b).

Under optimal conditions the skin can supply 80% to 100% of vitamin D requirements. Vitamin D_3 is synthesized in the skin from 7-dehydrocholesterol under the influence of ultraviolet B (UVB)

light. Use of sunscreen with a sun protection factor (SPF) of 8 excludes 95% of UVB radiation and severely limits vitamin D production (Glerup et al. 2000). Studies performed at a latitude of 42° N (north of Boston, Chicago, or Eugene, OR) indicate that the skin cannot produce any vitamin D in the winter months between November and March (Holick 2006a). Therefore, persons who regularly use sunscreen and those living at northern latitudes may have to rely solely on dietary sources of vitamin D. Darker skin pigmentation also limits the body's ability to make vitamin D from sun exposure (Calvo and Whiting 2003). Sensible sun exposure is defined as 5 to 10 min of exposure on the arms and legs or on the hands, arms, and face two or three times per week. Experts recommend exposure to sunlight of hands, face, and arms or of arms and legs for a period equal to 25% of what would be needed to cause a light pinkness to the skin (Holick 2004b). Excess sun exposure does not cause vitamin D toxicity because the ultraviolet radiation breaks down any surplus of vitamin D that is produced (Holick 2006b).

Methods of Assessment

The most useful index of vitamin D status is serum **25(OH)D,** which reflects both dietary intake of the vitamin and production in the skin due to sunlight exposure (Gibson 2005). Serum 25(OH)D is measured using competitive protein-binding assays and high-performance liquid chromatography (HPLC). While it is generally accepted that 25(OH)D is the best marker of vitamin D status, cutoff levels for deficiency, insufficiency, sufficiency, and toxicity are still uncertain. Some research suggests that an adequate serum 25(OH)D level for bone health is between 50 and 80 nmol/L, while many experts agree that 70 to 80 nmol/L is optimal (Dawson-Hughes et al. 2005). Concentrations below 12.5 nmol/L are associated with clinical signs of vitamin D deficiency, while levels above 370 nmol/L indicate toxicity (Holick 2006b). A number of factors influence serum concentrations of 25(OH)D, such as these:

- Season: Highest levels occur in late summer, lowest in late winter.
- Supplement use: Higher levels are found in people who take vitamin D supplements.
- Age and sex: Levels decrease with age and tend to be lower in women than in men.
- Latitude: People living at higher latitudes are exposed to lower levels of solar radiation, which decreases production of vitamin D in the skin.
- Levels of sun exposure: People of any latitude who get little or no sun exposure are at risk for low levels of 25(OH)D—a condition common in home-bound elderly persons; people who work indoors; and those who live in areas where the sky is overcast much of the time, particularly during the winter months.

Requirements

Table 13.2 lists the recommended AI values for vitamin D set by the IOM in 1997. The AI for vitamin D was based on intakes necessary to achieve normal ranges of serum 25(OH)D concentrations, assuming no vitamin synthesis in the skin. Although the topic is controversial, some recent evidence suggests that current AI levels

for vitamin D may not be set high enough. In a study of women who avoided sunlight exposure due to cultural dress habits, 60% were found to be vitamin D deficient despite consuming vitamin D at intakes three times greater than the AI (Glerup et al. 2000). Experts suggest that a daily intake of 15 μg/day (three times the current AI for people ages 1-50) of vitamin D_3 (cholecalciferol) is needed to reach a minimum serum concentration of 50 nmol/L (Dawson-Hughes et al. 2005). In order to attain a more optimal level of 75 nmol/L, 20 to 25 μg of vitamin D per day may be needed (Dawson-Hughes et al. 2005). Recent evidence suggests that many Americans are deficient in vitamin D. Deficiency seems to be more common in women than in men and more prevalent in African Americans than in whites. Dr. Holick (2002) reported that the prevalence of vitamin D deficiency is very high in African American women (42%) in comparison to white women (4.2%). Although women typically have lower nutrient intakes, vitamin D deficiency seems to be a problem in men as well; one-third of both genders, ages 18 to 29 and living in Boston, were measured as deficient (Tangpricha et al. 2002). Very few studies have measured serum 25(OH)D levels in American athletes. One investigation of 18 elite female gymnasts, ages 10 to 17, showed that 83% had serum vitamin D levels below ideal, and 33% were below the 50 nmol/L minimum threshold (Lovell 2008).

Requirements for vitamin D increase with age for four main reasons: (1) age-related changes in vitamin D conversion in the skin, (2) reduced absorption in the intestines, (3) decreased production of 25(OH)D by the kidneys, and (4) reduced exposure to sunlight with age (Gibson 2005). No evidence exists to suggest that physically active people have a higher vitamin D requirement than nonactive people. However, vitamin D is an important nutrient for athletes, not only for its role in maintaining bone health and preventing fractures, but also because it helps to maintain the immune system and moderate inflammatory responses (both of which are stressed in a trained individual). Meeting vitamin D requirements may be difficult for athletes who train indoors (e.g., figure skaters, gymnasts), live at higher latitudes, wear sunscreen habitually, have darker skin pigmentation, or fail to consume vitamin D–supplemented food products. Currently the Tolerable Upper Limit (UL) for vitamin D is set at 50 μg/day; however, some experts suggest revising the UL because recent data demonstrate that intakes of vitamin D as high as 100 to 250 μg/day are safe (Weaver and Fleet 2004).

Intakes

Several recent publications have indicated that many Americans are not meeting recommended intakes of vitamin D. Data from the National Health and Nutrition Examination Survey (NHANES III) and the Continuing Survey of Food Intakes by Individuals (CSFII) indicate that many women do not consume adequate amounts of vitamin D, with female teenagers and female adults consuming the lowest amounts of any group (Moore et al. 2004). Poor dietary intakes are even more pronounced in men and women ages 51 or older, who consume about 4.7 µg/day while the recommended levels are set at 10 µg/day (Moore 2005). Less than 10% of older adults, and no more than 2% of elderly people, meet the AI for vitamin D. With the minimal number of studies that have specifically examined the vitamin D intake of athletes, it appears that consumption follows the same inadequate trend as in the population as a whole. American collegiate soccer players and teenage male and female ice skaters on the national team have been found to consume about 2.5 µg/day of vitamin D (Clark et al. 2003; Jonnalagadda et al. 2004). This is well below the 5 µg/day AI. Athletes who spend many hours training indoors, habitually use sunscreen, and avoid consuming milk may be at risk for greater consequences as a result of poor vitamin D intakes. A majority of Americans are not consuming adequate vitamin D even with fortification of some food products.

Dietary Sources and Supplementation Products

Natural sources of vitamin D are limited to foods not often consumed in the typical American diet, like fatty fish and organ meats. Cod liver oil, salmon, sun-dried shiitake mushrooms, sardines, and tuna are all natural sources of vitamin D, although fortified milk, juice, yogurt, margarine, cheese, and cereal are also sources. The top two sources of vitamin D in the American diet are fluid milk and ready-to-eat breakfast cereals (Moore et al. 2005). Although only nonfat dry milk and evaporated milk are required to be fortified, many dairy products and other high-calcium foods can be fortified. The usual fortification level for milk is 2.5 µg (100 IU)/8 fl oz (or 100 IU/240 mL), but quality control is highly variable (Moore et al. 2005). Research indicates that cholecalciferol (previtamin D) is a more potent form of the vitamin than **ergocalciferol (vitamin D$_2$)**. Armas and colleagues (2004) demonstrated that cholecalciferol

elevates and sustains serum 25(OH)D levels to a considerably greater degree than does ergocalciferol. Therefore, if someone is considering use of vitamin D supplements, a product containing cholecalciferol is preferred because it requires fewer pills over time.

Vitamin D supplementation appears effective in preventing hip and spine fractures in the elderly and is an important therapeutic option in treating osteoporosis. Younger people may also need supplements if they have little exposure to the sun and poor dietary intakes of vitamin D. Consuming vitamin D–fortified orange juice appears to be an effective way to meet dietary needs, especially for those who are lactose intolerant. Because vitamin D is fat soluble (and therefore stored in the body), we must be aware that megadoses could cause toxicity. With that said, vitamin D intoxication is extremely rare, and research has shown that intakes as high as 100 to 250 µg/day (4000-10,000 IU/day) are safe (Weaver and Fleet 2004). Symptoms of vitamin D toxicity include hypertension, hypercalcemia, altered renal function, and calcification of nonbone tissue (Gibson 2005). There have been no reported cases of vitamin D intoxication due to consumption of food sources alone.

OTHER NUTRIENTS INVOLVED IN BONE METABOLISM

In addition to the nutrients already discussed, there are several others that play an important role in bone health.

Fluoride

Fluoride plays a critical role in the strengthening of bones and teeth. Fluoride replaces the hydroxyl portions of the hydroxyapatite crystal after mineralization of the skeleton, making it stronger and, in the case of teeth, more resistant to decay. **Fluorapatite** is the stabilized form of the apatite minerals in bone and teeth. The most significant sources of fluoride are fluoridated water, tea, and seafood. Short-term (two to three years), low-dose fluoride therapy can increase BMD in the spine and reduce vertebral fractures (Pak et al. 1994). Research suggests an optimal range for fluoride intake as demonstrated by the U-shaped relationship between fluoride content of water and prevalence of fractures (figure 13.7). In an epidemiological study, Li and colleagues (2001) found that prevalence of fractures was lowest

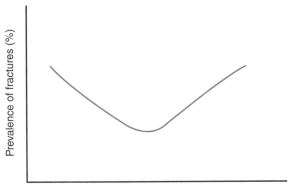

Figure 13.7 U-shaped relationship with prevalence of bone fractures. At very low and at very high water fluoride concentrations, there is a greater prevalence of fractures. A fluoride concentration of water that seems optimal for bone health is between 1.00 and 1.06 ppm.

Reprinted from Y. Li et al., 2001, "Effect of long-term exposure to fluoride in drinking water on risks of bone fractures," *Journal of Bone and Mineral Research* 16: 932-939.

in people who consumed water with 1.00 to 1.06 ppm of fluoride. Groups who consumed water with fluoride levels below 0.34 ppm and over 4.32 ppm had significantly greater fracture rates.

Energy and Protein

Adequate energy intake is critical for everyone, as macro- and micronutrients cannot be consumed in adequate amounts if energy intake is insufficient. Chronically low energy intakes hinder complete bone development and maintenance of healthy bone mass. This relationship between adequate energy and bone health plays an important interactive role in the "female athlete triad" (see "Female Athlete Triad and Osteoporosis," p. 416, and chapter 15).

Many physically active women restrict energy intake while maintaining demanding training schedules, thereby limiting energy availability. Ihle and Loucks (2004) have described a dose–response relationship between energy availability and bone turnover in young, exercising women. Severely lowering energy availability by both increasing physical activity and restricting calorie intake causes an uncoupling of bone formation and resorption in young, healthy, regularly menstruating women. Over time this uncoupling can lead to irreversible bone loss, and inhibition of bone formation may hinder young women from achieving optimal peak bone mass (Ihle and Loucks 2004). The relationship between energy restriction and

bone loss appears to apply to dieting postmenopausal women as well. Ricci and colleagues (2001) studied obese postmenopausal women who followed a moderate energy restriction weight loss program for six months. Six months of dieting led to an increase in bone resorption and loss of whole-body BMD. In contrast, bone resorption was not altered in premenopausal obese women following a similar six-month energy restriction diet (Shapses et al. 2001). No change in BMD of the whole body or spine was observed in the premenopausal women even after a 7% to 8% decrease in body weight. In fact, premenopausal women who supplemented with 1000 mg of calcium during their weight loss plan actually gained BMD at the spine. A negative energy balance in otherwise healthy athletic young women seems to initiate bone loss. Dietary restriction in postmenopausal women may also lead to bone loss. Premenopausal women who are dieting seem to be protected from bone loss, especially if they are supplementing with calcium. In summary, there appears to be a complex interaction between energy availability, hormonal status, and bone turnover in young and mature women. Athletes, particularly women, who are trying to lose weight should pay close attention to calcium intake and bone health.

Bone formation, growth, and maintenance are impossible without adequate protein. Proteins are a part of the collagen matrix of bone and make up the growth factors involved in bone formation. The effect of high dietary protein on bone health has been debated in the literature, with reports that a high protein intake can increase urinary calcium losses. Early researchers in this area speculated that bone was the source of elevated urinary calcium excretion during a high-protein diet. In 1997, Kerstetter and colleagues found that consuming a low-protein diet (0.7 g/kg body weight) caused an increase in serum PTH and $1,25(OH)_2D$, both of which exceeded the upper limits of normal. These two hormones work together to increase blood calcium levels. The elevated hormone levels suggest that a low-protein diet may decrease calcium absorption. A follow-up evaluation showed that 18% of calcium consumed is absorbed during a low-protein diet (0.7 g/kg). Absorption increases to 26% during a high-protein (2.1 g/kg) diet (Kerstetter et al. 1998). Therefore, it appears that an increase in intestinal calcium absorption as people follow a high-protein diet likely accounts for a majority of the observed increases in calcium excretion.

Many epidemiologic investigations have explored the relationship between protein intake

Highlight

Female Athlete Triad and Osteoporosis

Normal menstrual function is vital to the maintenance of bone health. The **female athlete triad** is a condition composed of menstrual irregularities, disordered eating patterns, and poor bone health. These conditions are closely related to one another. Disordered eating patterns can create a negative energy balance and lead to altered menstrual patterns, while both conditions contribute to the development of osteoporosis. Chapter 15 provides a complete description of this condition. We include a brief discussion here because of the direct links between low BMD, inadequate energy intake, low calcium intake, relatively high energy expenditure, and altered menstrual function.

The risk factors for development of osteoporosis include the following (Chesnut 1994):

- Gender (being female)
- Race: Caucasians and Asians have a greater risk
- Estrogen depletion (in women): postmenopausal state
- History of amenorrhea, anorexia nervosa, oligomenorrhea, delayed menarche, and so on
- Calcium deficiency
- Vitamin D deficiency
- Diminished peak bone mass at skeletal maturity
- Sedentary lifestyle
- Anorexia nervosa
- Family history of osteoporosis
- Testosterone depletion (in men)
- Aging
- Leanness (adipose tissue may be a source of postmenopausal estrogen production)
- Small frame
- Alcoholism
- Smoking
- Medication use (corticosteroids, excessive thyroid hormone, prolonged heparin usage)

A history of athletic-related menstrual dysfunction and disordered eating increases a woman's risk for developing osteoporosis. Significant bone loss is known to occur during periods of estrogen deficiency and poor dietary intake. The low circulating estrogen levels that accompany menstrual dysfunction in premenopausal athletes (or during menopause in mature women) lead to a decrease in bone formation, an increase in bone resorption, and consequent changes in serum calcium; the end result is bone loss. One major protective factor against osteoporosis in women is maintenance of normal menstrual function during the premenopausal phase of life. Bone loss that occurs with the female athlete triad may or may not be replaced if the condition is reversed. However, research does indicate that participation in impact loading-type sports, such as gymnastics, provides some protection against bone loss even with compromised menstrual status (Robinson et al. 1995).

and bone health. Much of this work has shown a positive relationship between protein intake and BMD (Teegarden et al. 1998; Kerstetter et al. 2000; Hannan et al. 2000). Paradoxically, these results conflict with an epidemiological investigation in which hip fracture was the primary outcome variable. In that study, low protein intakes were associated with lower fracture rates (Frassetto et al. 2000). At low protein intakes, intestinal calcium absorption is decreased, resulting in hormonal increases of PTH and vitamin D. At high calcium intakes, hypercalciuria results, and this may be at least partially explained by increased intestinal absorption. It is still not clear if the acute changes in calcium metabolism during low- or high-protein diets have any long-term impact on bone health. In conclusion, as with many dietary principles, there seems to be an optimal intake of protein that will be great enough to not alter calcium metabolism hormones but low enough to not cause large urinary calcium losses. Like most Americans, athletes are not at risk for low protein intakes except in cases of extreme dietary restriction.

Vitamins K and C

Vitamin K plays an important role in blood coagulation and is required for synthesis of osteocalcin. Osteocalcin is a protein produced by osteoblasts in bone tissue and is incorporated into the extracellular matrix of bone. Vitamin K is endogenously produced by bacteria in the digestive tract. Food sources of vitamin K include green leafy vegetables (e.g., spinach, kale), cruciferous vegetables (cabbage, brussels sprouts, broccoli), vegetable oils, and milk. The DRI for vitamin K is 100 μg/day for men and 90 μg/day for women over the age of 19. Epidemiological research on normally active populations suggests that poor vitamin K intakes are associated with an increased risk of fracture (Vermeer et al. 2004). Recent evidence suggests that there seems to be an improvement in bone health for people who supplement with calcium, vitamin D, and vitamin K. In a review article, Ryan-Harshman and Aldoori (2004) conclude that dietary intake of vitamin K less than 100 μg/day may not be optimal for bone health. A lack of evidence exists for evaluating vitamin K status or intake in athletic populations.

The function of vitamin C in bone health is related to its role in the formation of collagen. Epidemiological studies present conflicting results: Gunnes and Lehmann (1995) found that dietary vitamin C was positively related to forearm BMD in children and adolescents, yet Leveille and colleagues (1997) found no association between dietary vitamin C and BMD in postmenopausal women. However, it is logical that a severe vitamin C deficiency would alter collagen formation and thus affect bone health. Regular consumption of fruits, juices, and vegetables can easily provide adequate vitamin C.

EXERCISE AND BONE HEALTH

Hundreds of research articles have focused on exercise, physical activity, and bone health. In fact, some evidence suggests that weight-bearing activity has a greater impact on developing peak bone mass than does calcium intake (Welten et al. 1994). The American College of Sports Medicine's position stand, "Physical Activity and Bone Health," reviews much of the literature to date (Kohrt et al. 2004). It is clear that weight-bearing physical activity performed at all ages has favorable effects on the skeleton. The following summarizes important points from the review article by Kohrt and colleagues (2004).

- Children and adolescents may optimize bone mineral accrual by performing physical activity that generates high-intensity loading forces, such as gymnastics, resistance training, and plyometrics.
- Exercise-induced gains of bone mineral in children are likely sustained into adulthood, emphasizing that weight-bearing exercise during youth may have lifelong benefits for the skeleton.
- Many cross-sectional studies of adult men and women demonstrate that athletes have higher BMD than nonathletes. Bone mineral density values are greatest in gymnasts, weightlifters, and bodybuilders and lowest in swimmers.
- During adult life, age-related decreases in BMD can be prevented with regular weight-bearing physical activity.
- In order to preserve bone health during adulthood, one should participate in weight-bearing physical activities with moderate to high loading forces, two to five times per week, for 30 to 60 min.
- Benefits of high-intensity skeletal loading exercise may not be realized in athletes with dietary deficiencies or in female athletes with altered menstrual function.

Thus, it appears that physical activity and exercise can play health-promoting roles in bone formation and maintenance. However, proper hormonal, energy, and nutrient balance are critical to deriving the benefits of exercise for bone.

CHAPTER IN REVIEW

Calcium, phosphorus, magnesium, and vitamin D play critical roles in forming the bone matrix and in maintaining adult bone. Many adults in the United States do not consume the current recommended intake for calcium, and certain people may benefit from calcium supplementation. Vitamin D deficiencies can occur in individuals who spend little time outdoors, people who live at high latitudes, and athletes who train and compete indoors and fail to consume adequate dietary sources of vitamin D. Exercise and weight-bearing physical activity appear to have beneficial effects on bone maintenance in adults, but failure of women to maintain regular menstrual function can result in a reduction in bone mass and increase the risk for osteoporosis.

Key Concepts

1. Identify the primary nutrients associated with bone health.

In addition to energy intake, the primary nutrients associated with bone health are calcium, phosphorus, magnesium, vitamin D, fluoride, protein, vitamin C and vitamin K. The minerals play an important structural role in bone, while vitamin D acts as a hormone helping to assure calcium absorption and regulation in the body. Vitamin K is vital for the synthesis of osteocalcin and vitamin C is essential for collagen formation. Bone development is hindered by low energy intake, thus, adequate energy is important to assure that the macro and micronutrients important to bone are consumed. Protein intake is necessary since proteins are part of the collagen and noncollagen tissues, the bone matrix and the growth factors that regulate bone health.

2. Describe the five stages of the bone remodeling cycle. Which stages involve osteoclasts and osteoblasts?

The five stages of the bone remodeling cycle are activation, resorption, reversal, formation, and resting. Osteoclasts break down bone in the resorption phase, while osteoblasts build new bone in the formation phase.

3. Discuss the methods used to assess calcium status, identify calcium requirements and intakes of athletes, and identify sources of calcium and related supplementation products.

There is no satisfactory way to assess calcium levels directly. Assessment of bone can indicate long-term calcium status. Although calcium requirements are difficult to determine, DRI values have been established to help plan and assess diets for healthy people. Calcium intakes for some athletes and other people are lower than recommended, with milk and milk products being the most common sources of calcium in the United States. Athletes at risk for low calcium intakes are those with low energy intakes. Calcium supplements vary in absorbability and cost.

4. Describe the methods of assessment, the requirements, and the dietary sources of phosphorus.

Serum phosphorus levels are a general indicator of phosphorus status. The RDA for adult men and women is 700 mg/day, and phosphorus deficiencies are rare in the United States. Long-term excessive phosphorus intake is associated with bone loss. Phosphorus is found in most food and is particularly abundant in dairy products. The phosphorus intake in the United States is reported to be more than adequate.

5. Discuss magnesium's role in bone health.

Magnesium is the third most common mineral in bone. Magnesium is involved in bone mineralization and can act as a reservoir in bone to maintain magnesium for other bodily functions. Magnesium is abundant in food, and deficiencies are rare.

6. Describe the methods of assessment, the requirements, dietary sources, and supplementation products of vitamin D.

Vitamin D is a hormone involved in regulating serum calcium. The best marker of vitamin D status is serum total 25(OH)D. Vitamin D is supplemented in food and synthesized in the skin during exposure to ultraviolet light. Vitamin D requirements increase with age for several reasons. There is no evidence that active people require more vitamin D than sedentary individuals. Many Americans have suboptimal vitamin D intakes and low serum levels. If combined with limited sun exposure, this leads to insufficiency or deficiency. Vitamin D toxicity is very rare and cannot occur from sun exposure alone.

7. **Describe how fluoride, energy, and protein play a role in bone metabolism.**

Fluoride is a part of the hydroxyapatite crystals that strengthen teeth and bone. Significant sources of fluoride are fluoridated water, tea, and seafood. Low energy intakes result in low macro- and micronutrient intakes and prevent development and maintenance of healthy bone. Proteins are a critical part of collagen and noncollagenous tissues and of the growth factors involved in bone formation; they also are part of the bone matrix material.

Key Terms

1,25(OH)$_2$ vitamin D (calcitriol) 411
2,3-diphosphoglycerate (DPG) 409
25(OH) vitamin D or 25(OH)D (calcidiol) 412
7-dehydrocholesterol 411
achlorhydria 406
apoptosis 411
bone mineral content (BMC) 400
bone mineral density (BMD) 400
cholecalciferol (previtamin D$_3$) 411
cortical (or compact) bone 399
ergocalciferol (vitamin D$_2$) 414
female athlete triad 416
fluorapatite 414

formation 398
hydroxyapatite 401
insufficiency 412
osteoblast 398
osteocalcin 417
osteoclast 398
osteopenia 400
osteoporosis 400
phosphate loading 410
remodeling 398
resorption 398
secondary hyperparathyroidism 410
trabecular bone 399

Additional Information

Ervin RB, Wang CY, Wright JD, Kennedy-Stephenson J. Dietary intake of selected minerals for the United States population: 1999-2000. Advance data from vital and health statistics, no. 341. Hyattsville, MD: National Center for Health Statistics, 2004.

> This publication presents the most recent mineral intake data from the National Health and Nutrition Examination Survey, explaining calcium intake across different age groups, genders, and regions of the United States.

Institute of Medicine, Food and Nutrition Board. Dietary reference intakes: calcium, phosphorus, magnesium, vitamin D, and fluoride. Washington, DC: National Academy Press, 1997.

> This 1997 publication examined the nutrients important for bone health and set the Dietary Reference Intakes currently in use.

Gibson RS. Principles of nutritional assessment, 2nd ed. New York: Oxford University Press, 2005.

> This book provides a thorough review of nutrition assessment methods, including sections on calcium, phosphorus, and vitamin D.

Kohrt WM, Bloomfield SA, Little KD, Nelson MD, Yingling VR. American College of Sports Medicine position stand: physical activity and bone health. Med Sci Sports Exerc 2004;36:1985-1996.

> The paper is a position statement from the American College of Sports Medicine, providing guidelines on physical activity patterns important for improving bone health.

The Milk Matters Campaign: www.nichd.nih.gov/milk/

Milk Matters Campaign is a public health platform sponsored by the National Institute of Child Health and Human Development. It is designed to improve calcium intake among children and teenagers in order to help them build a strong and healthy skeleton.

Moore C, Murphy MM, Keast DR, Holick MF. Vitamin D intake in the United States. J Am Diet Assoc 2004;104:980-983.

This paper uses data from the National Health and Nutrition Examination Survey and the Continuing Survey of Food Intakes by Individuals to evaluate the American dietary intake of vitamin D.

National Institute of Arthritis and Musculoskeletal and Skin Diseases (NIAMS) Information Clearinghouse, National Institutes of Health: www.niams.nih.gov

The NIAMS disseminates general information, shares patient and professional education materials, and refers people to other sources of information.

National Osteoporosis Foundation (NOF): www.nof.org

The NOF is the premier nonprofit, voluntary health organization working to encourage lifelong bone health in order to lower the pervasive occurrence of osteoporosis and the related fractures. The NOF also works toward finding a cure for the disease by promoting research, education, and advocacy.

Weaver CM. Assessing calcium status and metabolism. J Nutr 1990;120:1470-1473.

This paper discusses the challenges of assessing calcium status and metabolism.

References

Anderson JJB. Nutritional biochemistry of calcium and phosphorus. J Nutr Biochem 1991;2:300-307.

Anderson JJB, Barrett CJH. Dietary phosphorus: the benefits and the problems. Nutr Today 1994(March/April):29-34.

Angus RM, Sambrook PN, Pocock NA, Eisman JA. Dietary intake and bone mineral density. Bone Min 1988;4:265-277.

Armas LAG, Hollis BW, Heaney RP. Vitamin D-2 is much less effective than vitamin D-3 in humans. J Clin Endocr Metab 2004;89:5387-5391.

Baron RE. Anatomy and ultrastructure of bone. In: Murray J, Favus MD. Primer on metabolic bone diseases and disorders of mineral metabolism, 4th ed. Philadelphia: Lippincott Williams & Wilkins, 1999;99-106.

Barr SI. Increased dairy product or calcium intake: is body weight or composition affected in humans? J Nutr 2003;133:245S-248S.

Baylink DJ, Jennings JC. Calcium and bone homeostasis and changes with aging. In: Hazzard WR, Bierman EL, Blass JP, Ettinger WH, Halter JB eds. Principles of geriatric medicine and gerontology. New York: McGraw-Hill, 1994;879-896.

Benardot D, Schwarz M, Heller DW. Nutrient intake in young, highly competitive gymnasts. J Am Diet Assoc 1989;89(3):401-403.

Beshgetoor D, Nichols JF. Dietary intake and supplement use in female master cyclists and runners. Int J Sport Nutr Exerc Metab 2003;19:166-172.

Bremner K, Bubb WA, Kemp GJ, Trenell MI, Thompson CH. The effect of phosphate loading on erythrocyte 2,3-bisphosphoglycerate levels. Clin Chim Acta 2002;323:111-114.

Calvo MS. Dietary phosphorus, calcium metabolism and bone. J Nutr 1993;123:1627-1633.

Calvo MS, Whiting SJ. Prevalence of vitamin D insufficiency in Canada and the United States: Importance to health status and efficacy of current food fortification and dietary supplement use. Nutr Rev 2003;61:107-113.

Chesnut CH. Osteoporosis. In: Hazzard WR, Bierman EL, Blass JP, Ettinger WH, Halter JB eds. Principles of geriatric medicine and gerontology. New York: McGraw-Hill, 1994;897-909.

Clark M, Reed DB, Crouse SF, Armstrong RB. Pre- and postseason dietary intake, body composition, and performance indices of NCAA division I female soccer players. Int J Sport Nutr Exerc Metab 2003;13:303-319.

Clarkson PM, Haymes EM. Exercise and mineral status of athletes: calcium, magnesium, phosphorus, and iron. Med Sci Sports Exerc 1995;27:831-843.

Dawson-Hughes B, Heaney RP, Holick MF, Lips P, Meunier PJ, Vieth R. Estimates of optimal vitamin D status. Osteoporos Int 2005;16:713-176.

Denke MA, Fox MM, Schulte MC. Short-term dietary calcium fortification increases fecal saturated fat content and reduces serum lipids in men. J Nutr 1993;123:1047-1053.

Ervin RB, Wang CY, Wright JD, Kennedy-Stephenson J. Dietary intake of selected minerals for the United States population: 1999-2000. Advance data from vital and health statistics, no. 341. Hyattsville, MD: National Center for Health Statistics, 2004.

Fischbach F. A manual of laboratory and diagnostic tests, 7th ed. Philadelphia: Lippincott, 2004.

Fleming KH, Heimbach JT. Consumption of calcium in the U.S.: Food sources and intake levels. J Nutr 1994;124:1426S-1430S.

Food Processor (software program), Version 10.0. ESHA Research, Salem, OR, 2006.

Forshee RA, Anderson PA, Storey ML. Changes in calcium intake and association with beverage consumption and demographics: Comparing data from CSFII 1994-1996, 1998 and NHANES 1999-2002. J Am Coll Nutr 2006;25:108-116.

Frassetto LA, Todd KM, Morris RC, Sebastian A. Worldwide incidence of hip fracture in elderly women: relation to consumption of animal and vegetable foods. J Gerontol A Biol Sci Med Sci 2000;55:M585-592.

Frost HM. Some effects of basic multicellular unit-based remodeling on photon absorptiometry of trabecular bone. Bone Min 1989;7:47-65.

Galloway SDR, Tremblay MS, Sexsmith JR, Roberts CJ. The effects of acute phosphate supplementation in subjects of different aerobic fitness levels. Eur J Appl Physiol 1996;72:224-230.

Gibson RS. Principles of nutritional assessment, 2nd ed. New York: Oxford University Press, 2005.

Glerup H, Mikkelsen K, Poulsen L et al. Commonly recommended daily intake of vitamin D is not sufficient if sunlight exposure is limited. J Intern Med 2000;247:260-268.

Goss F, Robertson R, Riechman S et al. Effect of potassium phosphate supplementation on perceptual and physiological response to maximal graded exercise. Int J Sport Nutr Exerc Metab 2001;11:53-62.

Gossel TA. Calcium supplements. U.S. Pharmacist 1991(Apr):26-32.

Gunnes M, Lehmann EH. Dietary calcium, saturated fat, fiber and vitamin C as predictors of forearm cortical and trabecular bone mineral density in healthy children and adolescents. Acta Paediatr 1995;84:388-392.

Hannan MT, Tucker KL, Dawson-Hughes B, Cupples LA, Felson DT, Kiel DP. Effect of dietary protein on bone loss in elderly men and women: The Framingham osteoporosis study. J Bone Min Res 2000;15:2504-2512.

Heaney RP. Bone Biology in Health and Disease. In: Shils ME, Shike M, Ross AC, Caballero B, Cousins R eds. Modern Nutrition in Health and Disease, 10th ed. Philadelphia, PA: Lippincott, Williams & Wilkins, 2006;1314-1325

Heaney RP, Dowell MS, Bierman J, Hale CA, Bendich A. Absorbability and cost effectiveness of calcium supplementation. Am Coll Nutr 2001;20:239-246.

Heaney R, Recker R. Distribution of calcium absorption in middle-aged women. Am J Clin Nutr 1986;43:299-305.

Heaney RP, Weaver CM. Calcium and vitamin D. Endocrinol Metab Clin 2003;32:181-194.

Holick MF. Too little vitamin D in premenopausal women: Why should we care? Am J Clin Nutr 2002;76:3-4.

Holick MF. Sunlight and vitamin D for bone health and prevention of autoimmune diseases, cancers, and cardiovascular disease. Am J Clin Nutr 2004a;80:1678S-1688S.

Holick MF. Vitamin D: importance in prevention of cancers, type 1 diabetes, heart disease, and osteoporosis. Am J Clin Nutr 2004b;79:362-371.

Holick MF. Vitamin D. In: Shils ME, Shike M, Ross AC, Caballero B, Cousins RJ eds. Modern nutrition in health and disease, 10th ed. Philadelphia: Lea & Febiger, 2006a:376-395.

Holick MF. Vitamin D: its role in cancer prevention and treatment. Prog Biophys Mol Biol 2006b;92:49-59.

Ihle R, Loucks AB. Dose-response relationship between energy availability and bone turnover in young exercising women. J Bone Min Res 2004;19:1231-1240.

Ilich JZ, Kerstetter JE. Nutrition in bone health revisited: a story beyond calcium. J Am Coll Nutr 2000;19:715-737.

Institute of Medicine (IOM), Food and Nutrition Board. Dietary reference intakes: calcium, phosphorus, magnesium, vitamin D and fluoride. Washington, DC: National Academy Press, 1997.

Jonnalagadda SS, Ziegler PJ, Nelson JA. Food preferences, dieting behaviors, and body image perception of elite figure skaters. Int J Sport Nutr Exerc Metab 2004;14:594-606.

Keller JI, Lanou AJ, Barnard ND. The consumer cost of calcium from food and supplements. J Am Diet Assoc 2002;102:1669-1671.

Kerstetter JE, Caseria DM, Mitnick ME, Ellison AF et al. Increased circulating concentrations of parathyroid hormone in healthy, young women consuming a protein-restricted diet. Am J Clin Nutr 1997;66:1188-1196.

Kerstetter JE, O'Brien KO, Insogna KL. Dietary protein affects intestinal calcium absorption. Am J Clin Nutr 1998;68:859-865.

Kerstetter JE, Svastisalee CM, Caseria DM, Mitnick ME, Insogna KL. A threshold for low-protein-diet-induced elevations in parathyroid hormone. Am J Clin Nutr 2000;72:168-173.

Klesges RC, Ward KD, Shelton ML et al. Changes in bone mineral content in male athletes—mechanisms of action and intervention effects. JAMA 1996;276:226-230.

Kohrt WM, Bloomfield SA, Little KD, Nelson MD, Yingling VR. American College of Sports Medicine position stand: physical activity and bone health. Med Sci Sports Exerc 2004;36:1985-1996.

Kreider RB, Miller GW, Schenck D et al. Effects of phosphate loading on metabolic and myocardial responses to maximal and endurance exercise. Int J Sport Nutr 1992;2:20-47.

Layman DK. The role of leucine in weight loss diets and glucose homeostasis. J Nutr 2003;133:261S-267S.

Leveille SG, LaCroix AZ, Koepsell TD, Beresford SA, Van Belle G, Buchner DM. Dietary vitamin C and bone mineral density in postmenopausal women in Washington State, USA. J Epidemiol Commun Health 1997;51:479-485.

Levenson DI, Bockman RS. A review of calcium preparations. Nutr Rev 1994;52:221-232.

Li YM, Liang CK, Slemenda CW et al. Effect of long-term exposure to fluoride in drinking water on risks of bone fractures. J Bone Min Res 2001;16:932-939.

Lin YC, Lyle RM, Weaver CM et al. Peak spine and femoral neck bone mass in young women. Bone 2003;32:546-553.

Lovell G. Vitamin D status of females in an elite gymnastics program. Clin J Sports Med 2008;18:159-161.

Lunar Corporation. Biochemical markers: variability high, predictive accuracy poor. Lunar News 1994(Dec):15-17.

Manore MM. Chronic dieting in active women: what are the health consequences? Women's Health Issues 1996;6:332-341.

Manore MM. Nutritional needs of the female athlete. Clin Sports Med 1999;18:549-563.

Minihane AM, Fairweather-Tait SJ. Effect of calcium supplementation on daily nonheme-iron absorption and long-term iron status. Am J Clin Nutr 1998;68(1):96-102.

Moore CE, Murphy MM, Holick MF. Vitamin D intakes by children and adults in the United States differ among ethnic groups. J Nutr 2005;135:2478-2485.

Moore C, Murphy MM, Keast DR, Holick MF. Vitamin D intake in the United States. J Am Diet Assoc 2004;104:980-983.

Morgan EF, Barnes GL, Einhorn TA. The bone organ system: form and function. In: Marcus R, Feldman D, Nelson DA, Rosen CJ eds. Osteoporosis. San Diego: Academic Press, 1996;3-26.

National Institutes of Health (NIH) Consensus Panel. Osteoporosis prevention, diagnosis, and therapy. JAMA 2001;285:785-795.

Nowson CA, Margerison C. Vitamin D intake and vitamin D status of Australians. Med J Aust 2002;177:149-152.

Pak CYC, Sakhaee K, Piziak V et al. Slow-release sodium fluoride in the management of postmenopausal osteoporosis. Ann Intern Med 1994;120:625-632.

Parikh SJ, Yanovski JA. Calcium intake and adiposity. Am J Clin Nutr 2003;77:281-287.

Pihlanto-Leppala A, Koskinen P, Piilola K, Yupasela T, Korhonen H. Angiotensin I-converting enzyme inhibitory properties of whey protein digests: concentration and characterization of active peptides. J Dairy Res 2000;67:53-64.

Reginster JY, Strause L, Deroisy R, Lecart MP, Saltman P, Franchimont P. Preliminary report of decreased serum magnesium in postmenopausal osteoporosis. Magnesium 1989;8:106-109.

Rianon N, Feeback D, Wood R, Driscoll T, Shackelford L, LeBlanc A. Monitoring sweat calcium using skin patches. Calcif Tissue Int 2003;72:694-697.

Ricci TA, Heymsfield SB, Pierson RN, Stahl T, Chowdhury HA, Shapses SA. Moderate energy restriction increases bone resorption in obese postmenopausal women. Am J Clin Nutr 2001;73:347-352.

Robinson TL, Snow-Harter C, Taaffe DR, Gillis D, Shaw J, Marcus R. Gymnasts exhibit higher bone mass than runners despite similar prevalence of amenorrhea and oligomenorrhea. J Bone Min Res 1995;10:26-35.

Rosen CJ, Tenenhouse A. Biochemical markers of bone turnover: a look at laboratory tests that reflect bone status. Postgrad Med 1998;104:113-114.

Ross EA, Szabo NJ, Tebberr IR. Lead content of calcium supplements. JAMA 2000;284:1425-1429.

Ryan-Harshman M, Aldoori W. Bone health: new role for vitamin K? Can Fam Phys 2004;50:993-997.

Shapses SA, Von Thun NL, Heymsfield SB et al. Bone turnover and density in obese premenopausal women during moderate weight loss and calcium supplementation. J Bone Min Res 2001;16:1329-1336.

Slawson DL, McClanahan BS, Clemens LH et al. Food sources of calcium in a sample of African-American and Euro-American collegiate athletes. Int J Sport Nutr Exerc Metab 2001;11:199-208.

Sojka JE, Weaver CM. Magnesium supplementation and osteoporosis. Nutr Rev 1995;53:71-74.

Suarez FL, Adshead J, Furne JK, Levitt MD. Lactose maldigestion is not an impediment to the intake of 1500 mg calcium daily as dairy products. Am J Clin Nutr 1998;68:1118-1122.

Szulac P, Delmas P. Biochemical markers of bone turnover in osteoporosis. In: Marcus R, Feldman D, Nelson D, Rosen C eds. Osteoporosis. San Diego: Academic Press, 2008;1519-1545.

Tangpricha V, Pearce EN, Chen TC, Holick MF. Vitamin D insufficiency among free-living adults. Am J Med 2002;112:659-662.

Teegarden D, Lyle RM, McCabe GP et al. Dietary calcium, protein, and phosphorus are related to bone mineral density and content in young women. Am J Clin Nutr 1998;68:749-754.

Teegarden D, Proulx WR, Martin BR et al. Peak bone mass in young women. J Bone Min Res 1995;10:711-715.

Thompson J, Manore MM. Nutrition: an applied approach. San Francisco: Pearson Education, 2005;309-344.

Thompson WG, Holdman NR, Janzow DJ, Slezak JM, Morris KL, Zemel MB. Effect of energy-reduced diets high in dairy products and fiber on weight loss in obese adults. Obesity Res 2005;13:1344-1353.

Tranquilli AL, Lucino E, Garzetti GG, Romanini C. Calcium, phosphorus and magnesium intakes correlate with bone mineral content in postmenopausal women. Gynecol Endocrinol 1994;8:55-58.

Vermeer C, Shearer MJ, Zitterman A et al. Beyond deficiency: potential benefits of increased intakes of vitamin K for bone and vascular health. Eur J Nutr 2004;43:325-335.

Weaver CM. Assessing calcium status and metabolism. J Nutr 1990;120:1470-1473.

Weaver CM. 2003 W.O. Atwater memorial lecture: defining nutrient requirements from a perspective of bone-related nutrients. J Nutr 2003;133:4063-4066.

Weaver CM, Fleet JC. Vitamin D requirements: current and future. Am J Clin Nutr 2004;80:1739S-80S

Weaver CM, Heaney RP. Calcium. In: Shils ME, Shike M, Ross AC, Caballero B, Cousins RJ. eds. Modern nutrition in health and disease, 10th ed. Philadelphia, PA: Lippincott, Williams & Wilkins, 2006;194-210.

Welten DC, Kemper HCG, Post GB et al. Weight-bearing activity during youth is a more important factor for peak bone mass than calcium intake. J Bone Min Res 1994;9:1089-1096.

Wiita BG, Stombaugh IA. Nutrition knowledge, eating practices, and health of adolescent female runners: A 3-year longitudinal study. Int J Sport Nutr 1996;6:414-425.

Wood RJ, Zheng JJ. High dietary calcium intakes reduce zinc absorption and balance in humans. Am J Clin Nutr 1997;65:1803-1809.

Yates AA, Schlicker SA, Suitor CW. Dietary reference intakes: the new basis for recommendations for calcium and related nutrients, B vitamins, and choline. J Am Diet Assoc 1998;98:699-706.

Zemel MB, Thompson W, Milstead A, Morris K, Campbell P. Calcium and dairy acceleration of weight and fat loss during energy restriction in obese adults. Obesity Res 2004;12:582-590.

CHAPTER 14

Nutrition and Fitness Assessment

Chapter Objectives

After reading this chapter you should be able to

- describe the characteristics of medical and health history questionnaires,
- discuss the methods used to assess energy and nutrient intakes,
- discuss the methods used to assess energy expenditure, and
- describe specific tests used to assess the components of fitness.

Tammy is a collegiate distance runner, participating in cross-country and track competitions. She is concerned about her performance: She has been very tired at practice and has not been performing her best during competition. (For more information about Tammy's fatigue, see "Case Study: Female Distance Runner Complaining of Fatigue" on p. 438.) Tammy wants to maintain a low body weight and a low percentage of body fat since she believes these characteristics will guarantee success in distance running. She wants to find ways to maximize her performance—and avoid body fat or weight gain—by maintaining healthy eating habits. How can you help Tammy maximize her health and performance? In addition to competitive athletes like Tammy, recreational athletes and untrained people also initiate diet or exercise programs (or both) and are interested in assessing their current nutrition and fitness status to maximize the benefits of a program. How can you assess a person's present status and design an optimal training program? How can you determine if someone's current program is working? In order to maximize an athlete's performance, you must be able to assess the person's status for health, nutrition, and physical performance. In this chapter, we review assessment techniques for nutrition and fitness. We briefly describe each technique, including its advantages and disadvantages. Appendixes E.1 through E.4 provide samples of some of the assessment techniques reviewed, a table of energy cost values for activities, and a table of recommended values for selected laboratory (i.e., blood) tests used to assess health status.

MEDICAL AND HEALTH HISTORY QUESTIONNAIRES

The American College of Sports Medicine (ACSM 2008) has recommended that certain components be included in a medical history and physical examination. These assessments are administered before exercise testing or before the beginning of an exercise program. The guidelines assist the exercise or nutrition professional in determining a person's level of risk and the extent to which medical evaluation is necessary. An important component of a medical history is the physical examination. Any untrained or detrained person should have a thorough physical examination before starting an exercise program. The physical examination should be performed by a licensed health professional (physician, nurse practitioner, or physician assistant) and may include the following:

- A 12-lead electrocardiogram
- Laboratory (blood and urine) assessments
- Vital signs (heart rate, blood pressure, temperature, ventilation)
- Heart sounds

The medical professional selects the tests to be conducted based on the client's medical history, risk factors, and disease symptoms. While a young, **apparently healthy** person does not require a 12-lead electrocardiogram prior to starting an exercise program, a 45-year-old man with elevated blood pressure should have this test. How often should someone have a thorough physical examination? The answer to this question is not simple, as the frequency of medical assessments should depend on an individual's age and health status. Typically it is recommended that a healthy person <30 years old have a thorough physical examination every two to three years. People aged 30 to 50 years should have an exam every 1.5 to 2 years; those >50 years should have an annual examination, including a stress test with a 12-lead electrocardiogram. The frequency of the examination and the screening tests to be conducted depend on the person's current health status and the physician's discretion.

Health history questionnaires help determine the presence of any current or potential health problems. Questionnaires should include the following:

- Demographic information (name, age, height, weight)
- Present medication status (ask for full drug name, dose, and frequency of administration for both prescription and over-the counter medications) and drug allergies
- Family history of disease
- History of illnesses and injuries
- Surgical history
- History of menstrual function (for females)
- Past and present health behaviors and habits
- Exercise history
- Diet history (including body weight fluctuations and history of eating disorders)

When designing your own health history form or administering a previously published form, always allow extra space for affirmative responses to the questions posed. Review a person's health history, and discuss it with that individual before you initiate any assessment procedures. Figure 14.1 provides an example of a general health history questionnaire appropriate to use with both untrained and active people. Use the information on the medical examination and health history form to determine a client's level of risk. The ACSM (2008) recommends categorizing an individual into one of three levels of initial risk stratification:

- Low risk: Younger individuals (men <45 years of age; women <55 years of age) who are asymptomatic and have no more than one risk factor for coronary artery disease (CAD) (see table 14.1 for the CAD risk factors)
- Moderate risk: Older individuals (men ≥45 years of age; women ≥55 years of age) or those who meet the threshold for two or more risk factors for CAD
- High risk: Individuals with one or more signs or symptoms of CAD or known cardiac, pulmonary, or metabolic diseases

Once you determine a client's level of risk, you can use that information to decide the safest course of action for fitness testing. A more detailed discussion of fitness testing is provided later in this chapter.

Personal Health History Questionnaire
That Can Be Administered to Active or Sendentary Individuals

Please complete this as accurately and completely as possible.

Name: _____ Age: _____ Sex: _____

Mailing address: _____

Phone number: (work) _____ (home) _____

Today's date: _____

Ethnic background (circle)

African American

Asian American

Caucasian

Hispanic American

Other

1. General Medical History

Circle one

Do you currently have any medical complaints?   Yes   No

(Please specify) _____

_____

Are you on any prescribed or over-the-counter medication?   Yes   No

(Please specify) _____

_____

2. Dietary History

What is the length of time you have maintained your present weight?

_____

Please describe any long-term weight changes you have experienced (e.g., lost 50 lb in 1982):

_____

Please describe your diet history. Make sure to specify if you participated in bingeing, crash diets, cyclic dieting, or were anorexic and/or bulimic:

_____

3. Exercise History

Do you participate in any form of regular exercise?   Yes   No

    a. What form of exercise?

    b. How many times per week?

    c. How long each session?

    d. How intensely do you exercise?

    e. How long have you been regularly training?

(continued)

Figure 14.1 Personal health history questionnaire that can be administered to active or sedentary individuals.

(continued)

4. Cardiorespiratory History

Do you have heart disease now?	Yes	No
Have you ever had heart disease?	Yes	No
Do you have a family history of heart disease?	Yes	No
Do you have a heart murmur?	Yes	No
Do you have occasional chest pains?	Yes	No
Have you ever fainted?	Yes	No
Do you have high blood pressure?	Yes	No
Do you have asthma or allergies?	Yes	No
Do you have any pulmonary (lung) problems?	Yes	No

Explain any Yes response(s) _____

_____

5. Musculoskeletal History

Do you have any muscle injuries now?	Yes	No
Have you had any muscle injuries in the past year?	Yes	No
Do you have muscle pains when you exercise?	Yes	No
Do you have any bone or joint injuries now?	Yes	No
Have you had any bone or joint injuries in the past?	Yes	No
Have you ever had swollen joints?	Yes	No

Explain any Yes response(s) _____

_____

6. General History

Have you had or do you have:

Adrenal disease	Yes	No
Hypoglycemia (low blood sugar)	Yes	No
Seizures	Yes	No
Diabetes	Yes	No
Kidney or bladder problems	Yes	No
Stomach ulcers	Yes	No
Menstrual irregularities (women only)	Yes	No

Explain any Yes response(s) _____

_____

Figure 14.1 *(continued)*

Table 14.1 Coronary Artery Disease Risk Factors

Risk factor	Defining criteria
Family history	Myocardial infarction, coronary revascularization, or sudden death before 55 years of age in father or male first-degree relative, or before 65 years of age in mother or other female first-degree relative
Cigarette smoking	Current cigarette smoker or someone who quit within the previous six months
Hypertension	Systolic blood pressure ≥140 mmHg or diastolic ≥90 mmHg, confirmed by measurements on at least two separate occasions, or on antihypertensive medication
Dyslipidemia	LDL-cholesterol >130 mg/dL or HDL-cholesterol <40 mg/dL; total serum cholesterol >200 mg/dL
Impaired fasting glucose	Fasting blood glucose ≥100 mg/dL confirmed by measurements on at least two separate occasions
Obesity	Body mass index (BMI) >30 kg/m² or waist girth >102 cm (40.2 in.) for men and >88 cm (34.6 in.) for women or waist/hip ratio ≥0.95 for men and ≥0.86 for women
Sedentary lifestyle	Persons not participating in a regular exercise program or not meeting the minimal physical activity recommendations from the U.S. Surgeon General's Report on Physical Activity and Health
Negative risk factor	High serum HDL-cholesterol (>60 mg/dL) (protective)

HDL = high-density lipoprotein; LDL = low-density lipoprotein.

Adapted from American College of Sports Medicine, 2008, *ACSM's health-related physical fitness assessment manual,* 2nd ed. (Philadelphia, PA: Lippincott Williams & Wilkins), 16-73; National Cholesterol Education Program, 2002, "Expert Panel on Detection, Evaluation, and Treatment of High Blood Cholesterol in Adults (ATPIII) final report," *Circulation* 106: 3143-3421.

ASSESSING ENERGY AND NUTRIENT INTAKE

A multitude of techniques are available to assess energy and nutrient intakes. To choose the most appropriate tool(s), first determine the type of information you need to obtain. Do you need to determine only a person's total energy intake, or do you also need to assess all macro- and micronutrient intakes? Is it critical to know the quality of protein and type of carbohydrates and fats the person consumes and when these foods are consumed? Knowing the answers to these questions will help you select the best tool(s). Remember that the techniques discussed in this chapter do not estimate the nutritional *status* of an individual but only energy and nutrient *intake*. To determine nutritional status, you must combine information on nutrient intake with other (e.g., biochemical, anthropometric, body composition, energy expenditure) methods. Collecting energy and nutrient intake information involves either *retrospective* methods (e.g., 24 h diet recalls, food frequency questionnaires, diet histories) or *prospective* methods (e.g., diet records, weighed food records, or direct observation of food intake). A combination of methods may provide the best

picture of a person's typical diet. For example, you may want to use a diet history or food frequency questionnaire to give you an idea of an individual's dietary habits, plus a diet record of current dietary practices.

Diet History

The diet history is often used with one of the diet assessment methods outlined in table 14.2. This table also lists advantages and limitations of the most commonly used assessment methods. The **diet history** is usually gathered through a questionnaire or an interview process. "Important Components of an In-Depth Diet, Training, Health, and Performance History" (p. 429) includes a suggested outline for an interview format, integrating diet, eating patterns, physical activity and training, and health and performance indices. The process is intended to help identify a client's nutrition problems or unique situations. It is especially important that you learn about the type, duration, and intensity of the activity in which the person is engaged. You may even want to have the individual keep 24 h activity records (see appendix E.2 for a sample form). This information will help you assess any energy or nutrition problems that may be associated with this person's activity level.

Table 14.2 Common Diet Assessment Methods and Their Advantages and Disadvantages

Type of method	Major advantages	Major disadvantages
24 h recall	• Respondent burden is low • Cost is low • Administration is easy	• Does not provide a good picture of an individual's dietary patterns • Relies on memory • May require a trained interviewer
Food frequency questionnaires	• Respondent burden is low • Cost is low • Administration is easy • Past dietary habits can be examined	• Are difficult to analyze • Rely on memory • Require validation of questionnaire
Food records, weighed food records, tape-recorded food records, photographed or videotaped food records, telephone food records	• A record of all foods consumed over the designated period is provided • Provides a better picture of current dietary habits and nutrient intakes than the other methods provide	• Entail high respondent burden • Require that individuals estimate measurements of food consumed • Are subject to change because individuals change what they normally eat during the recording period • May be costly to analyze • Require a trained interviewer or data recorder • May require provision of scales, camera, or tape recorder

Twenty-Four-Hour Dietary Recall

The **24-hour recall** is a quick and easy way to assess recent food intake. It requires that a person recall *in detail* all of the foods and beverages consumed during the previous 24 h period. The individual needs to know the serving sizes, preparation methods, and brand names of convenience foods or fast foods consumed. This method has serious limitations in that it does not give a picture of a person's "typical intake" unless repeated measures are done on different days of the week. This method is acceptable only when repeated 24 h recalls are done over a period of time. While Basiotis and colleagues (1987) found that energy intake could be reasonably assessed in *groups* of men and women over three days, an accurate assessment of the energy intake of *individuals* requires 27 to 35 days of data. An even longer period is required to accurately assess intake of nutrients, and many nutrients require records to be kept over 100 days—which is obviously prohibitive for both the client and the practitioner. Moreover, because this approach relies heavily on memory, it is not acceptable for young children or anyone with memory problems. Another source of error is that, during the assessment period, subjects may minimize poor food choices while emphasizing good food choices. The 24 h recall method is best

used with large populations or as a quick check to determine whether an individual is following suggested dietary recommendations.

Food Frequency Questionnaires

Food frequency questionnaires allow you to assess the typical dietary pattern in an athlete's life over a predefined period of time. The questionnaires contain lists of foods with questions regarding the number of times the foods are eaten during the specified period of time. The primary use of food frequency questionnaires is to rank individuals according to energy and nutrient intake (e.g., high vs. low intakes). Since food frequency questionnaires rely on self-assessments, they are not generally used to provide an accurate estimate of nutrient intakes. Both qualitative and semiquantitative questionnaires are available. **Qualitative** information includes only a list of typical foods that are eaten—information that provides a general indication of an athlete's dietary pattern or that helps you compare the consumption of certain types of food before and after a dietary intervention. **Semiquantitative** questionnaires are useful in determining the typical foods eaten and the quantity consumed. You can address concerns about specific nutrients (e.g., fats, carbohydrates) by using these types of questionnaires. It is important to use a questionnaire that has been demonstrated to be reliable for the given population. As there are no validated

Important Components of an In-Depth Diet, Training, Health, and Performance History

- Assessment of energy intake, energy expenditure, energy balance and availability, and changes along the annual training and competition plan
- Assessment of macronutrient and micronutrient intake and changes along the annual training and competition plan; quantity, quality, and timing of pretraining meal; intake during exercise; postexercise recovery foods and fluids; precompetition meal; traveling diet; history of inadequate intake before, during, and after training or competition
- Assessment of fluid balance and hydration: fluid intake before, during, and after exercise; daily fluid balance; urine color; thirst; estimation of sweating rate; extent of sodium loss (i.e., salty sweating); history of severe dehydration, heat illness, or hyponatremia
- Assessment of medications and herbal, sport, and dietary supplements and ergogenic aids: history and current use; performance and health effects; placebo effect; beliefs and knowledge regarding supplements
- Assessment of changes in appetite or intake: environmental conditions, training intensity and volume, competition preparation (carbohydrate loading), weight control, fatigue, illness or injury, eating disorder
- Psychological and eating disorder data: diet history and current dieting, history and current use of pathogenic weight control methods, history and current status of eating disorder and disordered eating, female athlete triad
- Assessment of eating patterns: frequency of eating and drinking at meals and before and after training; ethnic foods; eating rules; food purchasing; accessibility; preparation; planning; work, school, training schedule; characteristics of sport and cultural determinants of sport related to eating
- Assessment of physical activity and exercise training data: daily, weekly, and annual training and competition plan, coach and support staff, periodization and integration of diet into annual training and competition
- Assessment of anthropometric data: height and weight history, current weight, ideal body weight (athlete, coach, dietitian); body composition measures, % body fat, lean body mass, body composition goals (athlete, coach, dietitian); history of meeting weight and body composition goals; seasonal changes along training and competition plan and with changes in intake
- Assessment of diagnostic data: biochemical indices, resting metabolic rate, bone mineral density, intolerance and allergies, clinical problems (e.g., diabetes, dyslipidemia), history and current status of menstruation
- Assessment of fitness and performance data: aerobic and anaerobic tests, muscle strength and muscular endurance tests, sport-specific field tests, current performance level

questionnaires designed specifically for athletes or highly active people, the accuracy of existing questionnaires for these groups may be limited.

Diet Records

The diet record is probably the most frequently used method for assessing the energy and nutrient intakes of individuals. A food or **diet record** is a list of all foods and beverages consumed over a specified time, typically three to seven days. To more accurately predict energy and nutrient intakes, it is best if foods consumed are first weighed or measured, labels of convenience foods are saved, and labels of all supplements are copied. This method also allows the gathering of more in-depth information such as the times, places, feelings, and behaviors associated with eating. The dietitian or health care professional working with the person should review the diet record to ensure its accuracy. A primary drawback of this method is the tendency for individuals to change their "typical" eating habits on the days when they record food intake. Because this approach is also more time-consuming than 24 h recalls, its accuracy depends on the individual's cooperation and skill in properly recording foods.

How many days' consumption should be followed? Diet records of 3 to 14 days generally provide good estimates of energy and nutrient intake (Schlundt 1988). Within this range, reliability (precision) and validity (accuracy) appear to increase with each additional day up to seven days. Thus, a seven-day diet record during a period of typical food intake should give accurate data for energy, macronutrients, and most micronutrients. For most nutrients, there appears to be little advantage to recording diet records for more than two or three weeks. One advantage to the seven-day diet record is that it encompasses all the days of the week, including the dietary changes that frequently occur on weekends. The main disadvantage is that as the number of days increases, so does the respondent's burden. Note that for information on energy intake alone, at least three days of records are required to get an accurate

estimate for a *group* of people; *individuals* may need to record their intake over many more days. Discuss frankly with your client the limitations of recording dietary intake over an entire week.

Provide specific instructions to people before they use the 24 h recall or diet record method. The days chosen to be recorded should represent the clients' typical dietary and activity patterns. People may have to be trained to measure food portions or may need to practice using a diet scale. Guidelines for achieving accurate diet records are listed in "Instructions for Doing an In-Depth Diet Record." Clients should follow certain criteria when reporting dietary assessment data, as outlined in the two checklists on p. 431. A good rule of thumb: See that the methods are described to clients in sufficient detail that another researcher could duplicate the study design (Wheeler and Buzzard 1994).

Instructions for Doing an In-Depth Diet Record

Specific guidelines for keeping diet records should be included in the instruction sheet given to the client, and these instructions should also be reviewed verbally. The following are guidelines for clients who are recording foods in a food record.

1. Record items immediately after they are consumed. Use common measures, such as cups and tablespoons, to describe the amount consumed; and whenever possible, measure or weigh the food items being consumed.
2. Record all beverages and all items added to them, such as sugar and cream added to coffee. Include all sport beverages (Gatorade, Powerade, etc.), energy drinks (Red Bull, etc.), and the beverages (e.g., water, soda) taken with medications.
3. Include condiments, such as butter, margarine, mustard, mayonnaise, and salad dressing, even if they are low-fat or fat-free.
4. Completely describe the foods consumed (e.g., "whole wheat bread," "white turkey meat without skin," and "meatless spaghetti sauce").
5. Indicate how the food was prepared (e.g., "fried chicken," "broiled beef steak," "steamed broccoli").
6. Record all foods and beverages consumed as snacks, including brand names if possible.
7. Keep the food record diary sheet(s) accessible at all times so that items can be recorded immediately.
8. Write down any nutritional supplements (e.g., vitamins, minerals, food supplements) as well as any sport products (PowerBar, Gatorade, Clif Bar, etc.) consumed during training or a race. Keep the labels of these products and return them with the completed diary.
9. When using convenience foods, save the food labels and return them with the completed food diary.
10. Whenever possible, note the brand names of food items (e.g., canned foods, convenience foods, deli items).
11. If food is consumed at a restaurant or fast-food establishment, record the name of the restaurant and the product purchased. The more specific you can be, the better (e.g., "a McDonald's Big Mac with regular fries and regular Diet Coke").
12. Record all medications used, both over-the-counter and prescription.

Checklist for Reporting Dietary Intake Methodology: Guidelines for Specific Assessment Methods

Food Records and 24 h Recalls

- Designate the number of days recorded, which days, and whether days were consecutive.
- Describe any weighting algorithms used to account for day-of-the-week differences.

Food Frequency Methods (List-Based Diet Histories)

- Explain the purpose of the questionnaire (e.g., to rank individuals according to their intake of individual foods, food groups, or nutrients) and identify the nutrients of interest.
- Identify the population group (e.g., ethnicity and age range) used to develop and validate the questionnaire.
- Explain how the food list was developed.
- Indicate the number of foods and food groups in the food list.
- Indicate the level to which food consumption was quantified. If relevant, comment on respondent's ability to designate small, medium, or large servings.
- Describe the options available for specifying frequency of consumption.
- Indicate the average length of time required to complete the questionnaire.
- Describe any calibration studies designed to facilitate interpretation of the food frequency data.

Diet History Methods (Meal-Based Diet Histories)

- Indicate whether questions were open-ended or structured.
- Indicate the number of "typical" days accounted for as well as the extent of probing for variations in the usual eating pattern.
- Describe methods used to cross-check the history, such as a 24 h recall or food frequency checklist.

Food frequency questionnaires can be unquantified, semiquantified, or completely quantified. An unquantified method does not specify serving sizes; instead, the respondent indicates how many times the food is consumed per period of time (day, week, month). For example, a respondent may be asked "How often do you consume milk?" A semiquantified method provides typical serving sizes as the reference amount for determining frequency of consumption—for example, "How often do you consume an 8 oz glass of milk?" A completely quantified method allows the respondent to indicate any amount of food typically consumed as well as how often the food is consumed. Amounts are obtained through open-ended questions, usually prompted by an interviewer—for example, "When do you drink milk, and how much do you usually consume?"

From *Journal of the American Dietetic Association,* Vol 4, M.L. Wheeler and I.M. Buzzard, "How to report dietary assessment data," pgs. 1255-1256, Copyright 1994, with permission from Elsevier.

Checklist for Reporting Dietary Intake Methodology: Guidelines for All Assessment Methods

1. Describe the time frame of interest. Examples:
   - Usual intake over the last year, including seasonal variations
   - Defined period preceding disease incidence
   - Current intake (e.g., during the last week or month)

(continued)

Checklist for Reporting Dietary Intake Methodology   *(continued)*

2. Provide rationale for selecting the method used to collect dietary data.

   - If an existing method was used, cite published articles that describe the method and document its validity and reliability.

   - If an existing method was modified, describe key points of the original method and all modifications. Cite references to the original method, including validation and reliability studies.

   - If a new record was developed, describe the procedures used to develop and evaluate the new tool.

3. Describe the results of pretests of the selected assessment method conducted with either the target subjects or a similar population.

4. Describe procedures used to quantify portion sizes of foods eaten. Detail the use of the following:

   - Food scales
   - Household measuring cups or spoons
   - Rulers
   - Food pictures
   - Food models
   - Geometric shapes

5. Describe procedures used to analyze dietary data. If nutrients were calculated, this entails the following:

   - Identify the food consumption database used, by name, version number, and release date, and provide the name and location (city and state) of the database developer.

   - Evaluate the completeness of the database for the nutrients of interest.

   - Describe any modifications to the database.

   - Describe procedures for coding the data.

   - Describe quality control procedures for ensuring accurate calculations.

6. Indicate whether the assessment tool was administered by an interviewer or self-administered by respondents.

When Interviewer-Administered Methods Are Used

- Describe the minimum qualification of interviewers (e.g., registered dietitian, graduate degree in health science field).

- Describe training and certification procedures for interviewers.

- Indicate whether interviews were conducted in person or by telephone.

- Report the approximate length of the interview.

- Describe the level of detail solicited about food descriptions (e.g., type or brand of food; processing method, such as canned or dried; eating practices, such as trimming of meat or use of table salt; specification of recipe ingredients and other food preparation methods).

- Indicate whether the method used to query respondents for details about food intake was automated (interactive computer software that prompts for descriptive detail) or manual; describe any aids used for manual probing, such as checklist of details required for each food category.

When Self-Administered Methods Are Used

- Describe instructions or training provided to subjects on keeping good records or completing dietary questionnaires.

- Describe materials provided to help subjects describe foods (e.g., checklist of details required for each food category) or estimate portion sizes (e.g., food scales, household measures, or food models).

- Describe procedures used to collect additional information after the food records or questionnaires are completed.

From *Journal of the American Dietetic Association*, Vol 4, M.L. Wheeler and I.M. Buzzard, "How to report dietary assessment data," pgs. 1255-1256, Copyright 1994, with permission from Elsevier.

ASSESSING DAILY ENERGY EXPENDITURE

A plethora of methods are available to assess energy expenditure. These methods vary in their degree of accuracy, cost, and convenience. Unfortunately, the most accurate methods also tend to be the most costly and may also be the most time- and labor-intensive. As with the selection of any assessment tool, you must decide on the type of information you need in order to choose the most appropriate method. This section reviews several of the tools used to assess energy expenditure.

Behavioral Observation Records

Behavioral observation involves the recording of an individual's activity patterns by an observer. Recording forms have been developed so that a trained observer can use them to document various behaviors, types and levels of activities, and the time spent performing each activity (Baranowski et al. 1984; Hovell et al. 1978; Torún 1984; Wallace et al. 1985). Figure 14.2 includes an example of a recording form for a child's activities. Once the recording forms are completed, energy expenditure can be calculated using estimated energy cost values (Ainsworth et al. 1993, 2000). Table 14.3 lists the advantages and limitations of behavioral observation records and other assessments of energy expenditure (Vanhees et al. 2005; Ainslie et al. 2003). Although they are time-consuming and cumbersome, behavioral observation records are useful for studying activity levels of children and adults at work sites. In addition, there may be sports that are physiologically poorly understood and have not yet been measured. Thus, an initial assessment by the nutritionist might include a careful observation of the athlete engaging in a typical training session. Similar to what occurs with a behavioral observation record, the nutritionist monitors the types of activities, their intensities, and the time spent in the activity. For example, a snowboarder might be observed during a practice session in the half-pipe. The nutritionist would monitor the number of seconds or minutes required to complete a run (using a stopwatch), including the hiking or riding back up to the start. A heart rate monitor may provide data regarding the intensity. However, there are factors that could influence heart rate other than the physiological strain. These include environmental conditions, dehydration, and mental stress, which could be substantial in a high-risk sport such as snowboarding.

Motion Assessment Devices

The most commonly used **motion assessment devices** (instruments used to detect movement) are the pedometer and accelerometer. **Pedometers** are the most economical option and are typically worn on the ankle or clipped to a belt at the waist. Most new pedometers have a horizontal, spring-suspended lever that moves with the vertical acceleration or the up-and-down motion of the hips (Tudor-Locke et al. 2002) and are used to count the number of steps people take or to calculate the distance they have walked or run. Previous research has shown that while different brands of pedometers provide acceptable estimations of steps taken and distance walked, they can vary significantly across walking speeds (Bassett et al. 1996).

Accelerometers detect accelerations and decelerations of the body. The accelerations of the body during movement are theoretically in proportion to the forces generated by the muscles and are related to energy expenditure (Corder et al. 2007; Ainslie et al. 2003). **Single-plane** (or **uniaxial**) **accelerometers** detect acceleration exclusively in the vertical plane. The Caltrac is an example of a single-plane accelerometer. This device is worn on a belt that is attached firmly around the waist. Data output is in either kilocalories or movement counts. While the reliability of the Caltrac is good under controlled laboratory conditions, results are poorly reproduced in the field. The validity of the Caltrac is limited: Its estimation of energy expenditure during horizontal walking, running, and cycling is acceptable in many situations; but it does not accurately represent the energy cost of activities such as uphill or downhill running. **Triaxial accelerometers** detect acceleration in three dimensions. The reliability of these devices is good, and their output correlates highly with energy expenditure for activities such as level walking, running, and stepping. However, they may underestimate energy expenditure (Matthews and Freedson 1995) during activities such as walking uphill, weightlifting, and stationary cycling (Montoye et al. 1983). Chen and Sun (1997) developed two simple mathematical models that can significantly improve the estimation of energy expenditure over a wide range of activities using triaxial accelerometers.

Activity Comparison

Name *Jan Doe*   Day *Thurs*   7

Activity		Time	
Counselor	Camper	Counselor	Camper
Sleep		8.25 hrs.	9.0 hrs.
Easy			
Moderate			
warm-ups	warm-ups	15 min	15 min
weight training		30	
new games		15	
	basketball		30
Hard			
aerobics		45	
swimming	swimming	45	45
	tennis	45	45
run		15	
	basketball		45
	dance		60
Very hard			
dance		60	
	aerobics		45
	games		45

Figure 14.2 A form for recording physical activities of a child.

Reprinted with permission from *Research Quarterly for Exercise and Sport*, Vol. 56,161-165, Copyright 1985 by the American Alliance for Health, Physical Education, Recreation and Dance, 1900 Association Drive, Reston, VA 20191.

Table 14.3 lists the advantages and disadvantages of motion assessment devices. For a more detailed description of their reliability, validity, and mechanism of action, refer to the studies by Corder and colleagues (2007) and Vanhees and colleagues (2005). While pedometers and the Caltrac may be limited in their ability to accurately assess energy expenditure, they can be useful for indicating gross changes in activity level over time. Triaxial accelerometers show promise of accurate assessments of energy expenditure through ongoing modifications of the devices and through the use of mathematical models employed in calculations.

Published Activity Questionnaires

Several **activity questionnaires** have been designed to assess physical activity and energy expenditure. The simpler ones include single-item questions, while more complex questionnaires involve in-depth surveys done by an interviewer. Different questionnaires are designed to address activity over various time frames (e.g., single day, one month to one year, and as long as a lifetime). Kriska and Caspersen (1997) published an extremely useful review of activity questionnaires. This review includes the original reference, the

Table 14.3   Common Energy Expenditure (EE) Assessment Methods and Their Advantages and Disadvantages

Physical activity assessment method	Advantages	Disadvantages
Criterion methods		
Doubly labeled water	• Is an accurate and valid measurement of EE • Is applicable to children and adults • Induces no change in PA behavior in daily free-living conditions	• Is expensive • Requires expertise for analysis • Gives no indication of specific activities, only total daily EE • Is not appropriate for large-scale studies • Requires at least three days of recordings
Indirect calorimetry	• Is an accurate and valid measurement of short-term EE	• Is expensive • Is limited to laboratory setting • Measures PA indirectly
Direct observation	• Is best for recording type of PA and interpretation of the activities • Provides contextual information • Is applicable to children	• Is time-consuming • Is subject to reactivity of study participant • Is limited in monitoring time • Involves observer subjectivity
Objective methods		
Pedometer	• Is lightweight, portable (worn around waist) • Is simple and inexpensive • Is for free-living conditions	• Measures only walking or running steps; no recording of horizontal or upper body movements • Has limited validity for EE estimation • Gives no information on specific activity, only total daily PA
Accelerometer	• See Pedometer • Records accelerations in more than one plane and for extended periods • Indicates intensity of the movement; can measure a specific activity	• Has limited validity for EE estimation • Does not record horizontal or upper body movements, carrying a load
Heart rate monitor	• Is lightweight and portable • Is directly related to physiological response to PA • Enables detailed data recording over extended period; can measure a specific activity	• Measures EE, not PA • Is not suited to very low-intensity PA as heart rate is affected by nonactivity-related environmental factors; requires individual calibration of heart rate–PA relationship
Subjective methods		
Questionnaire	• Is applicable to epidemiological studies • Is valid for gross classification of PA level for a population (e.g., low, moderate, highly active)	• Has limited validity; provides no detailed information on PA; depends on subject's memory, interpretation • Is not suited for PA assessment at the individual level

* PA = physical activity; EE = energy expenditure.

Adapted, by permission, from L. Vanhees et al., 2005, "How to assess physical activity? How to assess physical fitness?" *European Journal of Cardiovascular Prevention and Rehabilitation* 12: 102-114.

actual questionnaire, reliability and validity data available for each questionnaire, instructions on administering the questionnaire, and sample calculations.

How do you know which questionnaire to use? First decide what information you want to obtain, and then find a questionnaire that can access this information using an assessment tool that applies as specifically as possible to the group or individual you are assessing. Questionnaires are available to assess energy expenditure in males, females, adolescents, adults, older adults, and various ethnic groups. For instance, you may have an older female client who wants to build lean mass and maintain bone. Since it is critical that she concentrate more on weight-bearing activities than on energy expenditure, you would look for a questionnaire that could assess these types of activities. As another example, if you work with many female clients, finding a questionnaire that documents household and childcare activities may significantly improve estimation of their energy expenditure.

To accurately represent energy expenditure, a questionnaire must provide the following information (Kriska and Caspersen 1997):

- Type of activity, including leisure, occupational, sport, and household activities
- Frequency, or the average number of sessions per time frame of interest
- Intensity of activities being performed
- Duration, or the average number of minutes per session during the time frame of interest

Table 14.3 lists the advantages and disadvantages of using questionnaires. Questionnaires are useful tools to determine energy expenditure and are helpful in classifying an individual's physical activity patterns. While the questionnaires available can be reliable and valid, the representation of energy expenditure obtained is always subject to some degree of error due to the use of standardized energy cost values. There are no published questionnaires designed specifically for athletes or highly active people, but several assess both occupational and leisure activities and provide information on high-intensity and sport-related activities.

Activity Records

Activity records can be used to estimate total daily energy expenditure or to estimate the energy

expended during specified activities (see appendix E.2 for sample activity record form). Chapter 5 discussed the application of the factorial method using activity records to estimate energy expenditure. Table 14.3 lists the advantages and disadvantages of using activity records. The energy expenditure values tabulated by Ainsworth and colleagues (1993, 2000) can be used to estimate energy expenditure for selected activities or for all activities performed over a 24 h period based on metabolic equivalents (METs) (see "What is a Metabolic Equivalent?"). Note that the accuracy of these methods is influenced by people's ability to record their activities correctly and by the degree to which the energy values used represent the actual energy expended (see "Energy Expenditure Values: Where Do They Come From?").

Doubly Labeled Water

We discussed the doubly labeled water technique in chapter 5. Table 14.3 reviews the advantages and disadvantages of this technique to allow for comparison with the other methods used to assess physical activity and energy expenditure.

FITNESS ASSESSMENT

How do we define fitness? While many people view being "fit" as having good cardiovascular endurance, this is only one of many components of physical fitness. We also know that as an individual increases fitness level, a number of metabolic parameters can improve (e.g., blood glucose, lipids, and blood pressure); however, there is no clear conceptual definition of fitness based on metabolic parameters alone. Currently, no one protocol exists that allows us to define fitness; thus, a number of fitness components are typically measured. The components of fitness we discuss in this section include

- flexibility,
- muscle strength (isometric, dynamic, and isokinetic),
- muscular endurance,
- cardiorespiratory fitness (also referred to as aerobic fitness),
- anaerobic fitness (also referred to as power), and
- body composition.

The extent to which people can maximize each component of fitness depends on the sport or

Highlight

Energy Expenditure Values: Where do They Come From?

A multitude of energy cost values are published in the research literature. How do you decide which values are most accurate and appropriate to use? Many researchers and practitioners use either their own laboratory values or values from a variety of sources in the literature. Until recently there was no standardized, comprehensive list of energy cost values. Ainsworth and colleagues (1993) published a Compendium of Physical Activities to assist researchers and practitioners with coding and estimating the energy cost of a wide variety of activities. More values from a variety of activities were added in 2000 (Ainsworth et al. 2000). Appendix E.3 illustrates the use of this compendium. Ainsworth and colleagues (1993) reported energy cost values in **metabolic equivalents (METs)** (see "What Is a Metabolic Equivalent?"); however, the data in appendix E.3 are expressed in kilocalories per kilogram of body weight per minute (kcal/kg BW per minute), and we also provide values for a given body weight to assist you with the calculations. While most of these energy cost values were derived using indirect calorimetry to measure oxygen consumption, some of the data were derived using imputed values. Note also that these data were derived from predominantly young adult subjects, which limits their usefulness for children or elderly people (Montoye et al. 1996). While the data are extremely useful to the researcher and practitioner, it is important to understand that these energy cost values will always introduce some degree of error into an estimation of energy expenditure.

Highlight

What Is a Metabolic Equivalent?

The abbreviation MET represents a metabolic equivalent, a unit of measurement that represents work rate, or oxygen uptake ($\dot{V}O_2$). One MET is equal to a $\dot{V}O_2$ of 3.5 mL $\cdot$ kg^{-1} $\cdot$ min^{-1}, which can be converted to kcal $\cdot$ kg^{-1} $\cdot$ hr^{-1}. The MET unit is generally used to refer to an individual's functional capacity. For instance, an individual with a maximal oxygen uptake ($\dot{V}O_2$max) of 60 mL $\cdot$ kg^{-1} $\cdot$ min^{-1} would have a functional capacity of 17 METs (60 / 3.5 = 17.1). The MET unit is also used to prescribe exercise intensity for training. If an individual with a $\dot{V}O_2$max of 17 METs wished to train at 70% of his or her $\dot{V}O_2$max, the training intensity would be 12 METs. One can design specific training intensities by referring to *ACSM's Guidelines for Exercise Testing and Prescription* (2006) and the work of Swain and Leutholtz (1997) and Gibala (2007).

activity in which they are engaged. A variety of tests are available to assess the level of fitness for each of the components listed, and there are standards available for comparison of an individual's performance with that of the general population. It is important to stress that these standards were developed on groups of individuals with heterogeneous fitness levels, which may limit the application of these standards to clients who deviate significantly from that population. While these tests are extremely useful for assessing the fitness level of the general population, their applicability to certain groups (e.g., athletes or individuals with limited mobility) needs to be determined on an individual basis. Excellent resources are available that describe the tests used in fitness assessment, give the normative performance values for each test, and list exercise prescription suggestions for each component of fitness (ACSM 2008; Heyward 2006; Howley and Franks 2003). The purpose of the following section is simply to familiarize you with the components of fitness and provide guidance for accessing information about the tests used in fitness assessment.

Case Study:
Female Distance Runner Complaining of Fatigue

The case of Tammy was introduced in the beginning of this chapter. Tammy has been complaining of fatigue and lackluster performance, and wants to maintain a low body weight and body fat percentage while concentrating on healthy eating habits. This case study is provided to illustrate how nutritional and energy expenditure assessment tools can be used with athletes and other clients. Tammy is a distance runner, competing in both cross-country and track. Her descriptive characteristics are as follows:

Age	19 years
Weight	107 lb (48.5 kg)
Height	59 in. (150 cm)
Body fat percentage (derived using hydrostatic weighing)	15.2%
Resting metabolic rate (measured using indirect calorimetry)	1200 kcal/day
Resting heart rate	42 bpm
Resting blood pressure	108/60 mmHg

Tammy has had problems with anemia in the past. Fasting blood samples were taken to assess her present iron status, and general chemistry screening and lipid panels were also completed at her request. The following table shows the results of those tests.

	Tammy's values	Normal values*
Hemoglobin	12.5 g/dL	12.0-16.0 g/dL
Hematocrit	38%	36-48%
Transferrin	300 mg/dL	250-425 mg/dL
Transferrin (% saturation)	38%	15-50%
Total iron-binding capacity	400 µg/dL	240-450 µg/dL
Ferritin	42 ng/mL	10-120 ng/mL
Glucose	75 mg/dL	62-110 mg/dL
Total cholesterol	146 mg/dL	<200 mg/dL
LDL-cholesterol	92 mg/dL	<100 mg/dL
HDL-cholesterol	55 mg/dL	<40 mg/dL
Triglycerides	75 mg/dL	<200 mg/dL

HDL = high-density lipoprotein; LDL = low-density lipoprotein.

Adapted, by permission, from F. Fischbach, 2004, *A manual of laboratory and diagnostic tests,* 7th ed. (Philadelphia, PA: Lippincott, Williams, and Wilkins); National Cholesterol Education Program, 2002, "Expert Panel on Detection, Evaluation, and Treatment of High Blood Cholesterol in Adults (ATPIII) final report," *Circulation* 106: 3143-3421.

Appendix E.4 provides a detailed list of typical clinical laboratory values. These results do not indicate any abnormal values for Tammy. Although Tammy complains of fatigue, neither anemia nor iron deficiency appears to be the culprit. Tammy completed weighed food records and activity diaries over a three-day period (representing two weekdays and one weekend day). Tammy's diet was analyzed using the Food Processor Plus nutrient analysis software (ESHA Research, Salem, OR); her total daily energy expenditure was estimated using the energy cost values reported by Ainsworth and colleagues (1993, 2000). Analysis of her activity records shows that Tammy requires approximately 2300 kcal/day to maintain her current weight. Her diet records show that her average energy intake for the three-day recording period was 2195 kcal/day.

Tammy's total energy intake appears slightly inadequate, providing 105 kcal/day less than necessary to cover her energy expenditure. This discrepancy is within the margin of error of the diet and activity assessment methods (see chapter 5), however; and since she is maintaining her body weight, it is assumed that her energy intake is adequate to meet energy demands. If this discrepancy were maintained over a prolonged period, it is possible that her body weight would drop and her performance would suffer due to inadequate energy intake. Tammy's average intakes of carbohydrate, protein, and fat are 58%, 16%, and 26% of total energy intake (kcal/day), respectively. While these percentages are within recommended intake range for a competitive athlete, she consumes an average of only 282 g (5.8 g/kg per day) of carbohydrate. This is less than the recommended carbohydrate intake (grams per kilogram BW per day) for a competitive endurance athlete during periods of high training and is probably a major contributor to her sluggish performance. An interview with Tammy also revealed that on race days she is nervous, is often nauseated, and does not eat well. She skips breakfast and consumes only 800 to 1000 kcal during a typical race day. After addressing these issues, Tammy was able to improve her performance and reduce fatigue by eating more complex carbohydrates on a regular basis and by consuming a sport drink on race days.

Flexibility Tests

Flexibility is defined as "the functional capacity of the joints to move through a full **range of motion (ROM)**" (ACSM 2008, p. 70). Achieving and maintaining appropriate flexibility are critical for optimal athletic performance, daily living activities, and prevention of injury. Flexibility is affected by many factors, including

- age;
- fitness level;
- excessive fatty or muscular tissue; and
- tightness of the joint capsule, muscles, tendons, and ligaments.

Flexibility tends to decrease with age due to structural and functional changes in the tissues surrounding the joint capsule. Excess body fat or very large muscles can also hinder flexibility. Inactivity leads to a shortening and tightening of connective and muscle tissues. While flexibility is an extremely important component of fitness, it is often neglected or ignored by people involved in fitness programs. People often feel rushed due to time constraints, leading them to minimize the time spent performing flexibility or stretching exercises. Many people, furthermore, are not properly trained to perform such exercises, which can lead to ineffective stretching and potential injury.

The ACSM (2008), Heyward (2006), and Liemohn (2003b) describe tests to assess flexibility about the major joints in the body. Liemohn (2003a) also reviews exercise prescription for flexibility, particularly of the lower back and hip—areas that are often associated with low back pain. Flexibility is typically expressed and measured relative to a particular joint. The flexibility of a specific joint depends on many variables including the muscles, tendons, ligaments, fascia, adipose tissue, and joint capsules; therefore, no measure exists for assessing whole-body flexibility. There is no single test that can assess one's flexibility.

The **sit-and-reach test** is one of the most common and widely accepted methods for measuring flexibility, as it represents the ROM of the hamstring, hip, and lower back (ACSM 2008). Exact procedures for the sit-and-reach test are described by the ACSM (2008), the Canadian Society for Exercise Physiology (2003), and the YMCA (2000). It is always important that the individual participate in a short warm-up and light stretching before performing the test in order to minimize the risk of injury. Normative values for the sit-and-reach test are shown in table 14.4.

In a clinical setting, ROM is typically calculated in degrees. The devices used include the Leighton flexometer, the goniometer, and the inclinometer. These enable a more precise measurement of individual joints; however, they require a highly trained tester. Protocols and standard norms

Table 14.4 Fitness Categories by Age Groups for Trunk Forward Flexion Using a Sit-and-Reach Box (cm)

Category	Age (years)									
	20-29		30-39		40-49		50-59		60-69	
Gender	M	F	M	F	M	F	M	F	M	F
Excellent	40	41	38	41	35	38	35	39	33	35
Very good	39	40	37	40	34	37	34	38	32	34
	34	37	33	36	29	34	28	33	25	31
Good	33	36	32	35	28	33	27	32	24	30
	30	33	28	32	24	30	24	30	20	27
Fair	29	32	27	31	23	29	23	29	19	26
	25	28	23	27	18	25	16	25	15	23
Needs Improvement	24	27	22	26	17	24	15	24	14	22

Note: These norms are based on a sit-and-reach box in which the "zero" point is 26 cm.

Source: Canadian Physical Activity, Fitness & Lifestyle Approach: CSEP-Health & Fitness Program's Health-Related Appraisal & Counselling Strategy, Third Edition, © 2003. Reprinted with permission from the Canadian Society for Exercise Physiology.

for each device have been summarized by Maud (1995, pp. 225-242). It is important to stress that the proper applications of these tests are critical to ensure the safety of the client. For instance, stretching exercises in which body position or limb movement causes excessive blood flow to the head and upper chest may be contraindicated in clients with hypertension.

Tests of Muscle Strength

Muscle strength is defined as the maximum amount of force exerted by a group of muscles. Muscle strength can be further delineated into three categories:

- **Isometric (static) strength:** Generation of force with no movement about a joint.
- **Isotonic (dynamic) strength:** Generation of force with movement about a joint. Isotonic contractions are further characterized as *concentric* (shortening of the muscle as it exerts tension) or *eccentric* (lengthening of the muscle as it exerts tension).
- **Isokinetic strength:** Generation of force at a constant speed throughout the entire ROM (also a component of dynamic strength).

Muscular strength is dependent on the muscle groups involved, the category of contraction (see the three categories in the preceding list), and the joint angle being tested. Therefore, there is no single test that can assess one's total body strength. However, it is still important to measure muscle force production to "assess muscular fitness, identify weaknesses, monitor progress in rehabilitation, and measure effectiveness of training" (ACSM 2008, p. 64).

Dynamometers are devices used to easily measure static strength. The common muscle groups tested include those involved in hand gripping and the leg and back muscles. The force generated from these tests is expressed as a maximal voluntary contraction (MVC) but is limited to the muscle and joint angle involved. These test protocols and normative values for static strength are described in detail by Heyward (2006) and Bond (2003).

Dynamic strength is measured using equipment that provides constant or variable resistance. Weight equipment (both machines and free weights) provides constant resistance. The **1RM test** (1-repetition maximum test) assesses the maximum weight a person can lift for one repetition of a particular movement. The maximum weight lifted is recorded and divided by the individual's body weight in pounds. Standard values are available for 1RM tests using the bench press (for upper body strength) and the leg press (for lower body strength) and are listed by ACSM (2008, pp. 65-67), Heyward (2006), and Bond (2003). Although the 1RM test has traditionally been used as the standard, multiple RM such as 4-, 8-, or 10RM may also be used as a safer alternative, especially in untrained populations. Variable resistance machines include isokinetic dynamometers manufactured by Cybex (including the Cybex II and Orthotron machines) (figure 14.3) and Hydra-Fitness (the Omnitron Total Power machine). Heyward (2006) has reviewed the average strength values for tests using the Omnitron machine.

Tests of Muscle Endurance

Muscular endurance is defined as the ability of a group of muscles to exert force repeatedly over a period of time. Simple field tests used to assess muscular endurance involve measuring the maximal number of curl-ups (crunches), push-ups, chin-ups, and bar dips one can perform without rest. The ACSM (2005, 2006) and Howley and Franks (2003) have published detailed descrip-

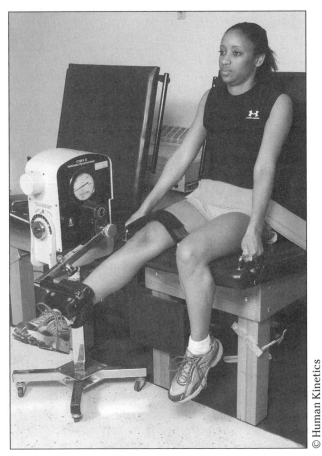

© Human Kinetics

Figure 14.3 Muscle strength can be tested using an isokinetic testing device that provides a constant speed throughout the entire range of motion.

tions of test protocols and performance values for these exercises. See tables 14.5 and 14.6 for fitness categories associated with push-up and curl-up tests. For a list of factors to consider regarding muscle strength and muscular endurance assessments, see "Using Muscle Strength and Muscular Endurance Tests."

Cardiorespiratory Fitness Tests

Assessing **cardiorespiratory fitness** encompasses testing the ability of the respiratory, cardiovascular, and skeletal muscle tissues to take in, deliver, and utilize oxygen while performing prolonged exercise of moderate to high intensity. **Maximal oxygen uptake ($\dot{V}O_2max$)** is considered the most valid measure of cardiorespiratory fitness. (For a discussion on the limitations of $\dot{V}O_2max$ to predict athletic performance, see "$\dot{V}O_2max$ and Athletic Performance," p. 443.) $\dot{V}O_2max$ is defined as the maximal amount of oxygen the body can use

Table 14.5 Fitness Categories by Age Group and Gender for Partial Curl-Up

Category	Age (years)									
	20-29		30-39		40-49		50-59		60-69	
Gender	M	F	M	F	M	F	M	F	M	F
Excellent	25	25	25	25	25	25	25	25	25	25
Very good	24	24	24	24	24	24	24	24	24	24
	21	18	18	19	18	19	17	19	16	17
Good	20	17	17	18	17	18	16	18	15	16
	16	14	15	10	13	11	11	10	11	8
Fair	15	13	14	9	12	10	10	9	10	7
	11	5	11	6	6	4	8	6	6	3
Needs improvement	10	4	10	5	5	3	7	5	5	2

Source: Canadian Physical Activity, Fitness & Lifestyle Approach: CSEP-Health & Fitness Program's Health-Related Appraisal & Counselling Strategy, Third Edition, © 2003. Reprinted with permission from the Canadian Society for Exercise Physiology.

Table 14.6 Fitness Categories by Age Groups and Gender for Push-Ups

Category	Age (years)									
	20-29		30-39		40-49		50-59		60-69	
Gender	M	F	M	F	M	F	M	F	M	F
Excellent	36	30	30	27	25	24	21	21	18	17
Very good	35	29	29	26	24	23	20	20	17	16
	29	21	22	20	17	15	13	11	11	12
Good	28	20	21	19	16	14	12	10	10	11
	22	15	17	13	13	11	10	7	8	5
Fair	21	14	16	12	12	10	9	6	7	4
	17	10	12	8	10	5	7	2	5	2
Needs improvement	16	9	11	7	9	4	6	1	4	1

Source: Canadian Physical Activity, Fitness & Lifestyle Approach: CSEP-Health & Fitness Program's Health-Related Appraisal & Counselling Strategy, Third Edition, © 2003. Reprinted with permission from the Canadian Society for Exercise Physiology.

Highlight

Using Muscle Strength and Muscular Endurance Tests

One must consider a number of factors when performing tests to assess muscle strength and muscular endurance. While many tests are simple to perform and score, each test should be selected not only for its convenience but also for its specific application to the client's activities. The following is a list of factors to consider when performing muscle strength and muscular endurance assessments:

- Be familiar with the advantages and limitations of the test and any related equipment. Muscle fitness testing is not completely reliable, and equipment often must be modified. Test results must be carefully interpreted in light of a test's limitations.

- Muscle fitness tests are specific to a given muscle group and the type of contraction being performed. There is no single test of whole-body muscle strength or endurance.

- The test results should be expressed in relative terms (e.g., relative to body weight or amount of lean body mass), as muscle fitness is related to both body weight and the amount of muscle mass. Expression of the results in relative terms also allows for comparison with other people performing the test.

- As tests of muscle fitness involve a maximal effort, every attempt should be made to control factors that affect maximal performance. This includes factors such as physical environment (e.g., temperature, humidity), time of day, the subject's motivation, medications that may affect performance, nutritional and hydration status, and amount of sleep.

- Select tests that the person is able to perform. For instance, some people may not be capable of lifting the lightest weight on a Universal machine when performing the 1RM bench press test. A multiple RM test may be needed, or modifications of the test may need to be developed.

- The standard values published for most tests of muscular fitness may be outdated and may not be applicable to your age category. Thus, these values may be invalid, unreliable, and inappropriate to use with many individuals.

Adapted from American College of Sports Medicine, 2006, *ACSM's guidelines for exercise testing and prescription*, 7th ed. (Philadelphia, PA: Lippincott Williams & Wilkins), 22-90; V.H. Heyward, 2006, *Advanced fitness assessment and exercise prescription*, 5th ed. (Champaign, IL: Human Kinetics).

during a given period of time and is calculated as the product of cardiac output and arterial-venous oxygen difference. $\dot{V}O_2$max is measured during an exercise test to volitional fatigue using open-circuit indirect calorimetry. Oxygen and carbon dioxide concentrations are measured during pulmonary ventilation and expiration. However, it is not always possible or appropriate to measure the $\dot{V}O_2$max of every client. The equipment needed to perform indirect calorimetry is usually available only in exercise physiology laboratories. Also, it may not be safe or accurate to have an untrained individual or client with multiple risk factors perform maximal exercise.

Tests have been developed to overcome these obstacles to assessing $\dot{V}O_2$max. $\dot{V}O_2$max can be predicted from submaximal exercise heart rates

and from maximal and submaximal exercise performance conducted either in the laboratory or on the field. Numerous protocols have been designed to predict $\dot{V}O_2$max using treadmills of various sizes (to accommodate runners, cross-country skiers with roller skis, and disabled athletes in wheelchairs), cycling ergometers, and rowing ergometers. Various walking, running, and stepping protocols can be used to test individuals in the field as well as to accommodate large groups of people. These include the Rockport 1-mile walk test, the 1.5-mile run test, and the McArdle step test. See ACSM 2008, Heyward 2006, and Howley and Franks 2003 for descriptions of specific testing protocols and normative values. Table 14.7 shows the $\dot{V}O_2$max values reported for populations ranging from highly fit

Highlight

$\dot{V}O_2$max and Athletic Performance

While $\dot{V}O_2$max is a good indicator of cardiorespiratory fitness, it is limited in its ability to predict athletic performance. In a heterogeneous group of individuals with variable activity levels, $\dot{V}O_2$max is highly correlated with cardiorespiratory fitness level and athletic endurance performance. However, in a group of highly trained athletes with homogeneous $\dot{V}O_2$max values, a variety of factors influence athletic performance. Some of these factors include

- economy of movement (e.g., running economy) (Conley and Krahenbuhl 1980),
- turnover of lactate (Costill et al. 1973; Messonnier et al. 1997),
- sport-specific biomechanical factors (e.g., push-off angle and trunk position in speed skating) (Van Ingen Schenau et al. 1996),
- ability to perform exercise for a longer duration at a higher percentage of $\dot{V}O_2$max (Costill et al. 1973), and
- ability to perform various skills and precision techniques specific to a given sport (e.g., soccer, basketball, synchronized swimming).

Table 14.7 Maximal Oxygen Uptake Measured in Healthy and Diseased Populations

Population	$\dot{V}O_2$ max $(mL \cdot kg^{-1} \cdot min^{-1})$ Men	Women
Cross-country skiers	82	66
Distance runners	79	62
College students	45	38
Middle-aged adults	35	30
Postmyocardial infarction patients	22	18
Patients with severe pulmonary disease	13	13

(cross-country skiers) to those limited by disease (pulmonary disease patients).

How do you decide whether it is safe to perform maximal or submaximal testing? And when is it necessary to have medical supervision during exercise testing? The ACSM (2006) has published guidelines to help answer these questions. Certain conditions have been identified as either **absolute** or **relative contraindications** to exercise testing (see p. 444). If an individual exhibits one or more absolute contraindications, exercise testing should not be performed for any reason until the

condition(s) is stabilized. For people exhibiting relative contraindications to exercise, the potential benefits of exercise testing must be weighed against the potential risks.

Physician supervision during exercise testing is recommended under certain conditions. It is *always* recommended during both submaximal and maximal testing of

- men older than 44 years,
- women older than 54 years,
- individuals with **known disease,** and
- individuals at **increased risk** (refer to table 14.1) who have one or more signs or symptoms of cardiopulmonary disease (see the list on p. 444).

A physician need not be present during submaximal testing of apparently healthy individuals or for those at increased risk who have no signs or symptoms of cardiopulmonary disease. Maximal exercise testing also can be performed without physician supervision in apparently healthy men younger than 45 years and women younger than 55 years.

Anaerobic Fitness Tests

Of all the components of fitness, the most difficult to assess may be anaerobic fitness. While many available tests are simple to perform, there is disagreement as to what the most appropriate

Contraindications to Exercise Testing

Absolute Contraindications

1. A recent significant change in the resting electrocardiogram, suggesting ischemia, recent myocardial infarction (within two days), or other acute cardiac event
2. Unstable angina
3. Uncontrolled cardiac dysrhythmias causing symptoms or hemodynamic compromise
4. Symptomatic severe aortic stenosis
5. Uncontrolled symptomatic heart failure
6. Acute pulmonary embolus or pulmonary infarction
7. Acute myocarditis or pericarditis
8. Suspected or known dissecting aneurysm
9. Acute systemic infection, accompanied by fever, body aches, or swollen lymph glands

Relative Contraindications

1. Left main coronary stenosis
2. Moderate stenotic valvular heart disease
3. Electrolyte abnormalities (hypokalemia, hypomagnesemia)
4. Severe arterial hypertension (systolic blood pressure of >200 mmHg or diastolic blood pressure of >110 mmHg or both) at rest
5. Tachydysrhythmia or bradydysrhythmia
6. Hypertrophic cardiomyopathy and other forms of outflow tract obstruction
7. Neuromuscular, musculoskeletal, or rheumatoid disorders that are exacerbated by exercise
8. High-degree atrioventricular block
9. Ventricular aneurysm
10. Uncontrolled metabolic disease (diabetes, thyrotoxicosis, or myxedema)
11. Chronic infectious disease (mononucleosis, hepatitis, AIDS)
12. Mental or physical impairment leading to inability to exercise adequately

Adapted, by permission, from American College of Sports Medicine, 2006, *ACSM's guidelines for exercise testing and prescription*, 7th ed. (Philadelphia, PA: Lippincott Williams & Wilkins), 50.

Major Symptoms or Signs Suggestive of Cardiovascular, Pulmonary, or Metabolic Disease*

1. Pain or discomfort (or other anginal equivalent) in the chest, neck, jaw, arms, or other areas that may be ischemic in nature
2. Shortness of breath at rest or with mild exertion
3. Dizziness or syncope
4. Orthopnea or paroxysmal nocturnal dyspnea
5. Ankle edema
6. Palpitations or tachycardia
7. Intermittent claudication
8. Known heart murmur
9. Unusual fatigue or shortness of breath with usual activities

*These symptoms must be interpreted in the clinical context in which they appear since they are not all specific for cardiopulmonary or metabolic disease.

Adapted from American College of Sports Medicine, 2006, *ACSM's guidelines for exercise testing and prescription,* 7th ed. (Philadelphia, PA: Lippincott Williams & Wilkins), 23-24.

method is and what the tests are actually measuring (Inbar et al. 1996). **Anaerobic fitness** is defined as the ability to perform very high-intensity exercise for relatively short periods of time (from a few seconds up to a few minutes). Various tests can determine anaerobic fitness from peak force, total work, peak muscle or blood lactate, and maximal accumulated oxygen deficit (MAOD), to name just a few. Again, there are a variety of protocols that can be performed either in the laboratory or on the field, including the Margaria step test, the vertical jump test, short sprints, cycle ergometer tests, and treadmill running.

The Wingate Anaerobic Test (WAnT) is the most widely used cycle ergometer test for assessing anaerobic capacity. Inbar and colleagues (1996) have published an entire book about the WAnT: what it measures, the equipment needed and procedures involved, factors that can influence the test, and normative values for various populations. One disadvantage of the WAnT is that it cannot assess the performance of a specific muscle or muscle groups—it is capable of assessing only the performance of combined muscle groups. Yet there are several advantages to using the WAnT to assess anaerobic fitness (Inbar et al. 1996):

- The test is highly reliable.
- The score is a valid indicator of supramaximal anaerobic capacity.
- The test is sensitive to changes in anaerobic fitness over time.
- It can provide information about peak power, muscle endurance, and muscle fatigability.
- It is simple to administer.
- It is inexpensive.
- It is noninvasive and can be used on many types of people, including those with disabilities.
- It can assess the performance of both upper and lower limbs.

Sport-Specific Performance Testing in Athletes

It is important to keep in mind that the basic fitness assessments presented in the preceding sections are valuable and that they provide good baseline measurements for all individuals. However, for athletes, there are additional sport-specific assessments that provide a better indication of performance and progress in a given

sport. Sport-specific performance testing can take place both in the laboratory and in the field. There are physiological requirements that are unique to each sport; therefore, special consideration should be given to maximize the specificity, relevance, and validity of the tests selected for a given sport. According to the Australian Sports Commission (2000, pp. xii-xiii), benefits of sport-specific performance testing in athletes include the following:

- Establishing an athlete's strengths and weaknesses
- Monitoring progress by repeating the tests at regular intervals
- Providing feedback and comparing performances on objective and relevant tests
- Educating the coaches and athletes
- Predicting performance potential or identifying individuals who may be suitable for certain sports

Specific laboratory and field protocols, as well as normative data for a variety sports, are described by the Australian Sports Commission (2000) and Baechle and Earle (2008).

Body Composition Tests

Body composition is defined as the relative proportion of fat and fat-free tissue in the body. According to ACSM (2008), assessment of body composition is important for establishing an ideal weight for health and physical performance, as well as for determining risk for diseases such as CAD, diabetes, hypertension, and hyperlipidemia. Tests for measuring body composition include anthropometry, bioelectrical impedance, hydrostatic weighing, and dual-energy X-ray absorptiometry (DXA). For more information and a description of the protocols, see chapter 7, "Body Composition."

CHAPTER IN REVIEW

Many techniques are available to assess nutritional and fitness status. The examples provided in this chapter are not exhaustive; we encourage you to thoroughly search the literature for the most appropriate test for a specific client or population. All tests have advantages and limitations that you must take into account when you review test results and when you explain the results to a client.

Key Concepts

1. Describe the characteristics of medical and health history questionnaires.

One important component of the medical history is a physical examination. The physical exam is particularly important for people who are untrained or detrained or who may have risks or symptoms for cardiovascular or metabolic diseases. A licensed health professional should select the tests to be performed during a physical exam. Health history questionnaires help to uncover current or potential health problems. The questionnaires should include questions about medication status, family history of disease, history of illness and injuries, menstrual history (of females), and diet and exercise history. Select fitness tests and prescribe exercises in light of a person's risk classification for coronary artery disease.

2. Discuss the methods used to assess energy and nutrient intakes.

Energy and nutrient intakes can be assessed with a variety of methods including retrospective methods (e.g., 24 h recall, food frequency questionnaires, and diet histories) or prospective methods (e.g., diet records, weighed food records, and direct observation). Each method has its advantages and weaknesses. Validity and reliability of these methods depend on a client's ability to accurately report dietary intake.

3. Discuss the methods used to assess energy expenditure.

Daily energy expenditure can be assessed using questionnaires, observation, self-report records, motion detection devices, and doubly labeled water. The accuracy of most methods depends on the applicability of published energy expenditure values to the actual activities reported. While doubly labeled water does not depend on the ability of the client or observer to accurately report activity or on the use of published energy values, this method is relatively expensive, requires highly specialized equipment, and cannot give an estimation of energy expenditure for a period of time less than one week.

4. Describe specific tests used to assess the components of fitness.

There are many components of fitness, and no single test can measure total body fitness. Components of fitness include flexibility, muscle strength, muscle endurance, cardiorespiratory fitness, and anaerobic fitness. While cost and convenience are important considerations, the reliability, validity, and applicability of assessment methods should also be critical concerns.

Key Terms

1RM test 440

24-hour recall 428

absolute contraindication 443

accelerometer 433

activity questionnaire 434

activity record 436

anaerobic fitness 445

apparently healthy 424

behavioral observation 433

body composition 445

cardiorespiratory fitness 441

diet history 427

diet record 429

dynamometer 440

flexibility 439

food frequency questionnaire 428

health history questionnaire 424

increased risk 443

isokinetic strength 440

isometric (static) strength 440

isotonic (dynamic) strength 440

known disease 443

Additional Information

American College of Sports Medicine: www.acsm.org

Publishes materials, including position statements, on physical activity, physical fitness, and other sports medicine and exercise science topics.

American College of Sports Medicine. ACSM's health-related physical fitness assessment manual, 2nd ed. Philadelphia: Lippincott Williams & Wilkins, 2008;16-73.

A manual to be used for the assessment of health-related components of physical fitness including preactivity screening and risk stratification.

President's Council on Physical Fitness and Sports: www.fitness.gov

Works with schools, clubs, recreation agencies, and employers on physical fitness and exercise program design and implementation. Produces informational materials on exercise; school physical education programs; corporate fitness; and physical fitness for youth, adults, and senior citizens.

The American Dietetic Association: www.eatright.org

Provides consumers and nutrition professionals with objective, credible food and nutrition information.

References

Ainslie P, Reilly T, Westerterp K. Estimating human energy expenditure: a review of techniques with particular reference to doubly labelled water. Sports Med 2003;33:683-698.

Ainsworth BE, Haskell WL, Leon AS, Jacobs DS Jr, Montoye HJ, Sallis JF, Paffenbarger RS Jr. Compendium of physical activities: classification by energy costs of human physical activities. Med Sci Sports Exerc 1993;25:71-80.

Ainsworth BE, Haskell WL, Whitt MC, Irwin ML, Swartz AM, Strath SJ, O'Brien WL, Bassett DR Jr, Schmitz KH, Emplaincourt PO, Jacobs DR Jr, Leon AS. Compendium of physical activities: an update of activity codes and MET intensities. Med Sci Sports Exerc 2000;32:S498-504.

American College of Sports Medicine (ACSM). Resource manual for guidelines for exercise testing and prescription, 5th ed. Philadelphia: Lea & Febiger, 2005.

American College of Sports Medicine (ACSM). ACSM's guidelines for exercise testing and prescription, 7th ed. Philadelphia: Lippincott Williams & Wilkins, 2006;22-90.

American College of Sports Medicine (ACSM). ACSM's health-related physical fitness assessment manual, 2nd ed. Philadelphia: Lippincott Williams & Wilkins, 2008;16-73.

Australian Sports Commission. Physiological tests for elite athletes. Champaign, IL: Human Kinetics, 2000.

Baechle TR, Earle RW. Essentials of strength training and conditioning, 3rd ed. Champaign, IL: Human Kinetics, 2008.

Baranowski T, Dworkin RJ, Cieslik CJ et al. Reliability and validity of self report of aerobic activity: Family Health Project. Res Q Exerc Sport 1984;55:309-417.

Basiotis PP, Welsh SO, Cronin FJ, Kelsay JL, Mertz W. Number of days of food intake records required to estimate individual and group nutrient intakes with defined confidence. J Nutr 1987;117:1638-1641.

Bassett DR Jr, Ainsworth BE, Leggett SR, Mathien CA, Main JA, Hunter DC, Duncan GE. Accuracy of five electronic pedometers for measuring distance walked. Med Sci Sports Exerc 1996;28:1071-1077.

Bond V. Muscular strength and endurance. In: Howley ET, Franks BD eds. Health fitness instructor's handbook. Champaign, IL: Human Kinetics, 2003.

Canadian Society for Exercise Physiology. The Canadian physical activity, fitness & lifestyle approach: CSEP-Health & Fitness Program's health-related appraisal and counseling strategy, 3rd ed. Ottawa, ON: Canadian Society for Exercise Physiology, 2003.

Chen KY, Sun M. Improving energy expenditure estimation by using a triaxial accelerometer. J Appl Physiol 1997;83:2112-2122.

Conley DL, Krahenbuhl G. Running economy and distance running performance of highly trained athletes. Med Sci Sports Exerc 1980;12:357-360.

Corder K, Soren B, Ekelund U. Accelerometers and pedometers: methodology and clinical application. Curr Opin Clin Nutr Metab Care 2007;10:597-603.

Costill DL, Thomason H, Roberts E. Fractional utilization of the aerobic capacity during distance running. Med Sci Sports Exerc 1973;5:248-252.

Fischbach F. A manual of laboratory and diagnostic tests, 7th ed. Philadelphia: Lippincott, 2004.

Gibala MJ. High-intensity interval training: a time-efficient strategy for health promotion? Curr Sports Med Rep 2007;6:211-213.

Heyward VH. Advanced fitness assessment and exercise prescription, 5th ed. Champaign, IL: Human Kinetics, 2006.

Hovell MF, Bursick JH, Sharkey R, McClure J. An evaluation of elementary students' voluntary physical activity during recess. Res Q Exerc Sport 1978;49:460-474.

Howley ET, Franks BD. Health fitness instructor's handbook, 4th ed. Champaign, IL: Human Kinetics, 2003.

Inbar O, Bar-Or O, Skinner JS. The Wingate anaerobic test. Champaign, IL: Human Kinetics, 1996.

Kriska AM, Caspersen CJ. A collection of physical activity questionnaires for health-related research. Med Sci Sports Exerc 1997;29:S3-S205.

Liemohn W. Exercise prescription for flexibility and low-back function. In: Howley ET, Franks BD eds. Health fitness instructor's handbook. Champaign, IL: Human Kinetics, 2003a.

Liemohn W. Flexibility and low-back function. In: Howley ET, Franks BD eds. Health fitness instructor's handbook. Champaign, IL: Human Kinetics, 2003b.

Matthews CE, Freedson PS. Field trial of a three-dimensional activity monitor: comparison with self report. Med Sci Sports Exerc 1995;27:1071-1078.

Maud PJ, Cortez-Cooper MY. Static techniques for the evaluation of joint range of motion. In: Maud PJ, Foster C eds.

Physiological assessment of human fitness. Champaign, IL: Human Kinetics, 1995;225-242.

Messonnier L, Freund H, Bourdin M, Belli A, Lacour J-R. Lactate exchange and removal abilities in rowing performance. Med Sci Sports Exerc 1997;29:396-401.

Montoye HJ, Kemper HCG, Saris WHM, Washburn RA. Measuring physical activity and energy expenditure. Champaign, IL: Human Kinetics, 1996.

Montoye HJ, Washburn R, Servais S, Ertl A, Webster JG, Nagle FJ. Estimation of energy expenditure by a portable accelerometer. Med Sci Sports Exerc 1983;15:403-407.

National Cholesterol Education Program (NCEP) Expert Panel on Detection, Evaluation, and Treatment of High Blood Cholesterol in Adults (ATPIII) final report. Circulation 2002;106:3143-3421.

Schlundt DG. Accuracy and reliability of nutrient intake estimates. J Nutr 1988;118:1432-1435.

Swain DP, Leutholtz BC. Metabolic calculations simplified. Baltimore: Williams & Wilkins, 1997.

Tudor-Locke C, Williams JE, Reis JP, Delores P. Utility of pedometers for assessing physical activity. Sports Med 2002;32:795-808.

Torún B. Physiological measurements of physical activity among children under free-living conditions. In: Pollitt E, Amante P eds. Energy intake and activity. New York: Liss, 1984;159-184.

Vanhees L, Lefevre J, Philippaerts R, Martens M, Huygens W, Troosters T, Beunen G. How to assess physical activity? How to assess physical fitness? Eur J Cardiovasc Prev Rehab 2005;12:102-114.

Van Ingen Schenau GJ, De Koning JJ, Bakker FC, De Groot G. Performance-influencing factors in homogeneous groups to top athletes: a cross-sectional study. Med Sci Sports Exerc 1996;28:1305-1310.

Wallace JP, McKenzie TL, Nader PR. Observed versus recalled exercise behavior: a validation of a seven day exercise recall for boys 11 to 13 years old. Res Q Exerc Sport 1985;56:161-165.

Wheeler ML, Buzzard IM. How to report dietary assessment data. J Am Diet Assoc 1994;4:1255-1256.

YMCA. YMCA's fitness testing and assessment manual, 4th ed. Chicago: YMCA of the USA, 2000.

CHAPTER 15

Nutrition and the Active Female

Chapter Objectives

After reading this chapter you should be able to

- understand the energy and nutrient requirements of active women and
- identify the components of the female athlete triad and discuss its prevention and treatment.

For most active females, including athletes, every day is a balancing act:

- When and what to eat? How much to eat?
- Should I supplement? If so, which supplement or supplements? How much? How often?
- How much should I exercise to maintain an optimal body weight for my sport or increase my competitive edge?
- When I am training harder, do I need more micronutrients?

Active women need to eat enough energy to maintain their fitness level and health; female athletes, moreover, need additional energy to maintain their competitive edge for training and competition. Yet many of these same women want to lose weight. In addition to the body weight issues these women deal with, they are bombarded with advertisements that tell them they need a host of other nutrients, supplements, and herbal preparations. How does one sort fact from fiction? What are the energy and nutrient needs of the active female? What nutritional factors are of greatest concern? This chapter is an effort to put into perspective the nutritional needs of active females, including female athletes. First, we address the energy requirements of active females and the importance of eating adequate energy for good health and performance. Second, we discuss the health consequences of restricting energy intake too dramatically. Next, we briefly address the major vitamin and mineral concerns for the active female. Finally, we discuss the components of the female athlete triad (energy availability, menstrual dysfunction, and bone health) and ways to detect and prevent this set of disorders.

ENERGY AND NUTRIENT REQUIREMENTS

In order to maintain body weight, female athletes of any age must consume enough kilocalories (kcal) to cover the energy cost of daily living, the energy cost of their sport, and the energy cost associated with building and repairing muscle tissue. Females of reproductive age must also cover the costs of menstruation and reproductive function, while younger females must cover the additional energy costs of growth.

Active females, like most women in our society, are often preoccupied with their body weights and shapes. Although their weights are often normal or even below normal by all medical or health standards, they still want to lose an extra 5 to 10 lb (2.3-4.5 kg). In addition, female athletes are frequently pressured by coaches, parents, peers, and themselves to weigh less. What are the health consequences of this type of dieting in the active female or the competitive female athlete? What are the potential health consequences if these behaviors are followed into the third, fourth, and fifth decade of life? What strategies can be used to help the active female identify and maintain a healthy body weight for her sport and throughout life? This section reviews the possible health consequences of chronic dieting or energy restriction in active females. Although these women usually do not have a clinical eating disorder, they nevertheless frequently engage in maladaptive dieting behaviors. Finally, we offer strategies for helping female athletes identify and maintain a healthy body weight throughout their athletic careers and their lives.

Health Consequences of Chronic Dieting

For most healthy women, "going on a short-term diet" should present few nutritional or long-term health problems. However, serious health problems may arise for the active female or the female athlete who *chronically* diets or restricts energy intake while expending high amounts of energy in exercise. In fact, the "female athlete triad" (discussed later in this chapter) is one example of a serious health consequence that can arise from chronic energy restriction in active females.

Poor Energy and Macronutrient Intakes

If an active female constantly restricts energy intake to less than 1600 to 1800 kcal/day, it is almost impossible to get adequate nutrients (protein, carbohydrate, essential fatty acids, vitamins, and minerals). Recreational athletes who exercise 6 to 10 h/week typically require 2200 to 2500 kcal/day for weight maintenance; competitive female athletes who exercise 10 to 20 h or more per week need at least 2500 to 2800 kcal/day to maintain body weight. Women involved in high-endurance sports (e.g., training for a competitive marathon or triathlon) may need as much as 4000 to 4500 kcal/day.

Active females with low energy intakes have protein and carbohydrate intakes below those recommended for active people. They do not eat enough protein to maintain and repair muscle tissue and to cover the cost of any protein used for energy during exercise. As mentioned in chapter 4, active individuals engaged in endurance activity need more protein (1.0-1.7 g protein per kilogram body weight) (Tarnopolsky 2004; "International Athletics Associations Federation Consensus Statement" 2007) than the **Recommended Dietary Allowance (RDA)** (0.8 g protein per kilogram body weight) (Institute of Medicine [IOM] 2002). When energy intake is low, moreover, carbohydrate levels are inadequate to replenish glycogen stores used during exercise. Most female athletes in training need ≥5 g carbohydrate per kilogram body weight to maintain glycogen stores. If activity is exceptionally high and training occurs on a daily basis, carbohydrate needs may be ~7 to 12 g of carbohydrate per kilogram body weight (Burke 2006). Many active females avoid fat either for weight loss or because they think fat is "bad" for their health. If fat intake is too low (<10-15% of energy intake), the intake and absorption of the fat-soluble vitamins and essential fatty acids may also be low. Finally, many female athletes with poor energy intakes complain of fatigue, frequent injuries, irritability, and poor athletic performance (Dueck, Manore, and Matt 1996). You often can reverse these complaints by having such a client follow two simple guidelines:

- She should increase her total daily energy intake (kcal/day) or decrease total energy expenditure (maybe add a rest day to her training routine) or both.
- She should be certain that she is in a state of positive energy balance before beginning any physical activity.

This means that she should be well fed *before* her daily workout. If she has a 3 p.m. workout, she may need to eat a 2 p.m. snack before going to the track or the gym. This snack helps provide the body with enough energy to fuel both the brain and the muscles during exercise. Frequently people who diet tend to restrict energy intake during the day and eat most of their kilocalories at the end of the day. An athlete who follows this pattern will come to her workout fatigued and unable to perform her best. Some of the symptoms of low energy intakes in active women are outlined in "How Do You Know If an Active Female Is Not Eating Enough?".

Poor Micronutrient Intakes

Active females with poor energy intakes frequently have poor vitamin and mineral intakes—especially calcium, iron, magnesium, zinc, and B-complex vitamins (Beals and Manore 1998; Manore 1999, 2000, 2002; Beals and Manore 2007). These micronutrients are especially important for active individuals and play an important role in energy production, hemoglobin synthesis, maintenance of bone health, and adequate immune function. Prolonged energy restriction combined with poor micronutrient intakes can place the female athlete at risk for poor nutritional status. This can result in decreased bone density, impaired immune response, menstrual dysfunction, anemia, poor exercise performance, and increased recovery time from injury. Which micronutrients are most likely to be deficient? What vitamin and mineral recommendations can you give to the active female?

Table 15.1 suggests intakes of vitamins and minerals for active women and compares them to the current RDAs or to **Dietary Reference Intakes (DRIs)** (IOM 1997, 1998, 2000, 2001). (See chapters 9-13 for detailed treatment of each of these nutrients.) Adequate intakes of B vitamins are necessary for energy production during exercise and for the prevention of anemia. About 10% to 60% of female athletes do not consume the RDA for the B vitamins; the most common deficiencies are in riboflavin, vitamin B$_6$, and folate (Billon

How Do You Know If an Active Female Is Not Eating Enough?

If a female athlete is not eating enough food, some of the following symptoms may occur:

- Hunger, irritability, and perhaps difficulty concentrating before or during her exercise routine. Sometimes she may even get shaky and light-headed. This may be the case especially if she exercises around 3 or 4 p.m. and has not eaten since lunch, or if she exercises before breakfast.
- Poor growth rates for young and adolescent female athletes. The diet must provide enough fuel for growth and menstruation, building and repair of muscle tissue, and exercise.
- Cessation of menstrual periods. This may be a sign that the body does not have enough energy to fuel both exercise and the reproductive functions of the body. An athlete does not have to have an eating disorder to stop having her period. Many female athletes stop menstruating if they are exercising hard and not eating enough food and kilocalories, even if they are making good food choices.
- Weight loss. This means that she is not providing enough fuel for both exercise and weight maintenance. If she is restricting energy intake and her exercise intensity is high, both muscle tissue and fat are being used for fuel.

Adapted, by permission, from M.M. Manore, 1997, "How do you know when you are eating enough?" *USA Gymnastics* 26(6): 8-9.

2006; Hansen and Manore 2006; Manore 2000, 2002; Woolf and Manore 2006, 2007). Research on folate status in active women is limited; but most studies show that when energy intakes are low, folate status is also low. For example, Ziegler and colleagues (2002) examined the folate status of 18 competitive female figure skaters and found that at least 22% to 35% of the skaters had low serum folate concentrations (<4 nmol/L) throughout the year (preseason, competition season, and off-season). During these same time periods, dietary intake of folate ranged from 175 to 302 μg/day, with the lowest intake levels present in the off-season. Mean energy intakes for these athletes were ~1600 kcal/day throughout the year. Exercise appears to increase the needs for certain B vitamins (Hansen and Manore 2006; Manore 2000; Woolf and Manore

Table 15.1 Recommended Daily Vitamin and Mineral Intakes for Active Premenopausal Women

Vitamin or mineral	Suggested intake or range of intakes for active women[1]	Current Recommended Dietary Allowance (RDA) or Dietary Reference Intake (DRI)[2]
Vitamins		
Thiamin	1.5-2.0 mg/day	1.1 mg/day (19-70+ years)
Riboflavin	2.4-3.0 mg/day	1.1 mg/day (19-70+ years)
Vitamin B$_6$	1.5-3.0 mg/day	1.3 mg/day (19-50 years)
Folate (Fe)	400 mg/day	400 mg/day (19-70+ years)
Vitamin B$_{12}$	2.4 mg/day	2.4 mg/day (19-70+ years)
Vitamin C[3]	400 mg/day	75 mg/day (19-70+ years)
Vitamin E[3]	200-400 IU/day	15 mg/day α-TE (14-70+ years)
Vitamin D[4]	10-20 μg/day (400-800 IU/day), especially if dietary intakes are low or exposure to sunlight is limited	5 μg/day (200 IU/day, 9-50 years) or 10 μg/day (400 IU/day, 50-70 years)
Minerals		
Iron	18 mg/day	18 mg/day (15-50 years)
Calcium	1300-1500 mg/day, especially for young athletes between the ages of 11 and 24 years and athletes with exercise-related amenorrhea	1000 mg/day (19-50 years)
Zinc	8 mg/day	8 mg/day (19-70+ years)
Magnesium	350-400 mg/day	310 mg/day (19-30 years) or 320 mg/day (31-70+ years)

FE = folate equivalents; TE = α-tocopherol equivalents. In general, 1 mg/day α-tocopherol = 1 α-TE = ~1 IU. Vitamin E comes in natural and synthetic forms (see your supplements for specifics). Conversions for these forms of vitamin E are as follows. *RRR*-α-tocopherol (natural or *d*-α-tocopherol): IU × 0.67 = mg *RRR*-α-tocopherol. Example: 100 IU = 67 mg. *all-rac*-α-tocopherol (synthetic or *dl*-α-tocopherol): IU × 0.45 = mg *RRR*-α-tocopherol. Example: 100 IU = 45 mg. Vitamin D: 1 IU of vitamin D is defined as the activity of 0.025 μg of cholecalciferol. 1 μg vitamin D = 1 IU. The activity of 25(OH)D is five times more potent than that of cholecalciferol; thus, 1 IU = 0.005 μg 25(OH)D. 1 μg cholecalciferol = 0.2 μg 25(OH)D.

[1] Anderson et al. (1998), Keith (2006), Joy et al. (1997); Manore (2000, 2002), Tang et al. (2007).

[2] Institute of Medicine (IOM), Food and Nutrition Board, Dietary Reference Intakes (DRIs) 1997, 1998, 2000, 2001.

[3] Linus Pauling Institute, Oregon State University. http://lpi.oregonstate.edu. Accessed December 2008.

[4] Heaney (2005) indicates that vitamin D toxicity is not seen at intakes equivalent to 10,000 IU/day (250 μg/day). The DRI Tolerable Upper Intake Level for vitamin D is 50 μg/day (2000 IU), which is considered too low to permit optimization of vitamin D status in the general population (Heaney 2005).

2006, 2007); thus, active females should consume at least twice the RDA for riboflavin and vitamin B$_6$ and at least the RDA for folate. If adequate intakes for these three B vitamins are achieved, intake should be adequate for the other B vitamins (thiamin, niacin, biotin, and pantothenic acid). Vitamin B$_{12}$ is usually of concern only for people who avoid animal foods or if gastrointestinal problems prevent absorption of the vitamin.

Antioxidant micronutrients (vitamins C, A, and E; β-carotene; selenium) help maintain cellular integrity and prevent tissue damage from the many pollutants in our environment and from internal sources of free radicals. Exercise increases the potential for tissue oxidation due to the higher oxygen consumption that occurs during exercise (Mastaloudis and Traber 2006).

Athletes who restrict intake of energy or fat may also be reducing their intake of fat-soluble vitamins—especially vitamin E, which is found in the fatty portion of foods and in many vegetable cooking oils. Vitamin C is found in citrus fruits and in some vegetables (e.g., tomatoes, broccoli, green and red peppers), while vitamin A and β-carotene are found in green, yellow, and dark green vegetables. If these foods are limited in the diet, the probability is high that the intake of these antioxidant vitamins will be low. Keith (2006) reviewed the research literature and found that 10% to 25% of female athletes consume less than two thirds the current 75 mg/day RDA for vitamin C. Intakes of antioxidant nutrients above the current RDA may be necessary for women who perform high-intensity exercise or who exercise in a highly polluted environment (see table 15.1) (Mastaloudis and Traber 2006; Keith 2006).

Chapters 11 and 12 discuss in detail the mineral requirements of active people. In this section we highlight the minerals that are of specific concern to active women, who generally are at increased risk for poor intakes of iron, calcium, magnesium, and zinc. This is due in part to the restriction of meat and dairy from the diets of many active women, especially those who restrict energy intake for weight loss. In fact, the reported incidence of iron depletion (stage I, low serum ferritin concentrations) in active females is quite variable and ranges from 15% to 60%, while iron depletion is seen in only 20% to 30% of the general female population. Iron is important for hemoglobin synthesis, and exercise may increase the loss of this mineral. Thus, female athletes should consume at least the 18 mg/day RDA for iron; if possible, some of this iron should be from heme iron sources (meat, fish, and poultry). If the heme iron is low or is absent in the diet, higher amounts of daily iron may be required. Iron status should be checked periodically and supplementation used only if warranted.

Calcium intake is also typically low in the diets of active women. Calcium is required for strong bones, along with adequate intakes of vitamin D and other bone-building nutrients such as protein, vitamin K, magnesium, and fluoride. The new DRI for calcium reflects the increased need for this nutrient in women of all ages (see chapter 13). Active women should strive to consume at least the DRI for calcium every day (table 15.1). If the diet is limited in dairy products, it is much more difficult to consume the required amounts of calcium from foods unless one uses fortified foods or selects other limited foods high in available calcium (e.g., sardines with bone). Milk is frequently fortified with vitamin D, which stimulates intestinal calcium absorption and is important for muscle health (Heaney 2007). Vitamin D levels are often low for people who consume little milk or fortified dairy foods and who have limited exposure to the sun. For the athlete who participates primarily in indoor sports (e.g., figure skating, hockey, volleyball, basketball, and gymnastics), exposure to the sun may be quite limited. This is especially true for people in northern climates where winter months may dramatically limit exposure to sunlight. For these people, dietary vitamin D supplementation or fortification in foods may be very important to maintain healthy bones. Currently, there is discussion of increased requirements of vitamin D to maintain good health (Cranny et

al. 2007; Tang et al. 2007; Reginster 2007; Heaney 2005, 2007); thus, the current RDAs for vitamin D may be too low (Raiten and Picciano 2004). Remember that adequate calcium and vitamin D intakes are very important for young females who are still laying down new bone. More than 90% of total **bone mineral density (BMD)** occurs by 17 years of age, with peak bone density occurring between the ages of 25 to 30 years (figure 15.1). It is imperative that all the micronutrients necessary for optimal bone growth be provided during this time. See "Calcium and Vitamin D Requirements of Active Women" on p. 454 and table 15.1 for more specific recommendations concerning calcium and vitamin D intake for active females.

If meat products are limited in a diet or if the diet is high in refined foods, zinc and magnesium intakes may be low. Zinc is especially important for building and repairing tissue, while magnesium is important for energy production during exercise. Active females should strive to consume at least the RDA for these nutrients (table 15.1). They should be careful not to oversupplement with minerals since mineral–mineral interactions may cause one mineral to block the absorption or transport of another. A good rule to follow is always to consume minerals at or near the RDA or DRI level unless a particular deficiency dictates otherwise.

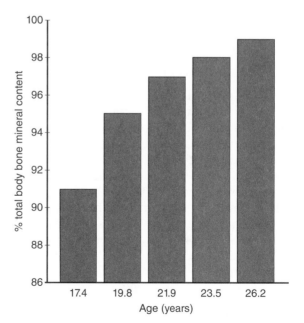

Figure 15.1 Total bone mineral content adjusted for age in young women.

Adapted from D. Teegarden, W.R. Proulx, and B.R. Martin, 1995, "Peak bone mass in young women," *Journal of Bone and Mineral Research* 10: 711-715.

Calcium and Vitamin D Requirements of Active Women

Females aged 9 to 18 years need to consume 1300 mg/day of calcium, while women aged 19 to 50 years need to consume 1000 mg/day. Women >51 years of age need 1200 mg/day of calcium to help maintain bone density during the postmenopausal years. Since milk and other dairy products are the primary source of calcium in the American diet, an athlete who does not use dairy products may need to supplement or use fortified foods, such as fortified soy milk or orange juice. Active females who already have poor bone density may need higher calcium intakes (e.g., 1000-1300 mg/day) (Nattiv et al. 2007).

Vitamin D is necessary for optimal intestinal absorption of calcium. Vitamin D is obtained in the diet or synthesized in the skin through exposure to sunlight (or both). In the past it was thought that exposure of hands, arms, and face to the sun for 5 to 15 min/day was adequate to provide sufficient amounts of vitamin D. We now know that a number of factors affect the amount of time needed for sun exposure to generate adequate vitamin D, including time of day, distance from the equator, skin color, and age (Heaney 2005). For active females who train or exercise primarily indoors or who live in northern latitudes, where exposure to sun is limited in the winter months, vitamin D status may be poor. These individuals may need to supplement with 400 to 800 IU of vitamin D and use vitamin D–fortified milk, margarine, or juices and consume other foods high in vitamin D (e.g., fatty fish such as salmon, tuna, mackerel, sardines), eggs, or fortified breakfast cereals or bars.

Current researchers have hotly debated the role of calcium and vitamin D in the prevention of osteoporosis. A resent meta-analysis by Tang and colleagues (2007) showed that 1200 mg/day of supplemental calcium, or a combined calcium (1200 mg/day) and vitamin D (800 IU/day) supplement, helped prevent osteoporosis in individuals 50 years or older. Another meta-analysis by Bischoff-Ferrari and colleagues (2004) also showed that supplementation of vitamin D (~400-1000 IU/day) reduced risk of falls in older individuals by more than 20%. This reduction in falls may be due to the role vitamin D plays in calcium absorption and muscle function (Heaney 2007). Thus, these two micronutrients are important at every stage of the life cycle to help keep bones healthy.

Decreased Resting Metabolic Rate and Total Daily Energy Expenditure

One effect of severe dieting or energy restriction is that it reduces **resting metabolic rate (RMR)**. During the dieting period, RMR declines to a greater extent than would be predicted based on decreases in total body weight and **fat-free mass (FFM)**. This means that total daily energy expenditure is reduced in people who chronically restrict energy intake. This decrease is compounded when heavy physical activity is combined with low energy intakes (Thompson et al. 1996; Manore and Thompson 2006). Moreover, the energy cost of digesting and metabolizing food declines when energy intake is restricted, thus further decreasing the total energy needs for the day. The end result of chronic energy restriction and high physical activity is that fewer kilocalories are required to maintain body weight in the dieting athlete than in a nondieting person of similar size and activity level.

This point was illustrated by Donnelly and colleagues (1994), who examined the effect of severe dieting (520 kcal/day) and exercise on RMR and FFM. Although this study was done in obese women, the results are applicable to nonobese people—especially active females of any size. This study is unique in that it used both aerobic and weight training exercise treatments. Sedentary women (n = 115) were randomly assigned to one of six dieting groups for a 12-week period. Each group was fed the same low-energy diet (520 kcal/day) for the entire 12 weeks, and the researchers monitored all the exercise. The treatments were as follows:

1. Diet-only group (control group): Did not exercise.

2. Diet + endurance exercise: Performed treadmill walking or cycling at 70% heart rate reserve, four days a week; exercise progressed from 20 to 60 min/day.

3. Diet + weight training: Performed six to eight repetitions at 70% to 80% of 1-repetition

maximum using five different weightlifting exercises, three days a week.

4. Diet + endurance exercise + weight training: Performed same weight training as group 3 and same endurance (aerobic) exercise as group 2.

5. Dieted for the first four weeks, added endurance exercise for the last eight weeks: For the first four weeks, did not exercise; for weeks 5 through 12, performed the same endurance (aerobic) exercise as group 2.

6. Diet + weight training for the first four weeks; endurance exercise added for the last eight weeks: For the first four weeks, performed same weight training as group 3; for weeks 5 through 12, continued the strength training but also performed the same endurance (aerobic) exercise as group 2.

All the groups lost weight; total weight loss did not differ among the groups and ranged from 16.7% to 22.3% of baseline body weight. In addition, changes in body fat were similar for all groups, with decreases ranging from 6.9% to 9.3%. Relative RMR (kilocalories per kilogram FFM per day) also decreased 1.6% to 9.3% over the treatment periods, but there were no significant differences among the groups. The greatest absolute decrease in RMR (down 240 kcal/day, which represented a 13.5% decrease) occurred in group 4—the dieters who did both endurance exercise and weight training ($p < 0.05$) (figure 15.2). However, the amount of FFM lost in this group was similar to that lost in the other five groups (9 lb or ~4 kg). These results illustrate that in the presence of severe energy restriction, exercise does not increase weight loss or slow the decrease of FFM or RMR compared to dieting without exercise. The group (group 4) with the highest exercise energy expenditure had the greatest absolute decrease in RMR during the 12-week dieting period. The body decreases RMR to conserve energy in the presence of severe negative energy balance (low energy intake and high energy expenditure).

A more reasonable approach to weight loss is to increase energy expenditure (~300-500 kcal/day, four or five days a week) using both endurance and strength training while making only moderate decreases in energy intake (~300-500 kcal/day). The actual decrease in energy intake should depend on age, sex, health, body size, and current energy intake and expenditure and can usually be achieved through alterations in food choices and serving sizes without counting kilocalories. This

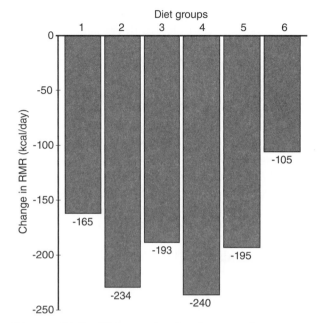

Figure 15.2 Changes in absolute resting metabolic rate (RMR) before and after a 12-week diet or diet plus exercise program. All groups followed a highly restrictive diet (520 kcal/day) for the entire 12 weeks. Group 1 = diet only; group 2 = diet + endurance exercise; group 3 = diet + weight training; group 4 = diet + endurance exercise + weight training; group 5 = diet only (first four weeks), then diet + endurance exercise (last eight weeks); group 6 = diet + weight training (first four weeks), then diet + weight training + endurance exercise (last eight weeks). Differences from baseline were statistically significant for each group, but differences between groups were not statistically significant.

Adapted from J.E. Donnelly et al., 1994. "Very low calorie diet with concurrent versus delayed and sequential exercise," *International Journal of Obesity* 18: 469-475.

more moderate approach minimizes decreases in FFM and RMR, while most of the weight lost is fat. However, it is important to remember that energy balance is dynamic and that individuals differ in how much energy they expend per kilogram FFM or body weight during physical activity. Thus, how quickly weight is lost may differ for individuals.

If a female athlete needs to lose weight, she should closely examine her current energy expenditure and intake. If she is already training hard, she should not increase her exercise and should attempt only moderate decreases in energy intake. If energy restriction is too severe, she will be fatigued, be irritable, have poor exercise performance and concentration, and be at increased risk of injury. She should be able to achieve small to moderate decreases in energy intake by altering food choices and serving sizes. Chapter 6 provides more detailed information on weight loss in athletes.

Poor Exercise Performance

The effect of chronic dieting on exercise performance or injuries has been examined in female athletes involved in aesthetic or lean-build sports (e.g., dancers, runners, gymnasts, and figure skaters) (Guest and Barr 2005; Sundgot-Borgen 1993, 1994). These individuals are constantly pressured to maintain a lean body for their sport, and many chronically diet to maintain a competitive weight. They are thinner and typically report higher incidence of maladaptive dieting behaviors than athletes participating in sports allowing more normal builds, such as basketball, volleyball, or downhill skiing (Beals and Manore 1994, 1998). Participants in lean-build sports report poorer energy intakes, higher rates of injury, less ability to concentrate, and longer recovery times from injuries than athletes in normal-build sports (Beals and Manore 1994, 1998, 2002). Poor physical performance can have a devastating psychological effect, especially if it is tied to team eligibility or scholarships. A number of psychological stresses are reported with severe dieting in athletes, including increased depression, obsession with food and body weight, increased incidence of binge–purge eating behaviors, increased stress of constantly trying to make weight or maintain an unrealistic body weight, and increased risk of developing an eating disorder (Beals and Manore 1994, 1998, 2002).

Strategies for Maintaining a Healthy Body Weight

One of the goals of the health professional is to help active females and female athletes to achieve and maintain a healthy body weight for their sport and for good health. The process begins by identifying what constitutes a realistic, healthy body weight based on genetic, physiological, social, sport, and psychological factors. A healthy weight is one that can be realistically maintained, allows for involvement in physical activity, and reduces risk factors for chronic disease. Strategies for helping active females identify and maintain a healthy body weight throughout the life cycle are listed on p. 457. Research shows that when pressure to achieve a weight goal is high, women attempt any weight loss method to achieve success, regardless

of health consequences. Any successful weight loss (e.g., fat loss) or weight maintenance program must address *changes in lifestyle* that can help athletes achieve and maintain a healthy weight for their sport without constantly dieting.

FEMALE ATHLETE TRIAD

The **female athlete triad** refers to the interrelationship among energy availability, menstrual status, and bone health (see figure 15.3). Each component of the triad spans a continuum from health to disease, and female athletes can have symptoms related to each component of the triad to different degrees. These disorders can manifest themselves through an eating disorder, disordered eating, or simply the inability to eat enough food; the result of inadequate energy intake can be amenorrhea and osteoporosis. These components are interrelated in etiology, pathogenesis, and consequences (Nattiv et al. 2007). The American College of Sports Medicine takes this triad of disorders quite seriously—see "American College of Sports Medicine (ACSM) Position Statement on the Female Athlete Triad," p. 459.

Active women, like most women in our society, are often concerned or even preoccupied with their body weight and shape. Their source of pressure is twofold: not only are they burdened by the general sociocultural demands placed on women to be thin; they are also expected to meet weight standards or body size expectations for their sport. Failure to meet these weight standards can result in severe consequences, such as being cut from the team, being given less participation with the team, or even being eliminated from competition. As the pressure to be thin mounts, active women may engage in disordered eating behaviors. This in turn may disrupt the menstrual cycle and result in menstrual dysfunction such as oligomenorrhea or amenorrhea. Without a normal menstrual cycle and adequate reproductive and metabolic hormones, which play an important role in bone and muscle health, a woman can experience decreases in BMD. The most severe cases lead to osteoporosis. Thus, for many female athletes, disordered eating is the event that leads to menstrual dysfunction, such as the absence of menstruation (amenorrhea), and poor BMD. Sports that emphasize leanness or a thin body build may place young girls or women at risk for the female athlete triad. Athletes who participate in the following sports may be at greater risk for the health issues of the triad:

Techniques to Help Active Individuals Identify and Maintain a Healthy Body Weight Throughout the Life Cycle

Emphasize Personal Health and Well-Being, Not Weight

- Focus less on the scale and more on healthy habits such as regular exercise, stress management, and making good food choices.
- Set realistic weight goals: What is the maximum weight for your height that would be acceptable? What is the maximum weight that will reduce the risk of chronic disease? What was the last weight you could maintain without constantly dieting?
- Mark progress by measuring changes in fitness level, health parameters (positive changes in blood pressure, glucose, lipids, etc.), and general well-being.
- Make lifestyle changes that help you maintain a healthy weight for yourself—not for your job, for your spouse, for your friends, or to prove a point.
- Understand that a number of factors have contributed to your current body size and shape, including genetics, the environment, current physical activity, eating behaviors, and habits. Thus, it is unrealistic to expect that you will respond to a diet and exercise program in exactly the same way as other individuals.

Change Diet and Eating Behaviors

- Do not constantly deprive yourself of favorite foods or set unrealistic dietary rules or guidelines.
- Make basic dietary changes that reduce energy intake, that fit into your lifestyle, and that you know you can achieve.
- Reduce fat intake, but remember that a lower-fat diet will not guarantee weight loss if you do not achieve a negative energy balance (reduced energy intake and increased energy expenditure).
- Eat more unprocessed foods, including whole grains, cereals, fruits, and vegetables.
- Make sure you consume adequate dietary fiber (>25 g/day).
- Do not skip meals and do not let yourself get too hungry.
- Eat something for breakfast. This will prevent you from being too hungry and overeating at lunch.
- Plan ahead and be prepared for when you might get hungry. Always have good food available for when and where you get hungry.
- Identify your own dietary weaknesses and plan a strategy for dealing with them.
- Remember, you are making lifelong dietary changes that will result in weight loss. You are not going on a diet that you will some day go off of.

Change Exercise Behaviors

- Start and maintain a regular exercise program, which includes both strength and aerobic exercise. This is an absolute requirement for the maintenance of a healthy body weight and FFM.
- Pick an activity or activities that you enjoy, including some that you can do on your own.
- Pick an activity that is inexpensive and does not require fancy equipment. This means that you will maintain your fitness program even when you are traveling and away from home.
- Find an exercise partner or exercise class to help you get started and motivate you. This will also help you get through the difficult days until exercise is a part of your lifestyle.
- Participate in group exercise activities whenever possible.
- Plan to include regular exercise and movement in your day: Add additional exercise by walking instead of driving, using stairs instead of the elevator, standing instead of sitting.
- Realize that you are making a lifetime change and a lifetime commitment to yourself for good health and weight management.

Adapted from M.M. Manore, 1996, "Chronic dieting in active women: what are the health consequences?" *Women Health Issues* 6: 332-341.

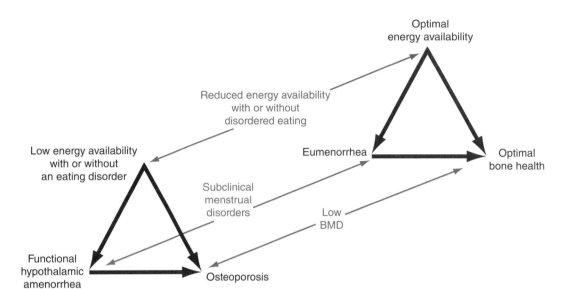

Figure 15.3 The female athlete triad. The spectrums of energy availability, menstrual function, and bone mineral density along which female athletes are distributed (thin arrows). An athlete's condition moves along each spectrum at a different rate, in one direction or the other, according to her diet and exercise habits. Energy availability, defined as dietary energy intake minus exercise energy expenditure, affects bone mineral density both directly via metabolic hormones and indirectly via effects on menstrual function and thereby estrogen (thick arrows).

Reprinted, by permission, from A. Nattiv et al., 2007, "American College of Sports Medicine position stand. The female athlete triad," *Medicine and Science in Sports and Exercise* 39(10): 1867-1882.

- Sports that have subjective performance scoring, such as dance, skating, diving, and gymnastics
- Endurance sports that emphasize a lean build or a low body weight (e.g., high power/weight ratio), such as long-distance running, cycling, and cross-country skiing
- Sports that require the athlete to wear body-contouring or body-revealing clothing, such as gymnastics, swimming, volleyball, aerobics, track, and dance
- Sports that require athletes to weigh in or that use weight-specific sport categories for participation, such as horse racing, martial arts, wrestling, and rowing
- Sports that emphasize a preadolescent body build for success, such as gymnastics, figure skating, and diving

Although participants in these sports may have an increased risk for developing one or more of the symptoms of the female athlete triad, it is important to remember that no sport is immune to this disorder.

The following sections outline each of the components of the female athlete triad and the serious health consequences associated with this syndrome.

Low Energy Availability

When the female athlete triad was introduced in 1997 (Otis et al. 1997), eating disorders was listed as the primary cause. We now recognize that decreased energy availability, whether caused by dieting, disordered eating, an eating disorder, or low energy intake, is the primary factor initiating the disorders of the triad. Thus, in this section we define and discuss low energy availability. We also address disordered eating and eating disorders, because both can lead to low energy availability and are a common problem in active women.

Energy availability is defined as dietary energy intake minus exercise energy expenditure (EEE). This is the amount of dietary energy remaining for exercise training after the energy required for all other physiological processes (cellular maintenance, thermogenesis, immunity, growth, reproduction, and activities of daily living) is subtracted. Because more energy is expended in FFM than in fat mass, it is also useful to normalize energy availability to FFM.

Highlight

American College of Sports Medicine (ACSM) Position Statement on the Female Athlete Triad

"Female Athlete Triad refers to the inter-relationships among energy availability, menstrual function and BMD, which may have clinical manifestations including eating disorders, functional hypothalamic amenorrhea and osteoporosis. With proper nutrition, these same relationships can promote robust health. Athletes are distributed along a spectrum between health and disease, and those at the pathological end may not exhibit all these clinical conditions simultaneously.

"Restrictive eating behaviours practiced by girls and women in sports or physical activities that emphasize leanness are of special concern. For prevention and early intervention, education of athletes, parents, coaches, trainers, judges, and administrators is a priority. Athletes should be assessed for the Triad at the pre-participation physical and/or annual health screening exam, and whenever an athlete presents with any of the Triad's clinical conditions. Sport administrators should also consider rule changes to discourage unhealthy weight loss practices. A multidisciplinary treatment team should include a physician or other health care professional, a registered dietitian (RD) and, for athletes with eating disorders, a mental health practitioner.

"The first aim of treatment for any Triad component is to increase energy availability by increasing energy intake and/or reducing exercise energy expenditure. Nutrition counseling and monitoring are sufficient interventions for many athletes, but eating disorders warrant psychotherapy. Athletes with eating disorders should be required to meet established criteria to continue exercising, and their training and competition may need to be modified. No pharmacological agent adequately restores bone loss or corrects metabolic abnormalities that impair health and performance in athletes with functional hypothalamic amenorrhea."

Reprinted, by permission, from A. Nattiv et al., 2007, "American College of Sports Medicine position stand. The female athlete triad," *Medicine and Science in Sports and Exercise* 39(10): 1867-1882.

Energy availability (EA) (kcal/kg FFM/day) = (EI − EEE) / FFM

where EI = energy intake (kcal/day) and EEE = exercise energy expenditure (kcal/day).

According to data collected in sedentary women, when energy availability is reduced below 30 kcal/kg FFM per day, the body suppresses reproductive function (Loucks and Thuma 2003) and bone formation (Ihle and Loucks 2004). This tends to restore energy balance and extend survival but impairs reproductive and skeletal health. "Calculating Energy Availability in an Active Female" on p. 460 shows how to calculate energy balance and availability and illustrates the differences between a sedentary and an active female of the same age and size.

Disordered Eating and Eating Disorders

The pressure to be thin is so pervasive in our society that it is difficult to differentiate normal from abnormal eating behavior. One fact on which eating disorder specialists agree is that dieting can lead to more severe forms of disordered eating. Thus, the pressure to be thin at any cost can lead some active females to develop disordered eating behaviors (Beals 2004; Beals and Houtkooper 2006). Eating behaviors form a continuum that can range from normal to clinically diagnosed abnormal behaviors. To be diagnosed with a clinical eating disorder, one must meet the criteria outlined by the American Psychiatric Association's (APA) *Diagnostic and Statistical Manual of Mental Disorders (DSM-IV)* (1994) and shown in "Diagnostic Criteria for Anorexia Nervosa, Bulimia Nervosa, and Eating Disorders Not Otherwise Specified (ED-NOS)" on p. 461.

The factors that trigger anorexia nervosa in a female athlete may differ from those that lead to the disorder in a nonathlete, and the early symptoms may differ from those in sedentary people since the disorder affects exercise performance

Calculating Energy Availability in an Active Female

Energy availability is the amount of dietary energy remaining for all other physiological functions after energy has been expended in exercise. When energy availability is too low, the body activates mechanisms that reduce the amount of energy used for cellular maintenance, thermoregulation, growth, and reproduction. For sedentary women, energy intakes ≤30 kcal/kg FFM per day may be the energy threshold below which menstrual dysfunctions occur. In the following we give the calculations for both energy balance and energy availability in an active and a sedentary female of similar size. One can be in energy balance, due to reductions in energy expenditure when energy intake is being restricted, but still have low energy availability.

Energy Balance

Total energy intake (EI) (kcal/day) = Total energy expenditure (TEE) (kcal/day).

Total energy expenditure is composed of the following factors added together: RMR, thermic effect of food (TEF), nonexercise adaptive thermogenesis (NEAT; e.g., activities of daily living), and EEE.

Negative Energy Balance

TEE (kcal/day) > EI (kcal/day).

Low Energy Availability

Total (EI) (kcal/day) – EEE (kcal/day).

The following are examples of low energy availability in a sedentary and an active female of the same age, height, and body composition:

Sedentary Female (20 Years)

Weight: 55 kg (121 lb).

Height: 155 cm (61 in.).

Body mass index = 23 kg/m^2.

Body composition: body fat = 20%; FFM = 44 kg.

EI = 2000 kcal/day.

TEE = 1974 kcal/day.

Energy balance = EI (2000 kcal) – Total EE (1974 kcal); [RMR (1374 kcal) + TEF (200 kcal) + NEAT (400 kcal) + EEE (0 kcal)].

Energy availability: EI (2000 kcal/day) – EEE (0 kcal/day) = 2000 kcal/day or 45 kcal/kg FFM per day.

Active Female Athlete (20 Years)

Weight: 55 kg (121 lb).

Height: 155 cm (61 in.).

Body mass index = 23 kg/m^2.

Body composition: body fat = 20%; FFM = 44 kg.

EI = 2000 kcal/day.

TEE = 2674 kcal/day (1974 + 700 kcal/day running).

EEE = 700 kcal/day running.

Energy Balance = EI (2000 kcal) – Total EE (2674 kcal); [RMR (1374 kcal) + TEF (200 kcal) + NEAT (400 kcal) + EEE (700 kcal)].

Energy Availability = EI (2000 kcal) – EEE (700 kcal) = 1300 kcal/day or 29.5 kcal/kg FFM per day; this means that only 1300 kcal/day is left for RMR (~1374 kcal), TEF (~200 kcal), and NEAT (~400 kcal), which is too low.

EEE = exercise energy expenditure.
RMR = resting metabolic rate.
FFM = fat free mass.

Diagnostic Criteria for Anorexia Nervosa, Bulimia Nervosa, and Eating Disorders Not Otherwise Specified (ED-NOS)

Below are the criteria for the major eating disorders typically seen in active females.

Anorexia Nervosa

- Refusal to maintain body weight at or above a minimally normal weight for age and height (e.g., weight loss leading to maintenance of body weight less than 85% of that expected; or failure to make expected weight gain during period of growth, leading to body weight less than 85% of that expected)

- Intense fear of gaining weight or becoming fat, even though considered underweight by all medical criteria

- Disturbance in the way in which one experiences one's body weight or shape, undue influence of body weight or shape on self-evaluation, or denial of the seriousness of the current low body weight

- In postmenarcheal females, amenorrhea (the absence of at least three consecutive menstrual cycles); a woman is considered to have amenorrhea if her periods occur only when she is given hormones (e.g., estrogen)

Bulimia Nervosa

- Recurrent episodes of binge eating

- Recurrent inappropriate compensatory behavior in order to prevent weight gain, such as self-induced vomiting; misuse of laxatives, diuretics, enemas, or other medications; fasting; or excessive exercise

- Occurrence of binge eating on average at least twice a week for three months

- Undue influence of body shape and weight on self-evaluation (the disturbance does not occur exclusively during episodes of anorexia nervosa)

Eating Disorders Not Otherwise Specified

In 1994, the APA added a new category of disordered eating called eating disorders not otherwise specified (ED-NOS). This category comprises disorders of eating that do not meet the criteria for any specified eating disorder, such as anorexia nervosa or bulimia nervosa. It is also frequently referred to as **subclinical eating disorders.** The criteria for ED-NOS are as follows:

- All the criteria for anorexia nervosa, except the individual has regular menses and weight is within normal range, although weight loss has occurred.

- All the criteria for anorexia nervosa, except that weight is within the normal range although weight loss may have occurred

- All the criteria for bulimia nervosa, except that the binge eating and the use of inappropriate compensatory behaviors occur less than twice a week or have a duration of less than three months

- Occurrence of the regular use of inappropriate compensatory behaviors in an individual with normal body weight after consumption of small amounts of food (e.g., self-induced vomiting after consumption of only two small cookies)

- Repeated chewing and spitting out of food, without swallowing the food

- Recurrent episodes of binge eating in the absence of the regular use of inappropriate compensatory behaviors characteristic of bulimia nervosa

Adapted from American Psychiatric Association, 1994, *Diagnostic and statistical manual of mental disorders (DSM-IV)*, 4th ed. (Washington, DC: American Psychiatric Association).

early on. But the diagnostic symptoms are the same for everyone:

1. People with anorexia nervosa have a "relentless pursuit of thinness" and a "refusal to maintain a body weight at or above a minimal level" that are prerequisites for diagnosis, yet the amount of weight loss required for diagnosis is variable (Garfinkel 2002). Because many female athletes are already lean and have low BMIs, the amount of weight they lose may be less than that observed in the nonathlete.

2. Individuals with anorexia nervosa have an intense fear of gaining weight or of becoming fat; even small amounts of weight gain trigger high stress and anxiety.

3. Individuals with anorexia nervosa also look at their body differently than healthy individuals and place a high value on a "thin" body type.

4. Amenorrhea is a criterion for diagnosis of anorexia nervosa and is due to hypothalamic dysfunction, which results from malnutrition.

Like anorexia nervosa, **bulimia nervosa** has specific characteristics that must be present for diagnosis:

1. There is an uncontrollable desire to overeat or binge on food; however, the quantity of food that constitutes a binge is difficult to define. For practical purposes, a "binge" is usually determined on an individual basis. For a small active female, what constitutes a binge might be quite different than what would constitute a binge for a larger, less active person.

2. Binge eating must also be characterized by a subjective sense of loss of control (Garfinkel 2002). This means that the person feels she cannot control the situation or prevent the binge once it has started.

3. The binge must occur within a discrete time period. This criterion is included to prevent the classification of "continual snacking" or "grazing" as a binge episode. It is less clear, however, how frequently binges must occur before an individual is classified as bulimic. The *DSM-IV* criteria designate that binges must occur on average at least twice a week for three months (APA 1994). An individual need not purge after the binge to be diagnosed with bulimia nervosa.

4. Like individuals with anorexia nervosa, people with bulimia nervosa are highly influenced by body shape and weight in their self-evaluation.

For the female athlete who is pressured to maintain a lean body weight, purging often follows a binge episode. This pattern of disordered eating may begin as an infrequent occurrence when the athlete must deal with unwanted food in a social situation. For example, the team is having a pizza party, and the athlete wants to join in the fun but feels guilty about eating so much food. Thus, what may begin as an isolated incident can develop into a daily event until the athlete is frequently purging after eating, regardless of the volume. Bingeing and purging behaviors can also be triggered by periods of dieting in which the athlete has deprived herself of adequate food and energy for some time or has engaged in other destructive weight loss behaviors (table 15.2). Whatever the factors that trigger the bingeing and purging, the athlete can quickly lose control of her ability to deal with food rationally. Not all athletes engage in vomiting to purge unwanted foods. They may use excessive exercise, laxatives, enemas, diuretics, or fasting to purge the unwanted kilocalories consumed in a binge. For example, after a binge, athletes may increase their daily mileage to equal the "calculated" energy content of the binge, or they may fast for a day or two until they feel they have purged the extra kilocalories (Garfinkel 2002). These destructive behaviors can have long-term health consequences; thus, female athletes need to be taught healthy weight loss or weight maintenance skills (or both) in order to prevent the development of an eating disorder. See "Techniques to Help an Active Individual Identify and Maintain a Healthy Body Weight Throughout the Life Cycle" on p. 457 for guidelines in helping an athlete identify and maintain an ideal body weight for good health and exercise performance.

Eating disorders not otherwise specified (ED-NOS) comprise a cluster of symptoms and abnormal eating behaviors that are not as well defined as those involved with anorexia nervosa or bulimia nervosa. Eating disorders not otherwise specified is diagnosed in an individual whose disordered eating behaviors are serious but do not easily fit into the diagnostic criteria for other eating disorders. Some of the behaviors you might observe are chronic dieting, extremely rigid eating behaviors, body dysmorphic disorder, and binge-eating disorder. The specific characteristics of ED-NOS are outlined in "Diagnostic Criteria for

Table 15.2   Disordered Eating Behaviors and Weight Loss Practices Frequently Used by Female Athletes and the Resulting Health Consequences

Dieting behavior	Health consequences
Fasting or starvation	Loss of lean body mass and bone mineral density (BMD); lower metabolic rate; increased risk of poor nutritional status; poor exercise performance.
Diet pills	Medical side effects such as rapid heart rate, anxiety, inability to concentrate, nervousness, inability to sleep, and dehydration. Any weight lost is quickly regained.
Diuretics (increase water loss from body)	Weight loss is primarily water, and weight is quickly regained once medication is stopped. Dehydration and electrolyte imbalance can be problems. Little fat is lost.
Laxatives (increase water loss from body and increase GI mobility)	Weight loss is primarily water, and weight is quickly regained once laxatives are stopped. Dehydration and electrolyte imbalance can be problems. Little fat is lost. Laxatives can be addictive.
Fat-free diet	Perhaps a lack of essential nutrients, especially fat-soluble vitamins and essential fatty acids. Total energy intake must still be reduced to produce weight loss. Many fat-free convenience foods are highly processed, with a high sugar content and few micronutrients unless they are fortified. Diet is difficult to follow.
Self-induced vomiting	Dehydration and electrolyte imbalances; gastrointestinal problems, especially irritation of the stomach and esophagus; erosion of dental enamel.
Sauna	Dehydration and electrolyte imbalances; weight regained quickly.
Enema	Dehydration and electrolyte imbalances; gastrointestinal problems.
Excessive exercise	Increased risk of overuse injuries, especially stress fractures in women.

GI = gastrointestinal.

Adapted from C.L. Otis, 1998, "Too slim, amenorrheic, fracture-prone: the female athlete triad," *ACSM's Health Fitness Journal* 2(1): 20-25.

Anorexia Nervosa, Bulimia Nervosa, and Eating Disorders Not Otherwise Specified (ED-NOS)" on p. 461.

It appears that many active women have atypical or subclinical eating disorders as evidenced by their preoccupation with food, kilocalories, body shape, and weight (Beals and Manore 1994, 1998, 1999, 2002; Fairburn and Walsh 2002; Sundgot-Borgen and Torstveit 2004). However, these women do not meet all the criteria necessary to classify them with a clinical eating disorder such as anorexia nervosa or bulimia nervosa (Sundgot-Borgen 1993, 1994; Sundgot-Borgen and Torstveit 2004), but may meet the criteria for ED-NOS. How do you know if a person has an atypical or subclinical eating disorder or ED-NOS? As previously mentioned, the APA recognizes certain atypical eating disorders such as ED-NOS (see p. 461). Women with an atypical eating disorder may or may not develop a clinical eating disorder, but they need to realize that their dieting behaviors can be harmful to their health (Fairburn and Walsh 2002). The trigger factors that may predispose an active woman to an eating disorder can include the following (Beals and Manore 1999; Beals 2004; Sundgot-Borgen 1994):

- Prolonged periods of dieting
- Frequent weight fluctuations
- A sudden increase in training volume and intensity
- A traumatic stressful event or high levels of stress (e.g., injury, loss of coach, stressful family event)
- Pressure placed on the female to maintain or achieve a low body weight

These trigger factors can be a warning to health professionals, coaches, and parents that an athlete is struggling with body image issues or may have a subclinical eating disorder that could progress to a more serious eating disorder. Active females with subclinical or atypical eating disorders are at risk for poor nutritional status since they generally restrict energy intake, frequently avoid animal products, and strictly limit their fat intake. Beals and Manore (1998) examined nutritional status in 24 female athletes classified as having a subclinical eating disorder compared to 24 control female athletes. Athletes with subclinical eating disorders had significantly lower energy, protein, and fat intakes, and many consumed less than

66% of the RDA for 8 (calcium, iron, magnesium, zinc, folate, niacin, vitamin B_6, and B_{12}) of the 11 micronutrients examined. Approximately half of the athletes with a subclinical eating disorder had one or more parameters indicating low iron status and had iron intakes that were less than the RDA. None of the control group had low iron intakes, yet some still presented with poor iron status. Five of the control athletes were in stage I iron depletion (low serum ferritin) compared to seven of the athletes with a subclinical eating disorder. Supplementation and fortified foods (sport foods and cereals) contributed significantly to the total micronutrient intakes of all the athletes, helping to improve overall nutritional status in spite of poor dietary intakes—yet the athletes with subclinical eating disorders were still not getting adequate energy and protein to sustain their high level of physical activity. Low energy intake levels in some female athletes become even more harmful if the athletes use excessive exercise to purge the body of unwanted energy intake.

Peterson and colleagues (1995) demonstrated how dieting and severe energy restriction in active people can increase the incidence of disordered eating behaviors. They examined the presence of bulimic weight loss behaviors in individuals enrolled in three weight management programs:

1. A military weight management program (n = 51)
2. A civilian weight management program (n = 53)
3. A comparison military (normal weight) group (n = 51)

The military weight management group consisted of U.S. Air Force (USAF) members who were mandated to enroll and required to lose weight or face possible administrative action or discharge. People in the civilian weight management group were volunteers. The study included both males (n = 78) and females (n = 77). Results showed that the military weight management group engaged in bulimic weight loss behaviors two to five times more often than the comparison groups. They engaged in vomiting, strenuous exercise, and use of the sauna or steam room for weight loss four times as often as the civilian weight management group. There was no statistically significant difference between men and women within the military weight management group in bulimic weight loss behaviors. For overeating behaviors, however, women engaged in binge eating twice as often as

men (males = 42%; females = 81%). Finally, more people (53%) in the military weight management group reported losing at least 10 lb (4.5 kg) in a month compared to the other groups (18%); yet more people from this group also regained at least 5 lb (2.3 kg) in the first week after the diet was over. At least 41% of the military weight management group reported such a gain, compared to only 27% in the civilian weight management group and 14% in the control group. The authors concluded that bulimic weight loss behaviors might develop in people who feel extreme pressure to lose weight. Thus, under pressures to lose weight or face possible discharge, these USAF members resorted to excessive and unhealthy weight loss measures. This study can easily be applied to female athletes who are required to lose weight to make the team or to please a coach or parent. When the pressure and stakes are high for weight loss to occur, female athletes frequently turn to harmful dieting practices to achieve their goal.

Menstrual Dysfunction

Diet and exercise can negatively affect reproductive and metabolic hormones; the most severe consequence is amenorrhea, in which reproductive hormones are severely suppressed. In the amenorrhea associated with anorexia nervosa, starvation is severe enough to shut down reproductive capabilities. Note, however, that an athlete need not have an eating disorder to sustain exercise-induced changes in her menstrual cycle. See "Normal Menstrual Cycle" for a description of a normal menstrual cycle and the hormonal changes that occur over a typical cycle. A growing body of evidence suggests that exercise-induced amenorrhea, as well as other reproductive hormone abnormalities seen in active women, may be due in part to periods of energy deficiency (Dueck, Manore, and Matt 1996; Loucks 2004; Fredericson and Kent 2005). Three factors contribute to inadequate energy availability in active females:

- High energy expenditure
- Low energy intake compared to energy expenditure
- High psychological and physical stress, which can reduce energy intake while increasing energy expenditure

Exercise-induced changes in the menstrual cycle may be an energy-conserving strategy to protect more important biological and reproductive

Normal Menstrual Cycle

The normal menstrual cycle is typically characterized by two phases that are separated by ovulation at midcycle (figure 15.4).

The beginning phase, or the **follicular phase,** is marked by the onset of menstruation. During this phase of the cycle, **follicle stimulating hormone (FSH)** plays an integral role in the recruitment of a single follicle. As the follicle grows, it begins to secrete **estradiol** (E), which acts in a positive feedback loop to stimulate the release of **luteinizing hormone (LH).** The end of the follicular phase is marked by ovulation, which typically occurs on days 15 through 18 and is characterized by a large increase in LH. The hormonal events associated with the follicular phase serve to ensure that ovulation and fertilization take place. After ovulation, the second phase of the cycle begins. This stage, called the **luteal phase,** is characterized by increases in ovarian production of estradiol and **progesterone** (Prog), which act in a negative feedback loop to inhibit LH and FSH release. After ovulation, the cells remaining after the egg is released from the follicle are called the **corpus luteum,** which produces estradiol and progesterone. These ovarian steroids play an integral role in preparing the uterus for implantation if fertilization occurs. Without fertilization, there is a rapid decrease in estradiol and progesterone as the corpus luteum becomes atrophied. The intricate series of hormonal events associated with normal menstrual function can be easily disrupted by physiological, metabolic, or psychological stress. Furthermore, the intensity of the stressor can have variable effects on the level and magnitude of disruption.

Reprinted, by permission, from C.A. Dueck, M.M. Manore, and K.S. Matt, 1996, "Role of energy balance in athletic menstrual dysfunction," *International Journal of Sport and Nutrition* 6: 165-190.

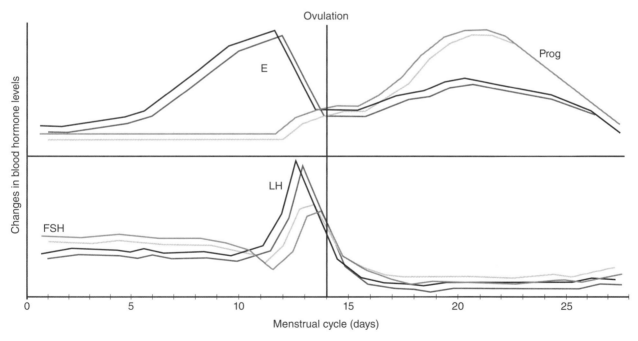

Figure 15.4 Normal menstrual cycle showing changes in plasma levels of hormones. Days 1 through 15 represent the follicular phase and days 15 through 28 represent the luteal phase; they are divided by ovulation at the midpoint of the cycle.

Adapted, by permission, from C.A. Dueck, M.M. Manore, and K.S. Matt, 1996, "Role of energy balance in athletic menstrual dysfunction," *International Journal of Sport and Nutrition* 6: 165-190.

processes (Dueck, Manore, and Matt 1996; Dueck, Matt et al. 1996). The prevalence of exercise-induced menstrual dysfunction may be as high as 50% in female athletes. Thus, the possibility that a female athlete may have some type of menstrual dysfunction should not be ignored (Nattiv et al. 2007). See "Common Types of Menstrual Dysfunction Seen in Active Women" on p. 467.

Researchers examining the effect of negative energy balance or low energy availability on the menstrual cycle and reproductive hormones have asked the following research questions:

- What is the role of dieting (energy restriction) alone on menstrual status?
- What is the role of exercise alone on menstrual status?
- What is the combined role of diet and exercise on menstrual status?

Energy deprivation can alter the hormonal profiles and the menstrual cycles of healthy women. The degree of menstrual dysfunction that occurs with dieting depends on a number of factors that can affect energy availability, such as the magnitude of the energy restriction, the body's level of energy reserves, and the initial hormonal status before dieting begins. In other words, if an individual already has some type of menstrual dysfunction, dieting may lead to amenorrhea more quickly than in someone who begins a diet with normal menstrual function. Kurzer and Calloway (1986) fed six healthy women (104-130% of ideal body weight) two diets differing only in energy intake. All subjects reported normal menstrual cycles during the nine months before beginning the study. The first diet provided a typical energy intake (40 kcal/kg body weight); the second provided 41% the intake of the first diet (17 kcal/kg body weight). Both diets lasted the length of the menstrual cycle plus one week; all subjects received their food daily from a metabolic unit. Weight loss on the low-energy diet ranged from 7.0 to 14.5 lb (3.2-6.7 kg) during the study. The two leanest women lost the most weight and became anovulatory and amenorrheic during this period. Thus, in this study the leanest subjects displayed the greatest menstrual dysfunction when placed on an energy-restrictive diet. Their bodies appeared to respond to low energy reserves in the presence of energy restriction by suppressing the ability for reproduction. This is supported by data showing that amenorrhea becomes more common during times of starvation.

Research also shows that energy restriction (e.g., low kilocalorie intake) plus exercise regimens severe enough to produce significant weight loss produces the greatest changes in menstrual function. Increasing energy expenditure while decreasing energy intake creates a negative energy balance, which requires the body to draw on energy reserves to cover the cost of exercise. This combination has a more negative effect on menstrual status than just exercise alone. Williams and colleagues (1995) illustrated this point while examining the effect of exercise—with and without energy restriction—on LH secretion. They studied four moderately trained normally menstruating women over three consecutive menstrual cycles during the follicular phase (refer to "Normal Menstrual Cycle" on p. 465 and to figure 15.4). Subjects experienced the greatest decrease in LH during the period of diet plus high exercise as compared to the other two periods (control period, high-exercise period). These results suggest that abrupt increases in training volume lead to a disruption in LH secretion if subjects are restricting energy and are in negative energy balance. Furthermore, only the period of diet plus high exercise produced significant weight loss, while weight was maintained in the high-exercise-only period. These results support the earlier work of Bullen and colleagues (1985), who reported that abrupt increases in physical activity resulting in weight loss (i.e., negative energy balance) are accompanied by a higher incidence of menstrual abnormalities than when exercise is accompanied by weight maintenance. To summarize, combined diet and exercise appears to have a more negative effect on menstrual status than just exercise alone or diet alone.

We now know that the menstrual dysfunction associated with sport is multifaceted, and that for any one individual a number of factors may be involved. However, the primary factor contributing to menstrual dysfunction appears to be low energy availability. In addition, several other lifestyle stressors have been identified as predisposing factors for the onset of menstrual dysfunction—including inadequate dietary habits, a history of weight fluctuations, a rigorous training regimen, and the social pressures associated with competition. In the past, researchers thought that inadequate body fat was the primary endogenous stressor contributing to amenorrhea (Frisch and McArthur 1974). Although there is no critical level of body fat required of all women for the maintenance of menstruation, one's level of body

Common Types of Menstrual Dysfunction Seen in Active Women

- **Luteal phase defects** are usually characterized by low estrogen concentrations early in the follicular phase with or without a shortened luteal phase length. Since the total menstrual cycle length may be normal, however, many women do not notice a change in menstrual status and report that they have normal menstrual cycles.

- **Anovulation** is the absence of ovulation, which can occur in the presence of menstrual bleeding; however, the menstrual cycle can be shorter (less than 21 days) or longer (35-50 days) than normal. Longer menstrual cycles are usually referred to as oligomenorrhea.

- **Oligomenorrhea** refers to irregular, longer menstrual cycles—for instance, a woman may have only six cycles per year instead of 12. Many active women have irregular cycles during periods of strenuous exercise training but return to more normal cycles when they reduce training levels. These individuals may ovulate infrequently or not at all, and reproductive hormones are usually suppressed.

- **Amenorrhea** is the absence of menstrual periods. **Primary amenorrhea** is the absence of menstruation by the age of 15 years in a girl who has secondary sex characteristics (American Society for Reproductive Medicine Practice Committee 2004), while **secondary amenorrhea** is the absence of the menstrual period after the beginning of menarche (Nattiv et al. 2007). These individuals do not ovulate, have low levels of estrogen, and lack the spike in LH that results in ovulation. The most common causes of amenorrhea are pregnancy and menopause. Both exercise- and anorexia nervosa–induced amenorrhea are forms of **hypothalamic amenorrhea.** This type of amenorrhea is characterized by a decrease in **gonadotropin releasing hormone (GnRH)** from the hypothalamus. Gonadotropin releasing hormone stimulates the pituitary gland to release LH, which in turn signals the ovaries to produce estrogen and progesterone. The result of depressed GnRH concentrations is that no ovulation or menstrual bleeding occurs.

fat stores cannot be totally ignored. Leptin, a hormone produced by the adipose tissue, appears to be a metabolic signal between fat stores and the hypothalamus (Thong et al. 2000). Leptin levels are highly correlated with body fat, and they decrease with weight loss. Finally, amenorrheic athletes have significantly lower leptin levels compared to eumenorrheic athletes (Thong et al. 2000). Thus, levels of body fat stores may be an important determinant in the etiology of athletic menstrual dysfunction. The total energy reservoir includes the amount of energy stored in glycogen and body fat and the energy consumed daily through food. This available energy must then be balanced against the daily energy expenditure. Athletes with the lowest energy stores may have less tolerance for low energy availability for an extended time and be at greater risk for developing menstrual dysfunction.

To more clearly demonstrate the effect that strenuous exercise has on menstrual function,

read "Case Study: Exercise-Associated Amenorrhea" on p. 468. Although the athlete in this study was not purposely restricting energy intake, her energy intake was not adequate to cover her high EEE. If an athlete presents with exercise-induced amenorrhea, one of the first steps in treating the disorder is to improve her energy availability by increasing her energy intake (250-350 kcal/day) and decreasing energy expenditure by 10% to 20% (Otis 1998).

Bone Health

The final component of the female athlete triad is bone health. If amenorrhea is allowed to persist, the resulting low or altered levels of reproductive and metabolic hormones can lead to loss of BMD. This in turn increases the risk of low bone mass or **osteoporosis,** both when the athlete is young and later in life. Reduced BMD also increases the risk of musculoskeletal injuries such as stress

Case Study: Exercise-Associated Amenorrhea

A 19-year-old amenorrheic runner reported the loss of menstrual function a year earlier when she switched from sprinting to distance events. After switching sports, she reported difficulty maintaining weight and had lost 6.5 lb (3 kg) during the previous track season. She complained of chronic fatigue, poor performance, and high frequency of illness and injury. She had been amenorrheic for 14 consecutive months before seeking help and participating in a research project designed to improve energy balance. Her running schedule at that time included morning and afternoon runs four days a week, and she lifted weights three days a week. She then began a 15-week nutrition and exercise intervention program designed to increase energy intake by 360 kcal/day (one can of a meal replacement per day) and to reduce energy expenditure by adding one day of rest per week. Here are her statistics for body weight, composition, and energy-nutrient intakes before and after intervention:

	Before intervention	After intervention (15 weeks)
Weight (kg)	48.2	50.9
Body mass index (kg/m²)	19.1	20.1
Body fat (%)	8.2	14.4
Total energy intake (kcal/day)[a]	3045	3683
Total energy expenditure (kcal/day)[a]	3200	3000
Energy balance (kcal/day) (intake − expenditure)[a]	−155	+683
BMD (% of age-matched norm for lumbar spine)[b]	111	113
Menstrual status[c]	Amenorrheic	Amenorrheic

[a] Estimates based on seven-day diet records and activity logs.
[b] Body composition and bone mineral density (BMD) measured by dual-energy X-ray absorptiometry.
[c] Normal menstrual status returned after the athlete had followed the intervention program for an additional three months.

Although the intervention program improved the young woman's energy balance, menstrual function did not return until she had followed the intervention program for an additional three months after the 15-week intervention. Hormonal changes during the 15-week intervention revealed increased fasting levels of LH and decreased cortisol. The athlete reported dramatic increases in performance and set personal best times in some of her events. She went on to receive a track scholarship from a major university.

Summary: This young woman had exercise-induced amenorrhea. She did not have an eating disorder, and her amenorrhea had not yet resulted in significant reductions in bone loss. Although her BMD was higher than age-matched norms, we do not know what her BMD could have been had she not been amenorrheic for 14 months. The athlete complained of weight loss and poor exercise performance. Improvement in energy balance and a small increase in body weight during a 15-week intervention period began to improve her reproductive hormonal profile. She reported improved exercise performance and reduced fatigue as a result of the intervention; however, an additional three months on the intervention program was required to bring about menses. This case study demonstrates that nonpharmacological treatment of exercise-induced amenorrhea can be successful if the athlete is willing to eat more, gain small amounts of weight, and reduce exercise training.

Adapted, by permission, from C.A. Dueck, M.M. Manore, and J.S. Skinner, 1996, "Treatment of athletic amenorrhea with a diet and training intervention program," *International Journal of Sport and Nutrition* 6: 24-40.

fractures. See chapter 13 for more detailed definitions and descriptions of osteoporosis. Note that in the context of the female athlete triad, the term "osteoporosis" is used loosely to represent the loss of bone mass or the decrease in bone deposition rather than the condition as strictly defined in chapter 13.

Amenorrheic athletes typically display reduced levels of estradiol and progesterone and have hormonal profiles more like those of postmenopausal women than those of their age-matched eumenorrheic counterparts (Drinkwater et al. 1984; Redman and Loucks 2005). Thus, despite the established positive effects of exercise training on bone, exercise may not be able to compensate entirely for the negative effects of estrogen, progesterone, and leptin deficiency. The estrogen deficiency observed in exercise-induced menstrual dysfunction may be different from that associated with menopause, in which bone becomes more sensitive to the calcium-mobilizing effect of parathyroid hormone (Kaufman et al. 2002). With menopause, a greater number of resorptive sites are established and a gradual loss of bone mass occurs. However, with exercise-induced amenorrhea, reproductive hormones may play only a small role in the reduced bone density (Kaufman et al. 2002). The primary contributors to low bone mass in these women may be low energy intake (Zanker and Swaine 1998) and low bone-building nutrients typically associated with malnutrition.

Research shows that lumbar BMD is reduced ~14% in amenorrheic athletes compared to eumenorrheic athletes (Dueck, Manore, and Matt 1996) and as much as 27% compared to that in sedentary women with normal cycles (Cann et al. 1984). However, not every amenorrheic athlete experiences decreased BMD. The effect of estrogen and energy deficiency on an athlete's BMD may depend in part on the workloads placed on the bone, how long she has been amenorrheic, how long her level of energy availability has been low, and the level of bone-building nutrients she consumes currently and has consumed in the past. With sufficiently high exercise stress, amenorrheic athletes may still be able to maintain BMD similar to or even higher than age-matched norms for a period of time (see "Case Study: Exercise-Associated Amenorrhea," p. 468). The degree to which exercise-induced amenorrhea influences BMD depends on a number of factors:

- Current age
- Age when amenorrhea occurred

- Length of time an individual has been amenorrheic
- Current body size and composition
- Type of exercise engaged in
- Dietary intakes of bone-building micronutrients
- Dietary and drug factors that decrease total body calcium levels
- Total energy intake, level of energy availability
- Baseline blood cortisol concentrations
- Genetics

Thus, despite the positive stimulus of exercise on bone, the hormonal and dietary changes associated with menstrual dysfunction compromise BMD and increase the risk for fracture. Brukner and Bennell (1997) reviewed 11 studies comparing stress fractures in female athletes with and without menstrual dysfunction. They found that the risk of stress fracture was much higher in athletes with menstrual dysfunction (52%) than in their eumenorrheic counterparts (28%) (figure 15.5). This increased risk of stress fracture not only jeopardizes a woman's athletic career but also increases her risk for bone fracture after menopause.

As already mentioned, not all data have shown reduced BMD in amenorrheic athletes compared to active eumenorrheic females. Wilmore and colleagues (1992) found no differences in lumbar

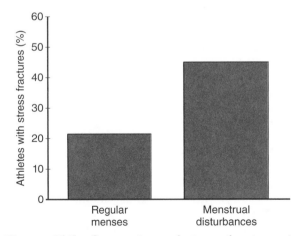

Figure 15.5 Comparison of stress fractures in athletes with and without menstrual disturbances in 11 cross-sectional studies.

Adapted from P. Brukne and K. P. Bennell, 1997, "Stress fractures in female athletes: diagnosis, management and rehabilitation," *Sports Medicine* 24: 419-429.

spine BMD between amenorrheic and eumenorrheic runners. Dueck, Matt, and colleagues (1996) even reported a higher BMD in the femoral neck of an endurance-trained amenorrheic athlete compared to her eumenorrheic teammates. Finally, Meyer and colleagues (2004) found no differences in BMD in oligo- or amenorrheic and eumenorrheic winter sport athletes at any skeletal site. These discrepancies illustrate the need to consider several important issues when interpreting bone density data. The development of peak bone mass is not determined solely by the levels of estrogen and progesterone during puberty and the ensuing 10 to 15 years of musculoskeletal growth and development. Bone mineral density is greatly influenced by genetics, dietary factors, and specific bone loading patterns experienced in a particular sport. For example, adequate intakes of energy, protein, calcium, vitamin D, vitamin K, and magnesium are all important for bone formation. Conversely, alcohol and smoking have negative impacts on bone.

The duration (e.g. number of years of participation) and type of sport in which an individual has participated may also affect the accretion of bone mass. Sports that significantly load the bones, such as gymnastics, stimulate BMD. Gymnasts appear to have significantly higher BMD than matched controls and other female athletes participating in endurance sports (Kirchner et al. 1995; Robinson et al. 1995; Creighton et al. 2001)—even when the gymnasts report menstrual dysfunction (Robinson et al. 1995). The actual BMD that these athletes *could* have achieved if menstrual dysfunction had not occurred is unknown. Remember, however, that even gymnasts can lose bone mass if amenorrhea persists for an extended period of time.

Treatment

Recognition and treatment of an athlete with one or more of the components of the female athlete triad (low energy availability, menstrual dysfunction, poor bone health) can be difficult, especially if the athlete is less than candid when questioned about the symptoms. For this reason, treating an athlete requires a multidisciplinary approach; the sports medicine team, sport dietitian, exercise physiologist, psychologist, coach, trainer, parents, friends of the athlete, and the athlete all must work together. If the athlete is having trouble with weight and body shape issues, dealing with these issues before they develop into something more serious is important. Table 15.2 outlines some

of the dieting practices and disordered eating behaviors that may precede the development of an eating disorder. You should learn to look for these symptoms in female athletes. Some of the warning signs that a female athlete may be at risk for developing one or more of the components of the female athlete triad are listed on this page.

If someone has one or more of the components of the female athlete triad, her level of participation in her sport should be determined by the treating health professional team and should be supported by the coach, the family, and the athlete. Every sports medicine team should have a standard procedure for preventing and treating disorders of the female athlete triad. "Case Study: Team Management Approach to Treatment of the Female Athlete Triad" (p. 471) outlines a **team management** approach to treating an athlete suffering from an eating disorder that has become severe enough to disrupt normal menstrual function and decrease bone density.

The decision to use hormone replacement treatment with a female athlete who presents with poor BMD is controversial but may still be appropriate if she is unwilling to change lifestyle factors that will restore menstrual function (Liu and Lebrun 2006). As with any health problem, prevention is the best treatment. It is imperative that the sports medicine team learn to recognize the risk factors of the female athlete triad and then begin to educate athletes, coaches, and parents about those risk factors.

Warning Signs of the Female Athlete Triad

1. Excessive dieting for weight loss, large fluctuations in body weight, or too much weight loss
2. Irregular or absent menstrual periods
3. Stress fractures, especially recurrent stress fractures
4. Self-esteem and mood that appear to be dictated by body weight and shape
5. Compulsive overexercise

Adapted from C.L. Otis, 1998, "Too slim, amenorrheic, fracture-prone: the female athlete triad," *ACSM's Health Fitness Journal* 2(1): 20-25; A. Nattiv et al., 2007, "The female athlete triad," *Medicine and Science in Sports and Exercise* 39(10): 1867-1882; M.M. Manore, L.C. Kam, and A.B. Loucks, 2007, "The female athlete triad: Components, nutrition issues and health consequences," *Journal of Sports Science* 25(S2):S61-S71.

Highlight

Case Study: Team Management Approach to Treatment of the Female Athlete Triad

A 20-year-old female gymnast returns from summer break, having lost 15 lb (6.8 kg) to reach a current weight of 85 lb (38.6 kg). Current body BMI is 15.6 kg/m², well below the typical BMI of gymnasts, which is 19 to 20 kg/m². She has not menstruated for four months. After two weeks of preseason conditioning, she comes to the training room with right shin pain. She reveals that she has been restricting her energy intake to 500 to 800 kcal/day and thinks the ideal body weight for her 62 in. (157.5 cm) frame is 75 lb (34.1 kg) (BMI = 13.75 kg/m²). Her coach, trainer, and team physician, however, believe that her ideal body weight is closer to 100 to 105 lb (45.5-47.7 kg). She reports that she had menarche at the age of 15 years and had fairly regular menstrual periods from age 16 years until four months ago. She has no history of bone or overuse injury.

Her physical exam reveals that she is quite thin, has facial and body lanugo (fine, soft hair that often appears in anorexia nervosa or starvation), but she has stable vital signs. An extremity exam reveals local tenderness to palpation on the midshaft of the tibia. Her laboratory results are normal except for low FSH and low estradiol, which are consistent with hypothalamic amenorrhea. A bone scan is positive for a tibia stress fracture.

Treatment: Proposed Role of a Sports Medicine Physician

First, obtain a more detailed history regarding the athlete's recent weight loss and psychological well-being, as well as her insight into the problem. After establishing a relationship with the athlete, confront her with the problem and facilitate getting her into a program involving a psychologist and sport dietitian who have expertise in working with disordered eating in athletes. Help her understand and agree to a written contract that details the steps she must take for continued participation in her sport. The focus of the contract is on optimal health and on helping the athlete to compete in a safe and healthy manner. For example, the contract may include specific increment goals for weight increases, such as 1/2 to 1 lb/week (0.5 kg), until she achieves the goal of an established healthy weight range.

Perform a more detailed physical exam and pelvic exam if the athlete has not had one recently. If the results of the medical exam are consistent with hypothalamic, hypoestrogenic amenorrhea, you might recommend oral contraceptive pills. You might recommend a calcium intake of 1500 mg/day and a vitamin D intake of 400 to 800 IU/day, and you should continue to monitor the progress of the athlete regarding her contract and her interactions with the sport dietitian and psychologist. Her training will need to change to non-weight-bearing activities because of her stress fracture, and her daily exercises will need to be monitored to ensure that her energy expenditure does not exceed her energy intake.

Treatment: Proposed Role of a Sport Dietitian

First, discuss with the athlete her weight history, her current weight, and what she wants to weigh. Since the optimal weight for a 62 in. (157.5 cm) gymnast is typically around 100 to 105 lb (45.5-47.7 kg), remind the athlete that her current weight of 85 lb (38.6 kg) is too low. Show her pictures of anorexic people and point out the muscle wasting that occurs with this disease. Also show pictures of healthy athletes and emphasize that the goal of treatment is to help her be lean, fit, healthy, and at peace with food. It is important to assure her that you are *not* trying to "fatten her up." You might want to take baseline body composition measurements to be used for future reference to show improvements in body composition as the woman rebuilds her body. It is important to discuss with her how she feels about her body and assure her that she is not fat, based on her body composition data. Discuss how food is not the problem but rather a symptom of some unhappiness in her life. Emphasize the importance of food to fuel the body and to provide adequate energy to cover the energy costs of daily living (e.g., 1200 kcal/day for sleep, 500 kcal/day for daily activities, 500 kcal/day for gymnastics). This should help her understand that her current energy intake of 500 to 800 kcal/day is far below her body's needs and can harm both her body and her ability to be a successful athlete. Calculate with her the grams of protein, fat, and carbohydrate she requires per day and design a healthy eating plan.

(continued)

This eating plan should *gradually* increase the athlete's energy intake to accommodate total energy expenditure and to improve weight gain. The initial amount of energy added per day may vary from as little as an extra 100 kcal per meal (e.g., a yogurt for breakfast, a banana for a preexercise snack, etc.) to an additional 400 to 500 kcal per meal. The integration of foods that the athlete avoids or considers forbidden should occur gradually so that she is not overwhelmed.

One goal of nutrition counseling is to move the athlete away from the fear that food is the fattening enemy and to help her see food as a fuel for her muscles so she can become a better athlete. You might ask her, "Are you training to improve your performance or to burn off kilocalories? What are you invested in? What are your goals? Do you think that you are ready to let go of the anorexia and be a healthy athlete?"

Another goal of nutrition counseling is to educate the athlete about the best ways to fuel her body. Make it clear that you can provide information, but that she must choose to put the information into practice. For example, if an anorexic athlete feels safe eating only broccoli, bagels, pretzels, and rice cakes, point out that there is little protein, calcium, iron, or zinc in these foods. All nutrients are important for top performance; and a balanced diet, complete with protein-rich foods and dairy products, can provide these nutrients.

Subsequent visits should include discussion of the athlete's fear of food and her drive to eat the perfect diet and have a perfect body. Make it clear to the athlete that she should discuss these issues in her sessions with the psychologist. Monitor the gradual increase in energy intake and food choices. Emphasize all the benefits of better eating habits—improvements in her energy level, health, sleeping ability, ability to concentrate, and body warmth, as well as better workouts. Although the approach used in nutrition counseling will vary from person to person, remember that many anorexic athletes are preoccupied with energy intake (kcal/day). Encourage the athlete to eat a variety of foods including some fat. You might also encourage her to eat with others. If she eats alone, she is more likely to talk herself out of eating enough. If she is with a supportive friend she trusts, she may feel safer eating all the food.

Treatment: Proposed Role of the Psychologist

First, it is important to find out what the athlete is struggling with in her life, such as relationships, career choices, or values. It is also helpful to identify the sources of stress in her life. Next, it is important to identify her motivation for treatment. Does she see a problem? Is she concerned? Or is she seeking treatment only because a coach, parent, or physician is forcing the issue? Does she see the treatment team members as resources or simply as authority figures? These are important questions that need to be addressed, since her view of the treatment and of the health care team can affect her compliance. For example, if she sees the physician or dietitian as authority figures, she may be very passive-aggressive toward them. The physician needs to know that the patient may not be motivated for treatment even if she is smiling in the office. She may have every intention of doing what she promises, but when she is by herself she may not eat as she's supposed to, or she may not report the times she's purging. She may do a lot of different things to cloak her behavior, like water-binge before an appointment at which she is being weighed. Anorexic athletes generally are not deceitful, but they can feel extremely threatened and may therefore hide maladaptive weight control behaviors. Treat each client as unique and develop individualized plans. Final note: The medical management team needs to communicate regarding the treatment of the athlete so that all are in agreement.

Return to Play

The athlete can return to team play or competition only after she has received clearance from the medical management team. Even after the stress fracture is healed, the athlete may need to continue cross-training with a gradual return to weight-bearing activities. The physician should continue to monitor her medical care and make sure that she is continuing to see the sport dietitian and the psychologist.

Adapted from E. Joy et al., 1997, "Team management of the female athlete triad. Part 2: Optimal treatment and prevention tactics," *Physician and Sportsmedicine* 25(4): 55-69.

CHAPTER IN REVIEW

There is increasing pressure on women, especially those in developed countries, to be thin or thinner. This pressure to achieve and maintain a low body weight leads to potentially harmful patterns of chronic dieting, which can affect long-term health. The health consequences of chronic dieting may include poor energy and nutrient intakes, poor nutritional status, decreased RMR and total daily energy expenditure, increased psychological stress, increased risk of developing a clinical eating disorder, and increased risk of exercise-induced amenorrhea. If the pressures to be thin are high,

a female athlete may develop the syndromes of the female athlete triad (disordered eating, amenorrhea, osteoporosis). Strategies to help active women get off the dieting bandwagon require the identification of an appropriate and healthy body weight, good eating and exercise habits, and techniques for maintaining these habits throughout the life cycle.

Female athletes need to be educated regarding the adverse effects of the female athlete triad. Athletes also need to know that a menstrual dysfunction can occur in the absence of an eating disorder. The most successful way to treat exercise-associated menstrual dysfunction, or the health problems of the female athlete triad, is to prevent them.

Key Concepts

1. Understand the energy and nutrient requirements of active women.

In active women, energy intake must cover the energy demands of daily living, exercise energy expenditure, reproductive function, building and repair of muscle tissue, and growth in young women. Active women frequently restrict energy intake to achieve a lean body for their sport or for social acceptance. If female athletes restrict energy intake too severely (especially in the presence of high energy expenditure), they increase their risks for one or more of the following health problems: poor macro- and micronutrient intakes, decreased metabolic rate, poor BMD, poor exercise performance, and one or more of the disorders of the female athlete triad.

2. Identify the components of the female athlete triad and discuss its treatment.

The female athlete triad is a serious syndrome that consists of three medical disorders frequently seen in active females: disordered eating and energy availability, menstrual dysfunction, and poor bone health. Each of these disorders exists on a continuum ranging from normal to severe. An athlete who has one disorder of the triad should be screened for the others. Treatment of the female athlete triad requires a multidisciplinary approach since it generally involves medical, nutritional, and psychological interventions plus changes in training and sport participation. Thus, depending on the severity of the problem, one or more of the following individuals or groups may be involved in the treatment: sports medicine team, sport dietitian, exercise physiologist, psychologist, coach, trainer, physical therapist, parents, and friends of the athlete. As with any health problem, prevention is the best treatment; thus, screening for the triad in active females is imperative.

Key Terms

amenorrhea 467

anorexia nervosa 459

anovulation 467

bone mineral density (BMD) 453

bulimia nervosa 462

corpus luteum 465

Additional Information

Beals KA. Disordered eating among athletes. A comprehensive guide for health professionals. Champaign, IL: Human Kinetics, 2004.

> This book addresses the nature and scope of disordered eating in athletes, effects of disordered eating, and methods for managing disordered eating in athletes.

Heaney RP. The vitamin D requirement in health and disease. J Steroid Biochem Mol Biol 2005;97:13-19.

> This paper provides an overview of the various functions of vitamin D in the body and the importance of vitamin D for health, especially for muscles and bones.

Manore MM. Dietary recommendations and athletic menstrual dysfunction. Sports Med 2002;32(14):887-901.

> An in-depth overview of how the energy and nutrient intakes of active eumenorrheic women differ from those of active amenorrheic women.

Nattiv A, Loucks AB, Manore MM, Sanborn CF, Sundgot-Borgen J, Warren MP. American College of Sports Medicine position stand. The female athlete triad. Med Sci Sports Exerc Oct 2007;39(10):1867-1882.

> The first position stand on the female athlete triad was written in 1997. This position stand is an update on the research literature since the first paper was written and focuses on components of the triad, mechanisms, assessment, and treatment.

References

American Psychiatric Association (APA). Diagnostic and statistical manual of mental disorders (DSM-IV), 4th ed. Washington, DC: American Psychiatric Association, 1994.

American Society for Reproductive Medicine Practice Committee. Current evaluation of amenorrhea. Fertil Steril 2004;82:266-272.

Anderson JJB, Stender M, Rondano P, Bishop L, Duckett AB. Nutrition and bone in physical activity and sport. In: Wolinsky I ed. Nutrition in exercise and sport. Boca Raton, FL: CRC Press, 1998;219-244.

Beals KA. Disordered eating among athletes. A comprehensive guide for health professionals. Champaign, IL: Human Kinetics, 2004.

Beals KA, Houtkooper L. Disordered eating in athletes. In: Burke L, Deakin V eds. Clinical sports nutrition. Sydney: McGraw-Hill, 2006;201-226.

Beals KA, Manore MM. The prevalence and consequences of subclinical eating disorders in female athletes. Int J Sport Nutr 1994;4:175-195.

Beals KA, Manore MM. Nutritional status of female athletes with subclinical eating disorders. J Am Diet Assoc 1998;98:419-425.

Beals KA, Manore MM. Subclinical eating disorders in physically active women. Clin Sports Med 1999;14(3):14-29.

Beals KA, Manore MM. Disorders of the female athlete triad among college athletes. Int J Sport Nutr Exerc Metab 2002;12:281-293.

Beals K, Manore MM. Nutritional considerations for the female athlete. In: Spurway N, MacLaren D eds. Advances in sport and exercise science series: nutrition and sport. Philadelphia: Elsevier, 2007;187-206.

Billon WE. Folate. In: Wolinsky I, Driskell JA eds. Sport nutrition: vitamins and trace minerals. Boca Raton, FL: CRC Press, 2006;93-110.

Bischoff-Ferrari HA, Bawson-Hughes B, Willet WW, Staehelin HB, Bazemore MG, Zee RY, Wong JB. Effect of vitamin D on falls. A meta-analysis. JAMA 2004;291:1999-2006.

Brukner P, Bennell K. Stress fractures in female athletes: diagnosis, management and rehabilitation. Sports Med 1997;24:419-429.

Bullen BA, Skrinar GS, Beitins IZ, Von Mering G, Turnbull BA, McArthur JW. Induction of menstrual disorders by strenuous exercise in untrained women. N Engl J Med 1985;1312:1349-1353.

Burke L. Nutrition for recovery and training and competition. In: Burke L, Deakin V eds. Clinical sports nutrition, 3rd ed. Sydney: McGraw-Hill, 2006;415-440.

Cann CE, Martin MC, Genant HK, Jaffe RB. Decreased spinal mineral content in amenorrheic women. JAMA 1984;251:626-629.

Cranny A, Horsley T, O'Donnell S, Weiler HA, Puil L, Ooi DS, Atkinson SA, Ward LM, Moher D, Hanley DA, Fang M, Yazdi F, Garritty C, Sampson M, Barrowman N, Tsertsvandze A, Mamaladze V. Effectiveness and safety of vitamin D in relation to bone health. Evidence report/technology assessment no. 158 (prepared by the University of Ottawa Evidence-based Practice Center under contract no. 290-02-0021). AHRQ pub. no. 07-E013. Rockville, MD: Agency for Healthcare Research and Quality, Aug 2007.

Creighton DL, Morgan AL, Boardley D, Brolinson PG. Weight-bearing exercise and markers of bone turnover in female athletes. J Appl Physiol 2001;90:565-570.

Donnelly JE, Jacobsen DJ, Jakicic JM, Whatley JE. Very low calorie diet with concurrent versus delayed and sequential exercise. Int J Obesity 1994;18:469-475.

Drinkwater BL, Nilson K, Chestnut CH III, Bremner WJ, Shainholtz S, Southworth MB. Bone mineral content of amenorrheic and eumenorrheic athletes. N Engl J Med 1984;311:277-281.

Dueck CA, Manore MM, Matt KS. Role of energy balance in athletic menstrual dysfunction. Int J Sport Nutr 1996;6:90-116.

Dueck CA, Matt KS, Manore MM, Skinner JS. Treatment of athletic amenorrhea with a diet and training intervention program. Int J Sport Nutr 1996;6:24-40.

Fairburn CG, Walsh TB. Atypical eating disorders (eating disorders not otherwise specified). In: Brownell KD, Fairburn DG eds. Eating disorders and obesity: a comprehensive handbook, 2nd ed. New York: Guilford Press, 2002;171-177.

Fredericson M, Kent K. Normalization of bone density in a previously amenorrheic runner with osteoporosis. Med Sci Sports Exerc 2005;37(9):1481-1486.

Frisch RE, McArthur JW. Menstrual cycles: fatness as a determinant of minimum weight for height necessary for their maintenance or onset. Science 1974;185:949-951.

Garfinkel PE. Classification and diagnosis of eating disorders. In: Brownell KD, Fairburn DG eds. Eating disorders and obesity: a comprehensive handbook, 2nd ed. New York: Guilford Press, 2002;155-161.

Guest NS, Barr SI. Cognitive dietary restraint is associated with stress fractures in women runners. Int J Sport Nutr Exerc Metab 2005;15:147-159.

Hansen CM, Manore MM. Vitamin B-6. In: Wolinski I, Driskell JA eds. Sport nutrition: vitamins and trace minerals. Boca Raton, FL: CRC Press, 2006;81-91.

Heaney RP. The vitamin D requirement in health and disease. J Steroid Biochem Mol Biol 2005;97:13-19.

Heaney RP. The case for improving vitamin D status. J Steroid Biochem Mol Biol 2007;103:635-641.

Ihle R, Loucks AB. Dose-response relationships between energy availability and bone turnover in young exercising women. J Bone Min Res 2004;19:1231-1240.

Institute of Medicine (IOM), Food and Nutrition Board, National Research Council. Dietary reference intakes for calcium, phosphorus, magnesium, vitamin D and fluoride. Washington, DC: National Academy Press, 1997.

Institute of Medicine (IOM), Food and Nutrition Board, National Research Council. Dietary reference intakes for thiamin, riboflavin, niacin, vitamin B-6, folate, vitamin B-12, pantothenic acid, biotin, and choline. Washington, DC: National Academy Press, 1998.

Institute of Medicine (IOM), Food and Nutrition Board, National Research Council. Dietary reference intakes for vitamin C, vitamin E, selenium and carotenoids. Washington, DC: National Academy Press, 2000.

Institute of Medicine (IOM), Food and Nutrition Board, National Research Council. Dietary reference intakes for vitamin A, vitamin K, arsenic, boron, chromium, copper, iodine, iron, manganese, molybdenum, nickel, silicon, vanadium and zinc. Washington, DC: National Academy Press, 2001.

Institute of Medicine (IOM), Food and Nutrition Board, National Research Council. Dietary reference intakes for energy, carbohydrate, fiber, fat, fatty acids, cholesterol, protein, and amino acids. Washington, DC: National Academies Press, 2002.

International Athletics Associations Federation Consensus Statement. Nutrition for athletics: the 2007 consensus statement of the IAAF. J Sports Sci 2007;25(S1):S1.

Joy E, Clark N, Ireland ML, Martie J, Nattiv A, Varechok S. Team management of the female athlete triad. Part 2: Optimal treatment and prevention tactics. Phys Sportsmed 1997;25(4):55-69.

Kaufman BA, Warren MP, Dominguez JE, Wang J, Heymsfield SB, Pierson RN. Bone density and amenorrhea in ballet dancers are related to a decreased resting metabolic rate and lower leptin levels. J Clin Endocrinol Metab 2002;87:2777-2783.

Keith RE. Ascorbic acid. In: Wolinsky I, Driskell JA eds. Sport nutrition: vitamins and trace minerals. Boca Raton, FL: CRC Press, 2006;29-46.

Kirchner EM, Lewis RD, O'Conner PJ. Bone mineral density and dietary intake of female college gymnasts. Med Sci Sports Exerc 1995;27:543-549.

Kurzer MS, Calloway DH. Effects of energy deprivation on sex hormone patterns in healthy menstruating women. Am J Physiol 1986;251:E483-E488.

Linus Pauling Institute (LPI), Oregon State University. http://lpi.oregonstate.edu. Accessed December 2008.

Liu SL, Lebrun CM. Effect of oral contraceptives and hormone replacement therapy on bone mineral density in premenopausal and perimenopausal women: a systemic review. Br J Sports Med 2006;40:11-24.

Loucks AB. Energy balance and body composition in sports and exercise. J Sports Sci 2004;22:1-14.

Loucks AB, Thuma JR. Luteinizing hormone pulsatility is disrupted at a threshold of energy availability in regular menstruating women. J Clin Endocrinol Metab 2003;88:297-311.

Manore MM. Chronic dieting in active women: what are the health consequences? Women's Health Issues 1996;6:332-341.

Manore MM. How do you know when you are eating enough? USA Gymnastics 1997;26(6):8-9.

Manore MM. Nutritional needs of the female athlete. Clin Sports Med 1999;18(3):549-563.

Manore MM. The effect of physical activity on thiamin, riboflavin, and vitamin B-6 requirements. Am J Clin Nutr 2000;72(2 suppl):598S-606S.

Manore MM. Dietary recommendations and athletic menstrual dysfunction. Sports Med 2002;32(14):887-901.

Manore MM, Kam LC, Loucks AB. The female athlete triad: components, nutrition issues and health consequences. J Sports Sci 2007;25(S2):S61-S71.

Manore MM, Thompson JL. Energy requirements of the athlete: assessment and evidence of energy efficiency. In: Burke L, Deakin V eds. Clinical sports nutrition. Sydney: McGraw-Hill, 2006;113-134.

Mastaloudis A, Traber MG. Vitamin E. In: Wolinsky I, Driskell JA eds. Sport nutrition: vitamins and trace minerals. Boca Raton, FL: CRC Press, 2006;183-200.

Meyer NL, Shaw JM, Manore MM, Dolan SH, Subudhi AW, Shultz BB, Walker JA. Bone mineral density of Olympic-level female winter sport athletes. Med Sci Sports Exerc 2004;36(9):1594-1601.

Nattiv A, Loucks AB, Manore MM, Sanborn CF, Sundgot-Borgen J, Warren MP. The female athlete triad. Med Sci Sports Exerc 2007;39(10):1867-1882.

Otis CL. Too slim, amenorrheic, fracture-prone: the female athlete triad. ACSM's Health Fit J 1998;2(1):20-25.

Otis CL, Drinkwater B, Johnson M, Loucks A, Wilmore J. American College of Sports Medicine position stand. The female athlete triad. Med Sci Sports Exerc 1997;29(5):i-ix.

Peterson AL, Talcott W, Kelleher WJ, Smith SD. Bulimic weight-loss behaviors in military versus civilian weight-management programs. Mil Med 1995;160:616-620.

Raiten DJ, Picciano MF. Vitamin D and health in the 21st century: bone and beyond. Executive summary. Am J Clin Nutr 2004;80(suppl):1673S-1677S.

Redman LM, Loucks AB. Menstrual disorders in athletes. Sports Med 2005;35(9):747-755.

Reginster JY. Calcium and vitamin D for osteoporotic fracture risk. Lancet 2007;370:632-634.

Robinson TL, Snow-Harter C, Taffee DR, Gillis D, Shaw J, Marcus R. Gymnasts exhibit higher bone mass than runners despite similar prevalence of amenorrhea and oligomenorrhea. J Bone Min Res 1995;10:26-35.

Sundgot-Borgen J. Nutrient intake of elite female athletes suffering from eating disorders. Int J Sport Nutr 1993;3:431-442.

Sundgot-Borgen J. Risk and trigger factors for the development of eating disorders in female elite athletes. Med Sci Sports Exerc 1994;26:414-419.

Sundgot-Borgen J, Torstveit MK. Prevalence of eating disorders in elite athletes is higher than in the general population. Clin J Sports Med 2004;14(1):25-32.

Tang BMP, Eslick GD, Nowson C, Smith C, Bensoussan A. Use of calcium or calcium in combination with vitamin D supplementation to prevent fractures and bone loss in people aged 50 years and older: a meta-analysis. Lancet 2007;370:657-666.

Tarnopolsky M. Protein requirements for endurance athletes. Nutrition 2004;20(7-8):662-668.

Teegarden D, Proulx WR, Martin BR. Peak bone mass in young women. J Bone Min Res 1995;10:711-715.

Thompson JL, Manore MM, Thomas JR. Effects of diet and diet-plus-exercise programs on resting metabolic rate: a meta-analysis. Int J Sport Nutr 1996;6:41-61.

Thong FS, McLean C, Graham TE. Plasma leptin in female athletes: relationship with body fat, reproductive, nutritional, and endocrine factors. J Appl Physiol 2000;88(6):2037-2044.

Williams NI, Young JC, McArthur JW, Bullen B, Skrinar GS, Turnbull B. Strenuous exercise with caloric restriction: effect on luteinizing hormone secretion. Med Sci Sports Exerc 1995;27:1390-1398.

Wilmore JH, Wambsgans KC, Brenner M et al. Is there energy conservation in amenorrheic compared with eumenorrheic distance runners? J Appl Physiol 1992;72:15-22.

Woolf K, Manore MM. B-vitamins and exercise: does exercise alter requirements? Int J Sport Nutr Exerc Metab 2006;16:453-484.

Woolf K, Manore MM. Micronutrients important for exercise. In: Spurway N, MacLaren D eds. Advances in sport and exercise science series: nutrition and sport. Philadelphia: Elsevier, 2007;119-136.

Zanker CL, Swaine IL. Bone turnover in amenorrheic and eumenorrheic women distance runners. Scand J Med Sci Sports 1998;8:20-26.

Ziegler P, Sharp R, Hughes V, Evans W, Khoo CS. Nutritional status of teenage female competitive figure skaters. J Am Diet Assoc 2001;101:374-379.

CHAPTER 16

Ergogenic Substances

Chapter Objectives

After reading this chapter you should be able to

- describe the issues surrounding the use of ergogenic substances,
- understand how to evaluate available ergogenic substances, and
- discuss one popular ergogenic aid.

Many people involved in fitness activities are familiar with various ergogenic substances. These substances have received extensive media attention over the last 20 years and include products such as anabolic steroids, ephedrine, caffeine, and creatine; there are also practices such as blood boosting. The use of ergogenic aids is widespread in the professional athletic community and is increasingly popular with youth and recreational athletes.

Why do people use ergogenic substances? How can the sport nutrition professional properly evaluate ergogenic substances? This chapter is not designed to review the ergogenic substances now available, as many books and research articles offer such information (e.g., Bahrke and Yesalis 2002; Antonio and Stout 2001; Juhn 2003; Nissan and Sharp 2003; Bemben 2005). In this text we have briefly reviewed a number of ergogenic aids (chapters 2, 3, 4, 8, and 11). The primary goals of this chapter are to review basic definitions of ergogenic substances and to address the following questions:

1. How prevalent is the use of ergogenic substances in active people?
2. What has contributed to the widespread use of ergogenic substances in our society?
3. What are the ethical implications of ergogenic substance use?
4. How can one effectively evaluate the efficacy of an ergogenic substance?

At the end of the chapter, we briefly review two of the most popular ergogenic substances, one legal (creatine) and one illegal (anabolic steroids), and discuss proposed mechanisms of action and evidence of effectiveness. We hope that you will gain the ability to review media claims and research studies with a critical eye—and that widespread critical evaluation of ergogenic substances will help reduce the flood of mythical information about them.

ERGOGENIC SUBSTANCES IN SPORT AND EXERCISE

Ergogenic substances can be defined as those "used to improve exercise and athletic performance by improving the production of energy" (Bucci 1993). Theoretically, there are potentially thousands of substances that could fit this definition. Certain drugs, carbohydrates, protein, fat, and vitamin or mineral supplements, in addition to other "nutritional" products (i.e., dietary supplements), can be defined as ergogenic based on their theorized or proven functions. You can think of ergogenic substances as essentially falling into two categories, ergogenic drugs and ergogenic supplements.

What is the difference between an ergogenic drug and an ergogenic supplement? The Food and Drug Administration (FDA) has specified that substances claimed to prevent, alleviate, or cure a physical or mental illness, or to affect the structure or function of the body, are classified as drugs (Cowart 1992; Lightsey and Attaway 1992). If a substance is classified as a drug, it is strictly regulated by the FDA. Drugs must go through rigorous clinical trials prior to approval, which costs a great deal of money and time. It is common for drugs to take several years to reach the market. Some drugs that have therapeutic value may also have ergogenic properties. These are a few of the most common ergogenic drugs:

- **Anabolic androgenic steroids:** Steroids are used illegally to increase muscle mass, strength, and power as well as recovery and endurance. Abuse of steroids has been associated with a number of long-term adverse health effects. They are particularly damaging for young athletes due to premature closing of epiphyseal (growth) plates.
- **Growth hormone:** Also known as somatropin, human growth hormone (HGH) is taken to enhance muscle size, strength, and performance. These claims have been difficult to confirm given the ethical constraints (i.e., low doses) in conducting controlled studies. Long-term consequences include acromegaly (enlarged jaw and nose), hypertension, muscle weakness, hyperlipidemia, cardiomyopathy, insulin resistance, and diabetes (Stacy et al. 2004; Tentori and Graziani 2007).
- **Erythropoietin (EPO):** EPO is a hormone produced mostly by the kidneys that stimulates the production of red blood cells. Therefore it is used by athletes to enhance oxygen transport and consequently performance. Side effects include hyperviscosity (thick blood), thrombosis, and hypertension (Gaudard et al. 2003).

If an ergogenic substance is not claimed to prevent, alleviate, or cure a disease, then it can be classified as a dietary supplement under the Dietary Supplement and Health Education Act (DSHEA) (see "The Dietary Supplement Health and Education Act"). As we will discuss later in the chapter, such substances are currently regulated rather loosely, putting the consumer at risk for a positive drug test as well as adverse health effects.

Doping in Sport

The use of ergogenic substances has a long history in sport. In the 1930s the term doping was used to refer to the use of any method of enhancing athletic performance (Boje 1939). Today, doping refers to the use of prohibited substances and to methods used to enhance athletic performance (World Anti-Doping Agency 2003). Doping in sport is banned not only in order to promote fair and equitable competition, but also in order to protect the health of athletes and preserve the integrity of sport (Hilderbrand et al. 2003; World Anti-Doping Agency 2003). In response to the need to control doping in sport, the World Anti-Doping Agency (WADA) was created in 1999 to coordinate and monitor doping throughout the world. In 2002, WADA defined the first World Anti-Doping Code. The code provides a uniform definition of doping and sanctions, as well as the athletes' and sport organizations' rights and responsibilities (WADA 2003). The definition of doping in the WADA Code is outlined on p. 480. The International Olympic Committee (IOC) and the U.S. Anti-Doping Agency (USADA) are just two of the organizations that have adopted the WADA Code.

Highlight

The Dietary Supplement Health and Education Act

Prior to passage of the DSHEA, supplements were regulated as foods "for special dietary use" under the Federal Food Drug and Cosmetic Act of 1938. In the 1970s, the FDA attempted to regulate the dose and quantity of vitamins and minerals in supplements, but was prevented from doing so by laws at that time. As a response to a need to regulate supplements yet provide freedom for the consumer to choose, DSHEA was passed in 1994. Dietary supplements were defined for the first time as follows:

"any product (other than tobacco) intended to supplement the diet that contains one of more of the following ingredients: a vitamin, mineral, herb or other botanical, an amino acid; or a concentrate, metabolite, constituent, extract; or a combination of any of these ingredients; and is intended to be taken by mouth as a pill, capsule, tablet, or liquid; and is labeled on the front panel as being a dietary supplement; and cannot be represented as a conventional food" (DSHEA 1994).

As you can see, this definition is extremely broad and open to interpretation.

Under DSHEA, guidelines for third-party literature (e.g., product pamphlets), labeling, quality control, and marketing claims were specified. As an example, you may have noticed that labels on supplements can legally include a **structure–function claim** (e.g., "promotes joint health"), but they cannot include the claim that they treat a disease (e.g., "treats osteoarthritis").

Safety guidelines were also outlined for dietary supplements and are summarized as follows:

- No premarket approval is required (unless product contains a new ingredient). A new ingredient is one marketed after October 15, 1994. Any ingredient in the market prior to DSHEA is assumed by the FDA to be safe.

- The burden of proof for unsafe supplements rests with the FDA.

- For a supplement to be considered unsafe, the FDA must prove that it presents "a significant or unreasonable risk of illness or injury under the conditions of use recommended or suggested on the label."

- Dietary supplements are regulated similarly to foods.

- Unlike drugs and food additives, supplements do not have to have undergone clinical studies to test safety, effectiveness, or interactions with other drugs.

What's the bottom line? The fact that a dietary supplement is sold in a store does not mean it is safe. Keep in mind that these safety regulations outlined by DSHEA are very different from those for pharmaceutical drugs, which undergo extensive testing before being put on the market. The safety of dietary supplements is monitored by the FDA, which is currently understaffed and has limited resources. Adverse events are often underreported, making it difficult for the FDA to remove supplements from the market.

Prohibited Substances

Many drugs and supplements, ergogenic and otherwise, are banned by organizations such as WADA and the National Collegiate Athletic Association (NCAA). Substances or methods that enhance (or have the potential to enhance) sport performance, that are harmful (or potentially harmful) to athletes, or that are unethical are included in the prohibited list. This list is revised every year. Table 16.1 provides a short list of substances that are banned by WADA and the NCAA. Notice that there are slight differences between the two lists. Athletes and professionals working with athletes should always consult the WADA and NCAA Web sites for the most current list of prohibited substances. While many other available substances are not banned, scientific experts and health practitioners have questioned the safety and ethics surrounding the use of these substances.

Prohibited Methods

While **banned substances** include drugs that may affect performance and may be harmful to the

World Anti-Doping Agency Code: Definition of Doping

As defined by the WADA Code (WADA 2003), doping encompasses one or more of the following:

- Presence of a prohibited substance or its metabolites or markers in an athlete's bodily specimen
- Use or attempted use of a prohibited substance or a prohibited method
- Refusing, or failing without compelling justification, to submit to sample collection after notification as authorized in applicable anti-doping rules or otherwise evading sample collection
- Violation of applicable requirements regarding athlete availability for out-of-competition testing including failure to provide required whereabouts information and missed tests which are declared based on reasonable rules
- Tampering or attempting to tamper with any part of doping control
- Possession of prohibited substances and methods
- Trafficking in any prohibited substance or prohibited method
- Administration or attempted administration of a prohibited substance or prohibited method to any athlete, or assisting, encouraging, aiding, abetting, covering up, or any other type of complicity involving an anti-doping rule violation or any attempted violation

Note: The code specifies strict liability, meaning that an athlete is responsible regardless of whether a violation was committed unknowingly or intentionally.

A complete explanation of the code can be found on the WADA Web site: www.wada-ama.org/en.

Table 16.1 Drugs Banned by the World Anti-Doping Agency (WADA) or National Collegiate Athletic Association (NCAA) or Both[1]

Substance	Examples
Stimulants	Caffeine,[2] ephedrine[3] (ephedra, ma huang), synephrine (Citrus aurantium, or bitter orange),[4] cocaine
Street drugs	Codeine, morphine, heroin, marijuana
Anabolic agents	Testosterone,[5] stanozolol, androstendione (Andro), dehydroepiandrosterone (DHEA), clenbuterol
Beta-2 agonists	Atenolol, metaprolol, propranolol
Diuretics and other masking agents	Furosemide, triamterene, acetazolamide
Peptide hormones and analogs	Growth hormone (HGH), insulin-like growth factor (IGF-1), erythropoietin (EPO)

[1] Complete lists of banned substances can be found at www.wada-ama.org/en/ and www.ncaa.org/wps/ncaa?ContentID=282
[2] Urine concentrations must exceed 15 μ/mL for NCAA. As of 2005, caffeine has not been banned by WADA.
[3] Urine concentrations must exceed 10 μg/mL for WADA.
[4] Not banned by WADA. Note: Phenylephrine and pseudoephedrine, found commonly in cold medications, are no longer banned by either organization.
[5] Ratio of total urine concentration of testosterone to epitestosterone must exceed 6.

With advancement of gene therapy, the method of **gene doping** has emerged as a threat to fair sport and the health of athletes. Gene doping is the nontherapeutic use or manipulation of cells, genes, or gene expression specifically for the enhancement of athletic performance. Gene doping is currently on WADA's list of prohibited methods (WADA 2007). Unfortunately, the gains that science has made to treat diseases such as muscular dystrophy with gene therapy have resulted in a desire on the part of healthy athletes to use the same technology to increase muscle size and strength and oxygen transport for the purposes of athletic enhancement.

In gene therapy, DNA or RNA is inserted into specific cells using a viral vector or direct injection. The inserted genetic material can then code for either a mutant or a missing gene or can inhibit an undesired gene. Studies using gene therapy have been conducted only in animals and in preliminary human trials. However, cloning of growth

individual, methods used to avoid detection of drug use are also banned. This includes methods such as tampering with samples and practices such as **blood boosting.** Blood boosting (formerly known as blood doping; the term doping is now associated with illegal use of recombinant EPO) is the practice of infusing extra red blood cells into the body in an attempt to increase oxygen-carrying capacity (Leigh-Smith 2004).

hormone, insulin-like growth factor (IGF-1), and EPO has been achieved, and in each case this has implications for sport performance (Trent and Alexander 2006).

Although the technology for gene doping is still in its infancy, the potential risks of gene doping are great. Not only will detection be difficult, but also the health consequences are disconcerting. For instance, if an athlete were able to gene dope with EPO, the increase in blood viscosity could cause a heart attack or even paralysis (Unal and Unal 2004). Unlike the situation with blood doping, in which red blood cell production returns to baseline after discontinuation of EPO, there would be a continuous increased production of red blood cells. An additional issue is that of therapeutic gene therapy. As technology improves, will athletes treated with gene therapy for health reasons be denied the opportunity to compete in sport? Currently, WADA is actively working on methods of detection and policies to address these issues.

Prevalence of Use

How prevalent is the use of ergogenic substances? This is a very difficult question to answer. The majority of information available is on anabolic steroid use. There are an estimated 1 to 3 million current or former steroids users in the United States (Kutscher et al. 2002). As the "win at all costs" mentality spreads to younger and younger athletes, so does the use of steroids. Data suggest that as many as 3% to 12% of high school males have abused steroids at some point in their lives (Yesalis et al. 1997). The most recent data from the Centers for Disease Control and Prevention (CDC) indicates that nationwide, 4% of high school students have taken steroids illegally at some time. The percentage is highest for 10th graders, at 5.2% (CDC 2006). The highest use of steroids in high schools continues to occur among football players, wrestlers, and track and field male athletes (Bahrke et al. 2000). Although illegal, steroid use has been reported in female athletes, but male athletes continue to be the most numerous users (Bahrke et al. 2000). This is of concern not only because of the potential long-term effects, but also because several studies have noted that steroid abusers are more likely to use cocaine, alcohol, and other drugs than nonusers of steroids (DurRant et al. 1993; Irving et al. 2002; Luetkemeier et al. 1995). Interestingly, NCAA athletes have reported lower rates of steroid use (1%) compared to other athletes, most likely due to random drug testing (Green et al. 2001b). Currently, only a few

high schools have implemented random drug testing, with mixed results (Goldberg et al. 2003).

Less is known about the prevalence of other ergogenic substances that athletes are taking. We do know that the use of ergogenic supplements is widespread in both young and adult athletes. Studies have shown that as many as 22% to 62% of high school athletes are using at least one supplement (Scofield and Unruh 2006; Sobal and Marquart 1994; Nieper 2005). The percentage is even higher in adults, collegiate athletes, and elite athletes. A study of people who exercise at gyms showed that 85% were using some type of supplement (Morrison et al. 2004). Recent studies have indicated supplement use in approximately 42% to 89% of college athletes (Jonnalagadda et al. 2001; Burns et al. 2004; Froiland et al. 2004). Similarly, in elite athletes, studies have shown that 51% to 88% use at least one dietary supplement (Corrigan and Kazlauskas 2003; Petroczi et al. 2007; Erdman et al. 2006). Of the supplements reported, multivitamin and minerals were the most popular among both athletes and nonathletes. According to National Health and Nutrition Examination Survey III, approximately 49% of those interviewed in the United States used a multivitamin and mineral supplement (Ervin et al. 1999). Recent studies conducted specifically in athletes have given even higher numbers (~73%) (Petroczi et al. 2007; Burns et al. 2004). Many athletes believe that the supplements are critical for optimal performance. Elite athletes and those involved in sports that emphasize muscle size (e.g., football, weightlifting, bodybuilding) report the greatest supplement use (Erdman et al. 2006; Sobal and Marquart 1994; Massad et al. 1995; Morrison et al. 2004).

An accurate estimate of the prevalence of ergogenic substance use by the general U.S. population is not available at the present time. While people may be willing to answer questions about vitamins and other nutritional supplement products, they are less open about their use of illegal or banned substances. Based on national sales of weight loss and ergogenic substances—$16.8 billion in 2005—it would appear that many people, not just athletes, are using these substances (*Nutrition Business Journal* 2006).

Reasons for Use

Why do athletes and nonathletes use ergogenic substances? While many athletes use these substances in an attempt to enhance performance, there are other reasons why even the general public may find them attractive:

- To improve physical appearance
- To prevent or treat injuries
- To treat or cure illness or disease
- To be accepted by peers
- To cope better with stress

Many of these substances are readily available and highly promoted in magazines and fitness facilities. A survey of 33 supplement companies showed that more than 800 performance claims were made for 624 supplements (Grunewald and Bailey 1993). Benefits attributed to these products include weight or muscle gain, increases in strength, loss of body fat, increases in energy and endurance, and enhanced recuperation. People with limited knowledge of sport nutrition, or people looking for a "magic bullet" to success, are among those susceptible to advertisers' claims. Even individuals with knowledge of proper nutrition may be tempted to try these products "just in case they might work" in an attempt to gain a competitive edge.

Ethical Issues

Williams (1994) suggested that there are three primary foundations on which individuals or groups can base their ethical decisions concerning use of ergogenic substances:

- The moral principles of a particular *school of thought*—for example, the Olympic ideal that athletes should succeed in sport through their own unaided efforts
- The rules of conduct recognized in certain *associations*—for example, rules of conduct defined by a specific sport organization, such as the IOC or the NCAA
- The moral principles by which an *individual* is guided

Williams observed that an athlete who wants to win at any cost will be driven to gain an unfair advantage, resulting in violation of the **ethics** of the Olympic ideal and the sport governing bodies. Even if the behavior of this athlete is consistent with his or her own personal ethics, it is contrary to the ethics put forth by the athletic governing organizations.

Is it acceptable for athletes to use any means available, including ergogenic substances, in order to gain the competitive edge? A simple answer to this question does not exist, and the ethical issues surrounding the use of ergogenic substances will be a heated topic of discussion for many years.

In a well-publicized survey conducted by *Sports Illustrated,* athletes were asked if they would use a banned substance if it was undetectable and they were guaranteed to win, and 98% said yes. The same athletes were asked if they would take the same substance if it allowed them to win for five years, even if taking it would result in death. Amazingly, over 50% still said yes (Bamberger and Yeager 1997). It is not surprising, then, that Smith and Perry (1992) found that many athletes consider ergogenic drugs an essential component of successful competition—most likely because in order to continue to set world records, athletes must find ways to push the limits of human performance. Because many record-setting athletes may be using these substances, the attitude prevails among other athletes that they also must use them to compete "fairly" with others.

It is unlikely that the use of ergogenic substances will ever disappear. Athletes will continue to find ways, many unethical, to be the very best in their sport. This situation appears similar to the nuclear arms race. Once one country has nuclear weapons, others feel they need them in order to protect themselves or to be competitive. Asking all countries to get rid of their weapons is ineffective because of the fear that some countries will secretly keep a few weapons. Since it is impossible to detect all ergogenic substances, these products will continue to be a part of many athletes' lifestyles.

Another important issue is whether it is ethical to use dietary supplements that are not banned or illegal. The WADA Code prohibits substances that have the potential to enhance sport performance, that may be harmful to the athlete, or that violate the spirit of sport. According to the code, many dietary supplements could fall under these specifications. Since some may actually improve performance, one has to question whether taking these substances is unethical. Should a dietary supplement be banned or its intake limited if it is found to enhance performance? While it is not within the scope of this text to answer this question, this issue should provide a lively debate topic in the classroom, at scientific meetings, and throughout the world of athletics.

EVALUATING ERGOGENIC SUBSTANCES

According to the companies that manufacture and market ergogenic substances, using their products will result in numerous physiological changes. These claims include not only improvements in performance-related characteristics but also reduced risk for diseases. Do these products meet the published claims? How do sport nutrition practitioners help laypeople evaluate the plethora of ergogenic products on the market? In this section, we discuss three areas in which one can evaluate ergogenic aids: marketing claims, research studies, and safety issues.

Marketing Claims

The primary goal of an advertisement is to present information about a product in a way that convinces consumers to purchase it. Unfortunately, this does not typically benefit the consumer. Under DSHEA (see p. 479), if a product qualifies as a dietary supplement, companies can use claims of nutritional support (structure–function claims) that link a nutrient and a deficiency or describe the effect of an ingredient on the body's structure,

function, or well-being. This is why you frequently see terms such as "promote" and "maintain" on supplement labels. Many athletes, and consumers in general, do not necessarily distinguish between structure–function claims and disease claims such as those legally made by drug manufacturers. Further, few realize that these claims are not premarket approved despite the disclaimer required on supplement labels. Manufacturers must be able to substantiate that any structure–function claim that is made is truthful and not misleading, but they do not need to provide this substantiation to the FDA (for labeling) or the Federal Trade Commission (for infomercials, Internet, and print or broadcast advertisements) unless asked.

Lightsey and Attaway (1992) reviewed the nine most common tactics manufacturers use to sell ergogenic substances (see "Nine Deceptive Advertising Practices Frequently Used to Market Ergogenic Aids"). It is clear that objective

---

Highlight

Nine Deceptive Advertising Practices Frequently Used to Market Ergogenic Aids

Due to the prevalence of the use of ergogenic aids, it is important for consumers, health professionals, and athletes to be aware of misleading advertising. Following are nine deceptive advertising practices highlighted by Lightsey and Attaway (1992):

1. General misrepresentation
   - Misuse of genuine research: Published research is taken out of context; conclusions are extrapolated beyond the published findings or applied in an unproven manner.
   - Claims that the product is university tested: If the study is legitimate and approved by a university, a specific professor may be named in the advertisement. The "research" is often conducted by a naive university staff member (not a trained researcher), with the firm controlling all aspects of the study. In some cases, the research has never been done.
   - Claims of endorsement by professional organizations: A member of a professional team may use the product, and the manufacturer uses this to suggest that the product is endorsed by the entire organization (which is frequently not the case).

2. Claims that the company is currently doing blind research work
   - This statement is commonly used in advertisements, but rarely is it true.
   - Firms are very seldom able to provide specific information about studies claimed to be in progress.

3. Research not available for public review
   - There is no rationale for "hiding" research information.
   - Consumers have the right to obtain documentation about performance claims.

(continued)

Nine Deceptive Advertising Practices   *(continued)*

4. Testimonials

 • These are based on the placebo effect. There is at least a 40% chance that a benign substance will enhance mental or physical performance.

 • Testimonials can be faked, bought, or embellished. Even if the testimonial is truthful, the benefit suggested by the person testifying may be a result of the placebo effect or coincidence.

5. Patents

 • Patents are not granted based on the effectiveness of a product; they only indicate distinguishable differences among products.

 • Patents do not demonstrate that a product is effective or safe, and it is possible to obtain a patent on no more than a theoretical model of a product. Sometimes no objective research has been conducted.

6. Inappropriately referenced research

 • References to unpublished research: Many of these studies have very poor research designs and lack adequate scientific control.

 • References to Eastern European research: Often there are no tangible research data; the research is not available for peer review; and it may be based upon unconfirmed reports or rumors.

 • Poorly controlled research: Ads quote only one published report that has not been verified by subsequent research. The availability of only one study indicates that the results are preliminary and that more studies are needed to substantiate the product.

 • Outdated research: Ads cite old research even though newer, appropriately controlled studies refute outdated claims.

 • Results taken out of context: Data are extrapolated from findings that have no relation to the product's effectiveness.

 • Publications not peer reviewed: References are to "studies" published in popular magazines or variety journals or directly distributed to the consumer. These studies are not adequately controlled or reviewed and should be considered invalid.

7. Media

 • Advertising companies use mass media marketing videos, and infomercials are popular tools. False claims in advertising are regulated by the Federal Trade Commission; the FDA regulates false labeling.

 • Publicity: Some communications are not recognizable as advertising (e.g., editorial comments, talk show interviews, and stories planted in the press). While publicity is not regulated as strictly as advertising, companies can be prosecuted if they use intentional deception to sell a product. Unfortunately, products are generally investigated only if they pose significant danger to the public.

8. Mail-order fitness evaluations

 • Most of these evaluations are too subjective to be of use to the consumer, and their accuracy should be questioned due to the generic nature of the information obtained.

 • They are provided only to convince consumers to buy products.

9. Anabolic measurements

 • Some companies use in-house methods (e.g., amino acid chromatography and nitrogen balance) to study changes in protein balance. The methods may be used inappropriately.

 • The manufacturer can claim that negative nitrogen balance occurred, supporting the use of the product, but fail to mention that this change is a normal response to training. Nitrogen balance returns to baseline levels or may become positive with further training. In addition, other nutritional factors can affect the results, and these factors may not be adequately controlled.

Adapted from D.M. Lightsey and J.R. Attaway, 1992, "Deceptive tactics used in marketing purported ergogenic aids," *National Strength and Conditioning Association Journal* 14(2): 26-31.

representation of these products is not available from the companies that sell them. The burden of proof that a substance does or does not work falls upon research scientists.

Research Studies

Understanding how to properly evaluate the literature on ergogenic substances will help sport nutrition professionals advise athletes about the products. It is unrealistic to expect the general public to possess the knowledge and to access the necessary resources to adequately evaluate ergogenic substances. One important role of the sport nutrition professional is to act as a conduit of reliable, accurate information about the substances that are available.

Butterfield (1996) reviewed the issues surrounding the evaluation of ergogenic substances, providing a list of criteria one should follow to evaluate the research literature (see "Criteria for Reviewing Research Literature on Ergogenic Substances" on p. 486).

Remember that many athletes care little, if at all, about the science or plausibility of a particular product. Their primary concern is whether the product enhances performance. In order to establish rapport with athletes and gain their respect and trust regarding your evaluation of an ergogenic substance, take the following steps (Butterfield 1996):

1. Assess the athletes' level of knowledge and belief about the product.

2. Do not demand that athletes stop using all ergogenic substances—you may come off as "out of touch," and they may not feel comfortable discussing products with someone who is adamantly against the use of all substances.

3. Accept practices that are not harmful or illegal—recommend changes *gradually*.

4. Assess the role that the substance plays in athletes' overall diets; determine if you need to address their dietary practices.

5. Focus on enhancing practices that are critical to performance.

6. Commend athletes for practicing sound nutrition principles.

7. Address questionable supplementing practices only after you have established trust and rapport with athletes.

Safety Issues

Many safe ergogenic products are available. They generally do not enhance performance in healthy, active individuals who regularly eat a well-balanced diet, but they may play a critical role in optimizing the nutritional and energy needs of many people who cannot regularly meet the demands of training and performance through diet alone. For instance, endurance runners generally benefit from the use of carbohydrate (e.g., glucose polymers, simple sugars) drinks and energy bars, while many female athletes with relatively low energy intakes benefit from multivitamin-mineral and calcium supplements.

Unfortunately, there are risks associated with the use of numerous ergogenic substances, particularly when people consume them in supraphysiologic doses. Note also that since dietary supplements are not subject to strict safety regulations, mass-marketed products are sometimes unsafe. The following risks are sometimes associated with use of ergogenic substances:

- Low energy intake: People attempt to compensate for poor energy and nutrient intakes by taking supplements. They fail to realize the necessity of consuming adequate energy derived from carbohydrates, protein, and fat. Food also supplies the essential micronutrients the body needs to function properly, many of which cannot be purchased in a bottle.

- Toxicity effects: Taking large doses of single micronutrients can lead to nutrient overload and toxicity symptoms, in addition to inhibiting the absorption of other nutrients. For example, large doses of zinc can inhibit the absorption of copper, and high intakes of folate can mask the signs of vitamin B_{12} deficiency or pernicious anemia. Individual supplements are commonly formulated with large doses of a particular nutrient, which can lead to toxic effects with regular consumption of the manufacturer's recommended dose. For example, most single vitamin B_6 supplements contain 50 mg per tablet, and the Tolerable Upper Intake Level for vitamin B_6 is 100 mg/day. Thus it is easy to see how an individual could take high amounts of the nutrient.

- Poor quality control: Despite the fact that DSHEA authorized the FDA to develop

Criteria for Reviewing Research Literature on Ergogenic Substances

Author

- Are the researcher and laboratory experienced and reputable?
- Is there any conflict of interest between the scientist or laboratory and the company making the product?

Abstract

- Is the abstract succinct, and does it accurately describe the objectives and results?
- Does the abstract include information that cannot be substantiated?

Research Design

- Is the purpose of the study based on scientifically valid (i.e., biologically plausible) information?
- Was the appropriate study design employed (e.g., double blind, placebo controlled)?
- Were subjects properly selected (e.g., gender, training status) and randomly assigned to treatment groups?
- Were confounding variables (e.g., prior diet, diet during intervention, exercise patterns) controlled as completely as possible?
- Do the researchers rely only on correlative relationships (with no cause-and-effect data available)?
- Is the sample size large enough to show a physiologically significant effect?
- Was a randomized, matched control group studied (or were subjects used as their own controls)?

Research Methods

- Were the methods used (e.g., performance tests) appropriate for the product being tested?
- Were the methods used reliable, and was the reliability of the methods reported?
- Were the methods sufficiently described or referenced so that they can be repeated?
- Were the statistics employed clearly specified and appropriate for the study design?

Results

- Were the results clearly presented in tables and graphs?
- Were statistically significant differences indicated?
- Do the results make sense, and are they appropriately applied to the original objectives?

Discussion

- Is the discussion presented objectively?
- Are both conflicting and similar data from other investigators presented?
- Are the limitations of the methods discussed, as well as the implications these limitations may have for the interpretation of the results?
- Are references other than the author's included?
- Are the final conclusions drawn directly from the data, and is speculation kept to a minimum?

Conclusion

- Is the conclusion specific to the purpose of the study?
- Is the conclusion consistent with the reported findings?

Adapted from G. Butterfield, 1996, "Ergogenic aids: evaluating sport nutrition products," *International Journal of Sport Nutrition,* 6: 191-197; P.K. Rangachari and S. Mierson, 1995, "A checklist to help students analyze published articles in basic medical sciences," *American Journal of Physiology* 268 (Adv Physiol Educ 13): S21-S25; W.M. Sherman and D.R. Lamb, 1995, "Introduction to ergogenic aids supplement," *International Journal of Sport Nutrition* 5: Siii-Siv.

current good manufacturing practices (CGMPs) for dietary supplements in 1994, the final rule specifying these guidelines was issued only recently, in 2007. The final rule for CGMPs is designed to ensure that supplements are manufactured consistently, specifically in relation to identity, purity, strength, and composition of the product. The final rule provides guidelines for the entire manufacturing process, from the design of the manufacturing plant to the final labeling of the product. The final rule specifically includes activities related to the following:

- Design and construction of manufacturing plants
- Cleaning
- Manufacturing operations
- Quality control procedures
- Final product testing
- Management of consumer complaints
- Maintenance of records
- The benefit for you as the consumer or educator is that once the final rule is implemented, you continue to have the freedom to purchase dietary supplements, *and* you can be more confident that a product is free from contaminants and that it contains what the label specifies. However, it should be noted that the CGMPs do not go into effect immediately. Depending on the size of the company, manufacturers will not be required to comply with the new CGMPs until 2010. In the meantime, some manufacturers have implemented their own quality control systems, but not all. Further, under the interim final rule, manufacturers may petition for an exemption from the requirement to test all of a particular ingredient (100% identity requirement). The complete CGMP final rule can be found at www.cfsan.fda.gov/~dms/dscgmps7.html.

It is important to understand that until the CGMP final rule is fully implemented, there are no required rigorous standards or manufacturing controls for supplements and no required safety testing. Consequently, there is no way to know if a product contains the ingredients listed on the label. As an example, Green and colleagues (2001a) evaluated 12 brands of over-the-counter androstenedione (Andro), a supplement taken to increase testosterone (Andro is now illegal). Eleven of the 12 brands did not meet labeling requirements. Most of the products contained less Andro than was stated on the label. However, more alarming was the finding that one product contained testosterone, a prescription steroid, and another contained almost twice the amount of Andro stated on the label (Green et al. 2001a).

Other quality control issues include contamination with harmful substances. The FDA has recalled various supplements for potentially toxic doses of vitamins A, D, B$_6$, and selenium (U.S. Department of Health and Human Services and FDA 2003). Other supplements have been found to contain impurities such as lead (Markowitz et al. 1994), *Digitalis lanata* (Slifman et al. 1998), salmonella, botulism, and glass (Department of Health and Human Services and FDA 2003). Once the CGMPs are in place, manufacturers will be required to test their products for impurities. Hopefully, this will reduce the risk of contamination and exposure to harmful substances.

Perhaps the most well-known studies concerning dietary supplement analysis are those conducted by the IOC. The IOC-accredited laboratory in Cologne, Germany, analyzed 634 dietary supplements from various countries. Products included vitamin and minerals, protein powders, and herbal products. Of these products, 15% were contaminated with anabolic steroids, and results for 10% were inconclusive (Dopinginfo.de 2000). In another IOC-accredited laboratory in Vienna, 12 of the 57 products tested contained anabolic steroids (Dopinginfo.de. 2000). It appears that athletes may be at risk not only for an unsafe and ineffective product, but for a positive drug test as well.

- Incomplete labels and untraceable products: Supplement labels must meet certain requirements. However, as already discussed, because of quality control issues the label may not reflect what is actually in the product (Green et al. 2001a; Department of Health and Human Services and FDA 2003; Markowitz et al. 1994; Dopinginfo.de. 2000). Further, if a supplement contains a proprietary blend or formula, legally the manufacturer does not have to declare the ingredients and their amounts. Only the total weight of all ingredients has to be listed. Many supplements contain proprietary blends, and we are left to guess what is in the blend.

- Illness and death: As there is currently minimal quality control of ergogenic products, these substances may contain contaminants or may react in an additive or synergistic way with other products or medications a person is taking (Kleiner 1991). In some cases, the product itself may be poisonous or harmful. The stimulant ephedra has been banned due to its potentially fatal effect related to elevations in heart rate and blood pressure. Philen and colleagues (1992) found a plant, hydrangea, listed as an ingredient on some supplements. The leaves and buds of this plant contain cyanogenic glycosides, which could induce cyanide poisoning.

CHOOSING QUALITY ERGOGENIC SUBSTANCES

Because of the many potential risks associated with supplements, it is important to critically evaluate ergogenic substances prior to using or recommending them. However, evaluating the marketing, research, and safety of products can be a daunting task in the current regulatory environment. How do you decide what is safe and effective?

Third-Party Evaluations

Several organizations now offer third-party evaluations of dietary supplements. Independent testing of individual products is conducted (usually for a fee) to evaluate such quality control issues as labeling accuracy, purity, strength, and ability to dissolve. Table 16.2 lists some of these dietary

Table 16.2 Summary of Evaluation Programs

Evaluation includes	CL	NNFA GMP	NSF	USP
Label review				
Test of contents for quantity of ingredients	✓		✓	✓
Test of contents for contaminants	✓		✓	✓
Inspection of manufacturing	✓	✓	✓	✓
Test of dissolution	✓			✓
Test of disintegration	✓		✓	✓
Membership in organization required		✓		
Voluntary participation	✓	✓	✓	✓
Nonvoluntary participation	✓			
A certification or other mark provided on label	✓	✓	✓	✓
Information about products available on Web site	✓	✓	✓	✓
Fee paid by manufacturer for service	✓*	✓	✓	✓

CL = ConsumerLab.com; NNFA = National Nutritional Foods Association; GMP = good manufacturing practices; NSF = NSF International, USP = United States Pharmacopeia.

*Fee is for voluntary testing requested by the company.

Adapted from M.K. Whybark, 2004, "Third party evaluation programs for quality of dietary supplements," *Herbalgram* 64: 30-33.

Supplement Resources

Office of Dietary Supplements	http://dietary-supplements.info.nih.gov/
FDA Center for Food Safety and Applied Nutrition	www.cfsan.fda.gov
Adverse Event Reporting	www.fda.gov/medwatch
Federal Trade Commission (FTC)	www.ftc.gov/
National Center for Complementary and Alternative Health	http://nccam.nih.gov
ConsumerLab.com	www.consumerlab.com
United States Pharmacopeia (USP)	www.usp.org
National Nutritional Foods Association	www.nnfa.org
NSF International	www.nsf.org

supplement evaluation programs. For companies that use these services, you will find certifications or seals of approval on their products. A recent certification useful for athletes is the Certified in Sport by NSF International. This program also tests for banned substances. Keep in mind that third-party testing is expensive; the fact that a product is not on the list of certified products does not mean it is unsafe. However, if it is on the list, it meets the criteria set forth by the evaluator. Third-party evaluation programs and other helpful Web sites are shown on p. 488.

Australian Institute of Sport (AIS) Sports Supplement Program

In recent years, the Australian Institute of Sport has implemented a sport supplement program to ensure that athletes are using sport foods and supplements safely. A panel of experts evaluates current research on various supplements and categorizes them based on how safe and effective they are.

- Group A supplements: Sport foods and supplements that provide a useful and timely source of energy and nutrients or for which there is scientific evidence supporting improved performance
- Group B supplements: Newer supplements on which not enough scientific studies have been conducted, but that may provide a performance benefit as suggested by preliminary evidence
- Group C supplements: Supplements that have not been shown to improve sport performance or that may impair sport performance—most ergogenic substances fall under this category
- Group D supplements: Supplements that are banned or are at high risk of being contaminated with substances (e.g., steroids) that could cause a positive drug test

Table 16.3 provides a complete list of supplements included in each category. Included are each supplement's claims and efficacy based on current research findings. See "Tips for Choosing a Quality Supplement" for helpful hints on how to choose a quality supplement.

Highlight

Tips for Choosing a Quality Supplement

When evaluating supplements, here are a few things to consider:

- Check the name of the manufacturer or distributor. Supplements made by nationally known food and drug manufacturers are more likely to have strict quality control because they must have these procedures in place for their other products.

- Look for products with USP (United States Pharmacopeia), NSF International, or ConsumerLab. com certification marks. This means that the company follows standards required by these third-party evaluators. In addition, a company that is willing to undergo certification is most likely one that has good quality assurance in place.

- Contact the company for more information. Ask what quality control procedures and GMPs it uses. Ask if the company tests the final product for quality and purity and whether the product meets standards for disintegration and dissolution. You can also find out if the product has been involved in clinical studies.

- Look at the label. If it does not follow the DSHEA guidelines for labeling, chances are there are other quality control problems.

- Realize that "natural" does not necessarily mean safe.

Adapted from P. Kurtzweil, 1999, "An FDA guide to dietary supplements," *FDA Consumer.* pgs. 1-9; A. Sarubin-Fragakis and C. Thomson, 2007, *The health professional's guide to popular dietary supplements,* 3rd ed. (Chicago, IL: American Dietetic Association).

Table 16.3   Claims and Efficacy of Ergogenic Substances Categorized by the Australian Institute of Sport (AIS) Sports Supplement Program

Supplement	Description	Claim	Evidence
Group A supplements: These supplements have potential benefits for athletes			
Antioxidants	Nutrients such as vitamins A, C, E, and zinc that combat free radicals in the body	Help reduce oxidative damage that occurs from a sudden increase in training	May help reduce oxidative damage, but no consistent evidence of performance enhancement following antioxidant supplementation.
Bicarbonate	Body's most important extracellular buffer	Protects against free-floating ions (acidosis) after muscle activity	Has been shown to have a moderate effect on short high-intensity (1-10 min) exercise performance. Loading of 0.3 g/kg body weight 1 h prior to exercise is typically used. May cause gastrointestinal problems.
Caffeine	A substance that occurs naturally in the leaves, nuts, and seeds of a number of plants; other names include guarana, kola nut, yerba maté	Enhances endurance performance, "spares" the use of stored muscle glycogen	Originally thought to be "glycogen sparing," caffeine now is thought to act through central nervous system activation. Low caffeine (2-5 mg/kg body weight) has been found to improve endurance performance (>90 min). Recent studies have also shown a benefit for short (1-5 min) and prolonged (20-60 min) high-intensity exercise as well as team sports (e.g., soccer). Responses vary, and there is no evidence of a dose–response relationship for caffeine—that is, performance benefits do not increase with increases in the caffeine dose. Note: *Caffeine above a urinary threshold of 15 µg/mL (>9 mg/kg body weight) is banned by NCAA.*
Calcium	Mineral needed for bone growth and maintenance	Protects against osteoporosis and bone fractures	Well documented that adequate intakes of calcium (and vitamin D), particularly during adolescence and early adulthood, may help prevent osteoporosis. Supplements may be warranted for those with calorie restrictions, lactose intolerance, and impaired menstrual function.
Creatine	A naturally occurring compound found in large amounts in skeletal muscle as a result of dietary intake and endogenous synthesis from amino acids; provides a number of important functions related to fuel supply in the muscle	Performance enhancer; aids in gaining lean body mass	May be beneficial for repetitive short bouts of high-intensity exercise (e.g., resistance training, sprints). Loading typically results in an initial weight gain of ~2 lb. Individual responses vary. Long-term effects are unknown. Creatine is not recommended for those under 18 years.

Supplement	Description	Claim	Evidence
Electrolyte gels or capsules	Contain sodium and potassium, electrolytes commonly lost in perspiration	Provide for rapid rehydration, replace sweat losses	May be useful in situations involving large fluid losses ("making weight" or ultra-endurance activities) or for those with high sweat rates or high sodium losses. Note: Typical sport drinks contain insufficient levels of electrolytes for ultra-endurance events.
Glucosamine	Mild anti-inflammatory properties	"Supports" or "repairs" articular cartilage	The majority of research has been conducted on people with osteoarthritis. No evidence of efficacy in athletes with cartilage damage.
Iron	Essential trace mineral involved in oxygen carrying and immune function	Improves oxygen-carrying capacity	People with low caloric intake, vegetarians, females, pregnant athletes, and those adapting to altitude training are at risk for low iron status. Anemic athletes or those with reduced iron status may benefit from supplementation under supervision.
Liquid meal supplements	High-carbohydrate, moderate-protein, low-fat liquid or powder supplements	Easy and convenient meal replacement	May be helpful for athletes undergoing growth spurts, experiencing heavy training loads, or attempting to gain lean muscle mass.
Glycerol	Backbone of a triglyceride molecule	Causes hyperhydration, decreases heat stress, and improves performance	Evidence for increased water retention (hyperhydration) due to osmotic effect. Studies on thermoregulation and exercise performance have shown mixed results.
Multivitamin-mineral	Provides vitamins and minerals needed for physiological function	Ensures adequate intake of vitamins and minerals	May be warranted for those who restrict calorie intake; eat a limited variety of foods; or eat few fruits, vegetables, and whole grains.
Sport bars	Compact source of carbohydrate and protein with vitamins and minerals	Increase energy, improve performance, enhance recovery	Useful as a convenient, portable source of carbohydrate and protein. Composition is formulated to provide key nutrients (e.g., carbohydrate, protein) for recovery. More expensive than "real" foods.
Sport drinks	Carbohydrate-containing fluid (6-8%) with electrolytes (sodium, potassium)	Provide for rapid rehydration, maintain carbohydrate availability during exercise	Useful for exercise lasting ≥60 min for improved performance, rehydration. Designed for before, during, and after exercise. Should not replace plain water throughout the day.
Sport gels	Concentrated source of easily digestible carbohydrate	Maintain carbohydrate availability during exercise	Provide a practical way to ingest carbohydrate during exercise. Must be taken with water to maintain hydration. Some may contain caffeine, medium-chain triglycerides, or both. May cause gastrointestinal problems for some.

(continued)

Claims and Efficacy of Ergogenic Substances *(continued)*

Supplement	Description	Claim	Evidence
Group B supplements: These supplements need further research on athletes			
Colostrum	Protein-rich substance secreted in breast milk in the first few days after a mother has given birth; usually from cow sources	Improves exercise performance and recovery, increases lean muscle mass	No consistent improvement in athletic performance.
Glutamine	An important fuel source for immune cells; plays a major role in protein metabolism	Maintains or boosts immune function, inhibits protein breakdown	No conclusive evidence that illness is prevented in healthy athletes or that supplementation affects protein metabolism.
Hydroxy-β-methylbutyrate (HMB)	Metabolite of the essential amino acid leucine	Decreases protein breakdown, improves muscle mass, and increases strength	Possibly small effects on lean-body mass and strength, particularly in untrained individuals.
Melatonin	Hormone that regulates circadian rhythms	Promotes sleep, decreases jet lag	Some evidence for use as a sleep aid and attenuation of jet lag. May cause headache and dizziness.
Probiotics	Live microbes	Promote a healthy intestine and immune system, prevent diarrhea	Studies in athletes have not supported claims. Most supporting evidence is in the pediatric population, in which probiotics may attenuate diarrhea.
Ribose	A sugar naturally found in the diet, present in DNA and RNA	Increases the availability of energy in muscle cells	No significant evidence that supplementation enhances performance in well-trained athletes.
Group C supplements: These supplements have little to no evidence as to effectiveness			
Branched-chain amino acids	Essential amino acids	Enhance recovery, decrease protein breakdown, increase lean muscle mass; delay fatigue in endurance exercise	Little evidence for recovery and protein breakdown. No evidence for increasing lean muscle mass. Appears to offer no benefit in delaying fatigue compared to adequate carbohydrate intake during exercise.
Carnitine	Substance used in fatty acid transport	Leads to fat reduction and weight loss	Not effective.
Chromium picolinate	Trace element that enhances insulin action	Increases muscle mass, decreases fat	Not effective for performance. May be useful for diabetics with low chromium status, under medical supervision.
Coenzyme Q_{10}	Part of the electron transport chain in the mitochondria	Improves performance, reduces fatigue	Not effective, and in some studies has been found to impair performance.
Cordyceps	Chinese mushroom or synthetic compound	Reduces fatigue, enhances performance	No effect on endurance or exercise performance.
Ginseng	An adaptogen from the Araliaceae plant family	Improves immunity, endurance, strength	Not effective.
Inosine	Nucleoside	Increases ATP stores, improves strength and performance	Not effective.
Nitrous oxide supplements	Formed from the amino acid L-arginine	Increase blood flow to muscles, promote muscle growth	Not effective. Infusion studies with L-arginine have shown improved blood flow in heart disease patients.

Supplement	Description	Claim	Evidence
Oxygen boosters	Liquid oxygen supplement	Reduce fatigue, increase energy and mental clarity	No evidence.
Pyruvate	Product of the metabolic pathway that breaks down carbohydrate (glycolysis)	Promotes weight loss, spares glycogen	Limited research and evidence.
Rhodiola rosea	Adaptogen; Alpine plant found in Siberia and China	Reduces fatigue, improves endurance	Not effective for exercise performance.
Fish oil	Polyunsaturated fatty acids high in omega-3 fatty acids	Increases endurance	Not effective for improved endurance; anti-inflammatory.
Medium-chain triacylglycerols (MCT)	Fat that is easily absorbed through the bloodstream; derived from coconut oil	Increase fat utilization, spare glycogen	Not effective. May cause gastrointestinal problems.
Group D supplements: These supplements are banned, illegal, or both			
Androstenedione	Precursor (prohormone) to testosterone	Increases testosterone, muscle mass, and strength; decreases fat mass; enhances recovery	Not shown to increase testosterone. No evidence for increased strength or recovery.
Dehydroepi-androsterone (DHEA)	Precursor of testosterone and estradiol	Increases testosterone, increases muscle mass	Little evidence for exercise performance.
Ephedra (ma huang); related compounds: bitter orange, synephrine, Citrus aurantium	α- and β-adrenergic agonists	Burn fat, promote weight loss, enhance endurance	Not effective.
Tribulus terrestris	Increases output of luteinizing hormone	Increases testosterone synthesis, increases muscle size and strength	Not effective.
Other herbal prohormones: chrysin, indole-3-carbinol, gamma-oryzanol, yohimbine, smilax, and mummio	Products that act on the synthetic pathways of either testosterone or estrogen	Increase testosterone concentration, increase muscle size and strength	Not effective.
Human growth hormone (HGH)	Increases gene expression, protein synthesis, fat breakdown, and bone synthesis	Enhances muscle size and strength, increases exercise performance	No evidence at recommended doses.
Anabolic steroids	Synthetic substance related to testosterone	Increase muscle mass, strength, and recovery	Limited evidence due to ethical issues concerning research on steroids.

Information complied from Australian Institute of Sport and Sport Nutrition. Available: www.ais.org.au/nutrition/SupOverview. asp.; J. Antonio and J. Stout, 2001, *Sports supplements* (Philadelphia:, PA: Lippincott, Williams, and Wilkins).

REVIEW OF TWO ERGOGENIC SUBSTANCES

This section briefly reviews two popular ergogenic substances, creatine and anabolic steroids. Creatine is a legal dietary supplement that is not banned by any athletic organization. Conversely, anabolic steroids are illegal and are a prohibited substance in sport. We will not discuss all of the studies involving these two substances. Rather, our purpose is to familiarize you with proposed mechanisms of action and to discuss whether they are effective. Additional references are included that provide more in-depth information about creatine and anabolic steroids.

Creatine

One of the most popular supplements taken to enhance sport performance is creatine. Numerous anecdotal reports on the effectiveness of creatine supplementation have prompted researchers to formally study its mechanism of action and review its effects on performance.

What Is Creatine?

Creatine phosphate (also called phosphocreatine, or PCr) occurs predominantly in skeletal muscle. The term "creatine" actually refers to free creatine in the muscle or to the supplement form of creatine. Creatine is obtained in part from the diet; meat is the predominant dietary source. The liver and pancreas also synthesize creatine from the amino acids argninine, glycine, and methionine. Synthesized creatine is then transported to the skeletal muscle. About 95% of the body's creatine pool is found in skeletal muscle, with the remainder in brain, kidney, liver, and testes (Hunter 1922; Myers and Fine 1915). Creatine can also be taken in supplement form—creatine monohydrate is the form studied in relation to exercise performance.

How Does Creatine Work?

Phosphocreatine is a reservoir of high-energy phosphate bonds. Phosphocreatine serves to resynthesize adenosine triphosphate (ATP), as shown in the following reaction (Hunter 1922):

$$PCr + ADP + H+ \leftrightarrow ATP + Creatine.$$

At rest, approximately 60% of creatine is in the form of PCr (Greenhaff 1997). Creatine and PCr function together to maintain ATP availability; they also buffer hydrogen ion accumulation during muscular contraction. Creatine has been linked with exercise performance due to its role in ATP regeneration. Depletion of PCr is thought to be one primary contributor to muscle fatigue during intense contractions, as its depletion causes adenosine diphosphate (ADP) concentration to increase; excess ADP inhibits crossbridge formation in the muscle, causing fatigue. In theory, creatine supplementation would be beneficial to performance by delaying depletion of PCr and the rate of ADP accumulation and by increasing PCr resynthesis during recovery (Greenhaff 1997). There is also some evidence that creatine may increase gene expression of type I and II myosin heavy chain skeletal muscle fibers, directly inducing muscle hypertrophy (Willoughby and Rosene 2001; Deldicque et al. 2008). Further, the osmotic gradient of creatine has been found to increase cellular swelling, resulting in enhanced glycogen stores (Robinson et al. 1999). Thus, creatine may enhance sport performance through several potential mechanisms.

Does Creatine Supplementation Enhance Performance?

While many ergogenic products do not influence exercise performance, creatine does appear to enhance exercise performance in some instances. Creatine supplementation increases the PCr content of muscle, particularly in type II, or fast-twitch, muscle fibers (Casey et al. 1996). The result of PCr enhancement is that force or work output can be sustained during maximal exercise, and this is especially true during repeated bouts of exercise.

Numerous papers have addressed the impact of creatine supplementation on performance. Creatine supplementation has been shown to improve sprint performance in swimming, running, cycling, soccer, and ice hockey (Balsom et al. 1995; Grindstaff et al. 1997; Kreider et al. 1998; Ziegenfuss et al. 2002; Cox et al. 2002; Jones et al. 1999) and to increase work performed during resistance exercise (Earnest et al. 1995; Kreider et al. 1998; Volek et al. 1999). Some researchers, however, have found no effect of creatine supplementation on exercise performance, particularly with continuous endurance exercise (Deutekom et al. 2000; Burke et al. 1996; Jones et al. 2002). Reasons for the discrepancies among these studies may include differences in prescribed creatine dose, differences among the subjects (e.g., presupplementation creatine status, skill level), and differences among specific exercise protocols and recovery periods.

The potential ergogenic effect of creatine is highly variable among individuals and is highly dependent on the initial muscle content of creatine (Volek and Rawson 2004). Greenhaff (1995) reported that there is a limit to the amount of creatine that muscle tissue can store. Long-term supplementation with creatine does not result in exceeding this maximal capacity. People with the lowest presupplementation creatine content (e.g., vegetarians and vegans) benefit most from supplementation in that they have a greater increase in muscle creatine content and show greater performance improvements (Volek and Rawson 2004). Thus, individuals who are already taking creatine supplements do not benefit from larger doses. Taking 20 g/day for five days is reported to be effective and has minimal risks for healthy individuals. Smaller doses for longer periods of time (3-5 g/day for one month) may also be effective (Bemben and Lamont 2005). Taking larger doses for longer periods may simply be a waste of money (Greenhaff 1995).

Creatine supplementation, while considered safe, may not be without risk. Anecdotal reports have included adverse effects such as kidney damage and muscle cramps. The only published account of adverse effects to date was about renal dysfunction in a British soccer player (Pritchard and Kaira 1998). In contrast, Poortmans and Francaux (1999) found that long-term oral creatine supplementation (i.e., 10 months to five years) had no adverse effect on the renal function of nine athletes. More research is needed to determine the safety of long-term and high-dose creatine supplementation, particularly in adolescents. Currently, creatine is not recommended for those under 18 years of age. Athletes in weight-class sports such as wrestling also need to be aware of the increased weight gain associated with creatine supplementation. The intracellular osmotic load of creatine may increase weight by as much as 2 to 4 lb (~1-2 kg) initially (Bohn et al. 2002).

Anabolic Steroids

Anabolic steroids are probably the best known of the illegal ergogenic substances. Media reports of athletes testing positive for anabolic steroids are not infrequent. Surprisingly, little research has supported the efficacy of anabolic steroids for improved sport performance despite anecdotal evidence to the contrary. This is largely due to

methodological issues that we will consider in this section.

What Are Anabolic Steroids?

Anabolic androgenic steroids are synthetic derivatives of the male hormone testosterone. "Anabolic" refers to promoting skeletal growth, and "androgenic" refers to the male sex characteristics (deepened voice, hair growth). There are several synthetic steroids; some are more anabolic and others more androgenic. Typically, athletes abusing steroids use multiple steroids (called stacking) at gradually increasing doses (called pyramiding) for 7- to 14-week cycles (Hartgens and Kuipers 2004).

Anabolic steroids have an interesting history and are perhaps among the first, and certainly the best-known, ergogenic aids in modern sport. The sporting implications were first noted in 1889 when Charles Edouard Brown-Sequard injected himself with dog and guinea pig testicle extract and announced at a scientific meeting that he "had increased physical strength and intellectual energy" (Foster and Housener 2004, p.334). In the 1930s, synthetic testosterone was synthesized to treat hypogonadism. When it was discovered that steroids could increase skeletal muscle in lab animals, athletes began to take notice. Steroid use became widespread in bodybuilders and weightlifters. In 1974, the IOC became the first organization to ban synthetic steroids, and others followed. The 1976 Montreal Olympic Games introduced the first drug testing for steroids. It was not until 1990 that the U.S. Congress passed the Anabolic Steroid Control Act, which made nonprescription steroids illegal to use and distribute. Athletes were able to avoid positive drug tests by using tetrahydrogestrinone (THG), a designer steroid that was undetectable at the time (Kutscher et al. 2002; Hartgens and Kuipers 2004).

How Do Anabolic Steroids Work?

Anabolic steroids may increase muscle size and strength in the following ways:

1. Increased protein synthesis from increased androgen receptor expression (Sheffield-Moore et al. 1999; Kadi et al. 2000) and gene expression of anabolic hormones such as insulin-like growth factor 1 (IGF-1) (Lewis et al. 2002)

2. Decreased protein breakdown through competition with catabolic hormones such as cortisol and other glucocorticoids for androgen binding sites (Hickson et al. 1990)

3. Increased number of muscle fibers through the activation of satellite cells (myoblasts that do not mature into mononuclei) (Kadi et al. 1999; Eriksson et al. 2005)

4. Psychological effects such as increased aggression, which may allow an athlete to train harder and longer (Yates 2000)

Do Anabolic Steroids Enhance Performance?

Whether steroids are effective or not was a matter of scientific debate for years. Multiple studies in humans showed no effect on strength, endurance, or recovery. However, ethical and methodological issues may account for this. For example, existing research studies used single anabolic steroids, in contrast to the real-life common practice of stacking more than one steroid. Doses in research are also much lower than those used by athletes. It would be unethical to test subjects at high doses of anabolic steroids when there are known health risks. Lastly, the mode of exercise and duration of anabolic steroid use vary widely in the studies that do exist.

The most evidence exists for improved strength performance with use of anabolic steroids. As noted in a review by Hartgens and Kuipers (2004), strength gains of 5% to 20% have been seen in studies evaluating the effects of anabolic steroids on strength performance. Of the 28 studies reviewed, 18 showed significant strength improvement. Even so, many of these studies had the methodological problems discussed here. The landmark paper by Bhasin and colleagues (1996) was the first definitive "proof" that steroids work. In this well-controlled study, testosterone in combination with resistance training was found to produce the greatest strength gains, followed by testosterone alone, compared to exercise alone and to no exercise. Other studies have shown a dose-dependent relationship between testosterone and leg power (Storer et al. 2003) and increased arm circumference and isokinetic force (Hartgens and Kuipers 2004).

In terms of endurance performance, there are very few data on the effects of anabolic steroids on endurance, and the data that exist have shown no effect (Hartgens and Kuipers 2004). Theoretically, anabolic steroids would be expected to increase endurance performance via increased EPO. Some animal studies have been promising. Georgieva and Boyadjiev (2004) performed a study on rats and found that anabolic steroids combined with submaximal training increased submaximal run-ning endurance more than training alone. However, there was no change in oxygen-carrying capacity, $\dot{V}O_2$max, or running economy. Currently, no human data suggest that anabolic steroids are helpful for enhancing endurance performance (Hartgens and Kuipers 2004).

Many athletes also take anabolic steroids for enhanced recovery. Again, there are many testimonials, but few supporting data. Most of the studies have been conducted in animals and have looked at indirect markers of recovery (creatine kinase, heart rate, etc.). As an example, Tamaki and colleagues (2001) found that protein synthesis increased following a bout of resistance exercise in rats.

Regardless of whether steroids work or not, athletes must weigh the risks and ethics of abusing steroids. Use of steroids presents acute and long-term health problems. Steroid use has been associated with a wide range of health consequences including dermatologic, reproductive, cardiovascular, hepatic, neoplastic, and psychological problems (Evans 2004; Hartgens and Kuipers 2004; Parssinen and Seppala 2002; Wu 1997). Perhaps the most serious side effects are those that are irreversible. For example, adolescents may stunt their linear growth through premature epiphyseal (growth plate) closure (Wu 1997).

In summary, evidence appears to be sufficient to support hypertrophy-induced gains in muscle strength and power with use of anabolic steroids. However, data are limited on endurance sport performance and are unconvincing with respect to recovery. In any case, with the large number of testimonials available and with professional athletes winning on steroids, it would be difficult to tell an athlete that anabolic steroids do not work. Education on the harmful side effects and safe alternatives for increasing muscle growth may be a better strategy.

CHAPTER IN REVIEW

Ergogenic substances include any substance used to enhance performance and increase energy production. Significant ethical and legal implications are related to the use of ergogenic substances, making this topic highly controversial. A plethora of substances are advertised to enhance performance and alter body composition. While many are harmless and ineffective, others may lead to health risks. You should be able to critically evaluate these substances and to assist the general public in assessing the true effectiveness and safety of these products.

Key Concepts

1. Describe the issues surrounding the use of ergogenic substances.

Ergogenic substances are used with the sole intention of artificially increasing performance in competition. Many ergogenic substances are banned due to safety concerns and ethical issues, yet their use appears widespread among athletes. Reasons for use include potential improvements in performance and body composition, prevention and treatment of injuries, and stress reduction. The ethical issues surrounding the use of ergogenic substances are highly controversial, and it is unlikely that use of these products will ever be eliminated.

2. Understand how to evaluate currently available ergogenic substances.

Thoroughly investigate all marketing claims. To adequately evaluate published research, you must assess (1) the quality of the investigators and of the laboratory; (2) the research design and the methods used; (3) the accuracy and appropriateness of the results; and (4) the appropriateness of the conclusion in light of the data. In addition, you should be aware of the risks associated with ergogenic substances, including poor dietary practices, potential toxicity, poor quality control, incomplete labels, and untraceable products. Always investigate reports of illness or death in a person who has been taking an ergogenic product, since in some cases even athletes' physicians or families are not aware that they are taking supplements. Report suspected adverse events to the FDA. One of the biggest issues with dietary supplements is underreporting of harmful side effects of these products.

3. Discuss popular ergogenic aids.

Creatine is a widely used ergogenic product. Creatine can improve sprint performance for some people in certain sports, and in some cases can increase the work performed during resistance exercise. Additional studies of creatine that are currently under way should help to clarify its influence on athletic performance.

Anabolic steroids are illegal and have long-term health consequences. Ethical and methodological issues have limited clinical research on the effects of anabolic steroids on exercise performance. However, the available data suggest that they improve strength and power performance but have little effect on endurance and recovery.

Key Terms

anabolic androgenic steroid 478

banned substance 479

blood boosting 480

creatine 494

creatine monohydrate 494

creatine phosphate 494

current good manufacturing practices (CGMPs) 487

Dietary Supplement Health and Education Act (DSHEA) 478

doping 478

ergogenic drug 478

ergogenic substance 478

ergogenic supplement 478

erythropoietin (EPO) 478

ethics 482

gene doping 480

growth hormone 478

phosphocreatine (PCr) 494

structure–function claim 479

World Anti-Doping Agency (WADA) 478

Additional Information

Burke L. Sport foods and supplements. In: Practical sports nutrition. Champaign, IL: Human Kinetics, 2007.

> This chapter provides a discussion of the regulatory issues surrounding sport foods and supplements and highlights some of the most common sport supplements.

Maughan RJ, King DS, Lea T. Dietary supplements. J Sports Sci 2004;22:95-113.

> This article reviews the theory and efficacy of some of the most commonly used sport supplements.

Sjöqvist F, Garle M, Rane A. Use of doping agents, particularly anabolic steroids, in sports and society. Lancet 2008;371(9627):1872-1882.

> This article reviews the prevalence, historical use, side effects, detection, and prevention of doping agents such as anabolic steroids and EPO.

Australian Institute of Sport Sports Supplement Program: www.ausport.gov.au/ais/nutrition/supplements

> This Web site provides general information on sport supplements as well as fact sheets for individual supplements.

References

Antonio J, Stout J. Sports supplements. Philadelphia: Lippincott Williams & Williams, 2001.

Bahrke MS, Yesalis CE. Performance-enhancing substances in sport and exercise. Champaign, IL: Human Kinetics, 2002.

Bahrke MS, Yesalis CE, Kopstein AN, Stephens JA. Risk factors associated with anabolic-androgenic steroid use among adolescents. Sports Med 2000;29(6):397-405.

Balsom PD, Söderlund K, Sjödin B, Ekblom B. Skeletal muscle metabolism during short duration high-intensity exercise: influence of creatine supplementation. Acta Physiol Scand 1995;1154:303-310.

Bamberger M, Yaeger D. Over the edge. Sports Illustrated 1997;70:325-329.

Bemben MG, Lamont HS. Creatine supplementation and exercise performance. Sports Med 2005;35(2):107-125.

Bhasin S, Storer TW, Berman N, Callegari C, Clevenger B, Phillips J et al. The effects of supraphysiologic doses of testosterone on muscle size and strength in normal men. New Engl J Med 1996;335:1-7.

Bohn AM, Betts S, Schwenk TL. Creatine and other nonsteroidal strength-enhancing aids. Curr Sports Med Rep 2002;4:239-245.

Boje O. Doping. Bulletin of the health organization of the league of nations 1939;8:439-469.

Bucci L. Nutrients as ergogenic aids for sports and exercise. Boca Raton, FL: CRC Press, 1993:xv.

Burke LM, Pyne DB, Telford RD. Effect of oral creatine supplementation on single-effort sprint performance in elite swimmers. Int J Sport Nutr 1996;6:222-233.

Burns RD, Schiller MR, Merrick MA, Wolf KN. Intercollegiate student athlete use of nutritional supplements and the role of athletic trainers and dietitians in nutrition counseling. J Am Diet Assoc 2004;104:246-249.

Butterfield G. Ergogenic aids: evaluating sport nutrition products. Int J Sport Nutr 1996;6:191-197.

Casey A, Constantin-Teodosiu D, Howell S, Hultman E, Greenhaff PL. Creatine supplementation favourably affects performance and muscle metabolism during maximal intensity exercise in humans. Am J Physiol 1996;271:E31-E37.

Centers for Disease Control and Prevention (CDC). Youth risk behavior surveillance: United States, 2005. MMWR 2006;55(SS5):1-122.

Corrigan B, Kazlauskas R. Medication use in athletes selected for doping control at the Sydney Olympics. Clin J Sports Med 2003;13:33-40.

Cowart VS. Dietary supplements: alternatives to anabolic steroids? Phys Sports Med 1992;20(3):189-198.

Cox G, Mujika I, Tumility D, Burke L. Acute creatine supplementation and performance during a fixed test simulation match play in elite female soccer players. Int J Sport Nutr Exerc Metab 2002;12:33-46.

Deldicque L, Atherton P, Patel R, Theisen D, Neilens H et al. Effects of resistance exercise with and without creatine supplementation on gene expression and cell signaling in human skeletal muscle. J Appl Physiol 2008;104:371-378.

Deutekom M, Beltman JGM, de Ruiter CJ, de Koning JJ, de Haan A. No acute effects of short-term creatine supplementation on muscle properties and sprint performance. Eur J Appl Physiol 2000;82:223-239.

Dietary supplement health and education act of 1994 (DSHEA). 1994. No. Pub L No. 103-417, 108 Stat 4325.

Dopinginfo.de. Analysis of non-hormonal nutritional supplements for anabolic-androgenic steroids: an international study, 2000. www.dshs-koeln.de/biochemie/rubriken/07_info/07_020320e.pdf

DurRant RH, Rickert VI, Ashworth CS, Newman C, Slavens G. Use of multiple drugs among adolescents who use anabolic steroids. New Engl J Med 1993;328:922-926.

Earnest CP, Snell PG, Rodriguez R, Alamada AL, Mitchell TL. The effect of creatine monohydrate ingestion on anaerobic power indices, muscular strength and body composition. Acta Physiol Scand 1995;153:207-209.

Erdman KA, Fung TS, Reimer RA. Influence of performance level on dietary supplementation in elite Canadian athletes. Med Sci Sports Exerc 2006;38(2):349-356.

Eriksson A, Kadi F, Malm C, Thornell LE. Skeletal muscle morphology in power-lifters with and without anabolic steroids. Histochem Cell Biol 2005;124(2):167-175.

Ervin RB, Wright JD, Kennedy-Stephenson J. Use of dietary supplements in the United States, 1988-1994. Vital and health statistics series 11: data from the National Health Survey, 1999;244(i-iii):1-14.

Evans NA. Current concepts in anabolic-androgenic steroids. Am J Sports Med 2004;32(2):534-542.

Foster ZJ, Housner JA. Anabolic-androgenic steroids and testosterone precursors: Ergogenic aids and sport. Curr Sports Med Report. 2004;3: 334-341.

Froiland K, Koszewski W, Hingst J, Kopecky L. Nutritional supplement use among college athletes and their sources of information. Int J Sport Nutr Exerc Metab 2004;14:104-120.

Gaudard A, Varlet-Marie E, Bressolle F, Audran M. Drugs for increasing the oxygen transport and their potential use in doping. Sports Med 2003;33(3):187-212.

Georgieva KN, Boyadjiev NP. Effects of nandrolone decanoate on VO2max, running economy, and endurance in rats. Med Sci Sports Exerc 2004;36(8):1336-1341.

Goldberg L, Elliot DL, MacKinnon DP, Moe E, Kuehl KS, Nohre L, Lockwood CM. Drug testing athletes to prevent substance abuse: background and pilot study results of the SATURN (Student Athlete Testing Using Random Notification) study. J Adolesc Health 2003;32(1):16-25.

Green GA, Catlin DH, Starcevic B. Analysis of over-the-counter dietary supplements. Clin J Sport Med 2001a;11:254-259.

Green GA, Uryasz FD, Petr TA, Bray CD. NCAA study of substance use and abuse habits of college student-athletes. Clin J Sport Med 2001b;11:51-56.

Greenhaff PL. Creatine and its application as an ergogenic aid. Int J Sport Nutr 1995;5:S100-S110.

Greenhaff PL. The nutritional biochemistry of creatine. J Nutr Biochem 1997;8:610-618.

Grindstaff PD, Kreider R, Bishop R, Wilson M, Wood L, Alexander C, Almada A. Effects of creatine supplementation on repetitive sprint performance and body composition in competitive swimmers. Int J Sport Nutr 1997;7:330-346.

Grunewald KK, Bailey RS. Commercially marketed supplements for bodybuilding athletes. Sports Med 1993;15(2):90-103.

Hartgens F, Kuipers R. Effects of androgenic-anabolic steroids in athletes. Sports Med 2004;34(8):513-554.

Hickson RC, Czerwinski SM, Falduto MT, Young AP. Glucocorticoid antagonism by exercise and androgenic-anabolic steroids. Med Sci Sports Exerc 1990;22(3):331-340.

Hilderbrand RL, Wanninger R, Bowers LD. An update on regulatory issues in antidoping programs in sport. Curr Sports Med Rep 2003;2:226-232.

Hunter A. The physiology of creatine and creatinine. Physiol Rev 1922;2:586-599.

Irving LM, Wall M, Neumark-Sztainer D, Story M. Steroid use among adolescents: findings from project EAT. J Adolesc Health 2002;30:243-252.

Jones AM, Atter T, George KP. Oral creatine supplementation improves multiple sprint performance in elite ice-hockey players. J Sports Med Phys Fit 1999;39(3):189-196.

Jones AM, Carter H, Pringle JSM, Campbell IT. Effect of creatine supplementation on oxygen uptake kinetics during submaximal cycle exercise. J Appl Physiol 2002;92:2571-2577.

Jonnalagadda SS, Rosenbloom CA, Skinner R. Dietary practices, attitudes, and physiological status of collegiate freshman football players. J Strength Cond Res 2001;15(4):507-513.

Juhn MS. Popular sports supplements and ergogenic aids. Sports Med 2003;32(12):921-939.

Kadi F, Bonnerud P, Eriksson A, Thornell LE. The expression of androgen receptors in human neck and limb muscles: effects of training and self-administration of androgenic-anabolic steroids. Histochem Cell Biol 2000;113(1):25-29.

Kadi F, Eriksson A, Holmner S, Thornell LE. Effects of anabolic steroids on the muscle cells of strength-trained athletes. Med Sci Sports Exerc 1999;31:1528-1534.

Kleiner SM. Performance-enhancing aids in sport: health consequences and nutritional alternatives. J Am Coll Nutr 1991;10(2):163-176.

Kreider RB, Ferreira M, Wilson M et al. Effects of creatine supplementation on body composition, strength, and sprint performance. Med Sci Sports Exerc 1998;30:73-82.

Kurtzweil P. An FDA guide to dietary supplements. FDA Consumer 1999;1-9.

Kutscher EC, Lund BC, Perry PJ. Anabolic steroids: a review for the clinician. Sports Med 2002;32(5):285-296.

Leigh-Smith S. Blood boosting. Br J Sports Med 2004;38:99-101.

Lewis MI, Horvitz GD, Clemmons DR, Fournier M. Role of IGF-I and IGF-binding proteins within diaphragm muscle in modulating the effects of nandrolone. Am J Physiol Endocrinol Metab 2002;282(2):E483-E490.

Lightsey DM, Attaway JR. Deceptive tactics used in marketing purported ergogenic aids. Natl Strength Cond Assoc J 1992;14(2):26-31.

Luetkemeier MJ, Bainbridge CN, Walker J, Brown DB, Eisenman PA. Anabolic-androgenic steroids: prevalence, knowledge, and attitudes in junior and senior high school students. J Health Educ 1995;6(1):4-9.

Markowitz SB, Nunez CM, Klitzman S, Munshi AA, Kim WS, Eisinger J et al. Lead poisoning due to hai ge fen. The porphyrin content of individual erythrocytes. JAMA 1994;273(1):24-25.

Massad SJ, Shier NW, Koceja DM, Ellis NT. High school athletes and nutritional supplements: a study of knowledge and use. Int J Sport Nutr 1995;5:232-245.

Morrison LJ, Gizis F, Shorter B. Prevalent use of dietary supplements among people who exercise at a commercial gym. Int J Sport Nutr 2004;14:481-492.

Myers VC, Fine MS. The metabolism of creatine and creatinine. VII. The fate of creatine when administered to man. J Biol Chem 1915;21:377-383.

Nieper A. Nutritional supplement practices in UK junior national track and field athletes. Br J Sports Med 2005;39:645-649.

Nissen SL, Sharp RL. Effect of dietary supplements on lean mass and strength gains with resistance exercise: a meta-analysis. J Appl Physiol 2003;94:651-659.

Nutrition Business Journal. Sports nutrition and weight-loss VI, Sep 2006;1-12.

Parssinen M, Seppala T. Steroid use and long-term health risks in former athletes. Sports Med 2002;32(2):83-94.

Petroczi A, Naughton DP, Mazanov J, Holloway A, Bingham J. Limited agreement exists between rationale and practice in athletes' supplement use for maintenance of health: a retrospective study. Nutr J 2007;6:34-41.

Philen RM, Ortiz DI, Auerbach SB, Falk H. Survey of advertising for nutritional supplements in health and bodybuilding magazines. JAMA 1992;268(8):1008-1011.

Poortmans JR, Francaux M. Long-term oral creatine supplementation does not impair renal function in healthy athletes. Med Sci Sports Exerc 1999;31:1108-1110.

Pritchard NR, Kaira PA. Renal dysfunction accompanying oral creatine supplements. Lancet 1998;351(9111):1252-1253.

Rangachari PK, Mierson S. A checklist to help students analyze published articles in basic medical sciences. Am J Physiol 1995;268(Adv Physiol Educ 13):S21-S25.

Robinson TM, Sewell DA, Hulman E, Greenhaff PL. Role of submaximal exercise in promoting creatine and glycogen accumulation in human skeletal muscle. J Appl Physiol 1999;87:598-604.

Sarubin-Fragakis A, Thomson C. The health professional's guide to popular dietary supplements, 3rd ed. Chicago: American Dietetic Association, 2007.

Scofield DE, Unruh S. Dietary supplement use among adolescent athletes in central Nebraska and their sources of information. J Strength Cond Res 2006;20(2):452-455.

Sheffield-Moore M, Urban RJ, Wolf SE, Jiang J, Catlin DH, Herndon DN, Wolfe RR, Ferrando AA. Short-term oxandrolone administration stimulates net muscle protein synthesis in young men. J Clin Endocrinol Metab 1999;84(8):2705-2711.

Sherman WM, Lamb DR. Proceedings of the Gatorade Sports Science Institute Conference on Nutritional Ergogenic Aids: Introduction. Int J Sport Nutr 1995;5:Siii-Siv.

Slifman NR, Obermeyer WR, Aloi BK et al. Contamination of botanical dietary supplements by digitalis lanata. New Engl J Med 1998;339:806-810.

Smith DA, Perry PJ. The efficacy of ergogenic agents in athletic competition: part II. Other performance-enhancing agents. Ann Pharmacother 1992;26:653-659.

Sobal J, Marquart LF. Vitamin/mineral supplement use among athletes: a review of the literature. Int J Sport Nutr 1994;4:320-334.

Stacy JJ, Terrel TR, Armsey TD. Ergogenic aids: human growth hormone. Curr Sports Med Rep 2004;3:229-233.

Storer TW, Magliano L, Woodhouse L, Lee ML, Dzekov C, Dzekov J, Casaburi R, Bhasin S. Testosterone dose-dependently increases maximal voluntary strength and leg power, but does not affect fatigability or specific tension. J Clin Endocrinol Metab 2003;88:1478-1485.

Tamaki T, Uchiyama S, Uchiyama Y, Akatsuka A, Roy RR, Edgerton VR. Anabolic steroids increase exercise tolerance. Am J Physiol Endocrinol Metab 2001;280(6):E973-E981.

Tentori L, Graziani G. Doping with growth hormone/IGF-1, anabolic steroids or erythropoietin: is there a cancer risk? Pharm Res 2007;55:359-369.

Trent RJ, Alexander IE. Gene therapy in sport. Br J Sports Med 2006;40:4-5.

Unal M, Unal DO. Gene doping in sports. Sports Med 2004;34(6):357-362.

U.S. Department of Health and Human Services and Food and Drug Administration (FDA). Current good manufacturing practice in manufacturing, packing, or holding dietary ingredients and dietary supplements: proposed rule. Fed Register 2003;68(49):12162-12163

Volek JS, Duncan ND, Mazzetti SA et al. Performance and muscle fiber adaptations to creatine supplementation and heavy resistance training. Med Sci Sports Exerc 1999;31:1147-1156.

Volek JS, Rawson ES. Scientific basis and practical aspect of creatine supplementation for athletes. Nutrition 2004;20:609-614.

Whybark MK. Third party evaluation programs for quality of dietary supplements. Herbalgram 2004;64:30-33.

Williams MH. The use of nutritional ergogenic aids in sport: is it an ethical issue? Int J Sport Nutr 1994;4:120-31.

Willoughby DS, Rosene J. Effects of oral creatine and resistance training on myosin heavy chain expression. Med Sci Sports Exerc 2001;33:1674-1681.

World Anti-Doping Agency (WADA). World Anti-Doping code, 2003. www.wada-ama.org/en.

World Anti-Doping Agency (WADA). World Anti-Doping code 2008 prohibited list, 2007. www.wada-ama.org/en.

Wu FCW. Endocrine aspects of anabolic steroids. Clin Chem 1997;43(7):1289-1292.

Yates WR. Testosterone in psychiatry: risks and benefits. Arch Gen Psychiatry 2000;57:155-156.

Yesalis EC, Barsukiewicz CK, Kopstein AN, Bahrke MS. Trends in anabolic-androgenic steroid use among adolescents. Arch Pediatr Adolesc Med 1997;151:1197-1206.

Ziegenfuss TN, Rogers M, Lowery L, Mullins N, Mendel R, Antonio J, Lemon P. Effect of creatine loading on anaerobic performance and skeletal muscle volume in NCAA division I athletes. Appl Nutr Invest 2002;18:397-402.

Appendix A

Nutritional Recommendations

Appendix A.1 Vegetarian Diet Pyramid

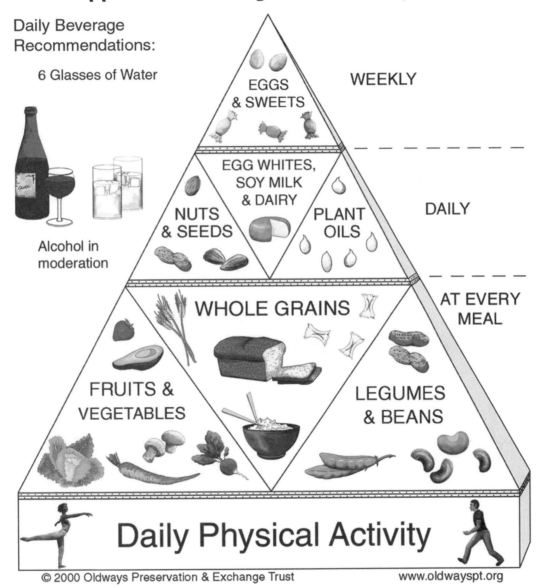

Daily Beverage
Recommendations:

6 Glasses of Water

Alcohol in
moderation

EGGS & SWEETS — WEEKLY

EGG WHITES, SOY MILK & DAIRY

NUTS & SEEDS

PLANT OILS — DAILY

WHOLE GRAINS — AT EVERY MEAL

FRUITS & VEGETABLES

LEGUMES & BEANS

Daily Physical Activity

The healthy traditional vegetarian diet pyramid reflects vegetarian dietary traditions associated with good health. It is one of a group of food pyramids developed in a series of conferences—Public Health Implications of Traditional Diets—that consider diverse traditions around the world. These pyramids, a principal objective of the conferences, are intended to stimulate greater dialogue and interest in cultural models for healthy eating and to provide the basis for effective healthy eating guidelines. This vegetarian diet pyramid is subject to revision in light of ongoing nutrition research.

Appendix A.2 Healthy Traditional Asian Diet Pyramid

Daily Beverage Recommendations:

6 Glasses of Water or Tea

Monthly

MEAT

SWEETS

Weekly

EGGS & POULTRY

FISH & SHELLFISH or DAIRY

Optional Daily

Sake, Wine, or Beer in moderation

VEGETABLE OILS

FRUITS

LEGUMES, SEEDS & NUTS

VEGETABLES

Daily

RICE, NOODLES, BREADS, MILLET, CORN & OTHER WHOLE GRAINS

Daily Physical Activity

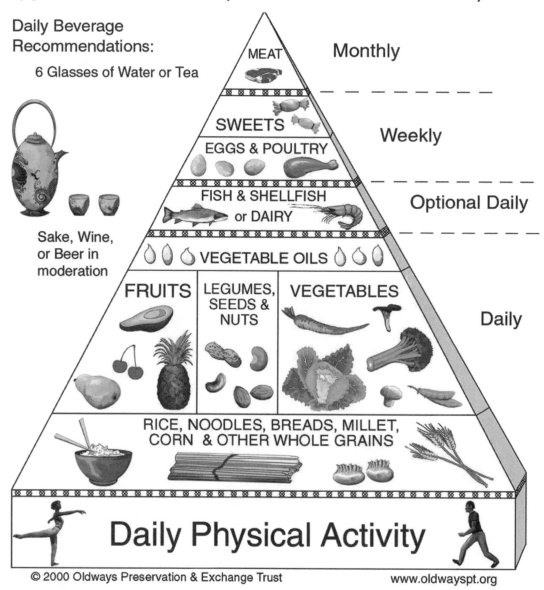

© 2000 Oldways Preservation & Exchange Trust   www.oldwayspt.org

© 2000 Oldways Preservation & Exchange Trust. Available: http://oldwayspt.org

502

Appendix A.3   Healthy Traditional Latin American Diet Pyramid

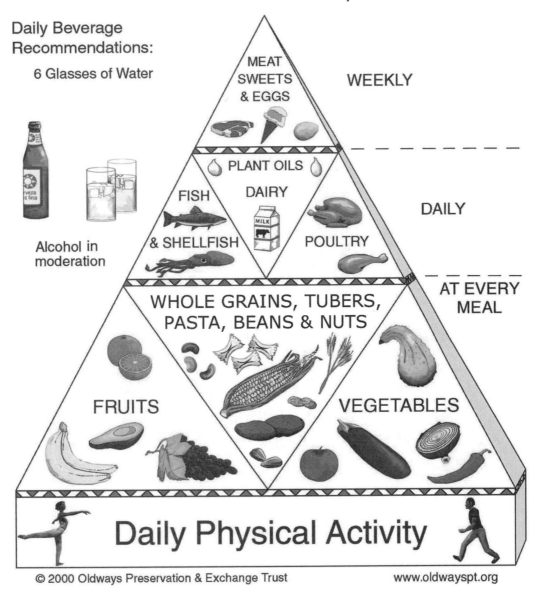

Daily Beverage Recommendations:

6 Glasses of Water

Alcohol in moderation

MEAT SWEETS & EGGS

WEEKLY

PLANT OILS

FISH & SHELLFISH

DAIRY

POULTRY

DAILY

WHOLE GRAINS, TUBERS, PASTA, BEANS & NUTS

AT EVERY MEAL

FRUITS

VEGETABLES

Daily Physical Activity

© 2000 Oldways Preservation & Exchange Trust   www.oldwayspt.org

Alcohol may be consumed by adults in moderation and with meals, but consumption should be avoided during pregnancy and whenever it would put the individual or others at risk.

© 2000 Oldways Preservation & Exchange Trust. Available: http://oldwayspt.org

Appendix A.4 Healthy Traditional Mediterranean Diet Pyramid

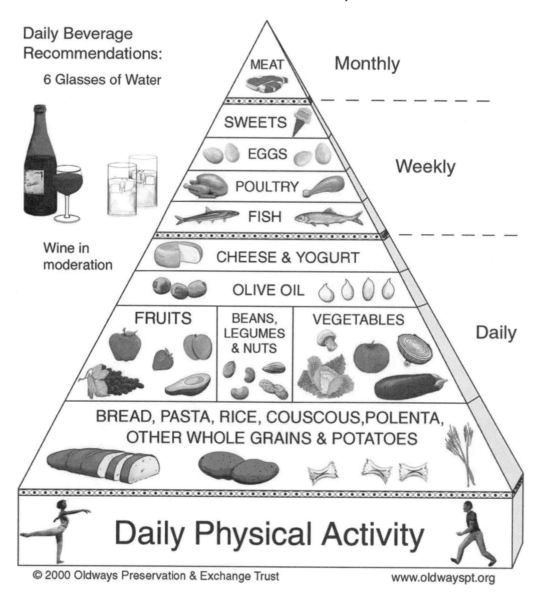

© 2000 Oldways Preservation & Exchange Trust

www.oldwayspt.org

© 2000 Oldways Preservation & Exchange Trust. Available: http://oldwayspt.org

Appendix A.5 Physical Activity, Nutrition, and Fitness Resource List

Physical Activity and Fitness Resource List

Centers for Disease Control and Prevention (CDC)
www.cdc.gov

National Center for Chronic Disease Prevention and Health Promotion
www.cdc.gov/nccdphp/index.htm

U.S. Department of Health and Human Services
www.dhhs.gov

National Institutes of Health (NIH)
Healthy People 2010
Office of Disease Prevention and Health Promotion
www.healthypeople.gov

National Institute of Arthritis and Musculoskeletal and Skin Diseases Information Clearinghouse
www.niams.nih.gov

National Diabetes Information Clearinghouse
www.diabetes.niddk.nih.gov

National Heart, Lung and Blood Institute (NHLBI)
Health Information Center
www.nhlbi.nih.gov

National Institute on Aging
www.nia.nih.gov

Office of Minority Health Resource Center
www.omhrc.gov

President's Council on Physical Fitness and Sports
www.fitness.gov

American Alliance for Health, Physical Education, Recreation and Dance
www.aahperd.org

American College Health Association
www.acha.org

American College of Sports Medicine (ACSM)
www.acsm.org

American Heart Association (AHA)
www.americanheart.org

Boys & Girls Clubs of America (BGCA)
www.bgca.org

National Disability Sports Alliance
www.ndsaonline.org

Disabled Sports USA
www.dsusa.org

National Recreation and Park Association
www.nrpa.org

YWCA of the USA
www.ywca.org

Nutrition Resource List

U.S. Department of Agriculture (USDA) Food and Nutrition Information Center
http://fnic.nal.usda.gov

Food and Nutrition Service (FNS)
www.fns.usda.gov

Food Safety and Inspection Service
www.fsis.usda.gov

Agricultural Research Service (ARS)
www.ars.usda.gov

Food and Drug Administration (FDA)
Center for Food Safety and Applied Nutrition
http://vm.cfsan.fda.gov

National Center for Education in Maternal and Child Health (NCEMCH)
www.ncemch.org

Indian Health Service
www.ihs.gov

National Institutes of Health (NIH)
National Institute of Diabetes and Digestive and Kidney Diseases
www.niddk.nih.gov

National Institutes of Health (NIH)
National Cancer Institute Cancer Information Service
www.cancer.gov

NIDDK Weight-control Information Network (WIN)
www.win.niddk.nih.gov

American Association of Retired Persons
www.aarp.org

American Cancer Society (ACS)
www.cancer.org

American Diabetes Association (ADA)
www.diabetes.org

The American Dietetic Association (ADA)
www.eatright.org

American School Food Service Association
www.schoolnutrition.org

American School Health Association
www.ashaweb.org

Center for Science in the Public Interest
www.cspinet.org

Appendix B

Artificial Sweeteners and Fat Replacers

Appendix B.1   Common Low- and Reduced-Kilocalorie Sweeteners Currently Used or Proposed for Use in the United States

acesulfame K (potassium)—Acesulfame K (brand names Sunnet and Sweet One) is a non-kcal sweetener (white, odorless, crystalline structure) that was discovered in Germany in 1967. It is 200 times sweeter than sugar (sucrose) and may be blended with other low-kcal sweeteners in foods. Acesulfame K is not metabolized by the body and is excreted by the kidneys unchanged. It is most frequently used in baked goods, frozen desserts, dry beverage mixes, instant coffee and tea, chewing gum, candies, oral hygiene products, and breath mints.

aspartame—Aspartame, a nutritive sweetener made from two amino acids (L-phenylalanine and L-aspartic acid), was discovered in 1965. Like acesulfame K, aspartame is 200 times sweeter than sugar. Although aspartame is made up of amino acids, so little is needed to sweeten products that it is considered calorie free even though it has 4 kcal/g. Since aspartame is composed of amino acids (a dipeptide), it is digested like protein and broken down to its components. This artificial sweetener has a sugar-like taste and actually enhances some flavors when added to products. When aspartame is combined with other low-kcal sweeteners, the effect is synergistic, that is, greater than the sum of the effects of the individual sweeteners. Aspartame is typically not used in products exposed to high temperatures because the amino acids are denatured by heat and lose their sweetening ability. Individuals with phenylketonuria (PKU) should restrict their intake of aspartame since it contains phenylalanine. Aspartame is most frequently used

as a tabletop sweetener and in carbonated soft drinks, gum, breakfast cereals, and other dry products. Currently it is found in more than 6000 products and is consumed around the world by over 200 million people. Aspartame is sold under the brand name NutraSweet. As a tabletop sweetener it is packaged and sold under the brand name Equal. More information on aspartame can be found in the "FDA Statement on Aspartame" at www.cfsan.fda.gov.

cyclamate—Cyclamate is a nonnutritive sweetener discovered in 1937 that is 30 times sweeter than sucrose. In general, it is not metabolized and is excreted from the body unchanged. The most common use of cyclamate is as a tabletop sweetener and in sugar-free beverages and sodas. Although it is widely used in over 50 countries, cyclamate was banned in the United States in 1970 due to safety concerns. The Food and Drug Administration (FDA) Cancer Assessment Committee reviewed the scientific research on cyclamates and concluded in 1984 that cyclamates were not carcinogenic. The National Academy of Sciences reconfirmed this decision in 1985. Currently there is a petition before the FDA to reapprove cyclamate in the United States.

neotame—Like aspartame, neotame is derived from the two amino acids aspartic acid and phenylalanine, which are uniquely joined together to form a dipeptide. Neotame is approximately 7000 to 13,000 times sweeter than sugar and 30 to 40 times sweeter than aspartame. It is quickly metabolized to its components via normal metabolic processes. Like aspartame, it is used in a variety of products including soft drinks, puddings and fillings, baked goods, and candies. Neotame was approved by the FDA as a general-purpose sweetener in July 2002. It is also approved for use in Australia and New Zealand.

saccharin—Saccharin, a non-kcal sweetener discovered in 1879, and has been used in commercially available products since the early 1900s. This sweetener is not metabolized by the body and is excreted by the kidney unchanged. Saccharin is 300 times sweeter than sucrose and has a stable shelf life. Similar to what happens with aspartame, when saccharin is combined with other low-kcal sweeteners, they have a synergistic effect that is greater than the sum of the effects of the individual sweeteners. Saccharin is used in tabletop sweeteners and in a wide variety of foods and beverages such as soft drinks, jams, candies, dessert toppings, and salad dressings. It is also used in vitamins and in cosmetic and pharmaceutical products. Saccharin has an aftertaste, but when combined with other low-kcal sweeteners the aftertaste is reduced. Although the FDA proposed a ban in the United States pending further study of saccharin as a potential carcinogen, this ban never went into effect. In 1991, the FDA withdrew the proposed ban, and in 2000 the president signed federal legislation to remove the saccharin warning label that had been required on saccharin-sweetened foods and beverages since 1977. Saccharin continues to be used in 100 countries. It is sold under the brand name Sweet'N Low.

sorbitol—Sorbitol is a sugar alcohol formed through the hydrolysis of sugar. It is approximately 0.5 to 0.7 times as sweet as sugar (sucrose) and is used in special dietary foods, candies, and gum marketed to diabetics. The FDA reports a kilocalorie value of 2.6 kcal/g; thus, this sweetener provides some energy, but its energy content is lower than the 4 kcal/g found in sucrose. Excessive consumption of sor-

bitol (50-80 g/day) can cause gastrointestinal distress and have a laxative effect.

sucralose—Sucralose was discovered in 1976 and approved by the FDA in the spring of 1998 as a noncaloric sweetener for use in 15 food and beverage categories; categorization was expanded to that of a general-purpose sweetener in 1999. Because of the high stability and versatility of sucralose, it can be used in anything to which sugar would more traditionally be added. Sucralose is a disaccharide that is made from sucrose in a five-step process that selectively substitutes three atoms of chlorine for three hydroxyl groups in the sugar molecule. This result is a high-intensity sweetener that is 98% pure and is 600 times sweeter than sugar. The majority of ingested sucralose is excreted unchanged in the feces, and most of what is absorbed appears unchanged in the urine. Therefore, sucralose adds sweetness without adding calories. It can also be used as a tabletop sweetener in either packets or granular form or as a sugar substitute under the name SPLENDA.

xylitol—Xylitol is a sugar alcohol derived from fruits and vegetables (e.g., strawberries, carrots). It has the same sweetness and bulk as sucrose, but the energy content is 2.4 kcal/g. Xylitol is frequently used in chewing gums, gumdrops, hard candies, and pharmaceutical and oral health products.

References for Appendix B.1

Calorie Control Council. Low-calorie sweeteners, 2007. www.caloriecontrol.org. Accessed Dec 2007.

National Cancer Institute (NCI) fact sheet. Artificial sweeteners and cancer: questions and answers. www.cancer.gov/cancertopics/fs-keyword-search. Accessed Dec 2007.

U.S. Food and Drug Administration. Artificial sweeteners: No calories...sweet! FDA Consumer Magazine, July-Aug 2006. www.fda.gov/fdac/features/2006/406_sweeteners.html Accessed Dec 2008.

Appendix B.2 Types of Fat Replacers Currently Used in the United States

Names on the ingredient list	Foods that may contain fat replacers
The following ingredients may be added to replace or reduce the amount of fat required to make the product.	These foods can contain any combination of fat replacers to reduce or eliminate the amount of fat required to make the product.
Carbohydrate-based fat replacers Provide kilocalories similar to carbohydrate (1-4 kcal/g): Corn syrup solids, dextrin, hydrolyzed corn starch, maltodextrin, modified food starch, polydextrose (Litesse), tapioca dextrin, oatrim (Beta-Trim, TrimChoice) Provide negligible kilocalories (dietary fibers): Carrageenan, cellulose gel, cellulose gum, guar gum, inulin, pectin, sugar beet fiber or powder, fiber (Z-Trim, oat fiber, Ultracel)	Baked goods, candy, cheese, chewing gum, salad dressing, frozen desserts, gelatin, meat-based products, puddings, sauces, sour cream, yogurt
Protein-based fat replacers Microparticulated protein (Simplesse) or egg white and milk protein (K-Blazer, ULTRA-Bake), modified whey protein concentrate (Dairy-Lo)	Butter, cheese, sour cream, mayonnaise spreads, baked goods, salad dressings
Fat-based fat replacers Caprenin, olestra (Olean), salatrim (Benefat), mono- and diglycerides, emulsifiers (Dur-Lo)	Soft candy, candy coatings, chips, crackers

Descriptions of Carbohydrate-Based Fat Replacers

Dextrins, maltodextrins, tapioca dextrin, modified food starch: These are bland, nonsweet carbohydrates made from hydrolyzed starches, which can mimic the texture and mouth feel of fat because of their gel-like structure. These products can provide 1 to 4 kcal/g and can completely replace or partially replace the fat in food.

Oatrim: This is a beta-glucan (type of soluble fiber), derived from oat fiber, that can replace fat and supply the additional cholesterol-lowering benefit of oat bran. Oatrim provides 4 kcal/g.

Z-Trim: This noncaloric, bland mix of insoluble fiber is made from the crushed hulls of corn, oats, and rice. It can replace some of the fat and carbohydrate in foods such as chocolates, brownies, cheese, and ground beef.

Polydextrose: This is a nonsweet starch polymer made from food-grade dextrose and small amounts of sorbitol and citric acid. It can be used to replace up to one-half the fat in a product. Most polydextrose passes through the body undigested (5% to 10% is digested) and provides only 1 kcal/g. Polydextrose bulking agents are used in baked goods, puddings, hard and soft candies, chocolates, salad dressings, nutrition bars, frozen dairy desserts, syrups, chewing gums, jams, jellies, and spreads.

Microcrystalline cellulose: This product, made from wood pulp, is noncaloric and can be used to replace 100% of the fat in a product.

Gum: Gums are a type of dietary fiber that mimics the functional properties of fat when water is used to replace fat in foods. Gums are not digested except by gut bacteria, which makes their caloric contribution negligible.

Descriptions of Protein-Based Fat Replacers

Simplesse: This protein-based fat replacer is made by the NutraSweet Company and was approved for use in frozen desserts, mayonnaise, sour cream, salad dressings, refrigerated desserts, yogurt, and cheese. Simplesse is made from milk or egg white proteins (or both), water, sugar, pectin, and citric acid and supplies 1 to 2 kcal/g.

Descriptions of Fat-Based Fat Replacers

Olestra (Olean): Olestra is produced by Proctor and Gamble and is one of the most widely studied fat replacers on the market. It is formed by the esterification of sucrose with six to eight long-chain fatty acids from edible oils. Olestra is not sweet; it has the appearance, taste, texture, and mouth feel of fat and can be used in fried, cooked, and baked products. Olestra is currently approved for snack foods like chips and crackers. Because it is not digested, Olestra is calorie free, but it may reduce the absorption of fat-soluble vitamins and cause some gastrointestinal distress if consumed in large quantities. Vitamins A, D, E, and K are added to products made with olestra.

Salatrim (Benefat): Salatrim was developed by Nabisco and is sold by Cultor Food Science, Inc. It represents a family of reduced-fat triglycerides containing only 4 to 6 kcal/g compared the 9 kcal/g found in normal dietary fats. Salatrim is a real fat, made by combining short-chain fatty acids (either acetic, propionic, or butyric) and one long-chain fatty acid (stearic) to a glycerol backbone. The energy content is lower than that of regular fat because short-chain fatty acids contain only 4 kcal/g and stearic acid is not completely absorbed by the body. This fat is made in either liquid or solid form and is used to replace full fat in ice cream, cheese, sour cream, margarine, spreads, chocolate bars and chips, and cookies and snacks.

References for Appendix B.2

Calorie Control Council (CCC). Washington, DC. www. caloriecontrol.org Accessed Dec 2006.

Hudnall MJ, Conner SJ, Conner WE. Position of the American Dietetic Association: fat replacements. J Am Diet Assoc 1991;91:1285.

Appendix C
Energy Balance

Appendix C.1 Equations Used to Determine Energy Expenditure (kcal/min) From Indirect Calorimetry

Weir (1949)[a]

$kcal/min = 3.941 \ (\dot{V}O_2 \ [L/min]) + 1.106 \ (\dot{V}CO_2 \ [L/min])$

$kcal/min = 3.941 \ (\dot{V}O_2 \ [L/min]) + 1.106 \ (\dot{V}CO_2 \ [L/min]) - 2.17 \ (g/min \ urinary \ N)$
where $\dot{V}O_2$ = oxygen consumed; $\dot{V}CO_2$ = carbon dioxide produced.

Consolazio and Colleagues (1963)

$kcal/min = 3.78 \ (\dot{V}O_2 \ [L/min]) + 1.16 \ (\dot{V}CO_2 \ [L/min]) - 2.98 \ (g/min \ urinary \ N).$

Peters and Van Slyck (1946)

$kcal/min = 3.82 \ (\dot{V}O_2 \ [L/min]) + 1.22 \ (\dot{V}CO_2 \ [L/min]) - 2.01 \ (g/min \ urinary \ N).$

Jequier and Colleagues (1987)

$kcal/min = [4.686 + 1.096 \ (NPRQ - 0.707)] \times NP\dot{V}O_2 + 4.60 \times P\dot{V}O_2$
where: NPRQ is the nonprotein respiratory quotient = $NP\dot{V}CO_2/NP\dot{V}O_2$;

$NP\dot{V}O_2$ is the nonprotein oxygen consumption (L/min);

$P\dot{V}O_2$ is the protein oxygen consumption (L/min);

$NP\dot{V}CO_2$ is the nonprotein CO_2 production (L/min);

$P\dot{V}CO_2$ is the protein CO_2 production (L/min);

$P\dot{V}O_2 = N \times 6.25 \times 0.996$ where N is the total urine nitrogen (g/min);

$P\dot{V}CO_2 = N \times 6.25 \times 0.774$;

$NP\dot{V}O_2 = \dot{V}O_2 - P\dot{V}O_2$;

$NP\dot{V}CO_2 = \dot{V}CO_2 - NP\dot{V}CO_2$.

When: NPRQ = 0.707, $NP\dot{V}O_2$ is entirely due to lipid oxidation, and the calorie equivalent of 1 L of oxygen consumed is 4.686 kcal (or 19.61 kJ).

[a] The difference in energy expenditure calculated by these two equations is less than 3%.

References for Appendix C.1

Consolazio CJ, Johnson RE, Pecora LJ. Physiological measurements of metabolic functions in man. New York: McGraw-Hill, 1963.

Jequier E, Acheson K, Schultz Y. Assessment of energy expenditure and fuel utilization in man. Ann Rev Nutr 1987;7:187-208.

Peters JP, Van Slyck DD. Quantitative clinical chemistry interpretations, vol. 1. Baltimore: Williams & Wilkins, 1946.

Weir JB. New methods for calculating metabolic rate with special reference to protein metabolism. J Physiol 1949;109:1-9.

Appendix C.2 Various Factorial Methods for Calculating Total Daily Energy Expenditure (TDEE)

1. Activity Factor Method 1

- Predict resting metabolic rate (RMR) using one of the prediction equations listed on p. 157.
- Multiply RMR by one of the following activity factors (AF).
- Use this method if you are using only one AF to estimate the whole day.

Factors for Estimating Daily Energy Allowance at Various Levels of Physical Activity for Men and Women (Ages 19-50 Years)

Level of activity	Activity factor (× RMR)	Energy expenditure (kcal · kg^{-1} · day^{-1})
Sedentary or confined to bed	1.2	25
Very light activity		
Men	1.3	31
Women	1.3	30
Light activity		
Men	1.6	38
Women	1.5	35
Moderate activity		
Men	1.7	41
Women	1.6	37
Heavy activity		
Men	2.1	50
Women	1.9	44
Exceptional activity		
Men	2.4	58
Women	2.2	51

The activity factor 1.3 × RMR is a minimum value, reflecting 10 h/day at rest and 14 h of very light activity. Thus, TDEE = RMR (AF).

Example: An active woman (age 41 years, height 163 cm, weight 64.4 kg, body fat 17.2%) exercises approximately 7.5 h/week in both aerobic activities and weight training. Use the Harris-Benedict equation to predict RMR (p. 157).

RMR = 655.1 + 9.56 (64.4 kg) + 1.85 (163 cm) − 4.68 (41 years) = 1380 kcal/day.

TDEE = 1380 kcal/day (AF)
      = 1380 (1.6) (using a moderate activity factor of 1.6)
      = 2208 kcal/day.

References for Method 1

Food and Nutrition Board, National Research Council, National Academy of Sciences. Recommended dietary allowances, 10th ed. Washington, DC: National Academy Press, 1989:27.

Zeman FJ, Ney DM. Applications of clinical nutrition. Englewood Cliffs, NJ: Prentice Hall, 1988:27.

2. Activity Factor Method 2

- Record typical 24 h activities; group amount of time spent in each activity according to the activity categories listed in the table on this page.
- Multiply the amount of time spent in each activity by the appropriate activity factor to calculate a weighted RMR factor. See following example.

- Average the weighted RMR factors to provide a mean activity factor for the day.
- Multiply the mean activity factor by RMR to provide TDEE.

Example: An active woman (age 41 years, height 163 cm, weight 64.4 kg, body fat 17.2%) exercises approximately 7.5 h/week in both aerobic activities and weight training. Activity factors are derived from the table on p. 512. This individual sleeps and rests for 9 h/day; works at a desk and cooks for a total of 9 h/day; does housecleaning, childcare, and walking for 5 h/day; and does aerobics for 1 h/day. RMR is estimated using the Harris-Benedict equation (p. 157).

Activities as multiples of RMR	Activity factor	Duration (h)	Weighted activity factor
Rest	1.0	9	9.0
Very light activity	1.5	9	13.5
Light activity	2.5	5	12.5
Moderate activity	5.0	0	0.0
Heavy activity	7.0	1	7.0
Total		24 h	42
Mean activity factor			1.75 (42 ÷ 24 h)

RMR = 655.1 + 9.56 (64.4 kg) + 1.85 (163 cm) – 4.68 (41 years).

TDEE = 1380 kcal/day (AF)

= 1380 (1.75) (using the estimated activity factor of 1.75)

= 2415 kcal/day.

Reference for Method 2

Food and Nutrition Board, National Research Council, National Academy of Sciences. Recommended dietary allowances, 10th ed. Washington, DC: National Academy Press, 1989:27.

3. Combination Method: General and Specific Activity Factors

- Record typical 24 h activities. Divide activities into two categories: general activities (record amount of time spent walking, sitting, reading, resting, etc.) and specific activities (e.g., record amount of time spent, running 60 min at an 8 mph (12.8 km/h) pace, lifting weights for 30 min, or cycling 15 miles [24 km] at a 20 mph [32 km/h] pace).
- Estimate RMR from one of the equations on p. 157.
- Determine a general activity factor (GAF) for the time the individual is not participating in specific activities. Multiply this activity factor by predicted RMR.
- Determine the amount of energy expended in the specific activities; this is called the specific activity factor (SAF). Use the table provided in appendix E.3 on p. 528 to do this. This table gives the amount of energy expended in mL · kg^{-1} · min^{-1}. Multiply this number by the kilogram body weight of the individual and the number of minutes spent in the activity.
- Add the GAF and SAF values (kcal/day), for example, RMR (GAF) + (SAF).
- Multiply the value by 10% to determine the thermic effect of food (TEF). Add this number to the value obtained in the previous step.
- TDEE = RMR (GAF) + (SAF in kilocalories) + 10% for TEF.

Example: A male long-distance runner (age 23 years, weight 80 kg, height 179 cm, body fat 13%) is a graduate student who trains 2 h/day. When he is not training, he is relatively sedentary and spends his time walking to class, sitting in class, studying, and working at the computer.

1. Determine RMR.

RMR = 66.47 + 13.75 (wt) – 5 (ht) – 6.76 (age) (use equation from p. 157)

RMR = 66.47 + 13.75 (80 kg) + 5 (179 cm) – 6.76 (23 years)

= 1906 kcal/day.

2. Determine energy expended for GAF by multiplying RMR by GAF. A GAF of 1.3 will be used (see table on p. 512, "Factors for Estimating Daily Energy Allowance at Various Levels of Physical Activity") since this individual is relatively inactive apart from the daily running.

   1906 kcal/day (1.3) = 2478 kcal/day.

3. Determine energy expended for SAF. These values are obtained from the table provided in appendix E.3.

60 min/day running 10 mph (6 min/mile) at 0.252 kcal $\cdot$ kg^{-1} $\cdot$ min^{-1}

   0.252 × 80 kg × 60 min = 1209 kcal.

60 min/day running 8 mph (7.5 min/mile) at 0.208 kcal $\cdot$ kg^{-1} $\cdot$ min^{-1}

   0.208 × 80 kg × 60 min = 998 kcal.

   Total energy spent in SAF = 2207 kcal/day.

4. Add values from steps 2 and 3. Thus, 2478 kcal + 2207 kcal = 4685 kcal/day.

5. Add cost of TEF at 10% to total energy needed (see step 4).

   TEF = 4685 × 10%

      = 468 kcal/day expended in TEF. Add this to the value in step 4.

6. TDEE = RMR (GAF) + SAF (kcal/day) + 10% TEF
      = 2478 kcal + 2207 kcal + 468 kcal

      = 5153 kcal/day required to cover energy expenditure.

4. Specific Activity Factor Method

- Determine all activities in a 24 h period. It is best if 24 h activities can be recorded for seven days and then averaged.
- Using the energy expenditure table in appendix E.3, calculate the number of calories expended in each activity the subject engaged in (kcal $\cdot$ kg body weight^{-1} $\cdot$ min^{-1}).
- Add calories expended in each activity over the 24 h period. This should give you TDEE.

Example: A male long-distance runner (age 23 years, weight 80 kg, height 179 cm, body fat 13%) is a graduate student who trains 2 h/day. When he is not training, he is relatively sedentary and spends his time walking to class, sitting in class, studying, and working at the computer.

Activity	Duration of activity (h)	Energy expenditure (kcal $\cdot$ kg^{-1} $\cdot$ min^{-1})	Total energy expended in activity (kcal/day)
Sleeping	7	0.020	672.0
Sitting quietly	6	0.021	604.8
Walking, normal pace	1.5	0.080	576.0
Standing quietly	1	0.027	129.6
Cleaning	0.25	0.058	69.6
Cooking	0.25	0.048	57.6
Eating (sitting)	1	0.023	110.4
Lying at ease	2	0.022	211.2
Playing the piano	1	0.040	192.0
Typing at computer	2	0.031	297.6
Running 6 min/mile	1	0.252	1209.6
Running 7.5 min/mile	1	0.208	998.4
Totals	24 h		5129 kcal/day

Thus, TDEE for this individual using the specific activity method is 5129 kcal/day. Many computer programs (e.g. Food Processor Plus, ESHA Research, Salem, OR) calculate TDEE using this method.

Appendix C.3 Effect of Exercise on Resting Metabolic Rate (RMR) in Trained Versus Untrained Young Men

Reference	Subjects	Mean V̇O₂max (mL · kg⁻¹ · min⁻¹)	Mean RMR (kcal/kg FFM)	% diff. in RMR	Significant difference
Almeras et al. 1991	CC skiers ($n = 7$)	NA	26.75	5.2%	NS
	Controls ($n = 8$)	NA	25.36		
Broeder et al. 1992	Trained ($n = 10$)	70.1	30.17	3.4%	NS
	Controls ($n = 21$)	41.1	29.47		
Bullough et al. 1995	Trained ($n = 8$)	62.9	27.73↑ flux day	16% (a)	$p < 0.01$
	Controls ($n = 8$)	43.0	23.27		
Byrne and Wilmore 2001	Aerobic trained ($n = 21$)	49.2	29.92	–	NS
	Controls ($n = 20$)	31.4	30.83		
Byrne and Wilmore 2001	Resistance trained ($n = 20$)	45.0	29.49	–	NS
	Controls ($n = 20$)	31.4	30.83		
Gilliat-Wimberly et al. 2001	Trained ($n = 18$)	NA	32.06	1.3%	NS
	Controls ($n = 14$)	NA	31.99		
Horton and Geissler 1994	Trained ($n = 10$)	(b)	26.75	5.3%	NS
	Controls ($n = 10$)	(b)	25.33		
Poehlman et al. 1988	Trained ($n = 9$)	70.5	28.32	11.0%	$p < 0.05$
	Controls ($n = 9$)	53.0	25.20		
Poehlman et al. 1990	Trained ($n = 22$)	60.2	26.50	4.2%	$p < 0.05$
	Controls ($n = 20$)	50.4	25.40		
Tremblay et al. 1983	Runners ($n = 8$)	69.2	34.12	4.8%	NS
	Controls ($n = 8$)	47.7	32.48		
Tremblay et al. 1986	Runners/skiers ($n = 20$)	68.4	26.95	5.4%	NS
	Controls ($n = 39$)	50.8	25.50		

NA = not available.
NS = not significant.

(a) Differences between groups found only when trained group was in a high flux period (exercising at least 90 min/day at 75% V̇O₂max) and compared to untrained subjects who were in a no-exercise state. No differences were found between groups when trained subjects were in a low flux period (no exercise for three days). Values estimated from paper.

(b) Subjects were classified as sedentary or highly active on the basis of their habitual exercise patterns.

References for Appendix C.3

Almeras N, Mineault N, Serresse O, Boulay MR, Tremblay A. Non-exercise daily energy expenditure and physical activity patterns in male endurance athletes. Eur J Appl Physiol 1991; 63:184-187.

Broeder CE, Burrhus KA, Svanevik LA, Wilmore JH. The effects of aerobic fitness on resting metabolic rate. Am J Clin Nutr 1992;55:795-801.

Bullough RC, Gillette CA, Harris MA, Melby CL. Interaction of acute changes in exercise energy expenditure and energy intake on resting metabolic rate. Am J Clin Nutr 1995;61:473-481.

Byrne HK, Wilmore JH. The effects of a 20-week exercise training program on resting metabolic rate in previously sedentary, moderately obese women. Int J Sport Nutr Exerc Metab 2001;11:15-31.

Gilliat-Wimberly M, Manore MM, Woolf K, Swan PD, Carroll SS. Effects of habitual physical activity on the resting metabolic rates and body compositions of women aged 35 to 50 years. J Am Diet Assoc Oct 2001;101(10):1181-1188.

Horton TJ, Geissler CA. Effect of habitual exercise on daily energy expenditure and metabolic rate during standardized activity. Am J Clin Nutr 1994;59:13-19.

Poehlman ET, McAuliffe TL, VanHouten DR, Danforth E. Influence of age and endurance training on metabolic rate and hormones in healthy men. Am J Physiol 1990;259:E66-E72.

Poehlman ET, Melby CL, Badylak SF. Resting metabolic rate and postprandial thermogenesis in highly trained and untrained males. Am J Clin Nutr 1988;47:793-798.

Tremblay A, Cote J, LeBlanc J. Diminished dietary thermogenesis in exercise-trained human subjects. Eur J Appl Physiol 1983;52:1-4.

Tremblay A, Fontaine E, Poehlman ET, Michell D, Perron L, Bouchard C. The effect of exercise-training on resting metabolic rate in lean and moderately obese individuals. Int J Obesity 1986;10:511-517.

Appendix C.4 Effect of Exercise Training on Posttraining Resting Metabolic Rate (RMR) in Previously Untrained Individuals

Reference	Subjects and type of training	Pretraining RMR (kcal/kg FFM)	Posttraining RMR (kcal/kg FFM)	% RMR difference (post-pre ÷ pre)[a]	Significant differences
Broeder et al. 1992	Males (n = 22): ET for 12 weeks	28.95	29.19	<1%	NS
Broeder et al. 1992	Males (n = 22): RT for 12 weeks	29.17	29.48	<1%	NS
Byrne and Wilmore 2001	Women: RT for 20 weeks (n = 10) or RT + walking (n = 9)	RT = 29.39 RT + walking = 30.35	RT = 29.20 RT + walking = 28.20	−4% −7%	NS $p \leq 0.05$
Goran and Poehlman 1992[b,c]	Males (n = 6) and females (n = 5): ET for 8 weeks	32.22	34.99	8.6%	$p < 0.01$
Keytel et al. 2001	Postmenopausal women (n = 9): ET for 8 weeks	33.08	34.32	9.4%	NS
Poehlman and Danforth 1991[b]	Males (n = 13) and females (n = 6): ET for 8 weeks	24.48	27.36	11.8%	$p < 0.01$
Tremblay et al. 1986[b]	Obese females (n = 8): ET for 11 weeks	26.64	28.51	7.0%	$p < 0.01$

ET= endurance trained; RT = resistance trained; NS= not significant.

[a] %RMR difference = post-training RMR-Pretraining RMR ÷ pretraining RMR. All RMR values are in kcal/kg.

[b] Subjects were >60 years of age.

[c] Relative RMR values estimated for graphs and tables.

References for Appendix C.4

Broeder CE, Burrhus KA, Svanevik LA, Wilmore JH. The effects of either high-intensity resistance or endurance training on resting metabolic rate. Am J Clin Nutr 1992;55:802-810.

Byrne HK, Wilmore JH. The effects of a 20-week exercise training program on resting metabolic rate in previously sedentary, moderately obese women. Int J Sport Nutr Exerc Metab 2001;11:15-31.

Goran MI, Poehlman ET. Endurance training does not enhance total energy expenditure in healthy elderly persons. Am J Phyisol 1992;263:E950-E957.

Keytel LR, Lambert MI, Johnson J, Noakes TD, Lambert EV. Free living energy expenditure in post-menopausal women before and after exercise training. Int J Sport Nutr Exerc Metab 2001;11:226-237.

Poehlman ET, Danforth E. Endurance training increases metabolic rate and norepinephrine appearance rate in older individuals. Am J Physiol 1991;261:E233-E239.

Tremblay A, Fontaine E, Poehlman ET, Mitchell D, Perron L, Bouchard C. The effect of exercise-training on resting metabolic rate in lean and moderately obese individuals. Int J Obesity 1986;10:511-517.

Appendix C.5 Effect of Type of Exercise and Exercise Intensity on Magnitude and Duration of Excess Postexercise Oxygen Consumption (EPOC)

Reference	Subjects: type of exercise training and fitness level	Exercise: intensity and duration	% EPOC or duration of EPOC (min or h)
Bahr et al. 1987	ET males ($n = 6$) $\dot{V}O_2$max = 54 mL · kg^{-1} · min^{-1}	70% $\dot{V}O_2$max for 20 min 70% $\dot{V}O_2$max for 40 min 70% $\dot{V}O_2$max for 80 min	5.1% at 12 h 6.8% at 12 h 14.4% at 12 h
Bahr and Sejersted 1991	ET males ($n = 6$) $\dot{V}O_2$max = 50 mL · kg^{-1} · min^{-1}	29% $\dot{V}O_2$max for 80 min 50% $\dot{V}O_2$max for 80 min 75% $\dot{V}O_2$max for 80 min	0.3 h 3.3 h 10.5 h
Bahr et al. 1992	Males ($n = 6$) $\dot{V}O_2$max = 49 mL · kg^{-1} · min^{-1}	2 min at 108% $\dot{V}O_2$max done 1 time 2 min at 108% $\dot{V}O_2$max repeated 2 times 2 min at 108% $\dot{V}O_2$max repeated 3 times	30 min 60 min 4 h
Bielinski et al. 1985	ET males ($n = 10$) $\dot{V}O_2$max = 63 mL · kg^{-1} · min^{-1}	50% $\dot{V}O_2$max for 3 h	O_2↑ 4-5 h post-ex; RMR↑ by 4.7% after 24 h
Brehm and Gutin 1986	ET subjects ($n = 8$) and controls ($n = 8$)	6.4 km/h walking for 2 miles	42 min
Braum et al. 2005	UT females ($n = 8$) controlled for MS	Weight training = 3 sets, 15 reps of 8 exercises at 65% 1-repetition max (1RM)	O_2 15%↑ at 30 min post-ex vs. 60 min; 60 min O_2 20%↑ vs. rest
Chad and Quigley 1989	UT females ($n = 5$)	55% $\dot{V}O_2$max for 90 min	O_2 still ↑ after 60 min
Chad and Quigley 1991	ET females ($n = 5$) and UT females ($n = 5$)	50% $\dot{V}O_2$max for 3 h 70% $\dot{V}O_2$max for 3 h	O_2 still ↑ after 3 h for both groups, but highest after 50% $\dot{V}O_2$max
Elliot et al. 1992	ET and RT males ($n = 4$) and females ($n = 5$) $\dot{V}O_2$max = 45-48 mL · kg^{-1} · min^{-1}	40 min cycling at 80% MHR; 40 min circuit training at 50% maximum repetition; 40 min heavy resistance at 80-90% at maximum repetition	↑10% 30 min post-ex (80% MHR) ↑19% 30 min post-ex (50%) ↑21% 30 min post-ex (80-90%)
Freedman-Akabas et al. 1985	ET subjects ($n = 12$) and controls ($n = 7$)	20 min at individual anaerobic threshold	Return to baseline by 40 min
Freedman-Akabas et al. 1985	ET males ($n = 4$) and females ($n = 3$)	40 min at 2 mph faster than anaerobic threshold	Return to baseline by 40 min
Fukuba et al. 2000	Females ($n = 5$)	70% $\dot{V}O_2$max for 60 min	8.6 L EPOC at 7 h (follicular) 8.9 L EPOC at 7 h (luteal)
Gillette et al. 1994	ET and RT males ($n = 10$) $\dot{V}O_2$max = 52 mL · kg^{-1} · min^{-1}	100 min weightlifting equaling 588 kcal; 64 min at 50% $\dot{V}O_2$max cycling equaling 536 kcal	5 h EPOC = ↑12.5% for weightlifting; ↑4.5% for cycling

Reference	Subjects: type of exercise training and fitness level	Exercise: intensity and duration	% EPOC or duration of EPOC (min or h)
Gore and Withers 1990a	ET males ($n = 9$) $\dot{V}O_2$max = 63 mL · kg⁻¹ · min⁻¹	30%, 50%, 70% $\dot{V}O_2$max at 20, 50, and 80 min	After 8 h EPOC only slightly ↑ (1-8.9%; mean = 4.8%)
Gore and Withers 1990b	ET males ($n = 9$) $\dot{V}O_2$max = 63 mL · kg⁻¹ · min⁻¹	30%, 50%, 70% $\dot{V}O_2$max at 20, 50, and 80 min	After 8 h, no EPOC after 30% $\dot{V}O_2$max ex; ↑EPOC for 50% and 70% $\dot{V}O_2$max ex
Jamurtas et al. 2004	Males ($n = 10$)	70-75% $\dot{V}O_2$max for 60 min; 40 sets of 8-12 reps at 70-75% 1RM	↑ after 24 h
McGarvey et al. 2005	ET males ($n = 12$; 30 years) $\dot{V}O_2$max = 49.7 mL · kg⁻¹ · min⁻¹	Interval cycling = seven 2 min intervals at 90% $\dot{V}O_2$max followed by 3 min at 30% $\dot{V}O_2$max. Continuous cycling = 30-32 min at 65% $\dot{V}O_2$max	2 h EPOC = ↑7.5-8.5% 2 h EPOC = ↑7.3-8.3%
Melby et al. 1992	RT males ($n = 6$)	40 min weightlifting	↑12% at 30 min and ↑6% at 60 min post-ex
Melby et al. 1993	RT males ($n = 13$)	90 min weightlifting	↑O₂ after 2 h by 11-12%; RMR↑ by 4.7-9.7% after 24 h
Osterberg and Melby 2000	RT females ($n = 7$)	100 min weightlifting	↑O₂ after 3 h by 13%; RMR↑ by 4.2 after 24 h
Pacy et al. 1985	Lean subjects ($n = 4$)	35-55% $\dot{V}O_2$max for 4 h	Return to baseline by 60 min
Sedlock et al. 1989	ET males ($n = 10$)	High intensity, short duration Low intensity, short duration Low intensity, long duration	33 min 20 min 28 min
Sedlock 1991a	Females ($n = 8$) $\dot{V}O_2$max = 40 mL · kg⁻¹ · min⁻¹	60% $\dot{V}O_2$max for 200 kcal	19 min
Sedlock 1991b	Females ($n = 7$), moderately ET	40% $\dot{V}O_2$max for 200 kcal 60% $\dot{V}O_2$max for 200 kcal	28 min 18 min
Smith and McNaughton 1993	ET males ($n = 8$) and females ($n = 8$)	40% $\dot{V}O_2$max for 30 min 50% $\dot{V}O_2$max for 30 min 70% $\dot{V}O_2$max for 30 min	27-31 min 36-42 min 39-48 min

ET = endurance trained; RT = resistance trained; UT = untrained; MHR = maximal heart rate; MS = menstrual cycle.

References for Appendix C.5

Bahr R, Gronnerod O, Sejersted OM. Effect of supramaximal exercise on excess postexercise O₂ consumption. Med Sci Sport Exerc 1992;24:66-71.

Bahr R, Ingnes I, Vaage O, Sejersted OM, Newsholme EA. Effect of duration of exercise on excess postexercise O₂ consumption. J Appl Physiol 1987;62(2):485-490.

Bahr R, Sejersted OM. Effect of intensity of exercise on exercise post-exercise O₂ consumption. Metabolism 1991;40:836-841.

Bielinski R, Schutz Y, Jequier E. Energy metabolism during the post-exercise recovery of man. Am J Clin Nutr 1985;42:69-82.

Braum WA, Hawthore WE, Markofski MM. Acute EPOC response in women to circuit training and treadmill exercise of matched oxygen consumption. Eur J Appl Physiol 2005;94:500-504.

Brehm BA, Gutin B. Recovery energy expenditure for steady state exercise in runners and nonexercisers. Med Sci Sports Exerc 1986;18:205-210.

Chad K, Quigley B. The effects of substrate utilization, manipulated by caffeine, on post-exorcise oxygen consumption in untrained female subjects. Eur J Appl Physiol 1989;59:48-54.

Chad KE, Quigley BM. Exercise intensity: effect on postexercise O$_2$ uptake in trained and untrained women. J Appl Physiol 1991;70(4):1713-1719.

Elliot DL, Goldberg L, Kuchl KS. Effect of resistance training on excess post-exercise oxygen consumption. J Appl Sport Sci Res 1992;6:77-81.

Freedman-Akabas S, Colt E, Kissileff HR, Pi-Sunyer X. Lack of sustained increase in VO2 following exercise in fit and unfit subjects. Am J Clin Nutr 1985;41:545-549.

Fukuba Y, Yano Y, Murakami H et al. The effect of dietary restriction and menstrual cycle on excess post-exercise oxygen consumption (EPOC) in young women. Clin Physiol 2000;20(2):165-169.

Gillette CA, Bullough RC, Melby CL. Postexercise energy expenditure in response to acute aerobic or resistive exercise. Int J Sport Nutr 1994;4:347-360.

Gore CJ, Withers RT. Effect of exercise intensity and duration on postexercise metabolism. J Appl Physiol 1990a;68(6):2362-2368.

Gore CJ, Withers RT. The effect of exercise intensity and duration on the oxygen deficit and excess post-exercise oxygen consumption. Eur J Appl Physiol 1990b;60:169-174.

Jamurtas AZ, Koutedakis Y, Paschalis V, Tofas T, Yfanti C, Tsiokanos A et al. The effects of a single bout of exercise on resting energy expenditure and respiratory exchange ratio. Eur J Appl Physiol 2004;92:393-398.

McGarvey, W., Jones, R., & Petersen, S. (2005). Excess postexercise oxygen consumption following continuous and interval cycling exercise. Int J Sport Nutr Exerc Metab, 15(1), 28-37.

Melby C, Scholl C, Edwards G, Bullough R. Effect of acute resistance exercise on postexercise energy expenditure and resting metabolic rate. J Appl Physiol 1993;75(4):1847-1853.

Melby CL, Tincknell T, Schmidt WD. Energy expenditure following a bout of non-steady state resistance exercise. J Sports Med Phys Fit 1992;32:128-135.

Osterberg KL, Melby CL. Effect of acute resistance exercise on postexercise oxygen consumption and resting metabolic rate in young women. Int J Sport Nutr Exerc Metab 2000;10:71-81.

Pacy PJ, Barton N, Webster JD, Garrow JS. The energy cost of aerobic exercise in fed and fasted normal subjects. Am J Clin Nutr 1985;42:764-768.

Sedlock DA. The effect of acute nutritional status on postexercise energy expenditure. Nutr Res 1991a;11:735-742.

Sedlock DA. Effect of exercise intensity on postexercise energy expenditure in women. Br J Sports Med 1991b;25(1):38-40.

Sedlock DA, Fissinger JA, Melby CL. Effect of exercise intensity and duration on postexercise energy expenditure. Med Sci Sports Exerc 1989;21:662-666.

Smith J, McNaughton L. The effects of intensity of exercise on excess postexercise oxygen consumption and energy expenditure in moderately trained men and women. Eur J Appl Physiol 1993;67:420-425.

Appendix D
Body Fat Percentages for Athletes

Sport	Level of competition			
Method	**Reference**	**Gender**	**% Fat ±SD**	**Age (years)**
Basketball	Collegiate postseason	Female	20.4 ± 0.9	20 ± 1
UWW[1]	Johnson et al. 1989			
	Collegiate	Female[4]	29.0 ± 5.2	19 ± 1
DXA[2]	Nichols et al. 1995			
	Not reported	Female	23.2 ± 3.4	—
Skinfolds	Mokha and Sidhu 1987			
	Collegiate	Female	24.4 ± 3.2	19 ± 1
BIA[3]	Nowak et al. 1988			
	U17 National Team	Female	18.0 ± 1.8	16 ± .4
Skinfolds	Bale 1991			
	Collegiate	Female	20.5 ± 2.3	20 ± 1
UWW	Siders et al. 1991			
	Collegiate	Male	10.6 ± 3.4	19 ± 1
BIA	Nowak et al. 1988			
	Collegiate	Male	7.7 (no SD)	Not reported
Skinfolds	Bolonchuk et al. 1991			
	Collegiate	Male	10.5 ± 3.8	21 ± 1
UWW	Siders et al. 1991			
Volleyball	Collegiate	Female[4]	27.1 ± 3.9	19 ± 1
DXA	Nichols et al. 1995			
	Not reported	Female	23.1 ± 3.6	—
Skinfolds	Mokha and Sidhu 1987			
	Collegiate	Female	20.9 ± 2.8	20 ± 1
UWW	Johnson et al. 1989			
Swimming	Collegiate (preseason)	Female	18.3 ± 3.6	19 ± 1
	(peak training)		15.7 ± 3.4	
UWW	Meleski and Malina 1985			
	Collegiate	Female	21.4 ± 3.4	19 ± 1
UWW	Sliders et al. 1991			
	National Team (synchronized)	Female	24.0 ± 4.8	20 ± 2
UWW	Roby et al. 1983			
	Collegiate	Female	22.2 ± 4.2	19 ± 1
UWW	Johnson et al. 1989			
	Collegiate	Male	14.3 ± 3.1	20 ± 1
UWW	Siders et al. 1991			
Distance running	Not reported	Female	19.7 ± 3.0	—
Skinfolds	Mokha and Sidhu 1987			
	Recreational	Female[4]	18.8 ± 1.7	23 ± 5
UWW	Phillips et al. 1993			
	Collegiate	Female	14.3 ± 4.3	21 ± 1
UWW	Johnson et al. 1989			
	Moderate mileage	Male	11.2 ± 1.6	32 ± 6
Skinfoldds	Lucia et al. 1996			
	Recreational	Male	10.5 ± 1.2	23 ± 4
UWW	Phillips et al. 1993			

(continued)

Body Fat Percentages for Athletes   *(continued)*

Sport		Level of competition			
	Method	Reference	Gender	% Fat ±SD	Age (years)
Gymnastics		Elite (and figure skaters)	Female[8]	17.5 ± 3.1	17 ± 1
	DXA and UWW[7]	Fogelholm et al. 1995			
		Collegiate	Female[4]	22.6 ± 3.7	19 ± 1
	DXA	Nichols et al. 1995			
		High school	Female	13.1 ± 1.4	15 ± 1
	UWW	Moffatt et al. 1984			
		Collegiate (preseason)	Female	21.4 ± 6.2	20 ± 3
		(postseason)		13.3 ± 5.9	
	Skinfolds	Vercryssen and Shelton 1988			
		Collegiate	Female	14.5 ± 3.5	19 ± 1
	UWW	Johnson et al. 1989			
Soccer		National	Female[4]	25.8 ± 3.0	18 ± 2
	DXA and UWW	Fogelholm et al. 1995			
		Collegiate, national, and professional	Male	9.1 to 15.7	17 to 27
	Not reported	Kirkendall 1985			
		Professional (team A)	Male	12.2 ± 2.4	26 ± 4
		Professional (team B)	Male	13.0 ± 2.5	23 ± 4
	Not reported	Maughn 1997			
Cycling		Professional	Male	9.4 ± 0.7	26 ± 2
	Skinfolds	Lucia et al. 1996			
		Amateur	Male	15.0 ± 3.0	55 ± 5
		Amateur	Male	15.0 ± 3.0	24 ± 6
	BIA	Giada et al. 1995			
Triathlon		Elite	Male	9.4 ± 0.5	26 ± 3
	Skinfolds	Lucia et al. 1996			
		European or World Champion	Male	8.2 ± 2.3	18 ± 2
	Skinfolds	Bunc et al. 1996			
		European or World Champion	Female	10.4 ± 2.6	17 ± 1
	Skinfolds	Bunc et al. 1996			
Power sports		High school	Male	16.8 ± 7.3	17 ± 1
	Skinfolds	Nindl et al. 1995			
		High school	Female	26.1 ± 5.6	16 ± 1
	Skinfolds	Nindl et al. 1995			
		Not reported (throwers)	Female	23.8 ± 3.5	—
	Skinfolds	Mokha and Sidhu 1987			
		Not reported (jumpers)	Female	19.2 ± 2.9	—
	Skinfolds	Mokha and Sidhu 1987			
Rowing		Elite (heavyweight)	Female	20.7 ± 4.0	26 ± 4
	UWW	Pacy et al. 1995			
		International winners	Male	6.5 ± 0.5	26 ± 0.6
	Not reported	Secher et al. 1983			
		International competitors	Male	8.3 ± 0.4	25 ± 0.5
	Not reported	Secher et al. 1983			
Wrestling		Collegiate	Male	9.8 ± 0.5	18 to 21
	Skinfolds	Enns et al. 1987			
		Collegiate	Male	10.9 ± 1.9	18 to 24
	Skinfolds	Song and Cipriano 1984			
		Collegiate	Male	11.4 ± 3.2	20 ± 1
	UWW	Siders et al. 1991			

Sport	Level of competition	Gender	% Fat ±SD	Age (years)
Method	**Reference**			
Football	Collegiate	Male	13.7 ± 4.2	20 ± 2
UWW	Siders et al. 1991			
	Collegiate	Male	12.4 ± 3.2	—
Skinfolds	Bolonchuk and Lukaski 1987			
	Collegiate (backs)	Male	7.3 to 13.8	—
Not reported	Pincivero and Bompa 1997			
	Collegiate (linemen)	Male	13.2 to 21.8	—
Not reported	Pincivero and Bompa 1997			
	Professional (backs)	Male	5.7 to 18.5	—
Not reported	Pincivero and Bompa 1997			
	Professional (linemen)	Male	15.5 to 18.7	—
Not reported	Pincivero and Bompa 1997			
Running/triathlon	Highly competitive	Female[4]	15.9 ± 1.3	31 ± 1
		Female[5]	16.0 ± 1.5	26 ± 2
DXA	Laughli and Yen 1996	Female	20.8 ± 1.1	20 ± 1
Swimming/running/ triathlon	Mixed (collegiate, local, and national)	Female	16.3 ± 1.7	34 ± 1
DXA	Ryan et al. 1996	Female[7]	22.6 ± 2.1	45 ± 1
Endurance training	Not reported	Male—young	10.9 ± 1.4	27 ± 1
		Male—middle aged	19.5 ± 3.4	52 ± 2
UWW	Meredith et al. 1989			
Swimming/Nordic skiing	Collegiate	Male	8.6 ± 0.2	27 ± 1
Skinfolds	Enns 1987			
Cross-country skiing	World-class	Male	12 ± 1	26 ± 2
	World-class	Female[6]	18 ± 3	25 ± 2
Deuterium dilution	Sjödin et al. 1996			
Ice hockey	Elite (professional)	Male	14.4 ± 0.6	24 ± 1
		Male	13.9 ± 0.7	25 ± 1
Skinfolds	Tegelman et al. 1996			
Field hockey	Not reported	Female	22.3 ± 4.1	—
Skinfolds	Mohka and Sidhu 1987			
Tennis	Collegiate	Female[4]	30.2 ± 3.5	22 ± 4
DXA	Nichols et al. 1995			
Ballet dancing	Classically trained	Female	16.4 ± 4.0	15 ± 1.6
UWW	Clarkson et al. 1985			
Baseball	Professional	Male	16.2 ± 3.2	26 ± 3
Skinfolds	Gury et al. 1985			
Rugby	National	Male	9.1 ± 2.7	28.1 ±3.1
Skinfolds	Maud and Schultz 1984			
Golf	Professional	Female	24.0 ± 4.0	33.3 ± 6.8
Skinfolds	Crews et al. 1984			

[1] Underwater weighing.
[2] Dual-energy X-ray absorptiometry.
[3] Bioelectrical impedence.
[4] Subjects reported to be regularly menstruating.
[5] Subjects reported to be amenorrheic.
[6] One subject reported to have prior history of anorexia nervosa.
[7] 80% of these athletes were postmenopausal.
[8] 25% of these athletes were oligomenorrheic; 17% were amenorrheic.

Appendix E

Nutrition and Fitness Assessment

Instructions for Recording Dietary Intake

The purpose of a multiple diet record is to provide a quantitative assessment of an individual's typical food intake. For active individuals, keeping food intake records over a typical training cycle, such as a week, is recommended to provide a better picture of an athlete's normal diet. If only three days are being recorded, it is typical to pick two weekdays and one weekend day to account for the potential differences in food intake during the week and on the weekend. To ensure that portion sizes are estimated correctly, a properly calibrated scale or measuring utensils should be used to weigh and measure foods. Additionally, participants must be trained to use the measuring tools properly. Participants should record foods consumed at home (providing labels and brand names when possible), as well as foods consumed in restaurants as accurately as possible. If the recording lasts longer than three days, participants should be encouraged to accurately record food and not change their diet to make recording simpler or to impress the dietitian or investigator.

Recording Procedures

1. Record all food and beverages consumed for the designated number of days, which is typically between 3 and 7. It is best to record on days that are typical of normal eating behaviors. Include all snacks, condiments (e.g. pickles, catsup, mayonnaise), energy or sport foods, bars and gels, candy, alcoholic beverages, and supplements or medications.

2. All snacks, meals, and beverages consumed away from home must also be recorded. Keep food labels from convenience or packaged foods.

3. When composite or mixed dishes are consumed, include all the components of the item when possible. For example, a turkey sandwich should be recorded as 2 slices of whole wheat bread, 1 tablespoon of mayonnaise, 1 slice of Swiss cheese, 1 lettuce leaf, and one large dill pickle slice.

4. Record time and place (e.g. home, restaurant, work) where meal, snack or drink was consumed.

5. Begin each day on a new recording form and include the date and day of the week.

6. If vitamin, mineral or other supplements are used, list the amount taken each day, the brand name, and label information. If possible, save the bottle for the dietitian or investigator to review.

Describing Foods and Drinks

For all foods recorded, provide the following details when possible:

1. Method of cooking (e.g. roasted, stewed, fried, baked, steamed)

2. Kind of food (e.g. raw or cooked; peeled or unpeeled; white or whole wheat; fresh, canned, frozen, or dried; 2%, 1%, nonfat or whole milk)

3. Brand names of all processed foods (e.g. Kraft Macaroni and Cheese, Post Grape Nut Flakes, Pacific Crest Organic Tomato Soup)

4. Include all condiments (e.g. pickles, mayonnaise, mustard, salad dressing).

5. Provide as much label information as possible and the brand name of any special items you consume (e.g. reduced sodium, calcium added).

6. Ethnic foods provide a special challenge. Give details such as where the food was purchased, how it was prepared and the brand name of the ingredients.

7. If a recipe is used to make mixed dishes, such as casseroles, baked goods, or sauces, provide the recipe to the dietitian or investigator while also recording the amount consumed.

8. Record the weight of cooked foods the way they are consumed (e.g. weight of cooked, not raw, pork chop). If the weight of an apple is recorded, subtract the weight of the uneaten core. Remove the peel from a piece of fruit before weighing (e.g. peel the banana before weighing).

9. Use household measures (cups or ounces) for liquids such as drinks, soups, broths, and sakes. Use measuring spoons (tablespoon, teaspoon) for items such as butter, peanut butter, jam, and sugar.

10. For meats, cheese, pies, and cakes, estimate the portion size in measured inches (e.g. a 1 inch cube of cheese or a 2 by 4 by 1 inch pork chop).

11. If the entire product or item is not eaten, only record the amount consumed.

Appendix E.1   Sample Food Intake Recording Form

Date _____ / _____ / _____   Day of the week _____

Food Intake Diary		Name:		
Time and Place (AM/PM)	Foods and beverages Include: fresh, frozen, low-fat, etc.	Amount	Method of preparation (baked, fried, broiled, etc.)	Food exchanges

Appendix E.2 Sample Recording Form for 24-Hour Activity Records

Name _____

Date _____

Minutes	0	5	1 0	1 5	2 0	2 5	3 0	3 5	4 0	4 5	5 0	5 5	6 0
AM 6													
7													
8													
9													
10													
11													
Noon													
PM 1													
2													
3													
4													
5													
6													
7													
8													
9													
10													
11													
Midnight													
AM 1													
2													
3													
4													
5													

Appendix E.3 Energy Cost Values for Various Activities

Activity	kcal/kgBW/min	Energy expenditure (kcal/min) for a specific body weight			
		50 kg (110 lb)	60 kg (132 lb)	70 kg (154 lb)	80 kg 176 lb)
Bicycling					
10-11.9 mph, leisurely	0.1	5.0	6.0	7.0	8.0
16-19 mph, racing	0.2	10.0	12.0	14.0	16.0
Conditioning exercise					
Stationary cycling, 100 W	0.092	4.583	5.5	6.417	7.333
Stationary cycling, 200 W	0.175	8.75	10.5	12.25	14.0
Hatha yoga	0.067	3.333	4.0	4.667	5.333
High-impact aerobics	0.117	5.833	7.0	8.167	9.333
Running					
12 min/mi	0.133	6.667	8.0	9.333	10.667
10 min/mi	0.167	8.333	10.0	11.667	13.333
8 min/mi	0.208	10.417	12.5	14.583	16.667
6 min/mi	0.267	13.333	16.0	18.667	21.333

Adapted from B.E. Ainsworth et al., 1993, "Compendium of physical activities: classification by energy costs of human physical activities," *Medicine and Science in Sports and Exercise* 25: 71-80; B.E. Farnsworth et al., 2000, "Compendium of physical activities: an update of activity codes and MET intensities," *Medicine and Science in Sports and Exercise* 32: S498-S504.

Appendix E.4   Commonly Reported Clinical Laboratory Values for Adults (Reference Ranges Can Vary; Refer to the Specific Laboratory Ranges Reported)

Test	Reference range	Purpose of test
Fasting glucose	62-110 mg/dL	Tests for diabetes
Glycosylated hemoglobin (HbA$_{1c}$)	4.0-6.7% (for nondiabetics)	Tests for diabetes and control of disease for diabetic client
Serum sodium	136-145 mmol/L	Detects changes in salt and water balance
Serum potassium	3.5-5.2 mmol/L	Detects acid–base and water imbalances
Serum chloride	96-106 mmol/L	Detects acid–base and water imbalances
BUN (blood urea nitrogen)	6-20 mg/dL	Gross index of renal function
Serum creatinine	0.8-1.2 mg/dL	Detects impaired renal function
Uric acid	3.4-7.0 mg/dL (men) 2.4-6.0 mg/dL (women)	Indicates renal failure, gout, and leukemia
Serum calcium (total)	8.8-10.4 mg/dL	Assesses parathyroid function, calcium metabolism
Inorganic phosphorus	2.7-4.5 mg/dL	Is evaluated in relation to calcium levels
Alkaline phosphatase	25-100 U/L	Is an index of liver and bone disease
GGT (glutamyltransferase)	7-47 U/L (men) 5-25 U/L (women)	Detects liver cell dysfunction and alcohol-induced liver disease
Bilirubin (total)	0.3-1.0 mg/dL	Evaluates liver function and hemolytic anemias
Serum glutamic-oxaloacetic transaminase (SGOT) or aspartate transaminase (AST)	14-20 U/L (men) 10-36 U/L (women)	Evaluates liver and heart disease
Serum glutamic-pyruvic transaminase (SGPT) or alanine transaminase (ALT)	10-40 U/L (men) 7-35 U/L (women)	Detects liver disease
Serum lactate dehydrogenase (LDH)	140-280 U/L	Used to confirm myocardial or pulmonary infarction in conjunction with other test results
Serum cholesterol	<200 mg/dL	Used to detect blood lipid disorders; potential risk factor for coronary artery disease
Serum triglycerides	<200 mg/dL	Detects potential coronary artery disease and measures body's ability to metabolize fat
HDL-C (high-density lipoprotein)-cholesterol	35-65 mg/dL (men) 35-80 mg/dL (women)	Assesses coronary artery disease risk; increased values are inversely proportional to disease
LDL-C (low-density lipoprotein)-cholesterol	<130 mg/dL	Assesses coronary artery disease risk
Total serum protein	6.0-8.0 g/dL	Detects liver and immune dysfunctions
Serum albumin	3.5-4.8 g/dL	Detects liver and immune dysfunctions

(continued)

Appendix E.4   *(continued)*

Test	Reference range	Purpose of test
Serum globulin	0.7-1.6 g/dL	Indicates chronic infections, liver and immune diseases, and leukemia and other cancers
Serum iron	65-175 μg/dL (men) 50-170 μg/dL (women)	Assists in diagnosis of various anemias and hemochromatosis
Total iron-binding capacity (TIBC)	250-450 μg/dL	Assists in diagnosis of various anemias, iron insufficiency, and hemochromatosis
Transferrin (% saturation)	10-50% (men) 15-50% (women)	Assists in diagnosis of various anemias, iron insufficiency, and hemochromatosis
Ferritin	20-250 ng/mL (men) 10-120 ng/mL (women)	Is a more sensitive test than iron or TIBC for diagnosing iron insufficiency or overload
Thyroid tests:		
T3 (triiodothyronine) uptake	25-35%	Assesses thyroid function
Serum T4 (thyroxine)	5.4-11.5 μg/dL	Assesses thyroid function
T7 index (free thyroxine)	1.5-4.5 (arbitrary units)	Assesses thyroid function
TSH (thyroid stimulating hormone)	0.4-4.2 μU/mL	Assesses thyroid function
WBC (white blood cell count)	4.5-10.5/μL	Indicates increased susceptibility to infection
RBC (red blood cell count)	$4.2\text{-}5.4 \times 10^6/\mu L$ (men) $3.6\text{-}5.0 \times 10^6/\mu L$ (women)	Detects anemia
Hemoglobin	14.0-17.4 g/dL (men) 12.0-16.0 g/dL (women)	Indicates severity of anemia
Hematocrit	42-52% (men) 36-48% (women)	Determines red cell mass and helps in diagnosing anemia
MCV (mean corpuscular volume)	82-98 fL (femtoliters)	Indicates volume of a single red blood cell; used in diagnosing anemia

Values from F.A. Fischbach, 2004, *A manual of laboratory and diagnostic tests,* 7th ed. (Philadelphia, PA: Lippincott, Williams, and Wilkins).

Index

Note: The italicized f and t following page numbers refer to figures and tables, respectively.

About the Authors

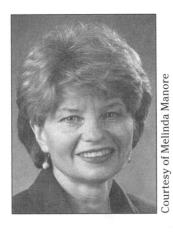

Melinda M. Manore, PhD, RD, CSSD, FACSM, is a professor in the department of nutrition and exercise sciences and a nutrition specialist in extension at Oregon State University. She has taught and conducted research in nutrition and exercise for more than 25 years. She is a highly regarded researcher, particularly in the nutrition needs of active women, and has written more than 60 research articles, 6 books, 20 book chapters, and numerous nutrition articles for health and nutrition professionals.

Dr. Manore is a member of several editorial boards of nutrition and exercise journals. She is a member of the American Dietetic Association (ADA) and several organizations within the ADA, including Sports Dietetics USA, Weight Control, the research practice groups, and Sports, Cardiovascular, and Wellness Nutritionists (SCAN). She is a member of the American Society of Nutrition, the American College of Sports Medicine (where she is a fellow), and the Obesity Society. She is also a founding member of Professionals in Nutrition for Exercise and Sport (PINES) and on the academic advisory board for the International Olympic Committee (IOC) diploma in sports nutrition. Dr. Manore is a certified specialist in sport dietetics (CSSD) from ADA. In 2001, she received an Excellence in Practice Award from the ADA.

In her leisure time, Dr. Manore enjoys hiking, walking, gardening, birding, and cooking.

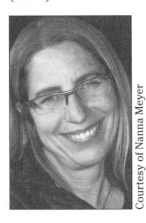

Nanna Meyer, PhD, RD, CSSD, is an assistant professor in health sciences at the University of Colorado. She has been working in sport nutrition as a scientist, clinician, and educator since 1996. She developed the sport dietetics emphasis degree at the University of Utah and recently obtained approval for a new graduate program in Sport Nutrition at the University of Colorado at Colorado Springs. Her primary research areas are the female athlete triad and nutritional issues in Olympic athletes. She also leads Professionals in Nutrition for Exercise and Sport (PINES), an international group that advances the field of study.

Dr. Meyer has been a member of the American College of Sports Medicine since 1992 and is a member of various other professional organization, including Sports Dietetics USA and Sports, Cardiovascular, and Wellness Nutritionists (SCAN), the American Dietetic Association, and the European College of Sport Science. Dr. Meyer is also a consultant for the United States Olympic Committee.

In her spare time, Dr. Meyer, who was a member of the Swiss ski team, likes to cross-country ski, alpine ski, run, cycle, and hike. She also enjoys modern art, reading, and writing.

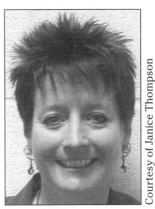

Janice L. Thompson, PhD, FACSM, is a professor of public health nutrition and head of the department of exercise, nutrition and health at the University of Bristol in the United Kingdom. She has spent more than 20 years conducting research and teaching at universities in areas related to nutrition, public health, exercise, and sport nutrition. In addition to coauthoring the first edition of *Sport Nutrition for Health and Performance*, she has authored three other textbooks on nutrition with Dr. Manore.

Dr. Thompson serves as the vice president of the American College of Sports Medicine and is a fellow of that organization. In 1997 she received an Excellence in Undergraduate Teaching Award from the University of North Carolina at Charlotte. In her leisure time, Dr. Thompson enjoys hiking, yoga, and cooking.

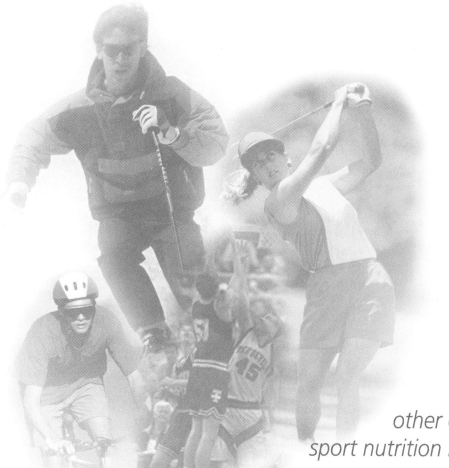

Dietary Reference Intakes (DRI)

Dietary Reference Intakes (DRIs): Tolerable Upper Intake Levels (UL[a]), Elements

Age (yr)	Sodium (mg/day)	Chloride (mg/day)	Calcium (mg/day)	Phosphorus (mg/day)	Magnesium (mg/day)[d]	Iron (mg/day)[b]
Infants						
6 mo	ND	ND	ND	ND	ND	40
7-12 mo	ND	ND	ND	ND	ND	40
Children						
1-3	1500	2300	2500	3000	65	40
4-8	1900	2900	2500	3000	110	40
Adults						
9-13	2200	3400	2500	4000	350	40
14-18	2300	3600	2500	4000	350	45
19-70	2300	3600	2500	4000	350	45
>70	2300	3600	2500	3000	350	45
Pregnancy						
≤18	2300	3600	2500	3500	350	45
19-50	2300	3600	2500	3500	350	45
Lactation						
≤18	2300	3600	2500	4000	350	45
19-50	2300	3600	2500	4000	350	45

[a] UL = The maximum level of daily nutrient intake that is likely to pose no risk of adverse effects. Unless otherwise specified, the UL represents total intake from food, water, and supplements. In the absence of ULs, extra caution may be warranted in consuming levels above recommended intakes.

[b] The ULs for magnesium represent intake from a pharmacological agent only and do not include intake from food and water.

ND = Not determinable due to lack of data of adverse effects in this age group and concern with regard to lack of ability to handle excess amounts. Source of intake should be from food only to prevent high levels of intake.

SOURCES: *Dietary Reference Intakes for Calcium, Phosphorous, Magnesium, Vitamin D, and Fluoride* (1997); *Dietary Reference Intakes for Thiamin, Riboflavin, Niacin, Vitamin B6, Folate, Vitamin B12, Pantothenic Acid, Biotin, and Choline* (1998); *Dietary Reference Intakes for Vitamin C, Vitamin E, Selenium, and Carotenoids* (2000); *Dietary Reference Intakes for Vitamin A, Vitamin K, Arsenic, Boron, Chromium, Copper, Iodine, Iron, Manganese, Molybdenum, Nickel, Silicon, Vanadium, and Zinc* (2001); and *Dietary Reference Intakes for Water, Potassium, Sodium, Chloride, and Sulfate* (2004). These reports may be accessed via http://www.nap.edu.

Adapted, by permission, from National Academies Press, 2006, Dietary reference intakes: Tolerable upper intake levels, elements. In *Dietary reference intakes: The essential guide to nutrient requirement* © 2006 by the National Academy of Sciences, Washington, D.C.